ESPES Manual of Pediatric Minimally Invasive Surgery

Ciro Esposito • François Becmeur
Henri Steyaert • Philipp Szavay
Editors

ESPES Manual of Pediatric Minimally Invasive Surgery

Springer

Editors
Ciro Esposito
Pediatric Surgery Unit
University of Naples Federico II
Naples
Italy

Henri Steyaert
Pediatric Surgery Unit
Queen Fabiola Children's University Hospital
Brussels
Belgium

François Becmeur
Pediatric Surgery Unit
Centre Hospitalier Universitaire de Hautepierre
Strasbourg
France

Philipp Szavay
Pediatric Surgery Department
Luzerner Kantonsspital
Luzern
Switzerland

ISBN 978-3-030-00963-2 ISBN 978-3-030-00964-9 (eBook)
https://doi.org/10.1007/978-3-030-00964-9

This Springer imprint is published by the registered company Springer Nature Switzerland AG
The registered company address is: Gewerbestrasse 11, 6330 Cham, Switzerland

To my wife, partner, and best friend, Marina, for her precious support and encouragement every day in the last 35 years

I love you

Ciro Esposito

I want firstly to dedicate this MIS book to the older generation of colleagues and friends who pioneered MIS in children and took us with them on board very early. But I will not forget all the sick children all over the world hoping that this book will help them to recover a beautiful smile.

Henri Steyaert

To all my friends and colleagues in pediatric surgery, many of them also authors of this book, who have been so inspiring, enriching, and supporting me.

Philipp Szavay

It was a pleasure to contribute to this book that will help us to clarify the state of the art for video surgery in children.

Next step will be robotic assistance for surgeons. New tools are and will be created to secure our procedures.

François Becmeur

Foreword

It is a pleasure for me to write the preface of this manual of pediatric MIS for two main reasons: first of all because I was involved in the field of Pediatric MIS Surgery from the beginning of its development in Europe at the beginning of the 1990s and second because one of the editors of this book, Ciro Esposito, was my trainee between 1991 and 1993, whom I also consider as my "surgical son."

Since nearly 10 years, the main goal of ESPES (European Society of Pediatric Endoscopic Surgeons) is education, and for this reason, to publish a manual of pediatric MIS techniques is an excellent idea.

At the beginning of laparoscopic area, we had to prove that pediatric laparoscopy offered some benefits to our patients. While some of you, as pioneers, paved the way and ignored the criticism of their colleagues, the others choose to watch with interest. And over the last 25 years, pediatric MIS made the transition from the "look what I can do" phase to a real validation of the MIS approach by randomized trials and comparisons of the open versus the scopic approach. Today, nearly everything, in pediatric surgery, can be done laparoscopically, retroperitoneoscopically, thoracoscopically, and even using robotic surgery.

The technique has evolved to a standard of care in many centers around the world. Even if many senior surgeons haven't learned the technique and therefore don't offer it to their patients, most surgeons in their team and in training are as confident with laparoscopy as they are with the open approach. Of course, the approaches have evolved over the years as well as the learning curve, but we can say now that MIS procedures are cost-effective operations that rarely take extra time to perform, even in some cases save time, and more importantly are part of our current practices.

This manual, then, serves as both an update of current practices and a real guide to the most common operations in pediatric. It covers the basics of anesthesia, instrumentation, and ergonomics and then reviews many of the more commonly performed laparoscopic, thoracoscopic, retroperitoneoscopic, and robotic pediatric procedures, including a review of the possibilities of prenatal treatment. While any book written about such a rapidly evolving technique may miss some of the very newest twists or modifications of technique, I am sure that most of the content will serve as a reference for many years. The format is designed to be readily accessible, and it will be certainly a must and a real opportunity for the new generation of pediatric surgeons.

CHU la Timone, Marseille, France Jean Michel Guys

Preface

The field of minimally invasive surgery in children and infants is rapidly growing and currently is considered the new frontier of pediatric surgery.

ESPES Manual of Pediatric Minimally Invasive Surgery (MIS) provides practicing pediatric surgeons and pediatric urologists with authoritative chapters that were written by recognized experts and cover all the aspects of pediatric MIS. The goal of the editors and the authors is simple: to provide the readers a unique resource consisting of practical and technically oriented chapters focused on all the aspects of pediatric laparoscopy, retroperitoneoscopy, and thoracoscopy.

ESPES Manual of Pediatric Minimally Invasive Surgery is based on a simple but important philosophy: give a practical and up-to-date resource for the practicing surgeon detailing the specific needs and special considerations surrounding the minimally invasive care of children.

We especially wanted to convey this information in an accessible and pleasing format.

Written by expert surgeons, each chapter has been carefully edited to maintain continuity in style and format while preserving the unique voice of the experienced and knowledgeable contributing author. In addition, this manual will serve as a useful reference for pediatric surgeons, pediatric urologists, general surgeons, and gynecologists. *ESPES Manual of Pediatric Minimally Invasive Surgery* is also specially designed to be used by surgical residents in pediatric surgery and urology rotation and chief residents who have chosen to obtain further specialized training in a pediatric surgery fellowship program.

This ESPES Manual is concise and easy to read, containing detailed and relevant information that can help you in taking care of the patient in your surgical practice using the more advanced MIS techniques. To cover all the aspects of minimally invasive surgery from the basis of MIS to the more advanced procedure as robotics or fetal surgery, the manual is divided into six parts: basics, chest, abdomen, urology, gynecology, and miscellanea.

The chapters give advice about room setup, patient positioning, as well as step-by-step descriptions of how each surgical procedure should be performed, including all technical aspects of the procedure, complications, and tip and tricks.

We are very impressed by the material present in this manual, and we are sure that the concepts outlined, if followed by the reader, will add to the value of minimally invasive care that we provide to our pediatric patients.

Enjoy this lecture and remember minimal incision, easy decision.

Naples, Italy Ciro Esposito
Strasbourg, France François Becmeur
Brussels, Belgium Henri Steyaert
Luzern, Switzerland Philipp Szavay

Contents

Part I Basics

Part II Chest

Part III Abdomen

Part VI Miscellanea

Part I

Basics

1 Equipment and Instruments

Raimundo Beltrà Picó

1.1 Introduction

Today, minimally invasive surgery (MIS) in paediatrics (MIPES: minimally invasive paediatric endoscopic surgery) is a consolidated and universally accepted surgical tool of indispensable use in our daily work.

The great, successful progress that this discipline has experienced in the last 20 years has been fundamentally due to the:

- Improvement of specialized anaesthetic techniques for paediatric endoscopic surgeries

Incessant achievement of highly sophisticated technological equipment and the continuous development of instruments designed specifically for these surgical techniques [1].

Equipment and instruments are designed to allow safe access to the child's anatomic cavity, to get and maintain a good working space, to see neatly inside the operating field and to perform all conventional manoeuvres in surgical techniques (grasping, dissecting, cutting, suturing, haemostasis, tissue sealing, etc.) with the same safety and efficacy as in open surgery.

MIPES surgeons must learn the principles and technical characteristics of the instruments and equipment at their disposal, without always depending on their technical team should an emergency arrive.

The next section will provide an overview of the basic equipment and instruments that should be available [2].

1.2 Description

1.2.1 Access: Cannulae and Trocars

Cannulae and trocars are used to pierce the anatomical cavity to enable the placement of telescope and surgical instruments.

Access by puncture with the well-known Veress needle (Fig. 1.1), while widely used in adult MIS, is generally discouraged in MIPES and even banned in many paediatric surgery services due to the high risk of damaging underlying structures.

The author discourages using this manoeuvre—and any other blind manoeuvres—in children and strongly recommends performing the first access through an open small incision. This allows for the safe introduction, under direct vision, of the first cannula, always with a blunt trocar inside (removable puncheon). By doing this, we create the first working port, preventing life-threatening complications of vascular or hollow viscus perforation [3].

R. B. Picó (✉)
Complejo Hospitalario Universitario Insular
Materno-Infantil, Las Palmas de Gran Canaria, Spain

C. Esposito et al. (eds.), *ESPES Manual of Pediatric Minimally Invasive Surgery*,
https://doi.org/10.1007/978-3-030-00964-9_1

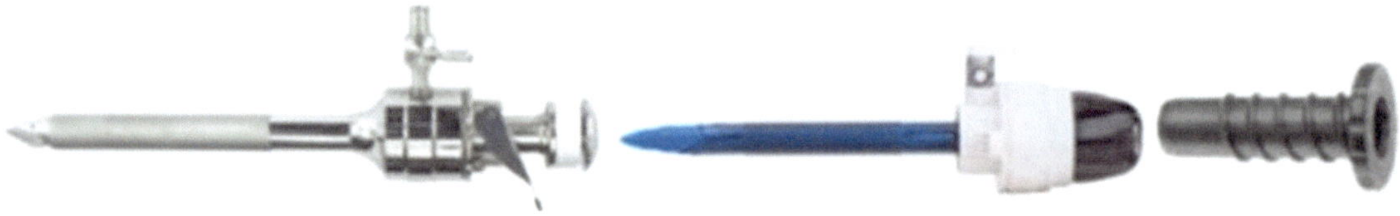

Fig. 1.1 Cannulae. From left to right: reusable. Disposable. Thoracoscopic

Once the first access port is created, we add as many working ports as strictly necessary, but limiting its number to the fewest possible.

Under direct vision through the lens placed in the first cannula, we can introduce any type of cannula with any type of trocar inside it, blunt or sharp, controlling at all times the entrance into the anatomical cavity, thus preventing accidental injuries.

As it happens with many other instruments used in MIS, cannulae and trocars are available in disposable, non-disposable or partially disposable forms (Fig. 1.1).

1.2.1.1 Disposable

Advantages

1. Clean, sterile, effective mechanisms
2. Easy storage, widespread, immediate availability
3. Later reuse in experimental surgery

Disadvantages

1. Purchase costs
2. Requires proper waste disposal after use

1.2.1.2 Reusable

Advantages

1. Allows multiple uses and thus can be amortized, implying a lower cost

Disadvantages

1. Needs to be cleaned, sterilized and packed.
2. Less availability units in stock.
3. Reliability decreases with each use.

1.2.1.3 Size

Diameter

- 2 mm
  The 2 mm instruments are fragile and bend easily, and grasping them firmly is difficult. Its use is quite limited and has few and very selected indications.
- 3.3 mm
  It is highly recommended in MIPES and its use is very widespread. There is a large choice of 3 mm instruments, both disposable and reusable. They are technically very reliable and allow performing in children most of the endo-surgical operations with complete safety. Handling of tissues is very delicate, and the scars left are aesthetically very satisfactory.
  On the other hand, vision with a 3 mm lens is not as accurate as with a 5 mm lens. Therefore, on many occasions it is more convenient to combine 3.3 mm cannulae with 6 mm ones.
- 6 mm
  Most 5-mm-diameter surgical instruments and accessories can be found nowadays.
- 11–12–15 mm
  They are sometimes necessary because some instruments such as staplers and retrieval bags are not available yet in a 5-mm-diameter size.

Length

- Cannulae of 60, 75, 100 and 110 mm are available.

The chosen length depends on the thickness of the wall of the child's anatomical cavity. It is advisable to insert the sheath as little as possible, so it occupies less space in an already limited working field, therefore allowing for a better instrumental manoeuvrability without interference.

1.2.1.4 "Luer" Lock Adapter

There are cannulae with and without an adapter to connect to the source of gas insufflation. There are also cannulae with a stopcock or with a rubber stopper that occludes the "luer" connection.

The heads of the cannulae that do not have a connector for the gas are less bulky than those that have it. Therefore, combining cannulae of both types helps to reduce the space occupied by them on the surface of the child.

1.2.1.5 Valve

There are cannulae with and without a valve to prevent gas leakages when the instrument is not inside the cavity. The valve should be easy to open for the removal of tissue samples.

1.2.1.6 Trocar

There are several types of awl tips:

- Sharp pyramidal. Very traumatic. Leakage of gas occurs easily.
- Sharp conical. Less traumatic as it dilates the tissues.
- Eccentric. Makes a slit-like hole and requires less force for insertion.
- Blunt conical. Ideal when a cannula is inserted using an open technique.
- With a small blade of a knife at the end of the trocar, which retracts as soon as the piercing resistance is lost.

1.2.1.7 Cannula Fixation

Dislodgment of cannulae due to the thinness of the child's body wall happens very often and becomes a great problem in MIPES.

Some cannulae have a screw-like structure on the outer surface. After a long operating time, they are not very effective and can often enlarge the diameter of the porthole.

There is a disposable cannula with an inflatable balloon at its end and a synthetic plate at the outside to be compressed against the wall. The disadvantage is that the part of the cannula inside the abdominal cavity is rather long, thereby limiting the working space.

A simple and useful way to fix the cannulae is to place a ring made from a silicone catheter, which fits well but can slide on its surface. It should be placed at the precise distance that we want the cannula to enter the cavity and should be fixed to the body wall with a suture, which can also be passed around the stopcock.

There is a type of cannula called Step™, available in 3–6–10–12 mm and in different lengths, which includes the cannula (with valve and stopcock), a blunt puncheon, a Veress needle with a length according to that of the cannula and a sheath formed by a mesh with 2–3 mm of outer diameter.

The mesh can be inserted through the first hole in its "open" mode or over the Veress needle in the next ports and under direct vision. Once the sheath is inside, the Veress needle is then removed leaving the sleeve in place. The cannula with the awl is then inserted through the sleeve, thereby radially dilating the sheath and stretching the orifice without tearing it.

Its advantages are:

- The tip of the cannula and trocar are protected by the mesh and don't damage the anatomical structures.
- The distended mesh adapts very well to the hole, providing a firm fixation.
- Cannulae of higher calibre can be introduced through the mesh, enlarging only the skin incision by a few millimetres.

1.2.1.8 Single Incision Laparoscopic Surgery (SILS)

For this MIPES modality, there are devices that consist of two rings, external and internal, connected to each other with a membrane in the shape of an hourglass. These devices can accommodate 3–4 ports and have a lateral connection for gas input. The device is normally inserted through the umbilicus [4] (Fig. 1.2).

1.2.2 Working Space: Insufflator

Both in the thorax and in the abdomen, the best way to get a good working space is through the insufflation of carbon dioxide (CO_2), the most commonly used gas.

CO_2 has the advantage of being rapidly absorbed by blood, is non-toxic and cost-effective and can be used with cautery.

Although in the thorax the simple entry of air through the cannula with the open stopcock

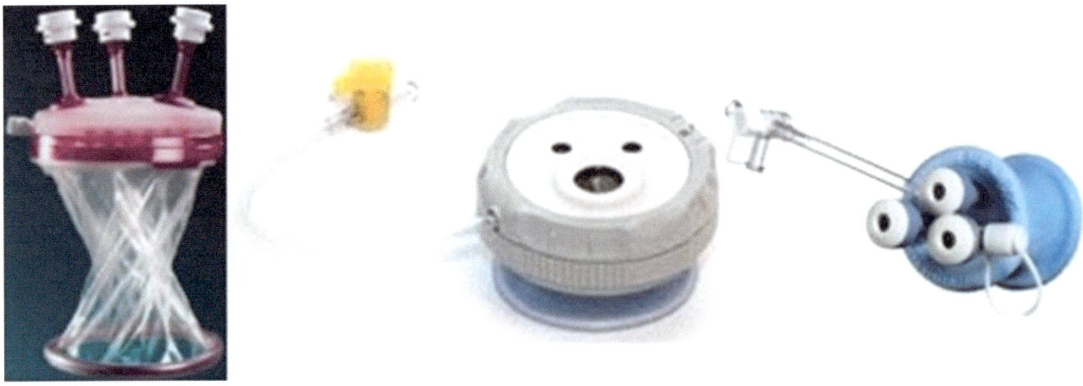

Fig. 1.2 SILS devices

collapses the lung, the positive pressure of the patient's ventilation reverses the collapse. Therefore, the working space is compromised, not allowing a comfortable and safe surgery.

Sufficient space in the chest can be created by inducing a pneumothorax with 3–6 mmHg CO2 pressure.

In the abdominal cavity, a good working space can be created using a pressure of maximum 8–10 mmHg and lower in small babies.

The main risks that appear when insufflating children's anatomical cavities with CO_2 arise from its high pressure and a maintained high flow [5, 6]:

- Negative effects on systemic and local hemodynamic, lung compliance and intracranial pressure (decreases venous return and cardiac output, increases heart rate, mean arterial pressure and systemic and pulmonary vascular resistance).
- A high flow rate when the pneumoperitoneum is created with the first cannula produces a sudden reduction of the venous return and compromises the adaptation of the cardiovascular system. Therefore, it is recommended using less than 1 L/min at the beginning.
- More than 2 L/min increases the tension of the diaphragm and produces scapular pain.
- High consumption of CO2 causes hypothermia.

The safety of the procedures depends on the quality of the insufflator. The surgeon must know well the characteristics of the insufflator before deciding which one to choose.

Recommended features:

- Automatic exsufflation valve in case of excessive pressure. External, to avoid cross-contamination.
- Safety maximum pressure adjustment with sound alarm.
- Automatic flow rate management according to leakages.
- Insufflation rate from 1 L/min.
- Current pressure, flow rates, volume and CO_2 remaining level of tank permanently displayed on screen.
- The gas used must be preheated and humidified under sterile conditions.
- Disposable filter between insufflator and sterile tube system towards the patient.

1.2.3 Visualization: Imaging System (Telescopes, Light Source, Cables, Camera Control Unit, Monitors, Video Recorder)

1.2.3.1 Telescopes

The telescope itself consists of an outer ring of optical fibres used to transmit light into the body and an inner distal-mounted core of rod lenses through which the images are relayed back to the camera where they get magnified for the surgeon. Different types of laparoscopes are available, different in terms of overall length, number of rods, diameter and angle of view.

Rigid telescopes are available in 2–3–5–10–12 mm with an ending angulation varying from 0° to 70°. The quality of visualization and light transmission of the telescope are inversely related to its diameter. 5 mm size is the most common choice in paediatrics. The author recommends starting MIPES with 5-mm-diameter telescopes and instruments of the same width. After gaining additional experience, the surgeon can decide whether smaller telescopes give them sufficient vision.

Regarding the angulation, it is advisable to use 30° telescopes for most operations because angled tips allow looking behind structures, around corners or below the surface of the abdominal wall.

There are new-generation rigid telescopes that enable three-dimensional (3D) procedures in conjunction with a 3D and high-definition (HD) camera.

5–10 mm HD telescopes with a flexible tip containing the chip are nowadays available.

To perform certain surgeries through a single port, there is the possibility of using a 10 mm, 0° operative laparoscope with a 6 mm working channel.

During surgery, fog, blood, saline or other materials can frequently obscure the scope lens. Various devices have been developed to solve this problem, including lens flushing systems, mechanical wipers, continuously flowing jets of air and mechanically spooled reels of transparent tape. A good alternative approach involves the use of a stainless steel shaker (sterilizable) with wet and warm gauze in the bottom with which one can effectively clean the tip of the telescope without damaging it. Angled lenses can also become dirty quicker due to increased contact with the intra-abdominal organs.

1.2.3.2 Light Source

Light may be the essence of endoscopic imaging, and it is the starting point of the imaging chain. HD endoscopy generally relies heavily on surgical light sources. Because HD cameras have lower sensitivity due to smaller pixel size, a powerful 300 W Xenon light source is frequently recommended. The light source should be set at maximum capacity in its non-automatic mode as modern cameras have a fast and automatic shutter built in. These HD cameras make use of the luminance signal derived from the video output to determine if the image is overexposed and adjust the intensity of the light source accordingly.

Ideal performance characteristics of the lighting system:

- Optimum intensity must adequately illuminate the operative field.
- Must ensure true-colour properties and brilliant image presentation.
- Sufficient brightness and contrast to discriminate healthy tissue from suspect ones that require treatment.

It should be noted that cold light does not exist. The temperature at the end of the light cable rises up to 225 °C within seconds and at the end of the telescope up to 95 °C within 15 min. A heat filter to reduce the amount of infrared light transmitted to the laparoscope is therefore required. The cable should therefore always be attached to the telescope, and one should never wipe the lens clean against surrounding tissues.

1.2.3.3 Cables

Light Cables

It is important to have good quality light cables adapted to the telescope that is being used, as the cables will provide the amount of light needed to illuminate the entire abdomen through a very small opening. The thickness of the cable should match the thickness of the light inlet of the telescope. Thick cables will not produce more light but more heat, while thin cables will not transport enough light.

A condensing lens is used to concentrate light from the bulb down into a narrow beam at the cable input, where it is transmitted to the laparoscope via a gel or fibre cable.

- Gel cables consist of a metal sheath filled with liquid crystal gel, terminated at each end with a quartz crystal.
- Fibre-optic cables are formed from tightly packed bundles of optical fibre, surrounded by several layers of protective flexible sheathing.

Both types of cable offer very high levels of light transmission but are somewhat fragile, and while gel cables can provide superior results in terms of brightness and colour temperature, they are also more prone to breaking due to the rigidity of the outer metal sheath.

Video Cables

Video cables have a great importance in video system of MIPES. They carry digital image data between the camera head, camera control unit (CCU), monitor(s) and recording devices.

The introduction of optical fibre provides an optimum cable solution as it has sufficient bandwidth for transmitting HD signals over long distances. This offers the opportunity to transmit other HD signals from imaging sources in a picture archiving and communication system (PACS).

An optical fibre for HD signal transmission can also be necessary for the development of HD imaging technology into integrated operating room systems.

1.2.3.4 Camera Unit

Camera Head

The camera consists of a lens, a prism and three sensors for acquiring the primary colours of the image. Some camera heads also incorporate an optical zoom for adjusting the image size (magnification). Due to better image performance, triple chip cameras have been generally accepted as the industry standard for endoscopic surgery. The primary advantage is the fact that colour reproduction is much more natural.

Image quality, however, will depend on the camera acquisition standard that's been put on a given system. Nowadays, we are moving from standard definition (SD) to HD video formats.

- Typical SD formats offer a 4:3 aspect ratio in 640 × 480 pixels image resolution.
- The 1080 HD format provides a 16:9 aspect ratio and 1920 × 1080 resolution. The speed at which the camera captures the images is expressed in frames per second (fps). In laparoscopic operations for HD endoscopy, 1080p60 (1080p at 60 fps) may be the highest standard readily available for acquiring and displaying images, and it offers a superior viewing experience for surgeons.

  Instead of circular images created by SD video camera lenses, with HD cameras surgeons can operate watching a monitor with full-screen images, as if they were watching movies, shows or sports events on a modern HD TV set. Wide-screen image acquisition increases the horizontal field of view (panoramic image) and decreases the vertical field of view. With laparoscopic instruments primarily entering the concept of view laterally, wide-screen 16:9 aspect ratios seem advantageous. Another positive effect is the fact that a telescope positioned further away from the site of surgical interaction catches less debris and smoke on the front window, improving image quality.

The quality of the cameras has been greatly improved over the years. Instead of a single chip that contains sensors for red, green and blue light embedded on a single silicon chip called a charge-coupled device (CCD), triple chip designs use a prism located in the camera head unit to split the incoming image into its red, green and blue components and direct those beams of light into three separate CCD chips. The resulting image can offer superior quality in terms of colour definition and clarity, but triple chip cameras are more expensive and heavier than single chip versions. Weight is a significant factor as the camera is typically mounted directly on top of the scope, so a heavier camera can make the instrument more difficult to manoeuvre.

The camera is attached via a rotating coupler, allowing the scope to be turned independently during use. This requires the camera to be held in the correct orientation throughout the procedure.

Lastly, a short mention about robotic 3D systems (discussed in more detail in Chap. 10). These systems use a pair of cameras and two different lenses working almost in parallel, but with a slight difference, to capture a stereoscopic image. Ocular disparity is the difference between the position between the left and the right eye in the human vision.

Camera Control Unit

The CCU connects various elements of the HD imaging chain, capturing and processing video signals from the camera head for display about the monitor, as well as for transfer to existing recording and printing devices.

The HD CCU must offer flexible output choices to ensure that the unit can continue to be used with HD equipment. The CCU should be able to accommodate both SD and HD inputs, and, conversely, it will have two digital video outputs:

- Digital video interface for the HD signal
- Serial digital interface for the SD signal

1.2.3.5 Monitors

The author recommends 26″ HD flat-panel monitors displaying images acquired in 16:9 format. Images in these characteristics enable surgeons to experience a more natural, panoramic vision, and, perhaps more importantly, visualization is much more in tune with human anatomy.

Our horizontal field of view is wider than our vertical field of view. Therefore, it is more natural and less fatiguing during procedures. Additionally, while we are viewing full-screen endoscopic images, trocars and hand instruments that normally approach the surgical area laterally are visible earlier with a 16:9 monitor than with 4:3 or 5:4 monitors.

1.2.3.6 Video Recorders

There is little doubt that with time all surgical operations recordings will have to be stored for a defined period of time as part of the patient's electronic chart.

Recording will also enable its use for studying, teaching and training of younger surgeons.

Normally, the recordings of endoscopic surgeries are made digitally on the hard disk of a computer. From there they can be organized for studying, reviewing or exhibiting.

Images can also be routed to a mounted screen, as it happens with 3D systems. In addition, video output can also be recorded and even viewed remotely through a live web stream, opening a range of opportunities in terms of remote and collaborative work.

At present, the trend in hospitals is to use modern and sophisticated systems that allow jointly storing data from different hospital units (recording of surgical interventions, electronic imaging studies). It is also possible to store non-image data, such as scanned documents that may be incorporated using standard formats like PDF.

Known as *picture archiving and communication system* (PACS), this medical imaging technology provides economic storage and convenient access to images from multiple modalities (source machine types). The universal format for PACS image storage and transfer is DICOM (Digital Imaging and Communications in Medicine).

A PACS consists of four major components:

- Imaging modalities such as X-ray plain films, ultrasound studies, computed tomography or magnetic resonance imaging
- Secured network for the transmission of patient information
- Workstation for interpreting and reviewing images
- Archives for the storage and retrieval of images and reports

Combined with available and emerging web technology, PACS has the ability to deliver timely and efficient access to images, interpretations and related data. PACS reduces the physical and time barriers associated with traditional film-based image retrieval, distribution and display.

1.2.3.7 What Will the Immediate Future Offer to Is?

Newer developments in laparoscopic technologies include virtual reality (VR) and augmented reality (AR) systems. VR systems rely solely on computer-generated images, while an AR system provides the surgeon with computer-processed imaging data in real time via dedicated hardware and software. The projection of AR is made possible by using displays, projectors, cameras, trackers or other specialized equipment. In AR systems, images of the patient, captured using X-ray, volumetric computerized tomography (CT) or other types of medical imaging technique, are overlaid onto the live feed from stereoscopic surgical cameras to create an enhanced 3D image that the surgeon can refer to during a procedure without the need to look away from the operating site. Although the technique has been used successfully in neurosurgery for a number of years, live AR laparoscopy is still in its infancy. However, both AR and VR systems have been used successfully in laparoscopic training applications [7].

1.2.4 Surgical Manipulation: Basic Working Instruments

1.2.4.1 Suction and Irrigation

The surgeon's vision during an endoscopic surgery can be hindered due to bleeding or smoke coming from ablation and resection procedures. Since blood absorbs light, even in areas far from the direct area that is being operated on, blood has to be removed to provide a clean visibility on the endoscopic monitor.

Moreover, biological debris that may remain after a surgery can lead to threatening sepsis complications in patients. Surgical suction pumps are also used to extract tissue and leakage of organic fluids and to irrigate water to wash the area.

Irrigation is also very important in endoscopic surgery for general washing, mechanical debridement of tissues and rupture of clots. However, it is advisable to try to avoid an abusive use of irrigation because once the operative field has become thoroughly wet, it is difficult to dry it again and this interferes with vision and dissection. This device can help surgeons to seek bleeding points (haemorrhage) by irrigating and sucking normal saline.

As an irrigation fluid, usually NaCl 0.9% is used. It must be sterile, preheated and kept warm.

Suction-irrigation pumps are available in one single device. They come in 3- and 5-mm-diameter and different lengths. They can be disposable o reusable.

Endoscopic suctioning instruments are relatively small, as they have to fit in the cannulae, yet they should be able to remove blood clots. The aspirating instrument therefore should have the largest possible opening at its end. Larger blood clots have to be mechanically fragmented before they can be aspirated. This means that the aspiration force should be quite high, but this will interfere with the working space by concomitant removal of the insufflated gas. High aspiration pressures will also result in aspiration of the surrounding tissues, thereby blocking the suction opening. This can be prevented to a certain extent by using short bursts of suction or by using a suction apparatus that has an automatic interrupter. The suction force should be easily adjustable.

There should be a control panel indicating:

- Suction pressure
- Rest volume of the suction bottle
- Irrigation pressure
- Rest volume of the irrigation bottle
- Temperature of the irrigation fluid

1.2.4.2 Retraction

Retractors used in adult MIS are not ideally suitable for MIPES due to their size once they are deployed within the anatomical cavity. As endoscopic retractors are not always within the viewing field, they can easily damage the surrounding tissues, particularly the liver and spleen.

The most popular is the one that opens like a fan, although its blades can be quite dangerous.

There is another less dangerous retractor, articulate and flexible, in the shape of a snake. Its main disadvantage is that a lot of its length has to be introduced in order to shape it properly and it thus takes up a lot of space.

The use of endoscopic swabs is usually useful and quite harmless to separate or move anatomical elements.

Sometimes an endoscopic grasping forceps can be used as a retractor. In anti-gastroesophageal reflux surgery, for example, the left lobe of the liver can be kept out of the way by inserting a grasping forceps through a cannula high in the epigastrium underneath the left lobe of the liver and grasping the most anterior part of the hiatus.

There are available internal magnetic graspers [DMG] (IMANLAP, Buenos Aires, Argentina) that grasp an intra-abdominal organ (gallbladder, appendix, gut) and, controlled by powerful external magnets, supply the necessary retraction/counter traction force to mobilize the organ. It can freely cruise the abdominal cavity according to the surgeon's need [8] (Fig. 1.3).

1.2.4.3 *Surgical Tools:* Dissect, Grasp, Hold, Cut, Suture

The MIS instruments are composed of a handle, the shaft and the specific work tip.

There are disposable and reusable instruments, usually high quality stainless steel made. The fundamental advantage of reusable models is their economic amortization with repeated uses. On the other hand, its main disadvantage is the difficulty to ensure adequate cleaning and sterilization since they could be a serious source of contamination and infections. Moreover, opening-closing mechanisms and scissors blades sharpness deteriorate with repeated uses and therefore lose their maximum effectiveness.

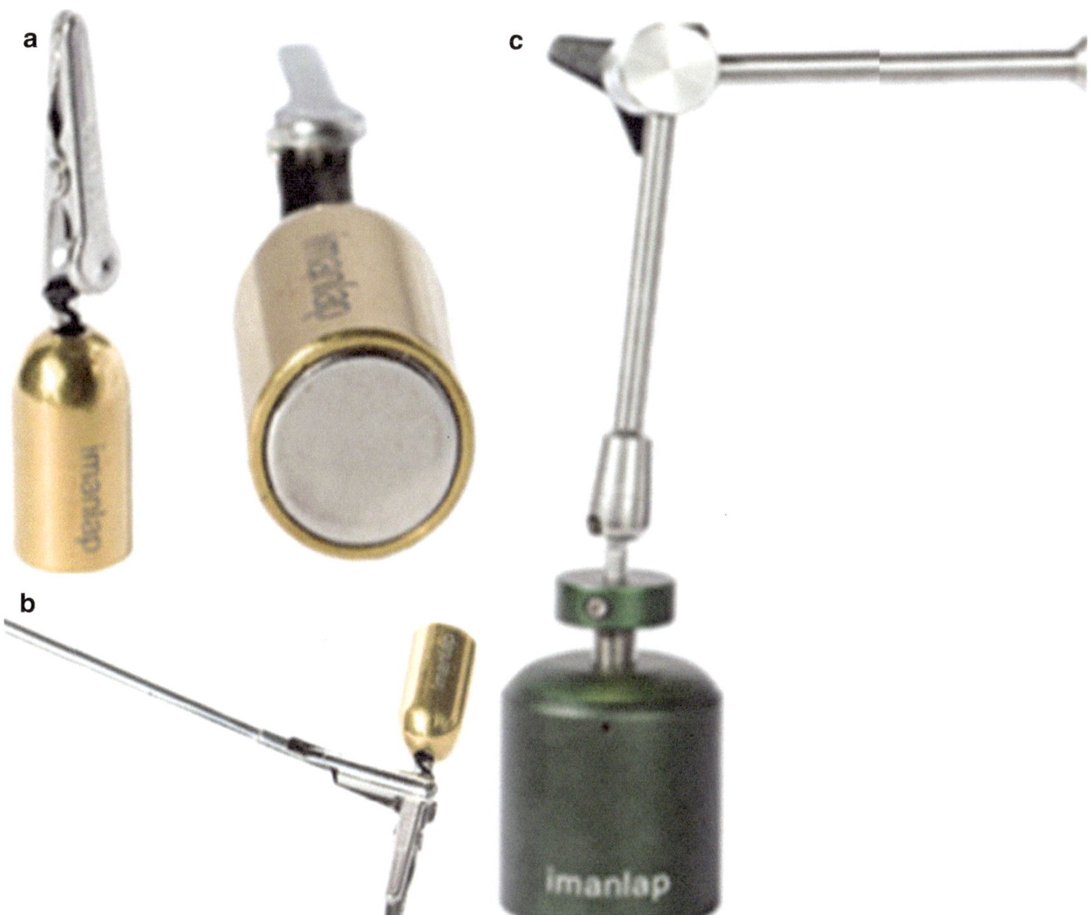

Fig. 1.3 (**a**) Dominguez magnetic graspers (DMG). (**b**) Thomas forceps are used to open the jaws of the DMG. (**c**) External magnet mounted on self-retaining retractor (By permission of Dr. M. Martinez Ferro)

There are different lengths, being the most appropriate in MIPES 24 cm and in older children 36. The two most used diameters in childhood are 3 and 5 mm.

There are many different handles, with the permanent idea of getting the best shape as possible for ergonomic rotating, grasping and locking abilities in a precise fashion. They are available with free opening mode or with an automatic ratchet that keeps them locked.

There are a wide variety of instrument tips available for multiple purposes, although not all have the same utility in terms of frequency and effectiveness. The following are the ones I consider the most commonly used:

1. Dissecting and grasping forceps
   - Kelly dissector
   - Maryland dissector
2. Grasping and holding forceps
   In MIPES, the use of atraumatic forceps is normally recommended. Traumatic clamps are limited to strong anatomic grasp, such as the diaphragm.
   To manipulate more delicate organs, such as exploring the intestine running through it, it is more appropriate to use a forceps with a broader atraumatic end.
   When forceps have to hold tissues for a longer period of time, it is advisable to use a handle with a ratchet in order to secure the holding grip.
   - Babcock
   - DeBakey
   - Standard
3. Scissors
   - Metzenbaum
   - Hook scissors (useful for cutting sutures and ligatures)
4. Needle holder
   Needle holders are usually made out of stainless steel and have straight axial designs that place the needle directly in line with the surgeon's hand to allow greater manoeuvrability and a more natural motion of the wrist when suturing. Various designs are available, but generally the jaws of the instrument are operated by means of an ergonomic spring-loaded palm grip on the handle. The grip is squeezed to open the jaws and released to close them. The needle is secured firmly in the jaws of the instrument by means of a ratcheted locking mechanism located in the handle.
   Needle driver jaws fall into one of four main categories: straight, curved left, curved right and self-righting.
5. Knot Pusher
   Normally, ligatures and tissue sutures are performed intracorporeally. In certain situations, for example, in the case of sutures with excessive tension, it may be advisable to externally make a self-slip Roeder knot or push a double knot inside until it is securely adjusted by means of a knot pusher.

1.2.4.4 *Haemostasis:* Clips, Staplers, Energy Sources

Clips

Clips are fast and effective for small- and medium-calibre vessels and for other small structures (cystic duct) (Fig. 1.4).

- Titanium [9]
  – 5 or 10 mm
  – Reusable one by one manual-pressure applier
  – Automatic single use device with multi-clip charges
- Non-absorbable polymer (Hem-o-lock™) [10]
  – Reusable one by one manual-pressure applier.
  – They are considered safer for larger vessels.

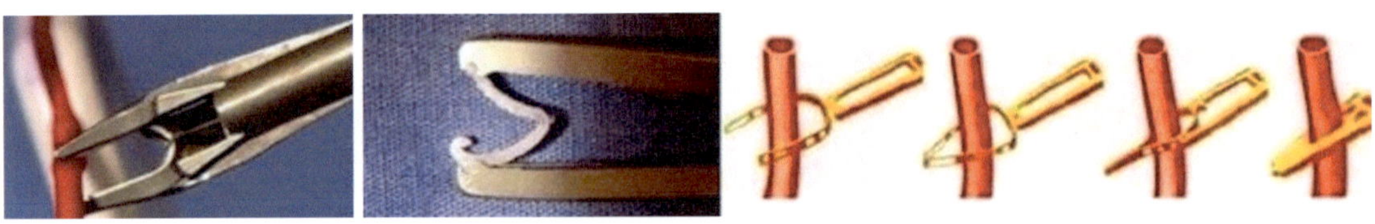

Fig. 1.4 Clips. From left to right: titanium, Hem-o-lock™ and Lapro-Clip™

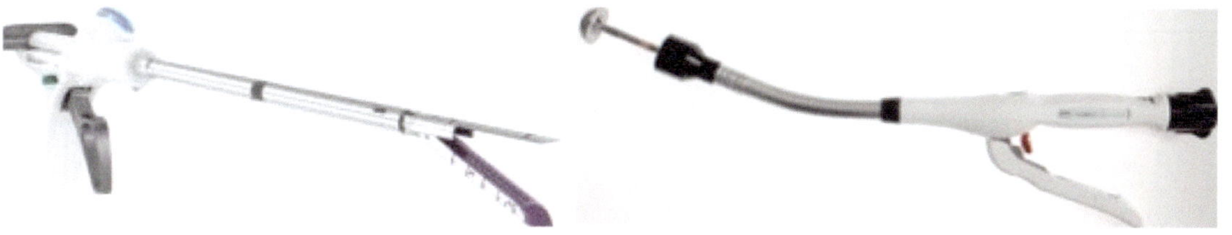

Fig. 1.5 Left: linear cutter-stapler. Right: circular stapler

- Absorbable dual-layer clip lock mechanism (Lapro-Clip™) [11]
  - Polygluconate inner track and polyglycolic acid outer track
  - Degrades via hydrolysis in 180 days (inner) and 90 (outer)

The last two are inert, nonconductive and radiolucent. They do not interfere with CT, magnetic resonance images (MRI) or X-ray diagnostics.

Staples

Staplers are safer in cases of much larger vessels such as splenic or renal artery/vein. They are also used for resecting the intestine and before performing an anastomosis. There are even specific staplers for end-to-end circular intestine anastomosis available (Fig. 1.5).

Staples cartridge lengths can be of 30, 35, 45 and 60 mm. The most important factor in staples is the height of the closed staple, because it must be able to contain the relevant tissue when closed. Each height adapts to the different tissues, such as the mesentery, which requires smaller staples, and vessels or gastrointestinal tissues, which require larger staples.

There are many different, but similar, endolinear mechanical suture devices available. The devices can be found in 5 and 10 mm diameters. All of them have an external rotation mechanism that facilitates their placement, and some of them are also articulated at the end of the suture.

Energy Sources [12, 13]

Monopolar High-Frequency Electro-Surgery (MHFE)

It can be used both to dissect tissues and to coagulate small vessels at the same time. Therefore, it is a very efficient and used instrument.

Various monopolar ends are available. In the author's experience, the 90° hook end is the most frequently used and is a good one as it allows for good vision even when the manipulation angle is small.

Warning
- If too high energy is delivered, it could cause faster cutting before coagulation is achieved.
- Insulation failure can cause collateral damage.
- Electrical over-scattering can cause distant electrical injuries.

Bipolar High-Frequency Electro-Surgery (BHFE)

The passive electrode and the active electrode are both located in each of the branches of the forceps. It coagulates only between the two branches of the instrument, minimizing electrical damage and other potential hazards of MHFE mentioned above. It has the disadvantage of being a noncutting instrument, which means that after coagulation, another instrument has to be used for cutting.

Advanced Alternative Energy Sources

The need for meticulous haemostasis and the tedium of vessel ligation in advanced cases has propelled the development of new energy source devices that have proved to be remarkably helpful in MIPES. However, surgeons do not always agree with the choice of the device that would be optimal for a particular procedure.

- Ultrasonic energy (Harmonic® shears and scalpel; Sonosurg) [14]
  The high-frequency vibration of tissue molecules produces stress and friction in the tissue,

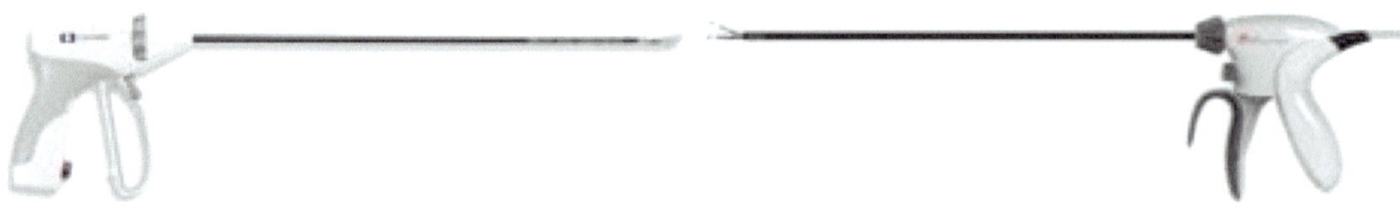

Fig. 1.6 Left: LigaSure™. Right: EnSeal®

which in turn generates heat and causes protein denaturation. Thus, coagulation and afterwards cutting are obtained.

- Electrical system with feedback (LigaSure™; EnSeal®)

  A low voltage is generated between the two branches of the instrument, which in turn is connected to a computerized system that measures the impedance of the tissue. The coagulation is produced by fusion of the collagen and elastin fibres (Fig. 1.6).
- Argon plasma coagulation

  It uses high-frequency electric current and ionized gas argon. The application of electric current on the gas releases a huge amount of heat resulting in a haemostatic jet. Its use is not too popularized and widespread.

1.2.4.5 Specimen Retrieval Bags

It is highly recommended to take anatomic specimens out of the body in an isolating bag in cases of:

- Infected tissue, to prevent contact with the body wall or in case of rupture during the manipulation, or gross contamination of the cavity
- Implantation of malignant cells in the port orifice or spilling of malignant or not malignant cells (splenic cells) inside the corporal cavity that may be hazardous

Currently marketed specimen retrieval bags can be found in diameters that range from 10 to 15 mm, with different capacity volumes and in their opening and closing technique [15].

1.3 Conclusion

There is generalized consensus that MIPES represents the recommended techniques for the majority of pathologies requiring surgical treatment, those settle in the abdominal, thoracic or retroperitoneal cavities.

Numerous breakthroughs in the design of instruments and advanced, highly sophisticated equipment make it essential for paediatric surgeons who want to advance safely in this field of surgery to know in detail the characteristics of the multiple devices and instruments that exist. In addition, surgeons should continuously learn about improvements and innovations of the most advanced endo-surgical techniques. That also requires being up-to-date on the continuous appearance of new products that outperform the previous ones.

The endoscopic surgeon should select a limited number of instruments to compose a standardized set. We cannot improvise or experiment during a surgery with the life or health of a child. From the first surgical use, we must already know perfectly the characteristics, proper use and, above all, possible risks or dangers derived from an inappropriate use or eventual collateral effect.

References

1. Spinelli G, Vargas M, Aprea G, et al. Paediatric anaesthesia for minimally invasive surgery in paediatric urology. Transl Pediatr. 2016;5(4):214–21.
2. Bax KNMA. Instrumentation in paediatric endoscopic surgery. In: Lobe TE, editor. Paediatric laparoscopy.

Georgetown: Landes Bioscience; 2003. p. 9–37. ISBN 1-57059-638-7.
3. Romain N, Michaud K, Brandt-Casadevall C, Mangin P. Fatal aortic injury during laparoscopy: report of two cases. Am J Forensic Med Pathol. 2003;24(1):80–2.
4. Krpata DM, Ponsky TA. Instrumentation and equipment for single-site umbilical laparoscopic surgery. Semin Pediatr Surg. 2011;20:190–5.
5. Gutt CN, Oniu T, Mehrabi A, et al. Circulatory and respiratory complications of carbon dioxide insufflation. Dig Surg. 2004;21:95–105.
6. Mitul AR, Sarin YK. Minimal access surgery in neonates. J Neonatal Surg. 2017;6:59.
7. Vávra P, Roman J, Zonča P, Ihnát P, Němec M, et al. Recent development of augmented reality in surgery: a review. J Healthc Eng. 2017;2017:4574172.
8. Padilla BE, Dominguez G, Millan C, Martinez-Ferro M. The use of magnets with single-site umbilical laparoscopic surgery. Semin Paediatr Surg. 2011;20:224–31.
9. Dell'Abate P, et al. Choledocholithiasis caused by migration of a surgical clip after video laparoscopic cholecystectomy. J Laparoendosc Adv Surg Tech A. 2003;13:203–4.
10. Cuaresma R, Benavides M, Buela E, Bignon H, Martínez-Ferro M. Uso de clips Hem-o-lock en apendicectomía laparoscópica de pacientes pediátricos (Use of Hem-o-lock clips in laparoscopic appendectomy in pediatric patients). Cir Pediatr. 2009;22:103–5.
11. Bo Lv X, Zhang JL, Shusheng L, Shuqiang L, et al. Absorbable polymeric surgical clips for appendicular stump closure: a randomized control trial of laparoscopic appendectomy with lapro-clips. Oncotarget. 2016;7(27):41265–73.
12. Harrell AG, Kercher KW, Heniford BT. Energy sources in laparoscopy. Semin Laparosc Surg. 2004;11(3):201–9.
13. Pantelić M, Ljikar J, Devecerski G, Karadzić J. Energy systems in surgery. Med Pregl. 2015;68(11–12):394–9.
14. Fitzgerald JEF, Malik M, Ahmed I. A single blind controlled study of electrocautery and ultrasonic scalpel smoke plumes in laparoscopic surgery. Surg Endosc. 2012;26(2):337–42.
15. Smorgick N. Laparoscopic specimen retrieval bags. J Obstet Gynaecol India. 2014;64(5):370–2.

2 Ergonomics in Minimally Invasive Surgery

Zacharias Zachariou

2.1 Introduction

Ergonomics is the science that studies human actions during labor. Results of ergonomic studies lead to the adaptation of the worker's environment by improving the work place, the equipment, and associated training programs. In minimally invasive surgery (MIS), ergonomics apply to the development of improved operational instruments, of optics with higher resolution, of the operating room (OR) environment, as well as of the surgeon's posture and workload [1, 2]. The number of MIS procedures is constantly increasing, and it is even expected that it will prevail open surgery. Although the clinical benefits of this technology are becoming more evident, the risk factors for the surgeon and her/his performance and the incidence of physical fatigue as well as the economic outcomes are still not completely clarified [3].

Since the introduction of MIS almost 30 years ago, this technique underwent advancements including improvement in instrument development as well as the resolution of cameras and monitors. Despite these significant advancements in MIS technology, ergonomics are still a big challenge, especially in conventional MIS, with a main issue remaining the disassociation between the visual and the working field. The lack of fixing tissues and the limited tactile sensations aggravate the working conditions. The strain on the surgeon due to operation theatre arrangements, instrument structure, operating table height, monitor position, etc. has a significant effect on the outcome of MIS in general. In addition, the evaluation of stress and strain to surgeons during MIS procedures is still technically very challenging. It is thus important that the awareness about these ergonomic challenges that MIS surgeons are facing today are addressed properly and serve as a basis before the actual training of the surgical procedures.

2.2 Operating Room and Its Components

The work in the OR has fundamentally changed since the development of MIS, and it is obvious that ergonomics had to be redefined in order to meet the requirements of this new technology. Lifting all equipment from the floor improves the functionality of the OR complex and minimizes occupational safety and health (OSH) risks as the movement of equipment towers is reduced and the floor is clear of cables and cords (Fig. 2.1). Additionally, the user controls all systems used from a central location within the sterile area reducing unnecessary movements in the OR.

Z. Zachariou (✉)
Department of Pediatric Surgery, Medical School, University of Cyprus, Nicosia, Cyprus
e-mail: zzach@ucy.ac.cy

C. Esposito et al. (eds.), *ESPES Manual of Pediatric Minimally Invasive Surgery*,
https://doi.org/10.1007/978-3-030-00964-9_2

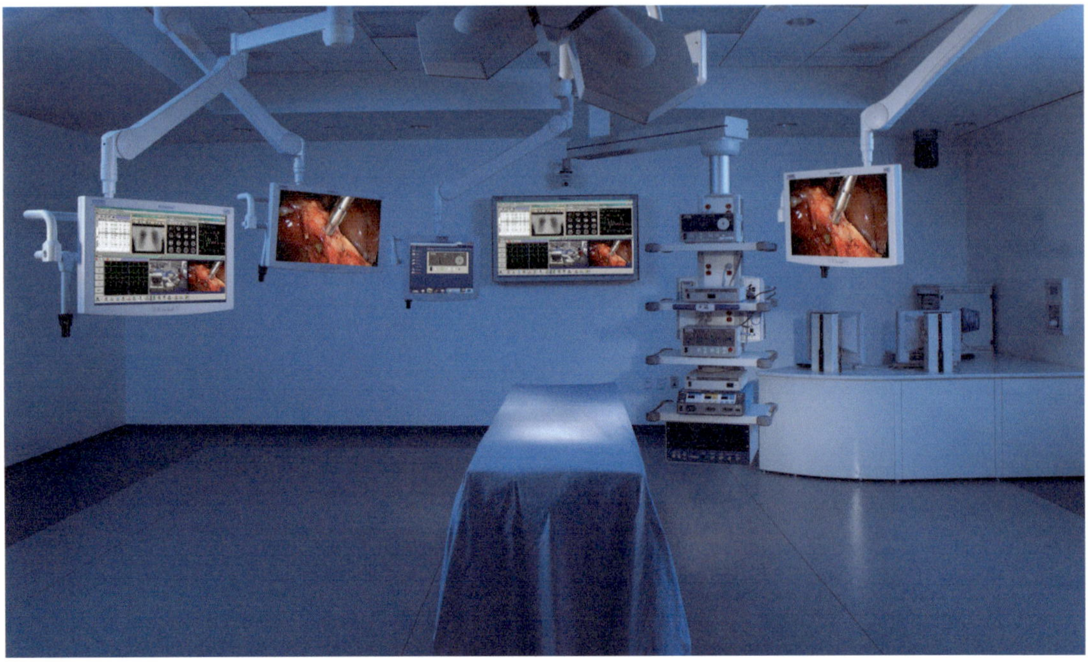

Fig. 2.1 Integrated operating room OR1™, KARL STORZ

During MIS procedures additional complex devices and complicated interfaces are placed in the OR between the patient, the surgeon, and the operation nurse. Appropriate ergonomics in the OR may increase safety, efficiency as well as comfort of the operating team, and by consequence the clinical outcome of the patient [1]. This can be achieved if the workplace organization ensures that every individual member of the surgical team has appropriate space and access to all equipment as the lack of balance in this respect leads inevitably to work overloads and injuries.

It is of utmost importance that the following considerations have to be taken into account when using the MIS equipment before and during surgical procedures:

- Operating table
  The operating table has to allow inclinations in the longitudinal as well as horizontal planes and enable tilts to the left and right. It should also enable kinking of the body on the level of the pelvis. The height of the operating table is essential and has to be adapted to the surgeon's individual height and position (standing or sitting). A table that is too high forces the surgeon to apply considerably more contraction of the body muscles in order to raise and hold the shoulders and elbows to compensate the high table. This can be tolerated for a short time, but if this position is maintained, it leads quickly to shoulder muscle fatigue.

  The table height that offers comfortable working conditions (about 64–77 cm above floor level) is when the MIS instrument handles are slightly below the level of the surgeon's elbows keeping the shoulders in a neutral position and the angle between the lower and upper arm during surgery is between 90° and 120° [4, 5] (Fig. 2.2).
- Monitor
  The monitor is the main visual contact between the patient and surgeon as the surgical scenarios are transmitted by this monitor. It is essential that the monitor is adjusted in its position already prior to surgery to avoid undesirable postures of the surgeon and the team in the whole for a long period of time. The monitor should be placed in such a manner that in the horizontal plane, it is in line

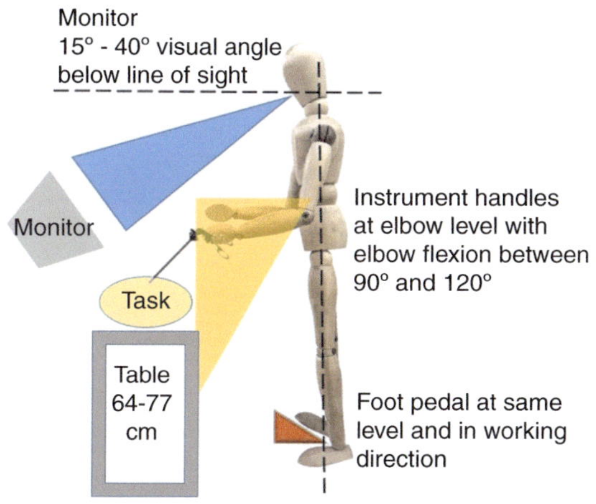

Fig. 2.2 Ergonomic position of OR equipment during MIS

with the surgeon and the forearm–instrument motor axis. In the sagittal plain, the monitor should be about 15° downward than the surgeon's eye level to ensure comfortable viewing, avoiding neck extension. The distance between the surgeon and monitor is highly dependent on monitor size, and it should be far enough to prevent extensive eye accommodation as well as extreme contraction of the extraocular muscles. It should be, however, close enough to avoid staring, resulting in loss of detail [6, 7]. An additional monitor near the operative field could offer additional benefits specially to accomplish precision tasks by improving hand–eye coordination [2, 7].

- Foot pedals
  Equipment like electrocauters, ultrasonic shears, laser, or other tissue welding/dividing instruments commonly need foot pedals to activate the instruments used during MIS. The lack of visual contact to the pedal results in an unbalanced position of the surgeon making the situation more difficult especially if more than one pedal is in use. The best solution is to replace them with hand controls. If not possible the pedals should be placed near the foot aligned in the same direction as the instrument in use and the monitor, thus enabling the surgeon to activate the device without twisting the body or leg. Pedals with a built-in footrest should be preferred.
- Theatre lighting
  In order to increase the contrast on the monitor, the lights in the OR are only dimmed and not completely switched off as working even in relative darkness may have a negative impact on the appropriate choice of similar instruments and safe handling of needles and scalpels as well and increase the risk of collision.

2.3 Patient Position

The position of the patient during MIS is usually supine with the arms of the patient in a position that does not interfere with the visual axis of the surgeon. This implies that the arms are tucked along the body at least unilaterally. The legs of the patients may be spread apart with the thighs extended below the pelvis in order to avoid instrument clash. Despite the abovementioned complex patient position, it is essential to prevent any compression of nerves.

2.4 MIS Instruments

The majority of the first-generation MIS instruments was offered by the industry in one standard size, which transmitted lower force compared to standard instruments, demanding higher muscular activity and effort from the surgeon to handle the tissue [8]. Nowadays most MIS instrument development is technology-driven and less designed for the physical and emotional comfort of the users, potentially leading to a user-unfriendly product design. The design of surgical instruments influences the performance of MIS procedures as it dictates the position of the surgeon's arms, hands, and fingers. Mainly the shape of the handle and the tool length are of great significance as non-ergonomic designs lead to discomfort and even to paresthesias of the thumb [9]. A possible solution for this problem is to use powered instruments, similarly used in staplers; however these are more expensive. Although there are different handle designs, it seems that instruments with axial handle lead to a more ergonomic posture for the wrist compared to a ring handle. Different instrument handles influence the task to be achieved. Pistol-type handles enable better performance in tasks that require force, while precision-type handles enable tasks that require precision [10].

In recent years efforts are made to improve and overcome the ergonomic limitations of MIS. One essential parameter to achieve this is by increasing the instrument's degrees of freedom. New instruments are more of devices with precision-driven and articulating instrument tips which increase the triangulation, thus improving the performance of surgical maneuvers. However, this development requires new manual skills and complementary knowledge of how to use them.

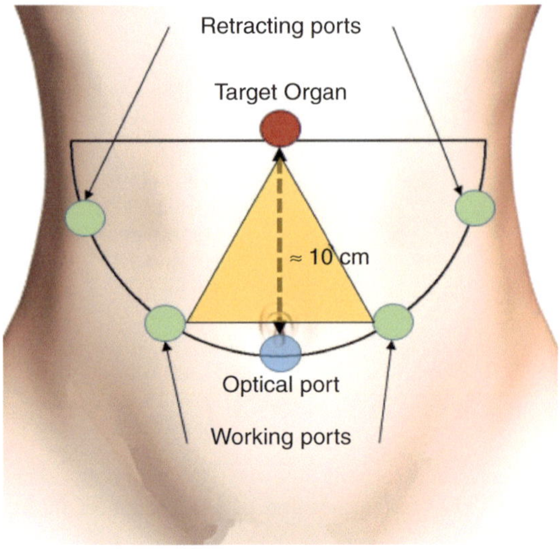

Fig. 2.3 Triangulation of the trocars

2.5 Trocar Placements

Although trocar placements are currently dictated by the surgeon's preference based on individual experience, defined ergonomic principles should be applied when possible. The trocars should be placed in triangular fashion as this configuration facilitates smooth instrument manipulation along with adequate visualization. In most of the procedures, the optical port should be placed about 10 cm from the target organ with two working ports on the same 10 cm arc on either side of the optical port allowing a working space at a 60°–90° angle. If necessary additional retracting ports could be placed more laterally to the working ports on the same arc (Fig. 2.3).

In certain cases, the target organ is on one side so that the optical port comes to lie on one side and the working ports on the other side of the target organ. This is defined as sectorization (Fig. 2.4).

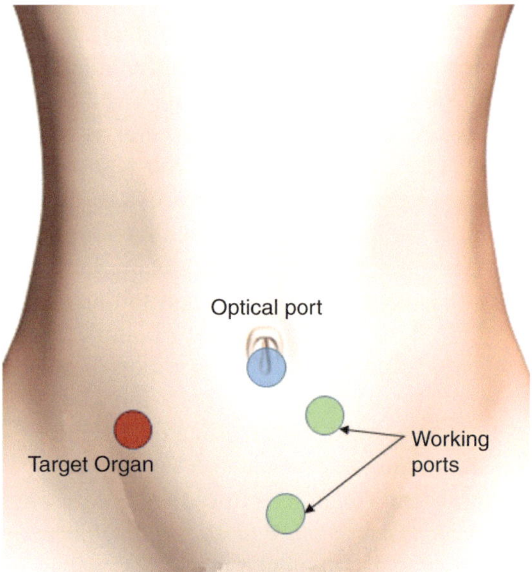

Fig. 2.4 Sectorization of trocars

Due to the limited length of the instruments, trocars have to be positioned in such a way that the tip of the instrument can reach the target organ without having to put the whole instrument in the trocar or sometimes to push the trocar all the way in the abdomen. This impairs the movement of the instrument making it less precise as well. The angles between the instruments are also a factor that, if chosen correctly, increases the performance and causes less fatigue for the surgeon. The trocars have to be positioned in defined distances from body landmarks in order to facilitate the optimal ergonomic manipulation, i.e., suture and knotting. The suggested positions within the triangulation principle are indicated in Fig. 2.5. Manipulation angles below 45° or above 75° are accompanied by increased difficulty and degraded performance. In addition, the intra-/extracorporeal (I/E) length ratio of the working instruments should be preferably close to 1:1. A direct correlation between the manipulation and the elevation angle influences ergonomics significantly. The optimal elevation angle which yields the shortest execution time and optimal quality performance is 60° (Fig. 2.6).

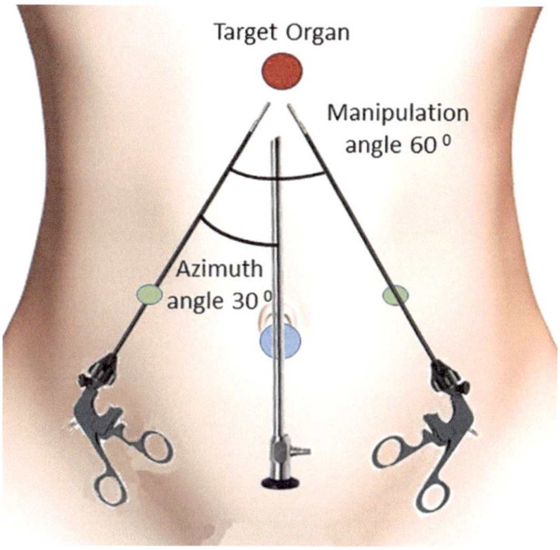

Fig. 2.5 Angles between instruments

2.6 Limited Degree of Freedom

A MIS procedure is performed by the surgeon using an instrument through a trocar. The movements of the surgeon's hand are transmitted through the incision point to the tip of the instrument. The degree of freedom (DoF) is defined by the potential for movement of the instrument either in one direction or around the instrument axis. While in open surgery the surgeon is allowed to work within the natural six DoFs (Fig. 2.7a), MIS instruments possess a motion constraint of four DoFs (Fig. 2.7b) [11]:

- 1st DoF—up/down (heave)
- 2nd DoF—rotation around instrument axis (roll)
- 3rd DoF—left/right (sway)
- 4th DoF—forward/backward (surge)

The limitation in the DoFs with MIS instruments makes handling of the target organ more difficult, which has to be compensated by experience and full application of ergonomic principles.

2.7 Disconnection of the Visual and Motor Axes

A three-dimensional spatial vision field and work performed in line with the person's visual axis are the features we naturally adopt during our

Fig. 2.6 Elevation angle, intra-/extracorporeal (I/E) length ratio

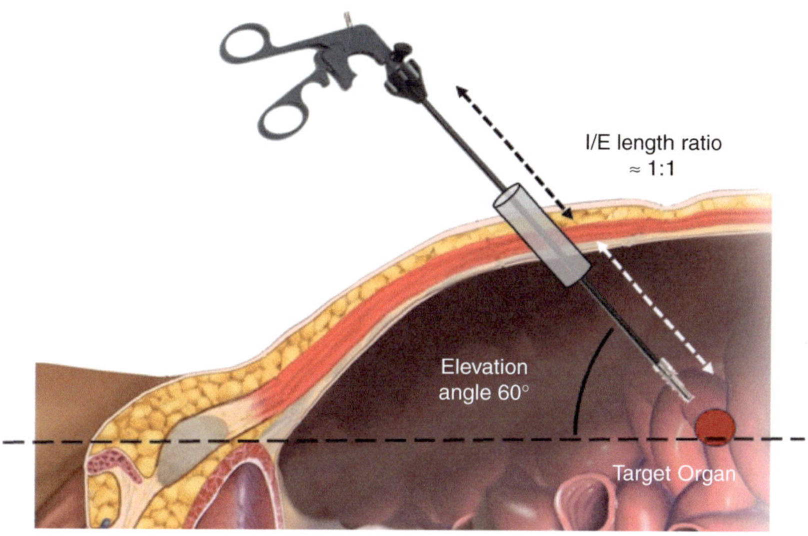

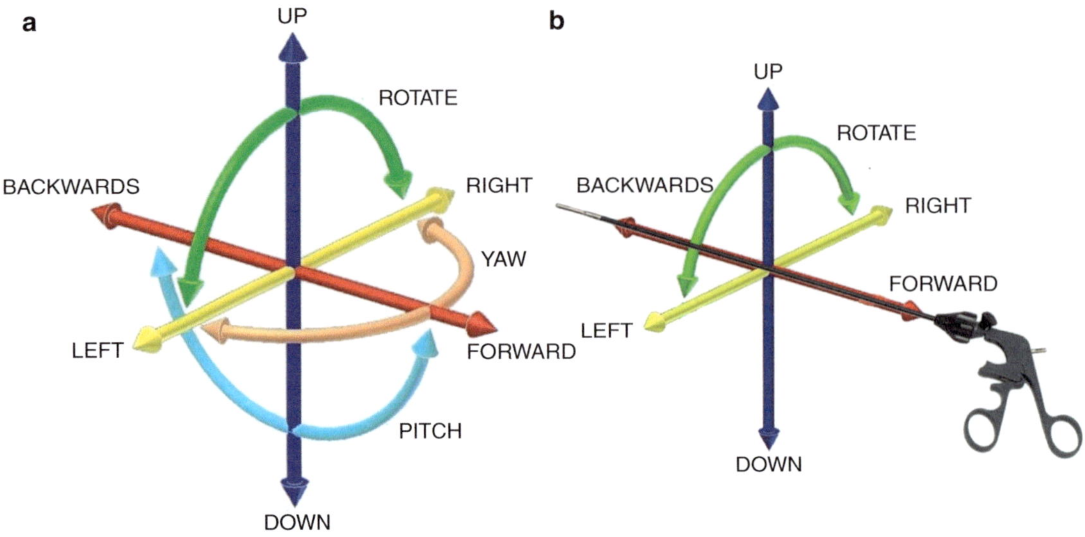

Fig. 2.7 Six degrees of freedom (**a**) vs four degrees (**b**) during MIS

actions. In MIS the visual field is reduced to bidimensional vision shown on the screen, causing confusion. This loss of the third dimension is associated with the loss of depth perception and reconstruction of space which is strongly limited especially if operating small children. During MIS the surgeon's motor actions are decoupled from the visual axis so that the surgeon is not able to directly look at the instruments. The hands and the surgical field at the same time and has to overcome the spatial separation of the axis of vision and the axis of the physical procedure by combining the two functions into one channeled approach. The surgeon has to concentrate more during MIS procedures, and this may decrease performance, leading to higher rates of error [1].

2.8 Diminished Tactile Feedback

Since childhood, we learn different skills and train to "see" not only with our eyes but also with our hands. We become competent and reach a high level of dexterity by achieving this dual job. During MIS procedures, the haptic and tactile feedback is conspicuously lacking as the long instruments manipulated through the access ports reduce the efficiency during the learning curve and result in an increased time of dissection [12]. However, through experience this tactile feedback can be partly regained by learning to "feel" using the instrument as an extended hand.

2.9 Hawthorne Effect

Since MIS was introduced, the Hawthorne effect was observed. It has been proven that every individual applies more caution and performs better whenever this individual is under observation of other people resulting in an immediate assessment of the performance. This results in a better score as compared with a situation where the person is unaware that an assessment is performed. This behavior contributes essentially to ergonomics; however, although beneficial for the patient, it results in a bias for the evaluation of ergonomics during MIS.

2.10 Body Posture

The specific arrangement of the equipment in the OR as the location of the monitor, operating table, foot pedals, and the design of surgical instruments determines to a large extent the surgeon's posture and the organization of the surgical team. The way surgeons interact not only in the operating

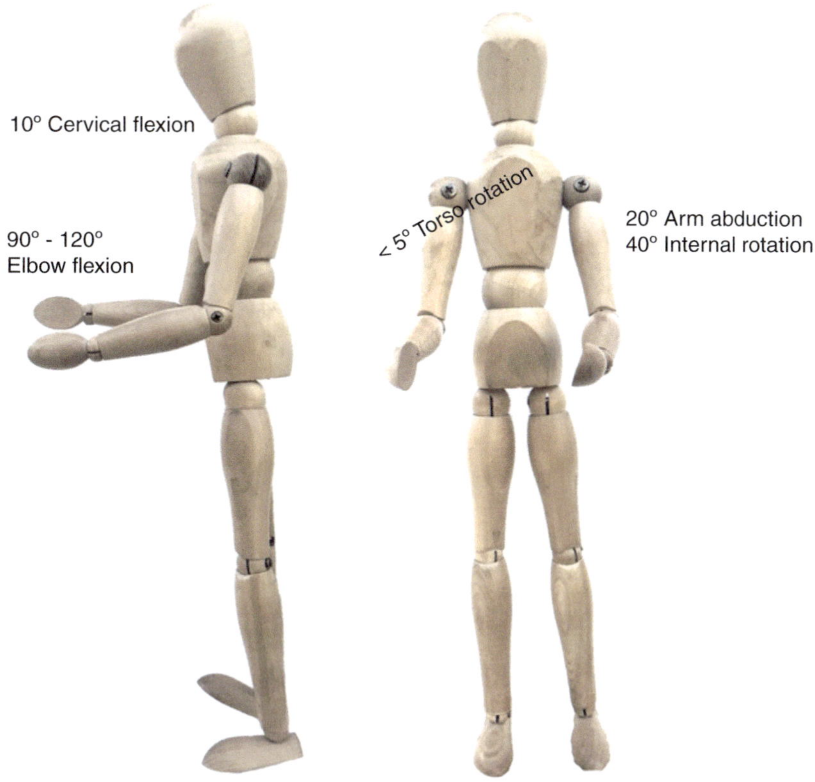

Fig. 2.8 Suggested surgeon's posture during MIS

field but also regarding their position and movements during MIS has changed radically. While during open surgery the surgeon moves the whole body in order to get a better view of the target organ, during MIS the only possibility to view the target organ is the visual contact to the monitor, resulting in certain ergonomic inconveniences with loss of freedom deriving from the static posture of the surgeon. Due to the fixed port position, which determines defined instruments motion, dexterity is limited. The surgeon is in an upright position with fewer movements of the torso and infrequent weight shifting. This behavior is ergonomically not correct. These limitations affect the surgeon's posture, which during MIS procedures is static, maintaining forced and somewhat awkward long-term postures. It has been demonstrated that muscles and tendons build up lactic acid and toxins when keeping the abovementioned postures. This body deviation from the neutral position is associated with increasing fatigue over time and increases the risk factor for musculoskeletal disorders [13].

The position considered ideal for MIS procedures is when the cervical spine has a slight flexion (10°) and the arms are slightly abducted (20°) and rotated inward (40°). The elbow should be bent at a 90°–120° angle. The torso can be minimally rotated, however, less than 5° (Fig. 2.8). The hands should grasp the instruments with the wrist slightly extended and with the distal interphalangeal joints almost extended, and the metacarpophalangeal and proximal interphalangeal joints fixed at 30°–50°. Fingers should be abducted, and the thumb should be opposed to the index finger [9, 14].

2.11 Ergonomics in Novel MIS Approaches

In order to improve medical outcomes as well as aesthetic results, novel MIS procedures have been developed. However, these innovative methods are connected with an increase of technical applications that result in new ergonomic challenges.

- Laparoendoscopic single-site surgery (LESS) This method leads to a reduction of the number and size of incisions. However, despite that LESS inherits the constraints of conventional laparoscopy, it creates new ergonomic restrictions such as reduced triangulation, lack of coordination, and external and internal instrument clashing [15]. Experienced surgeons performing a defined task were evaluated in respect of muscular activity and wrist and hand motion in comparison to conventional laparoscopy. Results showed that the LESS approach required greater level of muscular activity in the trapezius and forearm extensor muscles but better wrist position [16]. Generally, LESS is more stressful and physically demanding.
- Robotic surgery
  In addition to beneficial effects for the patient, robotic systems have been propagated as a potential solution to the limited ergonomics during conventional MIS through enhanced dexterity, maneuverability, stability, and accuracy. Surgeons with different experience levels in robotic surgery were assessed regarding their physical workload compared with conventional laparoscopy. The physical and cognitive ergonomics with robotic assistance were significantly less challenging [17]. This could even be confirmed in medical students performing sutures on porcine specimens [18]. Surgeons applying robotic surgery report less frustration and higher good mood using robotic assistance. High expenses, maintenance costs, and low case volume seem to be the main limitations of robotic surgery [19].
- Single-incision laparoscopic surgery (SILS)
  The ergonomics imposed by this approach are considerably different from those of multiport MIS. The main issues utilizing this technique are the narrow angulation of the instruments, the instrument crowding, and the limited traction/retraction possibilities [20]. A modification of the conventional ergonomics is mandatory as well as novel instrument designs such as handheld manipulators with seven DoFs.

Cutting-edge technologies that combine imaging with virtual and/or augmented reality as well as simulations could contribute to establish new techniques for more and more surgical procedures.

2.12 Methods for Ergonomic Assessment

Ergonomic assessments are of imminent importance in order to improve the medical outcome as well as the comfort of the surgeon which influences the medical result. The instruments applied for this assessment include:

- Body posture which is accessed with photogrammetry.
- 3-D motion tracking that quantifies movements by means of positional data obtained from sensors placed on the subject's body.
- Electrogoniometers are devices which measure electrical signals induced by flexion or rotation. Data gloves are equipped with this technology that allows recording movements of the fingers and wrist.
- Force platforms are used to analyze the body balance during static or dynamic situations.
- Mental workload evaluates the psychological burden of surgeons assessed by subjective techniques.
- Questionnaires focus on gathering information from a population of surgeons on specific issues that can identify elements where the abovementioned studies have to be performed to identify procedures to be improved.

2.13 Conclusion

Despite multiple patient advantages, MIS entails a number of ergonomic inconveniences for the surgeon. With the number of procedures and surgeons performing MIS increasing, it seems that the lack of ergonomic guidelines for MIS results in musculoskeletal disorders of the surgeon and decreasing performance. Despite this fact, additional costs related to ergonomics during MIS are considered not justified. The progress in ergonomics in MIS is not only dependent on the manufacturers that constantly try to reduce the production cost. Governments, reimbursement systems, as well as the surgeons themselves should be responsible for the development of ergonomics in MIS from the innovating idea to the final product. MIS provides patients with less trauma resulting in rapid recovery, however requires that surgeons work under new conditions that might increase complaints of surgeon fatigue and discomfort, leading to serious health problems. Since the cost-containment pressures demand more efficient surgery and MIS requires increased technological complexity, ergonomics have to be included in development and investment priorities.

The parameters that influence ergonomics are the static surgeon's posture, the adjustability of the operating table, the position of the equipment in use, and the design of MIS instruments. An ergonomic upgrade would alleviate these adverse conditions experienced by surgeons.

References

1. Supe AN, Kulkarni GV, Supe PA. Ergonomics in laparoscopic surgery. J Minim Access Surg. 2010;6:31–6.
2. Rogers ML, Heath WB, Uy CC, Suresh S, Kaber DB. Effect of visual displays and locations on laparoscopic surgical training task. Appl Ergon. 2012;43:762–7.
3. Fullum TM, Ladapo JA, Borah BJ, Gunnarsson CL. Comparison of the clinical and economic outcomes between open and minimally invasive appendectomy and colectomy: evidence from a large commercial payer database. Surg Endosc. 2010;24:845–53.
4. Berquer R, Smith WD, Davis S. An ergonomic study of the optimum operating table height for laparoscopic surgery. Surg Endosc. 2002;16:416–21.
5. Van Veelen MA, Kazemier G, Koopman J, Goossens RH, Meijer DW. Assessment of the ergonomically optimal operating surface height for laparoscopic surgery. J Laparoendosc Adv Surg Tech A. 2002;12(1):47–52.
6. Xiao DJ, Jakimowicz JJ, Albayrak A, Goossens RHM. Ergonomic factors on task performance in laparoscopic surgery training. Appl Ergon. 2012;43:548–53.
7. Van Det MJ, Meijerink WJHJ, Hoff C, Totté ER, Pierie JPEN. Optimal ergonomics for laparoscopic surgery in minimally invasive surgery suites: a review and guidelines. Surg Endosc. 2009;23:1279–85.
8. Forkey D, Smith W, Berguer R. A comparison of thumb and forearm muscle effort required for laparoscopic and open surgery using an ergonomic measurement station. In: 19th Annual International Conference of the IEEE Engineering in Medicine and Biology Society; 1997.
9. Matern U, Waller P. Instruments for minimally invasive surgery. Principles of ergonomic handles. Surg Endosc. 2009;13:174–82.
10. Berguer R. Ergonomics in laparoscopic surgery. In: Whelan RL, Fleshman JW, Fowler DL, editors. The SAGES manual of perioperative care in minimally invasive surgery. New York: Springer; 2005. p. 454–64.
11. Pérez-Duarte FJ, Sánchez-Margallo FM, Díaz-Güemes I, Sánchez-Hurtado MÁ, LucasHernández M, Usón J. Ergonomics in laparoscopic surgery and its importance in surgical training. Cir Esp. 2012;90:284–91.
12. Patkin M, Isabel L. Ergonomics, engineering and surgery of endosurgical dissection. J R Coll Surg Edinb. 1995;40:120–32.
13. Geng L, Sun C, Bai J. Single incision versus conventional laparoscopic cholecystectomy outcomes: a meta-analysis of randomized controlled trials. PLoS One. 2013;8(10):e765.
14. Matern U. Ergonomic deficiencies in the operating room: examples from minimally invasive surgery. Work. 2009;32:1–4.
15. Matos-Azevedo AM, Díaz-Guëmes I, Pérez-Duarte FJ, Sánchez-Hurtado MÁ, SánchezMargallo FM. Comparison of single access devices during cut and suturing tasks on simulator. J Surg Res. 2014;192(2):356–67.
16. Pérez-Duarte FJ, Lucas-Hernández M, Matos-Azevedo A, Sánchez-Margallo JA, Díaz Güemes I, Sánchez-Margallo FM. Objective analysis of surgeons' ergonomy during laparoendoscopic single-site surgery through the use of surface electromyography and a motion capture data glove. Surg Endosc. 2014;28:1314–20.
17. Lee GI, Lee MR, Clanton T, Clanton T, Sutton E, Park AE, et al. Comparative assessment of physical and cognitive ergonomics associated with robotic and traditional laparoscopic surgeries. Surg Endosc. 2014;28:456–65.
18. Stefanidis D, Wang F, Korndorffer JR, Dunne JB, Scott DJ. Robotic assistance improves intracorporeal suturing performance and safety in the operating room while decreasing operator workload. Surg Endosc. 2010;24:377–82.
19. Elhage O, Challacombe B, Shortland A, Dasgupta P. An assessment of the physical impact of complex surgical tasks on surgeon errors and discomfort: a comparison between robot-assisted, laparoscopic and open approaches. BJU Int. 2015;115(2):274–8.
20. Tang B, Hou S, Cuschieri SA. Ergonomics of and technologies for single-port laparoscopic surgery. Minim Invasive Ther Allied Technol. 2012;21(1):46–54.

3 Checklist and Preoperative Preparation

Jürgen Schleef, Sara Cherti, and Edoardo Guida

3.1 Introduction

Any kind of procedure can be divided in different steps. This is a standard rule for programming and performing operative procedures not only in surgery. Generally we talk about preoperative, intraoperative and post-operative steps. Each step has its own characteristics and principles. As in any procedural process, a standard approach is desirable. To guarantee this standardisation, the procedure is defined and divided in different steps, and the process needs to be well defined, described and reproducible. This reproducibility is absolutely necessary for guaranteeing a standard and gives the basis for any kind of evaluation on complications, outcome and results [1]. The basis for the preparation of a reproducible procedure is in most cases a checklist. Checklists are almost present in any kind of procedure not only in medicine. The checklist is the basis for guaranteeing the preparation of all single processes of a procedure.

This chapter is dealing with the preoperative preparations and the checklists used in this phase of operative procedures. We have to pay attention to different aspects, to a certain timeline, to technical requirements and to the role of all professionals involved. This is generally a very complex and dynamic situation [2].

J. Schleef (✉) · S. Cherti · E. Guida
Department of Paediatric Surgery and Urology, Institute for Maternal and Child Health—IRCCS Burlo Garofolo, Trieste, Italy
e-mail: jurgen.schleef@burlo.trieste.it

3.2 Preoperative Preparation

Preoperative preparation is essential for any kind of procedure. These can be divided in different steps:

- *Preoperative preparation of the OR*
- *Preoperative preparation of the team*
- *Preoperative preparation of the patient*

Each step is usually accompanied by a checklist.

3.2.1 Preoperative Preparation of the OR

Surgical procedures in endosurgery require a complex equipment in the operation theatre. This might also vary in respect to the type of surgery. Standard procedures need a checklist which facilitates the preparations and the standardisation. In our OR setting, we are using specific checklist for single standard surgeries like appendectomy, fundoplication, splenectomy, pyloromyotomy, laparoscopy for non-palpable testicles, lobectomy and transanal or laparoscopic-assisted

C. Esposito et al. (eds.), *ESPES Manual of Pediatric Minimally Invasive Surgery*,
https://doi.org/10.1007/978-3-030-00964-9_3

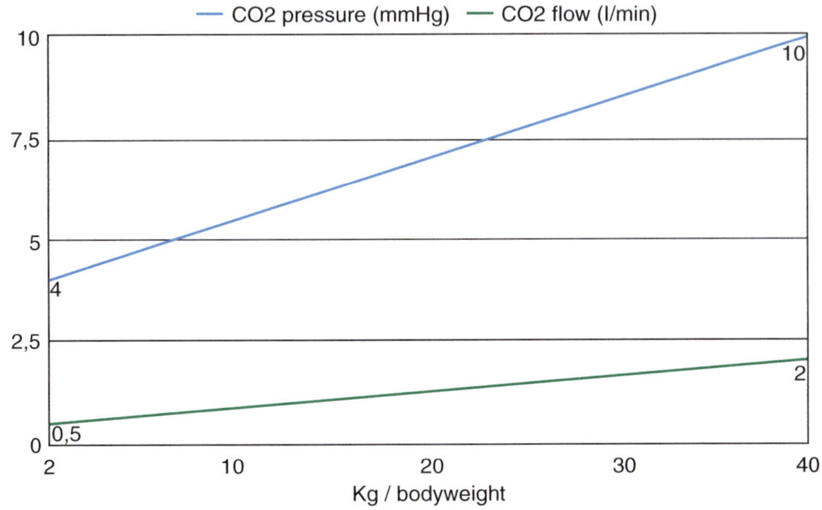

Fig. 3.1 Values of CO2 pressure (mmHg) and CO2 flow (L/min) related to the patient's weight

pull-through procedures. The following aspects have to be considered:

- Instrumentation (size, length, specific instruments, scope size and length)
- Setup of technology (position of the patient on the OR table; position of equipment, monitors, eventual special devices)
- Localisation of actors in the operation theatre (anaesthesiologist, surgeons, nurse)
- For the installation of the CO2 pneumoperitoneum, we are using since many years a diagram which adjusts the pressure in relation to the body weight of the patient. This general rule gives a standard value which is preset by the OR nurses and can be individually modified (Fig. 3.1).

An example for this short and basic checklist can be seen in Fig. 3.2, which is the checklist for the laparoscopic cholecystectomy. All these checklists are complementary to the joint commission standard checklist and protocols which are used for all kinds of procedures in the operation theatre but which do not pay attention to the specific aspects of endosurgical procedures.

3.2.2 Preoperative Preparation of the Team

The above-mentioned checklist is also providing information concerning the details of the procedure. Every procedure is described in detail, and specific conditions (e.g. suture material, stapler, endo equipments) are underlined. This description is performed together with nurses and surgeons. This kind of description is extremely important to guarantee a standard procedure and to facilitate the preparation and performance of surgery. All these checklists are constantly updated. Recently, also the anaesthesia team starts to rely on this checklist and information. In some procedures (e.g. lung resection), anaesthetists have to have a precise knowledge of the procedures and need a special preparation of the patient before surgery (selective blocking of the bronchus, Fig. 3.3).

3.2.3 Preoperative Preparation of the Patient

The preparation before surgery of the patient is an essential step. The introduction of fast-track procedure is reducing the time the patient is being recovered especially before surgery [3]. Many operations are performed in a day-surgery setting. The patient who is not requiring a pre-op recovery for special indications (transfusion, bowel preparation) is entering the hospital in the morning of the day of surgery. That means, all important steps (lab examination, cardiology consultation, consent forms, visit with the anaesthetist) have to be planed earlier usually during

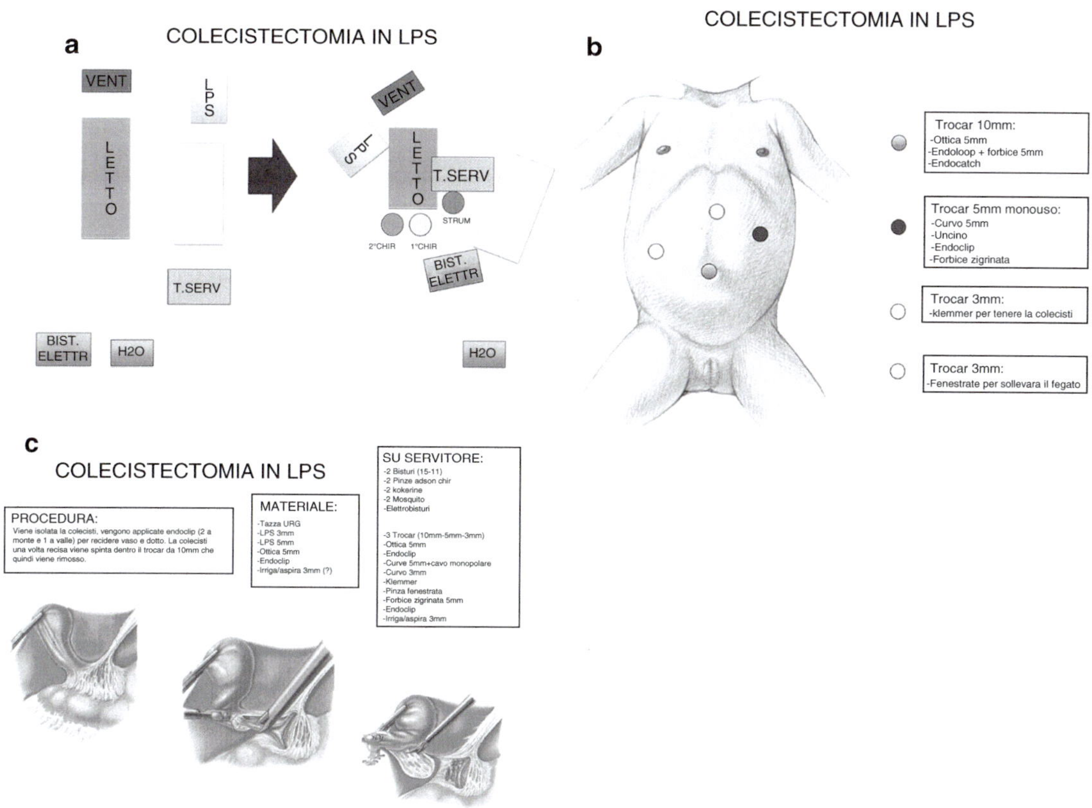

Fig. 3.2 Example of checklist and protocol used for laparoscopic cholecystectomy. (**a**) Layout of the operating room during the operation; (**b**) Laparoscopic trocars position; (**c**) Instruments description to perform laparoscopic cholecystectomy

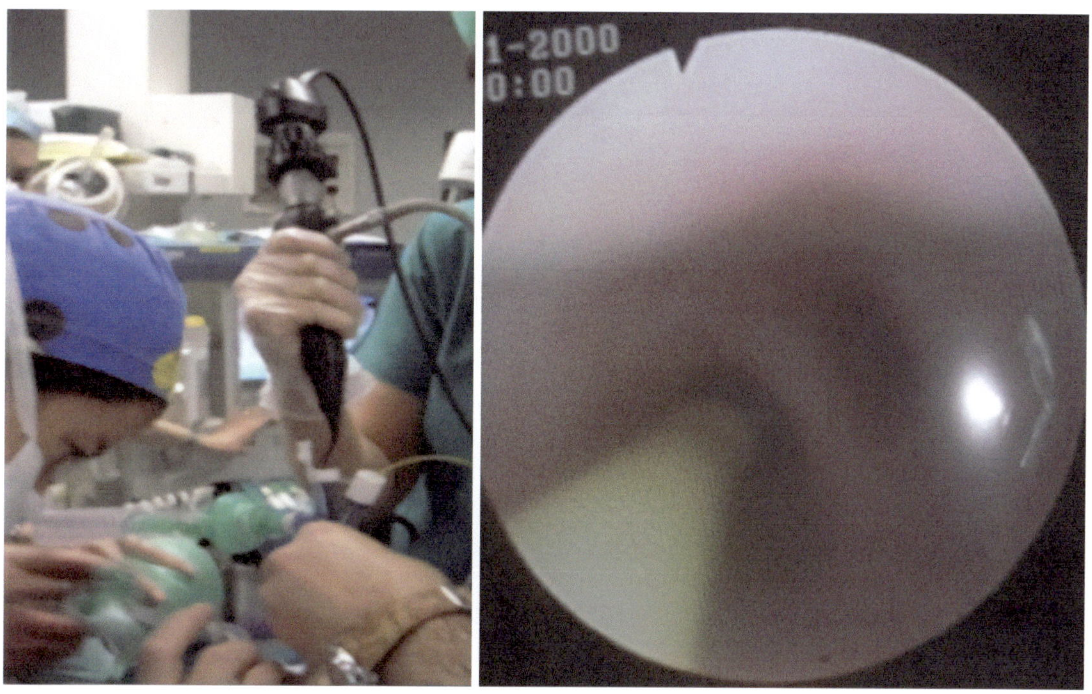

Fig. 3.3 Selective blocking of the bronchus performed by anaesthetist before lung surgery

an outpatient visit [4]. Patients and their parents have to be informed in advance and need all information concerning timing and location of visits and consultation. All patients are getting usually an information form with all necessary details. A phone number for further information or contacts in case of problems are given to parents and patients.

3.3 Conclusion

This brief overview should give some information for the organisation of the preoperative management in the hospital. Every hospital and every structure might have a detailed and self-developed schedule. In all structures organisation details might be different and should be considered. Nevertheless checklist and procedures have to be defined to standardise and organise surgery. After this step of preoperative measures, intra- and post-operative steps should be organised in a similar way and give some kind of continued organisation. We should keep in mind that legal aspects and problems are very often associated to missing.

References

1. Liu J, Zheng X, Chai S, Lei M, Feng Z, Zhang X, Lopez V. Effects of using WeChat-assisted perioperative care instructions for parents of pediatric patients undergoing day surgery for herniorrhaphy. Patient Educ Couns. 2018;19:0738–3991.
2. Gentry KR, Lepere K, Opel DJ. Informed consent in pediatric anesthesiology. Paediatr Anaesth. 2017;27(12):1253–60.
3. Schukfeh N, Reismann M, Ludwikowski B, Hofmann AD, Kaemmerer A, Metzelder ML, Ure B. Implementation of fast-track pediatric surgery in a German nonacademic institution without previous fast-track experience. Eur J Pediatr Surg. 2014;24(5):419–25.
4. Reismann M, Dingemann J, Wolters M, Laupichler B, Suempelmann R, Ure BM. Fast-track concepts in routine pediatric surgery: a prospective study in 436 infants and children. Langenbecks Arch Surg. 2009;394(3):529–33.

4 Basis of Laparoscopic Approach

Jozef Babala

4.1 Introduction

Laparoscopy is a visual examination of the abdominal cavity by means of a telescope, which is inserted through the abdominal wall.

The condition of laparoscopic surgery is that a space is created in the abdominal cavity by distending the abdominal wall, which allows the visualisation and instrument manipulation for diagnostic and therapeutic purposes.

The working space in the abdominal cavity is accomplished by gas insufflation (pneumoperitoneum) or by mechanical traction of the abdominal wall (gasless laparoscopy).

Mostly, the abdominal cavity is filled with CO2 gas, which creates capnoperitoneum. The gas is insufflated via closed technique with the Veress needle or open Hasson technique.

With the closed technique, after the initial creation of capnoperitoneum using the Veress needle, the first port is blind inserted and a telescope is placed in it. Further ports are inserted under direct vision; the number and layout are determined according to the type of the operation.

With the open Hasson technique, it is necessary to verify through the incision that we are safe in the peritoneal cavity and we insert the first port, create capnoperitoneum through it, and place a telescope in it. Further ports are inserted under direct vision; the number and layout are determined according to the type of the surgery.

In like manner, for the performance of single-incision laparoscopy (SILS), a special port is inserted via open technique through a greater incision.

J. Babala (✉)
National Institute of Children's Diseases,
Bratislava, Slovakia
e-mail: babala@dfnsp.sk

4.2 Preoperative Preparation

If the laparoscopic approach is indicated in a patient, it is necessary to consider the age and weight of the patient and cardiovascular, respiratory, and other risk factors. The surgeon must have cognisance of previous abdominal surgeries with respect to the occurrence of possible adhesions and also of enlarged organs (liver, spleen, dilated urinary bladder), and of potential pathological masses, such as tumours, inflammatory masses, aneurysms, and hernias.

In planning a less frequent and/or technically demanding operation, the surgeon will familiarise the team with the surgical procedure and technical requirements. This includes the position of the patient, position of the surgical team, position of the laparoscopic tower, location of the monitor/monitors, and specification of instruments.

In newborns and infants, preoperative degassing of the gastrointestinal tract is recommended. Where

C. Esposito et al. (eds.), *ESPES Manual of Pediatric Minimally Invasive Surgery*,
https://doi.org/10.1007/978-3-030-00964-9_4

the operation includes intestine opening (appendectomy, etc.), antibiotic prophylaxis is administered, which is carried out in the operating room after the intravenous cannula has been inserted.

A child patient is placed under general anaesthesia with relaxed muscles. Nasogastric tube as a prevention of aspiration when applying an increased intra-abdominal pressure is indicated in all patients [1, 2].

The urinary bladder should be emptied naturally before operation. After the patient has been placed under general anaesthesia, the urinary bladder can be emptied by means of Crede manoeuvre, and for demanding surgery, the insertion of a Foley catheter is recommended [3].

Immediately before the commencement of the operation, the function of instruments needs to be checked: light source, camera, and insufflator with a sufficient quantity of gas in the CO2 bottle. An open surgery instrument kit should be available in case conversion is necessary.

4.3 Positioning

For the laparoscopic approach, the position of the patient should be supine.

The Veress needle is usually inserted at the site where the primary cannula for the telescope will be placed [1]. The most frequent regions for access are transumbilical access and infra- or supra-umbilical access.

Access in pararectal lines may also be used. However, also other abdominal wall sites can be selected, provided that the physiological status is modified by post-operative scars, a tumour mass, or other abnormalities.

The position of the patient on the operating table can be longitudinal or transversal, which is suitable for newborns and infants (frog position).

For laparoscopic surgery, which requires an elevated position of the patient (splenectomy, adrenalectomy), the initial supine position is reached by supporting the patient and rotating the operating table.

For entry into the abdominal cavity, a cooperation is necessary between the surgeon and the assistant, who stand either on one side of the patient or opposite each other. Adequate visualisation can be obtained provided that the monitor is placed ergonomically opposite the surgeon.

4.4 Instrumentation

Laparoscopic kit components: insufflator with a well visible display and adjusted values of pressure (6–12 mmHg) and gas flow (low, medium, high). Light source and camera with white balance calibrated.

Veress needle with the mechanism of safety telescopic blunt-tip trocar. The sharp needle penetrates the abdominal wall, and the centrally placed blunt-tip trocar is extended after penetrating the resistance, thus protecting the intra-abdominal organs against injury. Initial pneumoperitoneum is created by CO2 insufflation through the hollow trocar with a hole at its end. Veress needles can be reusable or disposable.

Working ports are tubular cannulas with an extractable trocar. After placing the working port transparietally, the penetration trocar will be removed. The hollow cannula equipped with a valve mechanism against CO2 leak serves to access the abdominal cavity. In addition to the working access, the port also participates to maintain pressure in the distended abdominal cavity.

The diameter of most frequently used working ports is from 3.5 to 15 mm (the initial port for telescope entry 5 and 10 mm). Working ports can be reusable or disposable. Some disposable safety ports have a trocar that is equipped with a mechanism similar to the Veress needle; when after penetrating the abdominal wall, the sharp point is hidden in the extracted part of the blunt-tip trocar. Ports with a diameter of 12 and 15 mm with the possibility of valve reduction from 5 to 12 or up to 15 mm are available so that it is not necessary to replace the entire port when alternating instruments of various diameters. Ports with visual intraluminal control during insertion into the abdominal cavity are also available.

For purposes of initial incision or for the open access using the Hasson technique, conventional instrumentation is used. Monopolar coagulation used in open surgery should also be available.

4.5 Creation of Pneumoperitoneum: Technique

Creation of capnoperitoneum via closed method using the Veress needle—infra-umbilical approach.

Veress needle insertion. Using a scalpel, an incision is made that copies the inferior arc of the umbilical depression and is by 1–2 mm longer than the port diameter (Fig. 4.1). By blunt dissection the fascia is exposed and seized on the sides by means of Kocher forceps (towel clips or strong holding sutures can be used instead of the Kocher forceps). Ventral traction is used to elevate the anterior abdominal wall. A small longitudinal incision is made in the fascia for Veress needle entry (Fig. 4.2). Before insertion, the Veress needle must be checked for patency, and the telescopic safety trocar for functionality. The trocar is checked by leaning against a firm support and springing.

The needle is grasped at a distance of 4 cm from the tip, and while elevating the abdominal wall, the Veress needle is inserted perpendicularly through the fascia incision (Fig. 4.3). After the penetration into the abdominal cavity, with the "click" sound, the needle is directed at an angle of 45° into the abdominal cavity (Fig. 4.4). The correctness of Veress needle positioning is checked by the following manoeuvres. A free circular movement of the needle indicates the correct position. Then a syringe is connected and we try to aspirate the content (blood, enteric content, urine); if aspiration is not possible, 5–10 mL of

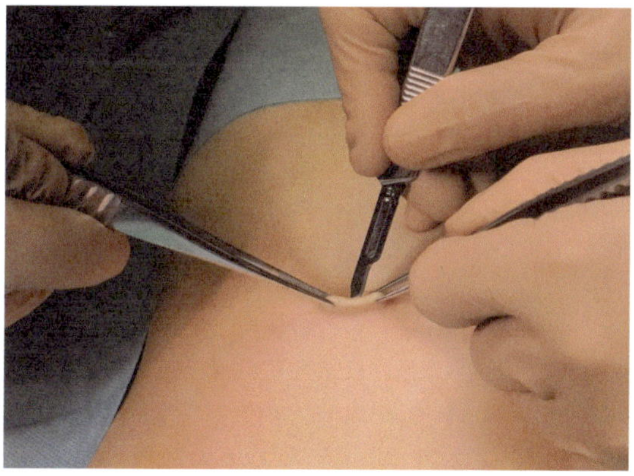

Fig. 4.1 The incision copies the inferior arc of the umbilicus (infra-umbilical approach)

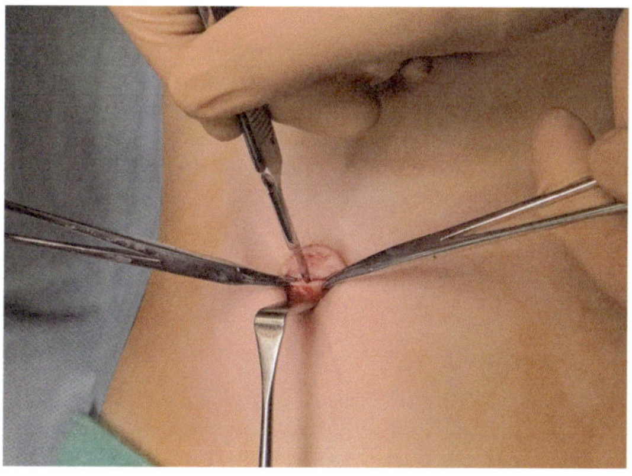

Fig. 4.2 A small longitudinal incision in the fascia for Veress needle entry

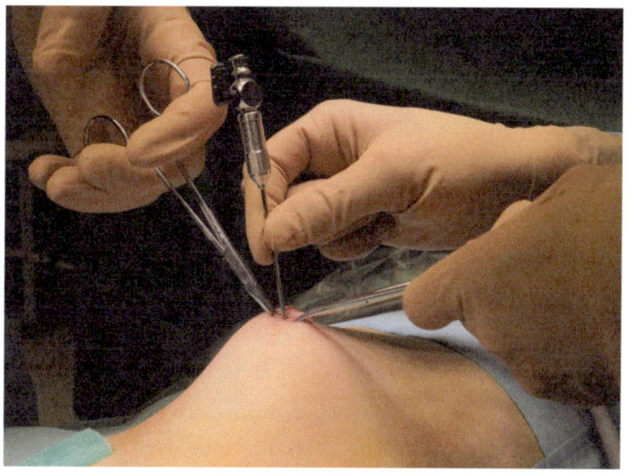

Fig. 4.3 The Veress needle is inserted through the fascia incision. Abdominal wall is elevated

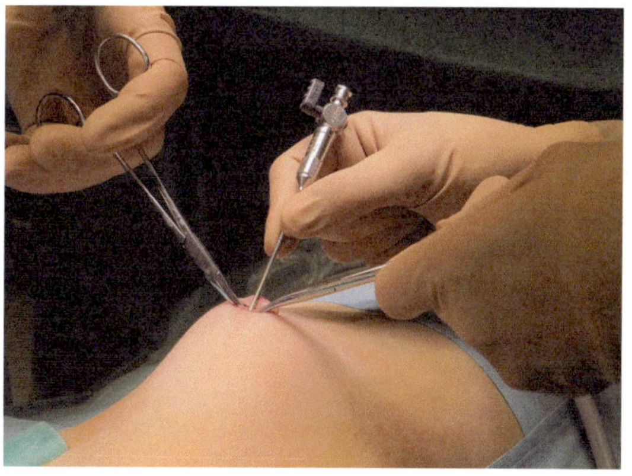

Fig. 4.4 The needle is directed at an angle of 45° into the abdominal cavity

saline is administered. Instillation should be free without resistance and without a possibility of subsequent aspiration.

Gas insufflation. The insufflation hose is connected to the Veress needle, and the peritoneal cavity is slowly insufflated (the initial values of gas flow are 100–500 mL/min, pressure 6–10 mmHg). If the pressure increases too quickly with a small volume of instilled gas and the abdominal cavity is not distended, the incorrect positioning of the insufflation cannula should be assumed. The gradual filling of the peritoneal cavity causes that it is distended symmetrically and a hyperresonant percussion is present above the liver. The gas flow is increased to 1–6 L/min, and we will wait until the real pressure value reaches the set value of pressure. In a child patient with a weight of 10 kg, this corresponds to a volume of 0.9 L of CO_2 [4].

Insertion of the primary working port (a cannula with a trocar). The first working port is usually inserted at the site of insufflation through Veress needle; the needle is extracted after the capnoperitoneum has been created. Working ports with a diameter of 5 and 10 mm are used most frequently. The valve for CO_2 insufflation on the cannula is checked whether it is closed. The cannula with the trocar is grasped so that the index finger acts as a break and prevents inadvertent deep penetration into the abdominal cavity (Fig. 4.5). The distended abdominal wall is maintained in an elevated position by pulling the Kocher forceps. The trocar tip is directed into the small incision in the fascia, and using twisting movement and concurrent pressure, it is inserted perpendicularly through the abdominal wall. While penetrating the abdominal wall, the cannula with trocar is tilted to an angle of 45° (Fig. 4.6). The sharp trocar is pulled out a little and the cannula is inserted deeper into the abdominal cavity. Gas leakage after the valve is opened for a short while indicates the correct insertion of the cannula. The trocar is removed and the telescope is introduced, which serves to visually verify free access to the peritoneal cavity. Subsequently, the cannula is attached to the CO_2 hose, and the space, to which the tip of the Veress needle and trocar was directed, is examined. Further, the accessible parts of the abdominal cavity are examined.

Capnoperitoneum creation by Hasson method using infra-umbilical approach. The open method is used when with the closed method there is a risk of damage to intra-abdominal organs. This includes patients after previous abdominal surgery with the occurrence of adhesions expected, and also newborns and infants with space limitation, where intra-abdominal pressure sufficiently high to safely insert the cannula and trocar cannot be created. Using a scalpel, an incision is made that copies the inferior arc of the umbilical depression and is by 1–2 mm longer than the port diameter. On the circumference of the incision in

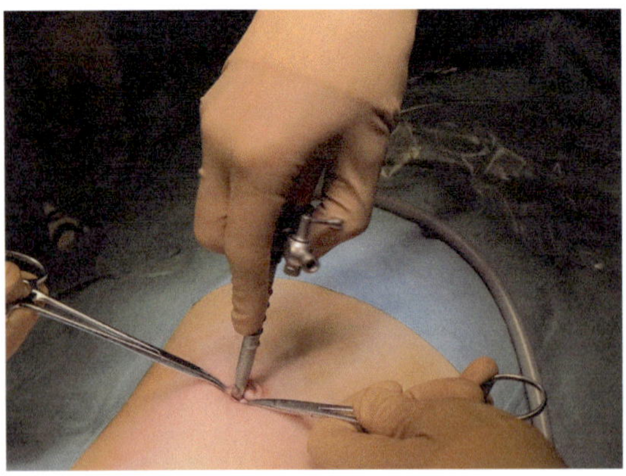

Fig. 4.5 The grasping of the cannula/trocar. The index finger acts as a break

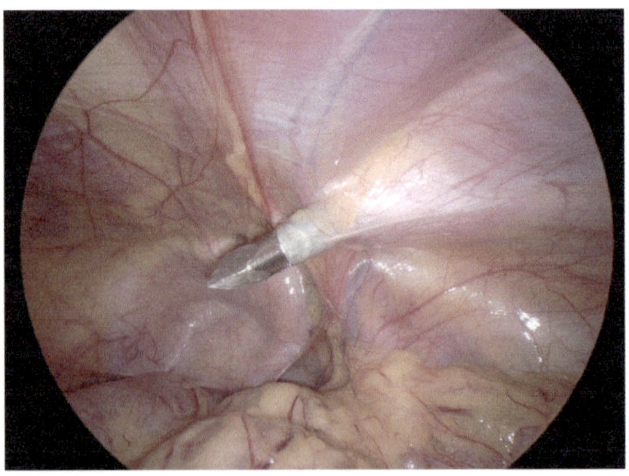

Fig. 4.6 The cannula with trocar is inserted perpendicularly through the abdominal wall and then is tilted to an angle of 45° into the peritoneal cavity

the fascia, a circular suture is placed serving to fix the cannula in the correct position and preventing gas leakage. In newborns, patience is needed for opening the elastic peritoneum between the developed embryonic structures—ductus urachus and obliterated umbilical artery. Once the peritoneal cavity has been opened, a cannula with blunt-tip trocar, or only a cannula without a trocar, is inserted into the opening and fixed by the prepared circular suture, which is also fixed at the insufflation valve of the cannula. Insufflation hose is attached and capnoperitoneum is gradually created. The patient is ready for a visual inspection of the accessible part of the abdominal cavity.

Introduction of working ports (secondary cannula). The placement and number of working ports are selected according to the type of surgery and standardised procedures or practice in individual workplaces. The ports are introduced in the initial phase of surgery; however, it is not a mistake to also add an access port during the surgery if the situation requires it. The ports are introduced through the skin incision by pressure and circular motion while visually checking the monitor. For ergonomic reasons, the insufflation hose can be moved to other port.

4.6 Port Extraction and Emptying of Capnoperitoneum

After the laparoscopic operation itself has been finished, the CO2 intraperitoneal pressure is decreased, and the operating field is inspected focusing on possible bleeding. If the situation requires it, some of the working ports can be used to insert an abdominal drain and place it specifically under visual control by means of a grasper. Subsequently, the secondary working ports are extracted taking note of possible bleeding into the peritoneal cavity after the cannula has been extracted. The insufflation hose is disconnected from the last/or primary cannula, the valve remains open, and light compression of the rib arches and abdominal wall is used to remove as much CO2 as possible. Then the cannula is extracted. If an organ or a tissue formation is extracted by means of an endobag, its extraction immediately follows the port. In some cases, incision in the fascia needs expanding. The defect in the fascia from the 10 mm port is closed by 2–3 non-absorbable sutures. Sufficient closure of the defect is verified by palpation, in particular in obese patients.

4.7 Tips and Tricks

Infra-umbilical or supra-umbilical incision is carried out in such a way that the surgeon and the assistant grasp the skinfold (the skinfold under or above the umbilicus) and straighten it between forceps. Incision is made on its top, which results in a perfect arch. Incision for the port is made by 1–2 mm wider than the cannula diameter. Thus, an adequate opening for free working port entry is created, preventing skin edge ischemisation. There is a difference between disposable and reusable ports. The disposable ones penetrate easily the abdominal wall thanks to their sharpness; with the reusable ones, it is sometimes necessary to make considerable effort to penetrate. When secondary ports are inserted in newborns, the elastic abdominal wall is resilient at low intra-abdominal pressure. The trocar tip should be directed into the cannula containing the telescope. While introducing the trocar/cannula, it is slightly pulled out. If we concentrate on the monitor looking for a site to introduce the cannula with trocar by means of the telescope and we lose orientation, we should look at the patient instead of the monitor for a while to correct the camera direction. During the visualisation of the secondary port entry, it is recommended that the telescope is rotated by 180° if angulated optics is used (usually 30° optics).

4.8 Discussion

The general principles for performing a laparoscopic operation have not changed significantly since the laparoscopic revolution began in the late 1980s [2]. In the 1990s, minimally invasive surgery was developed for infants and children. As technology has improved, we are now able to perform complex minimally invasive operations on our smallest, most vulnerable patients [5].

The contraindications for the laparoscopic approach are few. Primary contraindications include situations in which an adequate pneumoperitoneum cannot be created. Adhesions from previous procedures preclude adequate visualisation. Finally, patients with chronic lung disease and uncorrected cardiac disease may not be able to tolerate creation of a capnoperitoneum [2].

The gases that can be insufflated are CO2, N2O, air, and helium. Of these, the most commonly used gas is CO2 because of its inability to support combustion and high blood solubility, it is rapidly eliminated, and it has minimal potential of intravascular embolisation [4]. As regards the tolerance of intra-abdominal pressure, some authors recommend that the value of 6–10 mmHg should not be exceeded in child patients [1]. Other authors routinely use pressures of 12–15 mmHg without a worsening effect [2]. Children have a higher vagal tone, and sometimes a stimulus to the peritoneum by sudden distension of the peritoneal cavity or trocar penetration can lead to bradycardia and asystole [6, 7]. Intra-abdominal pressure is an important determinant for maintaining cardiovascular stability during laparoscopy [4]. The value of intra-abdominal pressure recommended for baby is 6 mmHg and for children is 12 mmHg because it has a minimal effect on cardiac index [7, 8]. Finally, a critical appraisal is warranted in regard to safety of surgery in neonates, as they fail to have cerebral autoregulation. As endoscopy may add additional risk factors, close monitoring is obligatory [9].

Another recommended procedure for first port introduction in infants is the vertical incision through the centre of the umbilicus with fascia opening by cutdown technique. The step cannula system is used, the expandable sleeve is introduced directly into the abdominal cavity and the cannula with blunt-tip trocar is inserted through it. The authors consider this method to be very safe. The defect in the fascia within the umbilical hernia can also be used as an entry [2].

The stab incision is recommended for secondary port introduction in newborns and infants. A transparietal puncture channel is created by scalpel point, and the laparoscopic instrument is introduced directly through it, without the use of a cannula, into the abdominal cavity [2].

The stab incision is on the rise, and during operation, we can avoid difficulties related to cannulas, such as cannula dislodgement, gas leakage, and instrument movement limitation [10].

With the increasing experience in paediatric endoscopic surgery, minimally invasive surgery (MIS) has been extended more and more towards infants and even neonates. A short self-retaining trocar sleeves were especially developed for neonatal surgery/paediatric laparoscopic surgery. The distal tip of the cannula enables fixation directly under the abdominal wall and prevents the cannula from slipping out of the abdominal wall [9].

Visual ports and smaller scopes via modified Veress needles are also available, but experience with children is limited [10, 11].

Bleeding from the port site should be avoided by translumination of the abdominal wall and by inserting the cannula with trocar out of vessel paths. If the visualisation is insufficient, bleeding from the abdominal wall from deep epigastric vessels may occur after the cannula has been introduced. We try to stop it by compression by changing the cannula position. For persistent bleeding, one of the possible methods is to introduce a Foley catheter through the cannula, insufflate the end balloon, and pull the catheter, thus compressing the injured site [1, 2].

Possible complications such as umbilical granuloma or instrumental problems belong to the classification 1st grade Clavien-Dindo, which authors report in 2.9% [12].

References

1. Najmaldin A, Guillou P. A guide to laparoscopic surgery. London: Blackwell Science; 1998.
2. Holcomb GW III. Principles of laparoscopic surgery. In: Holcomb III GW, Georgeson KE, Rothenberg SS, editors. Atlas of pediatric laparoscopy and thoracoscopy. Philadelphia: Saunders Elseviers; 2008.

3. Abdulhai S, Glenn IC, Ponsky TA. Inguinal hernia. Clin Perinatol. 2017;44(4):865–77. Philadelphia: Elsevier.
4. Gupta R, Singh S. Challenges in paediatric laparoscopic surgeries. Indian J Anaesth. 2009;53(5):560–6.
5. Wulkan ML, Lee H. Minimally invasive neonatal surgery. Clin Perinatol. 2017;44(4):xix. https://doi.org/10.1016/j.clp.2017.09.002. Philadelphia: Elsevier.
6. Sood J, Jain AK. Anaesthesia in laparoscopic surgery. In: Anaesthesia for laparoscopy in pediatric patients. 1st ed. New Delhi: Jaypee; 2007. p. 167–76.
7. Bozkurt P, Kaya G, Yeker Y, et al. The cardiorespiratory effects of laparoscopic procedures in infants. Anaesthesia. 1999;54:831–4.
8. Pennant JH. Anesthesia for laparoscopy in the pediatric patient. Anesthesiol Clin North Am. 2001;19:69–88.
9. van der Zee DC. Endoscopic surgery in children—the challenge goes on. J Pediatr Surg. 2017;52:207–10.
10. Marven SS, Godbole PP. Laparoscopy in children: basic principles. In: Godbole PP, editor. Pediatric endourology techniques. London: Springer; 2007.
11. Wong WSF. A safe optically guided entry technique using Endopath Xcel Trocars in laparoscopic surgery: a personal series of 821 patients. Gynecol Minim Invasive Ther. 2013;2:30–3.
12. Espositio C, Escolino M, Castagnetti M, Cerulo M, Settimi A, Cortese G, Turra F, Iannazzone M, Izzo S, Servillo G. Two decades of experience with laparoscopic varicocele repair in children: standardizing the technique. J Pediatr Urol. 2018;14:10.e1–7.

Basis of Retroperitoneoscopic Approach

5

Jean Stephane Valla, Agnese Roberti, Maria Escolino, and Ciro Esposito

5.1 Introduction

Minimally invasive surgery (MIS) has gained popularity in the last three decades due to numerous advantages and has evolved and made remarkable progress. Compared to the adult population, the application of this approach in the pediatric population was somewhat delayed [1, 2].

However, since its advent, the use of laparoscopy and later retroperitoneoscopy in pediatric urology has revolutionized the diagnosis and treatment of many pediatric urological diseases.

The aim of a retroperitoneal approach is to strictly adhere to the principles of open urology for benign lesions and to ensure a high level of cosmesis after the surgical incisions are made [3].

In particular, retroperitoneoscopy has been used with excellent results on children for a wide range of urological procedures such as in renal, adrenal, upper, and lower urinary tract surgery.

The main indications of the retroperitoneoscopic technique are:

- Nephrectomy to treat benign diseases such as multicystic or dysplastic kidneys causing renal hypertension, nonfunctioning kidneys associated with obstructive uropathy or VUR, xanthogranulomatosis, pyelonephritis, protein-losing nephropathy, and occasionally nephrolithiasis or nephropathy causing uncontrollable hypertension.
- Partial nephrectomy to treat renal duplication and a poorly functioning and chronically infected upper pole segment. The retroperitoneal approach has already been described for upper and lower pole nephrectomy.
- Dismembered pyeloplasty to treat ureteropelvic junction obstruction (UPJO) that is the most common disorder of the upper urinary tract in children.

The aim of this chapter is to describe the basis of technique and find out the benefits of retroperitoneoscopy in the main frequent urological diseases in children.

5.2 Preoperative Preparation

The parents give their informed consent to the procedure. This is essential in pediatric population because the reported benefits of a retroperitoneoscopic approach have not been firmly established.

J. S. Valla
Pediatric Surgery Unit, CHU Lenval, Nice, France

A. Roberti · M. Escolino · C. Esposito (✉)
Pediatric Surgery Unit, Department of Translational Medical Sciences (DISMET), University of Naples "Federico II", Naples, Italy
e-mail: maria.escolino@unina.it; ciroespo@unina.it

C. Esposito et al. (eds.), *ESPES Manual of Pediatric Minimally Invasive Surgery*,
https://doi.org/10.1007/978-3-030-00964-9_5

Children are prepared for surgery as usual without bowel preparation.

A standard anesthesia protocol is used after a premedication with midazolam: all children were mechanically ventilated after insertion of an appropriately sized endotracheal tube. Nitrous oxide is generally contraindicated to reduce bowel distension; a nasogastric tube is introduced for the same purpose, and a bladder catheter is inserted to quantify diuresis.

Preoperative antibiotic dose is given according to the etiology: not necessary in case of dysplastic multicystic kidney but necessary in case of destructed kidney by an obstructive or refluxing uropathy.

An intraoperative monitoring is performed with a pulse oximeter, a noninvasive blood pressure monitor, and an electrocardiogram; end-tidal carbon dioxide (ETCO2) was monitored through a capnogram.

5.3 Positioning

The procedure is performed with the patient placed in lateral decubitus position (Fig. 5.1).

This access has been demonstrated as reliable for a large number of indications particularly total nephrectomy, pyeloplasty, and pyelotomy [4–6]. Its direct access to the renal vessels without violating the peritoneal cavity is the main advantage of the lateral retroperitoneal method, and if an urgent open conversion is needed, it offers the best exposure to control great vessels.

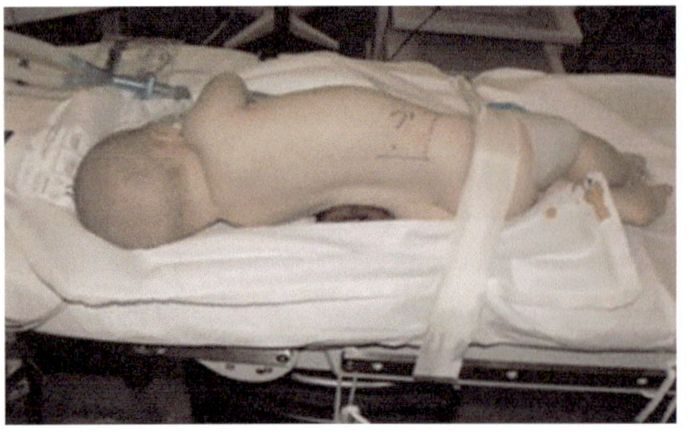

Fig. 5.1 Position of the patient

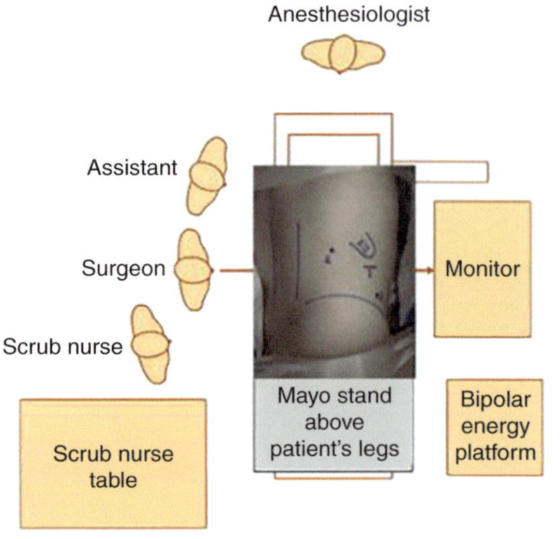

Fig. 5.2 Team position

Normally the surgeon and assistant face the back of the patient. The video column stands on the other side; the cables are fixed to the superior part of the operative field (Fig. 5.2). If a total ureterectomy is needed at the same time, the position of the surgeon and his assistant and the position of the video column may change during the procedure; the installation must be planned accordingly.

5.4 Instrumentation

The choice of the telescope and of the cannulas must be adapted to each case: for example, to remove a dysplastic multicystic kidney in a normal child less than 2 years of age, a 5 mm telescope and two 3 or 5 mm normal cannulas for operating device seem to be the good option. At the opposite, in order to remove a large hydronephrotic infected kidney in an obese teenager, there is no other way for the primary access than a quite large skin incision (15/20 mm) and the use of a large cannula with balloon for the primary access.

A plastic bag is fixed to the dorsal part of the patient and instruments are put away in this bag: monopolar hook, bipolar forceps, harmonic scalpel, and aspiration cannula.

In the recent years, thanks to the use of new hemostatic and synthesis devices that permit faster and safer procedures, the technique seems to be easier to perform.

5.5 Technique

5.5.1 Access in the Retroperitoneal Space

First port placement. We favor an open technique for primary retroperitoneal access. This is the key point of the technique because the majority of complications deal with access technique and the development of a working field [7]. After sterile preparation and draping, anatomical landmarks are palpated (11th and 12th ribs, iliac crest, sacrospinalis muscle), and the surgeon mentally localizes the lateral peritoneal reflection.

The skin incision (8–15 mm long) is made just below the 12th rib tip at the posterior axillary line, in the area where the muscular wall is the thinnest (Fig. 5.3). If the incision is oversized, resultant gas leak could be managed with large retaining sutures or large cannulas with fascial retention balloons. A muscle-splitting dissection is used to gain access into the retroperitoneal space; dissecting forceps, retractors, and Metzenbaum scissors are usually sufficient to bluntly divide the external oblique and internal oblique; after piercing the white transversalis fascia with the tip of scissors, the dissection is stopped when the yellow perirenal fat becomes visible. Two stay sutures are placed on each side of the muscular layers (2/0 short curved needle—semicircular 16 mm). In case of large (15 mm) incision, it is sometimes possible to recognize the Gerota's fascia, to incise it in order to begin CO_2 insufflation directly in the perirenal space; most often, the Gerota's fascia is not visible, so the working space is created in the retroperitoneal space, and the Gerota's fascia will be opened posteriorly in the following step.

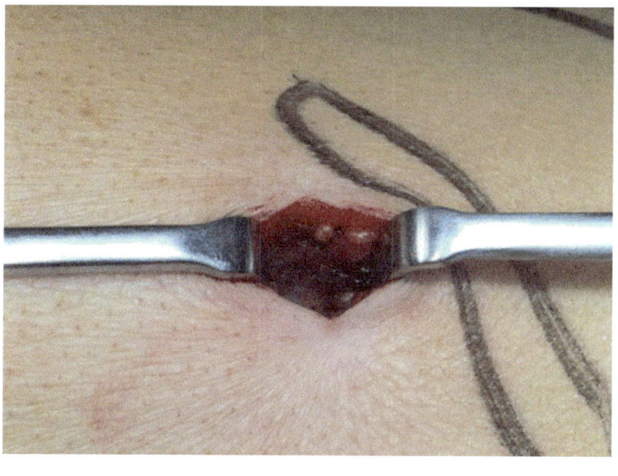

Fig. 5.3 Camera port is classically placed just below the tip of the 12th rib

Then a small gauze is introduced in the retroperitoneal space and manipulated carefully to create the space. The surgeon must keep the dissection in close touch with the posterior muscular wall to avoid peritoneal perforation. The primary blunt port (5–10 mm—disposable or reusable) is placed and secured to create a seal for the retropneumoperitoneum. CO_2 insufflation is started (8–10 mm in infant, 12–15 mm in children). A 0° or 30° lens is inserted. The working space, already created by the gauze, is progressively enlarged by moving the tip of the telescope, used as a palpator to free retroperitoneal fibrous tissues, behind the kidney. This allows to expose the anatomical landmarks: quadratus lumborum, psoas muscles, and posterior part of the kidney. The thick lateral and posterior abdominal wall, closely attached to the bony boundaries, cannot be distended by insufflation as well as the anterior abdominal wall; this explains why a good curarization is essential so a sufficient operating space can only be achieved by pushing away peritoneum and intra-abdominal organs and by dissecting the lateral peritoneal reflection at least to the anterior axillary line [8].

Placement of accessory ports. Two additional ports (3 or 5 mm) are placed under direct vision: the posterior port is introduced first, in the costospinal angle, at the junction of the lateral border of the erector spinae muscle with the underside of the 12th rib; the inferior port just above the iliac crest must not be placed too close to the iliac crest because the bony relief could restrict the device's mobility.

This port placement allows to achieve a triangulation of ports in order to maximize exposure and minimize instrument conflict in a small working space.

5.5.2 Exit of Retroperitoneal Space

After performing a procedure and after a possible extraction, the port and telescope are reintroduced to check the hemostasis at low pressure particularly near the hilum. If needed a drain is introduced through the inferior cannula; ports are removed under direct vision. The closure of fascia is easy because of the two stay sutures, placed at the beginning of the procedure. Port sites can be injected with bupivacaine and lidocaine. The skin is close with subcuticular stitches and/or adhesive strips.

5.6 Mains Procedures of Retroperitoneoscopic Approach

5.6.1 Pyeloplasty

5.6.1.1 Access in the Retroperitoneal Space

Dissection of the pyeloureteral junction (PUJ). The kidney is approached posteriorly and the renal pelvis first identified. The pyeloureteral junction (PUJ) is identified and minimally dissection is used to free the PUJ from connective tissue; small vessels are divided after bipolar electrocoagulation. If needed, a fourth trocar (3 mm) is inserted lateral to the lumbosacral muscles near the iliac crest. A stay suture of 5/0 polydioxanone is placed for traction at the PUJ. The anterior surface of the PUJ is cleared to identify any polar crossing vessels.

Section of PUJ. The renal pelvis is partly divided by scissors at the most dependent part, when light traction on the stay suture is helpful for manipulating the PUJ. Maintaining the traction, the ureter is partly divided and incised vertically for spatulation. The traction suture helps to mobilize the ureter so that the scissors can be in the axis of the ureter. The anterior surface of the kidney is left adherent to the peritoneum so that the kidney is retracted medially with no need for individual kidney retraction.

Anastomosis. The pelvi-ureteric anastomosis begins using 6/0 polydioxanone sutures and a tapered 3/8 circular needle. The first suture is placed from the most dependent portion of the pelvis to the most inferior point or vertex of the ureteric spatulation. The suture is tied using the intracorporeal technique with the knots placed outside the lumen. The same suture is used on the anterior wall of the anastomosis. The PUJ is maintained on traction and the suture line stabilized. A polyurethane JJ stent was inserted through the suture line to the bladder at the end of the anterior layer reconstruction, through trocar N° 3.

Fluoroscopy was used to assess the placement of the JJ stent in the urinary tract.

The stent remains indwelling for 4–6 weeks. Perirenal suction drainage is normally used [9, 10].

5.6.2 Total Nephrectomy

5.6.2.1 Access in the Retroperitoneal Space

Initial dissection and control of the renal hilum. At this time landmarks should be clearly visualized and especially the posterior part of the kidney, great vessels ureter. With the help of two atraumatic instruments (palpator or peanut grasper), the Gerota's fascia is largely opened (if not already done) along the posterior part of kidney.

Anterior dissection should be limited at the beginning to prevent peritoneal injury and the kidney from flapping ventrally. On the contrary if the anterior peritoneal adherences are kept intact, the kidney is automatically retracted anteriorly by the insufflation pressure and pushed to the top of the field, giving a good posterior access to the hilum; if this spontaneous retraction is not sufficient, a third operating device—usually 3 mm—could be introduced on the midaxillary line for retraction of the kidney in the upper part of the field.

Dissection with a hook or scissors cleans the artery and vein; they appear vertically; the renal vessels must be dissected in the inferior part of the field, where there is only one artery and one vein, and not too close to the kidney hilum where the vessels divide into several branches. Vessels do not need to be taken at their origin with the aorta and vena cava, but a sufficiently wide area of exposure (at least 1 cm) to allow safe control on each side is necessary.

Countertraction using the nondominant hand is useful to create a large window around the vein and artery. If the search for renal vessels proves difficult, the ureter may serve as a lead; the ureter is easy to discover in the retroperitoneal space, and its dissection up to the kidney leads to the renal vessels.

Vascular control. The artery is controlled first. Many kinds of hemostasis could be used according to the anatomical situation and the vessel's diameter such as monopolar coagulation with hook in case of tiny vessels, bipolar coagulation, harmonic scalpel, ligasure in case of mid-sized vessels, and extracorporeal ligature or clip in case of large vessels.

Specimen dissection. Dissection using electrocautery or ultrasonic scalpel continues from caudal to cephalad. Polar vessels could be encountered at that time; a careful dissection allows to recognize them and to manage them according to their size. The upper pole dissection allows to separate the kidney and adrenal gland using an avascular plane. Lastly the anterior part of the kidney is completely freed and the kidney is totally mobilized.

Ureteral management.

- In case of non-refluxing or atrophic ureter, the ureterectomy could be limited to the lumbar part, and a ligature is not necessary. Just cut it.
- On the other hand, in case of refluxing or dilated ureter, a total ureterectomy is essential to avoid postoperative complications due to the stump [11].

Specimen removal. The benign nature of most pediatric renal diseases enables removal without concern for spillage. The specimen's extraction is of variable difficulty according to its volume. In case of multicystic dysplastic kidney, after puncture of all the cysts, the extraction is very easy; in the same manner in case of small kidney or kidney with very thin cortex, the extraction can be performed without morcellation. Large specimen can be extracted after enlargement of the 10 mm hole, with or without the use of an endobag and morcellation. If a low incision (inguinal or Pfannenstiel) is needed for another purpose, the kidney can be extracted through it (Fig. 5.4).

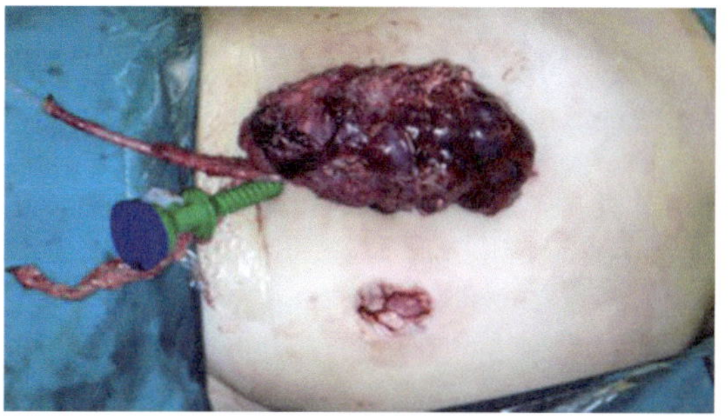

Fig. 5.4 A distal ureteral stump and left kidney are removed via a groin incision

5.6.3 Partial Nephrectomy

Upper pole nephrectomy: The first step is to locate the two ureters and provide access to the posterior surface of the renal hilum. Dissection is continued as far as the renal sinus to identify the vessels supplying the upper pole. These small-caliber vessels are ligated or coagulated and then sectioned.

The ureter of the upper renal moiety is then sectioned and drawn toward the diaphragm, which most closely represents the plane of parenchymal section.

Section of the renal parenchyma is performed with scissors and monopolar electrode or with an ultrasonic scalpel. The resection margin is carefully inspected; if there is any doubt about a possible opening of a lower pole calyx, saline, with or without methylene blue, is injected via the ureteric catheter: if the leak is confirmed, caliceal suture is performed with 5/0 absorbable suture material; otherwise no suture is performed on the resection margin. Biological adhesive is applied to the section [12].

The next step consists of ureterectomy, which is extended inferiorly beyond the pelvic inlet, carefully avoiding damage to the blood supply of the remaining ureter. The constantly dilated upper pole ureter is treated in the same way as via open surgery: section, aspiration for the contents in the case of obstruction, or ligation by Endoloop in the case of reflux (e.g., in the case of prior endoscopic incision). A Redon drain is systematically left in place.

Lower pole nephrectomy: Ureteral section of the lower pole ureter is not necessary; usually there are numerous vascular branches. The parenchymal section is more easy because the healthy hypertrophic upper pole pushes down the demarcation line and presents it in the right plane, perpendicular to the scalpel.

5.7 Postoperative Care

In the postoperative period, the patients can keep a normal decubitus.

They can restart full oral feeding few hours after surgery. The analgesic requirement (paracetamol every 6 h) is generally limited to the first 24 postoperative hours.

In case of drainage, the drain is removed at day 1 or day 2 post-op. An ultrasound is performed at 1 week and 1 month post-op to check the lumbar area. The following annual controls are focused on the remaining kidney.

5.8 Tips and Tricks

- ***Dense perirenal adhesions***: Ten years ago at the beginning of our experience, dense perirenal adhesions due to previous nephrostomy, repeated perinephritis, and xanthogranulomatous pyelonephritis were considered as contraindication for retroperitoneoscopic nephrectomy. Now, we try a retroperitoneoscopic attempt and most of the time we succeed [13].
- ***Horseshoe/ectopic kidneys***: We and others [14] have performed nephrectomy for horseshoe or ectopic sigmoid kidney, using the same lateral approach or a modified 45° flank position. Aberrant vascular anatomy is common in these cases, and a careful dissection and clamping before division are mandatory especially in case of ectopic sigmoid kidney. The ultrasonic scalpel is very useful to cut between healthy and destructed parenchyma.

  Sometimes the kidney is "invisible" before operation. If it is suspected to be located in the lower part of the abdomen, it seems preferable to use an intraperitoneal approach [15]. But if the "invisible" kidney is suspected to be located around the normal place, the retroperitoneal approach could be successfully used as in one of our cases.
- ***Giant hydronephrosis***: The destructed kidney with giant hydronephrosis is usually soft with low pressure in it. A careful open approach allows to avoid entering the renal cortex or pelvis during the initial trocar placement. After having dissected the posterior part, decompressing the renal pelvis with an aspiration needle under visual control greatly improves exposure of anatomical elements, and a large working space is naturally created.

5.9 Discussion

Retroperitoneoscopic surgery in children is feasible and safe if performed by well-trained surgeons. Between transperitoneal and retroperitoneal approach, the choice should be made according to each case; however, in our opinion, a pure pediatric urologist would favor the retroperitoneoscopic access to reach the upper urinary tract and the kidney, because this is the "natural" way even if it is more difficult to learn at the beginning.

Operative urological minimal access surgery has recently expanded its range of indications due to improved laparoscopic technology and an increased interest in minimally invasive therapeutics. In other words, the indications have evolved from diagnostic procedures 20 years ago to ablative procedures 10 years ago and now to reconstructive surgery [3].

Nowadays, minimally invasive surgery for pediatric nephrectomies is established as routine practice. Transperitoneal and retroperitoneal are the two approaches for performing either total or partial nephrectomy. During transperitoneal laparoscopy, the surgeon must mobilize the hepatic flexure of the colon in order to expose the right kidney and the splenic flexure to expose the left kidney. This approach is easier compared to retroperitoneoscopy, since it allows plenty of space, but it has an inherent risk of adhesion formation or intestinal perforation. Faster access and easier dissection of the parenchyma can be achieved with the retroperitoneal approach [1].

As for the repair of ureteropelvic junction obstruction, the retroperitoneal approach is now an acceptable method. The cosmetic result is superior in retroperitoneoscopy, and the need for reoperation is also reduced in comparison with the transperitoneal approach [1].

In conclusion, it is possible to state that retroperitoneoscopy is the technique of choice for reaching the urinary tract in children, as it can be performed safely and effectively in children. Still, this procedure is more challenging and requires excellent imaging of the retroperitoneal space, especially when partial nephrectomies are involved.

Retroperitoneoscopic approach offers several potential advantages. The main advantage is its more direct and rapid exposure without peritoneal cavity transgression and without dissection and handling of intraperitoneal structures which could be injured during these maneuvers.

The working space is not obscured by intestinal loops; therefore, the risk of postoperative paralytic ileus, shoulder pain, omental evisceration, and intestinal adhesions is eliminated.

References

1. Antoniou D, Karetsos C. Laparoscopy or retroperitoneoscopy: which is the best approach in pediatric urology. Transl Pediatr. 2016;5(4):205–13.
2. Esposito C, Valla JS, Yeung CK. Current indications for laparoscopy and retroperitoneoscopy in pediatric urology. Surg Endosc. 2004;18(11):1559–64.
3. Valla JS. Retroperitoneoscopic surgery in children. Semin Pediatr Surg. 2007;16(4):270–7.
4. El Ghoneimi A, Valla JS, Steyaert H, Aigrain Y. Laparoscopic renal surgery via a retroperitoneal approach in children. J Urol. 1998;160:1138–41.
5. Franks M, Schneck FX, Docimo SG. Retroperitoneoscopy in children. In: Caione P, Kavoussi LR, Micali R, editors. Retroperitoneoscopy and extraperitoneal laparoscopy in pediatric an adult urology. Springer; 2003. p. 103–18.
6. Gaur DD. The accurate placement of the balloon for retroperitoneal dissection by the percutaneous method, insuring that it expands in the right plane. BJU Int. 1999;84:1095.
7. Peters GA. Complications of retroperitoneal laparoscopy in pediatric urology: prevention, recognition and management. In: Caione P, Kavoussy LR, Micali R, editors. Retroperitoneoscopy and extraperitoneal laparoscopy in pediatric and adult urology. Springer; 2003, p. 203–10.
8. Micali S, Caione P, Virgini G, Capozza N, Scarfini M, Micali F. Retroperitoneal access in children using a direct vision technique. J Urol. 2001;165:1229–32.
9. Turrà F, Escolino M, Farina A, Settimi A, Esposito C, Varlet F. Pyeloplasty techniques using minimally invasive surgery (MIS) in pediatric patients. Transl Pediatr. 2016;5(4):251–5. https://doi.org/10.21037/tp.2016.10.0.
10. El-Ghoneimi A, Farhat W, Bolduc S, Bagli D, McLorie G, Aigrain Y, et al. Laparoscopic dismembered pyeloplasty by a retroperitoneal approach in children. BJU Int. 2003;92(1):104–8; discussion 108.
11. Esposito C, Escolino M, Corcione F, Draghici IM, Savanelli A, Castagnetti M, et al. Twenty-year experience with laparoscopic and retroperitoneoscopic nephrectomy in children: considerations and details of technique. Surg Endosc. 2016;30(5):2114–8. https://doi.org/10.1007/s00464-015-4472-7.
12. Lee RS, Retik AB, Borer JG, Diamond DA, Peters CA. Pediatric retroperitoneal laparoscopic partial nephrectomy: comparison with an age matched cohort of open surgery. J Urol. 2005;174:708–11.
13. Merrot T, Ordorica Flores R, Steyaert H, Ginier C, Valla JS. Is diffuse xanthogranulomatous pyelonephritis a contra-indication to retroperitoneoscopic nephroureterectomy? Surg Laparosc Endosc. 1998;8:366–9.
14. Leclair MD, Camby C, Capito C, De Windt A, Podevin G, Heloury Y. Retroperitoneoscopic nephrectomy of a horseshoe kidney in a child. Surg Endosc. 2003;17:1156.
15. Yeung CK, Liu KW, Ng WT, Ttan HL, Tam YH, Lee KH. Laparoscopy as the investigation and treatment of choice for urinary incontinence caused by small "invisible" dysplastic kidney with infrasphincteric ureteric ectopia. BJU Int. 1999;84:324.

Basis of Thoracoscopic Approach

6

Piergiorgio Gamba, Alba Ganarin, and Miguel Garcia Magne

6.1 Introduction

Thoracoscopy has now reached an excellent level even in neonatal and pediatric age. There are many procedures that can be performed; for many of them, thoracoscopic approach has actually proved its superiority compared to traditional surgery in terms of shorter days of hospitalization, less postoperative pain, reduction of scarring, and long-term complications (i.e., scoliosis, thoracic deformities) [1, 2]. The long-term effects (as well as laparoscopy) of the use of CO_2 in the neonatal age are still to be assessed. Even more than in laparoscopy, thoracoscopy requires greater collaboration with the anesthesiologist (see *Anesthesia in pediatric MIS* chapter). Another limit of thoracoscopic approach concerns the mobility of trocars and surgical instruments within the small pediatric intercostal spaces.

6.2 Indications

Currently technological advances, more skilled and experienced surgeons, and introduction of more efficient and standardized techniques allowed to expand significantly the spectrum of indications for thoracoscopic procedures [3].

In Tables 6.1 and 6.2, the relation between difficulty level, location within the thoracic cavity, possible procedures, and suggested patient's position is shown.

6.3 Contraindications

Nowadays the development of better instrumentation and improvement in surgical techniques reduced drastically the number of contraindications to perform thoracoscopy. Surgeon experience and patient clinical conditions are fundamental at the time of deciding the surgical approach [4].

Absolute. These comprehend conditions that prevent adequate visualization of the thoracic space and/or serious respiratory compromising:

- Severe respiratory distress which requires alternative forms of ventilation: inability to tolerate single-lung ventilation, contralateral pneumonectomy, high positive-pressure ventilation
- Giant anterior mediastinal masses that compromise respiration
- Severe hemodynamic instability

Relative. Do not discard thoracoscopy but must be carefully planned:

P. Gamba (✉) · A. Ganarin · M. Garcia Magne
Pediatric Surgery Unit, Department of Woman's and Children's Health, University of Padua, Padua, Italy
e-mail: piergiorgio.gamba@unipd.it

C. Esposito et al. (eds.), *ESPES Manual of Pediatric Minimally Invasive Surgery*,
https://doi.org/10.1007/978-3-030-00964-9_6

Table 6.1 Description of the possible indications described as low/moderate level of difficulty, location of the pathology, and possible positioning of the patient

Difficulty level	Location	Procedures	Position
Low/moderate	Intrathoracic	Pleural diagnostic evaluation	SLD, MPP, MSP
		Evacuation of hemothorax/empyema	SLD
		Mechanical or chemical pleurodesis	SLD, MPP, MSP
		Bleb resection	SLD, MPP, MSP
		Lung biopsy: interstitial lung disease, metastatic and fungal lesions	SLD, MPP, MSP
		Sympathectomy	SLD, MSP
		Transdiaphragmatic liver biopsy	MSP
	Mediastinum	Pericardial drainage	MSP
		Pericardial window	MSP
		Mediastinal tumor biopsy	SLD
		Mediastinal node biopsy	SLD

SLD standard lateral decubitus, *MPP* modified prone position, *MSP* modified supine position

Table 6.2 Description of the possible indications described as high level of difficulty, location of the pathology, and possible positioning of the patient

Difficulty level	Location	Procedures	Position
High (expert surgeons)	Intrathoracic	Trauma evaluation	SLD, MSP
		Decortication	SLD
		Lobectomy: infectious diseases, cavitary lesions, bullous disease, lobar emphysema, congenital adenomatoid malformations and tumors	SLD, MSP
		Resection of sequestration	MPP, SLD
		Diaphragmatic plication	SLD, MSP
		Congenital diaphragmatic hernia	SLD
		Anterior spine procedures: anterior spinal fusion for severe scoliosis	SLD
	Mediastinum	Vagotomy	MPP
		Thoracic duct ligation	MPP
		Patent ductus arteriosus ligation	SLD
		Esophageal myotomy	MPP
		Esophageal atresia repair	MPP
		Tracheoesophageal fistula ligation	MPP
		Bronchogenic cyst surgery	MPP, SLP
		Neurogenic tumor resection	MPP
		Benign esophageal tumor resection	MPP
		Aortopexy	MSP
		Thymectomy	MSP
		Insertion of cardiac and diaphragmatic pacemaker	SLD, MSP

SLD standard lateral decubitus, *MPP* modified prone position, *MSP* modified supine position

- Previous thoracic surgery
- Pleural adhesions caused by previous widespread infections
- Coagulopathy
- Large tumors or extended pulmonary metastasis

6.4 Preoperative

(a) Equipment

Basic thoracoscopy equipment has no significant difference with laparoscopy instrumentation. Basic instrument set must be used in case of a thoracoscopic procedure:

- According to the size and weight of the patients, 3–5 mm instruments must be available.
- Trocars: valved trocars allow to insufflate low-pressure CO2 to help collapse the lungs. This is particularly useful in smaller children in whom complete lung exclusion cannot be acquired. Trocar length must be decided according to the size, age, and weight of patient, in small and thin patients 50–70 mm. Blunt-tipped trocars reduce the chance of causing lungs or tissue injury during introduction due to thin chest wall. Because of the little thickness of children's chest walls, trocars must be fixed to it during long procedures in order to avoid them to slip during manipulation. Sometimes it could be indicated also to use instruments without trocars.
- Optics: 2.7 or 5 mm optics depending on age and weight of patients; 10 mm optics can be used in children of 8 years or more. The most commonly used scopes are 0° or 30°, but other angles as 45° or 70° might as well be used in particular situations in order to improve visibility.
- Basic set: grasper, curved dissectors, curved scissors, forceps, irrigator/aspirator, cautery device, needle holder, clip applier, monopolar/bipolar cautery.
- Disposable equipment: endoloops, hemostatic clips (5–10 mm).

Nevertheless, evolution in techniques, surgeon's ability and experience, and procedure's level of difficulty are just some factors that might require the use of special instruments such as harmonic scalpel (Ultracision®, Ethicon), LigaSure™ (Covidien), endoscopic ultrasound, argon beam coagulator, and endoscopic stapler (5–12 mm).

(b) Imaging

Preoperative imaging is essential for surgical planning since adequate imaging allows an accurate positioning of the patient, therefore better access points to the lesion area.

Depending on the nature of the pathology, different imaging techniques might be used: MRI scans are useful in cases of vascular lesions or masses involving the spinal canal, CT scans for masses and infiltrates, US for the largest fluid collections, or even X-ray in cases of pneumothorax. If possible, 3D reconstruction imaging is extremely helpful for the surgeon.

(c) Positioning, room set-up, and trocar placement

Depending on the procedure that will be performed, the patient has to be positioned correctly, in order to obtain the wider field of view and the best access to the anatomical structures of interest. The unaffected lung and the other structures must be kept out of the operative field; for this purpose the patient will be positioned so that these structures are located below the area of interest. In the photos are shown the three principal positions used for thoracoscopy. In Fig. 6.1 the patient is in a standard lateral decubitus position with operative side up and the ipsilateral upper limb flexed above patient's head. In this position the surgeon can dominate the entire pleural cavity, which makes this position the best choice for procedures such as lung biopsy and pleurodesis [5, 6]. In Fig. 6.2 the patient is in a prone modified position

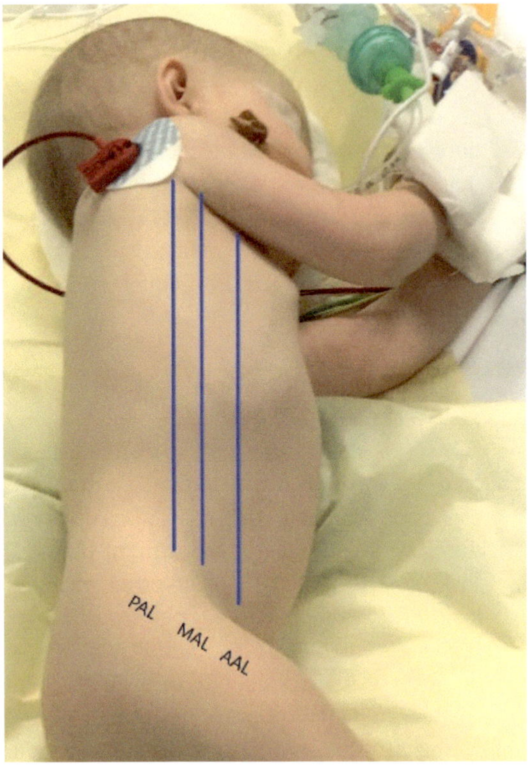

Fig. 6.1 Patient in standard lateral decubitus position. *PAL* posterior axillary line, *MAL* midaxillary line, *AAL* anterior axillary line

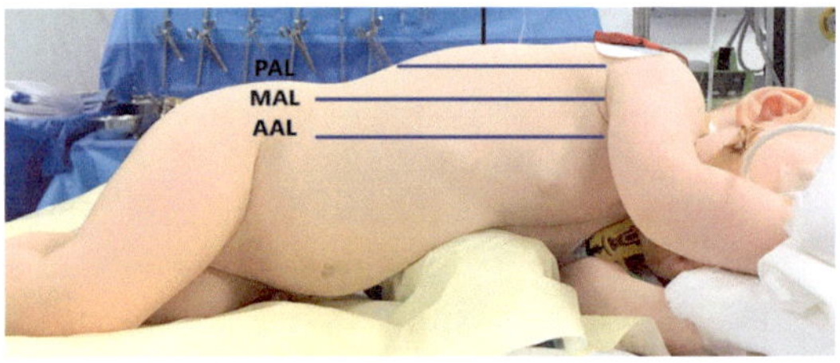

Fig. 6.2 Patient in modified prone position. *PAL* posterior axillary line, *MAL* midaxillary line, *AAL* anterior axillary line

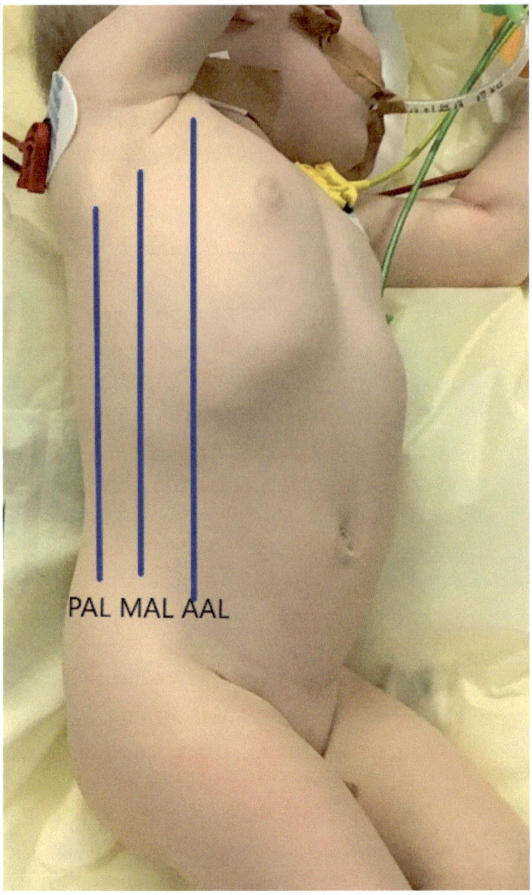

Fig. 6.3 Patient in modified supine position. *PAL* posterior axillary line, *MAL* midaxillary line, *AAL* anterior axillary line

with affected side slightly elevated. This position allows the surgeon the best access to the posterior mediastinal structures. Finally, in Fig. 6.3, the patient is in a supine position with affected side slightly elevated. This position provides an excellent view of the anterior mediastinum. Once the patient is secured, he can be moved in the Trendelenburg or reverse Trendelenburg position and rotated in order to achieve the best operative view and ergonomics for the surgeon. It is mandatory to have a monitor on both sides of the operating table, with one of it standing in line with the surgeon and the other in line with the assistant or the scrub nurse. The surgeon and the assistant stand normally in front of the operative area, with the scrub nurse positioned on the other side. In order to obtain the best operative view and working space, it is essential to correctly position the patient and choose the right placements of ports in the intercostal spaces. In general, a camera port and two operative ports may be sufficient to perform many thoracoscopic procedures; an additional port can be placed for retraction. In Figs. 6.1, 6.2, and 6.3 the sites to place the trocars depending on patient's position are shown: in lateral decubitus position, the camera port is placed along the midaxillary line (Fig. 6.1); if the lesion is localized in the posterior mediastinum, then the port should be placed along the anterior axillary line (Fig. 6.2). When approaching the anterior mediastinum, the camera port should stay along the posterior axillary line (Fig. 6.3). Normally, the camera port will be placed between and above the two operative ports.

(d) Anesthesia

Considering the complexity of pediatric patients and the pathologies treated, knowledge of the surgical plan and surgeon's experience alone won't guarantee success unless they are combined with an optimal relationship with the anesthesiology team.

Anesthetic features that comprehend double lung/single-lung ventilation will be discussed at the *Anesthesia in pediatric MIS* chapter.

6.5 Postoperative

The complexity of postoperative care depends on the difficulty of surgery. Patients who underwent biopsy, limited resection, or observation can be monitored at the surgical ward, without intensive special care. In some cases, after a 24-h time observation, these patients can be ready for discharge [7, 8]. Chest tubes can be removed in the first postoperative day once the pneumothorax resolves. Heavy nonabsorbable suture is used to secure the tube to the skin followed by application of an occlusive, adherent dressing. Thoracoscopic approach allowed to reduce muscle stretching resulting in a significant reduction in postoperative pain, allowing the patient to regain effective deep breathing; likewise, the injection of local anesthetics at trocar sites before insertion followed with an IV painkiller in the immediate postoperative period allows fast and efficient pain management. An adequate pain management and an early and aggressive pulmonary toilet help in reducing the incidence of postoperative pneumonias and other pulmonary complications. It hasn't been proved that thoracoscopic approach may not reduce significantly hospitalization time, but it surely reduces general morbidity and postoperative pain [9, 10].

6.6 Complications

(a) Intraoperative

- Conversion to open thoracotomy: the decision of converting to an open procedure should not be considered as a complication, unless a significant technical mistake was made.
- Tension pneumothorax during insufflation or initial air introduction.
- Significant bleeding from a vessel or parenchymal injury, most of the times it can resolve without conversion.
- Gas (air or CO2) embolism.
- Diaphragmatic or subdiaphragmatic organ lesions from port or instrument insertion
- Cardiac arrhythmias: due to use of cautery near to the heart, vagus nerve, or pericardium.

(b) Postoperative

- Air leak/persistent pneumothorax is one of the most common postoperative complications; luckily it can be considered a self-limited problem once a chest tube suction/drainage is positioned. Any thoracoscopic procedure, in which an air leak or accumulation of pleural fluid is anticipated, requires placement of an intercostal chest tube. Tubes sizes may range from 12 to 28 Fr, depending on the size of the patient and can be placed under direct vision (via one of the port sites) in order to evacuate pneumothorax. According to the possibility of air leak, the tube may be connected to a low-pressure suction system or a water seal. Tubes can be removed when lungs stay fully expanded for 24/48 h and fluid drainage is minimal (less than 2.5 mL/Kg per day) [11].
- If leaks persist the possibility of a bronchopleural fistula might be considered; in this case a re-exploration, thoracoscopically, is needed.

References

1. Bax KN, Georgeson KE, Rothenberg SS, Valla J, Yeung CK. Endoscopic surgery in infants and children. Berlin: Springer Science & Business Media; 2008.
2. Fortmann C, Schwerk N, Wetzke M, Schukfeh N, Ure BM, Dingemann J. Diagnostic accuracy and therapeutic relevance of thoracoscopic lung biopsies in children. Pediatr Pulmonol. 2018;53(7):948–53.
3. Gamba P, Midrio P, Betalli P, Snijders D, Leon FF. Video-assisted thoracoscopy in compromised pediatric patients. J Laparoendosc Adv Surg Tech A. 2010;20(1):69–71.
4. Holcomb GW. Thoracoscopic surgery for esophageal atresia. Pediatr Surg Int. 2017;33(4):475–81.
5. Lacher M, Kuebler JF, Dingemann J, Ure BM. Minimal invasive surgery in the newborn: current status and evidence. Semin Pediatr Surg. 2014;23(5):249–56.
6. Najmaldin A. Principles of minimally invasive surgery. In: Burge DM, Griffiths DM, Steinbrecher HA, et al., editors. Paediatric surgery, vol. 14. 2nd ed. London: Hodder Arnold; 2005. p. 115–9.
7. Najmaldin A, Rothenberg S, Crabbe D, Beasley S. Operative endoscopy and endoscopic surgery in infants and children. Boca Raton: CRC Press; 2005.
8. Rothenberg SS, Middlesworth W, Kadennhe-Chiweshe A, Aspelund G, Kuenzler K, Cowles R, et al. Two decades of experience with thoracoscopic lobectomy in infants and children: standardizing techniques for advanced thoracoscopic surgery. J Laparoendosc Adv Surg Tech A. 2015;25(5):423–8.
9. Saxena AK, Höllwarth ME. Essentials of pediatric endoscopic surgery. Berlin: Springer Science & Business Media; 2008.
10. Spitz L, Coran A. Operative pediatric surgery. Boca Raton: CRC Press; 2013.
11. Yamataka A, Koga H, Ochi T, Imashimizu K, Suzuki K, Kuwatsuru R, Suzuki K, et al. Pulmonary lobectomy techniques in infants and children. Pediatr Surg Int. 2017;33(4):483–95.

Basics of Paediatric Robotics

7

Azad Najmaldin, Thomas Cundy, Donatella Di Fabrizio, and Naved Alizai

7.1 Introduction

Robot-assisted surgery has been introduced to address some of the difficulties encountered with the introduction of minimal invasive surgery (endoscopic surgery) and extend the capability of surgeons.

In the late 1990s, Cadière from Brussels reported the feasibility and safety of robotic-assisted laparoscopic approach in adult general surgery. In 2001, Meininger et al. from Frankfurt published the first robot-assisted procedure in a child. Since then, increasing numbers of surgeons have reported the feasibility and success of robotic techniques in an increasingly wide range of paediatric subspeciality fields including urology, hepatobiliary and gastrointestinal, cardiovascular, thoracic and cervical surgery [1–3]. The application of robot-assisted single-port surgery has also been described.

Although robotic radical prostatectomy is established as standard practice in many adult urology settings in the developed world [4], the role of robotics in other adult surgical specialities and paediatric surgery is still being defined. Many paediatric surgical units around the world have developed their robotic programmes as part of a wider multidisciplinary university hospital services. To the best of our knowledge, we established the first independent paediatric robotic programme in Leeds, UK, using the da Vinci system in early 2006. In Leeds Children's Hospital, robot-assisted pyeloplasty, nephrectomy, partial nephroureterectomy, some bladder procedures, pelvic procedures in DSD, rectopexy, fundoplication, Heller's myotomy, partial and total splenectomy, cholecystectomy and liver cysts and choledochal cysts with hepaticojejunostomy are routinely performed in all ages with noticeably low morbidity rates and promising short- and long-term outcomes [5]. The number and types of the procedures performed with robotic assistance and the numbers of robotic surgeons continue to expand.

This chapter highlights the basics of robot-assisted surgery in children.

7.2 Advantages and Limitations of Robotics in Children

Paediatric surgery is characterised by a wide variety in pathology, procedures and patient size. Most operations are complex and reconstructive in nature. For these reasons, paediatric surgery demands high-quality operating view, dexterity and precision.

The three-dimensional panoramic high-resolution view, with depth perception and

A. Najmaldin (✉) · T. Cundy · D. Di Fabrizio
N. Alizai
Leeds Teaching Hospitals, Leeds, UK
e-mail: azad.najmaldin@nhs.net; naved.alizai@nhs.net

C. Esposito et al. (eds.), *ESPES Manual of Pediatric Minimally Invasive Surgery*,
https://doi.org/10.1007/978-3-030-00964-9_7

independent control of a stable visual field with increased magnification, contributes to a greatly enhanced ability to identify and manipulate tissue with improved precision as compared to conventional manual endoscopic or even what the open-technique surgery allows. The intuitive nature of the system and increased freedom of movement provided by the multijointed robotic instruments and motion scaling augment the surgeon's manual dexterity and control. Other significant advantages of the system include the near-normal restoration of native hand-eye co-ordination and noticeably superior ergonomics and comfortable seated posture, which are particularly important for the operator and in complex or prolonged surgical procedures. These characteristics make the robot a superior operating tool for the paediatric surgeon. The system has alleviated the need for a human camera assistant. Consequently the manpower in the operating room can be reduced, and costs of operating may be rationalised in this regard. Using the three-armed da Vinci robot platform, the senior author (AN) has successfully completed several robotic-assisted procedures with the scrub nurse alone (Fig. 7.1).

Laboratory-based studies indicate an initial steep learning curve when first using the robot, which plateau sooner for robotics when compared with conventional manual endoscopic surgery. Moreover, surgeons with experience in endoscopic surgery acquire robotic skills sooner than surgeons who have no experience [6, 7]. Some surgeons have successfully established a comprehensive robotic practice in children with little if any prior experience in manual laparoscopy or thoracoscopy [8]. The learning curve conversion and complication rates are comparable to, or lower than, manual endoscopic surgery [8–10].

There can be no doubt that the robotic system provides technological solutions that overcome many difficulties inherent with conventional endoscopic surgery. Robotic technology is described as a tool to "democratise" minimally invasive surgery, enabling more surgeons to become facile with complex endoscopic techniques and offer the benefits of laparoscopy and thoracoscopic approaches to their patients. However, robot-assisted surgery is not without limitations. The system has a near-complete lack of tactile (haptic) feedback. The operator relies

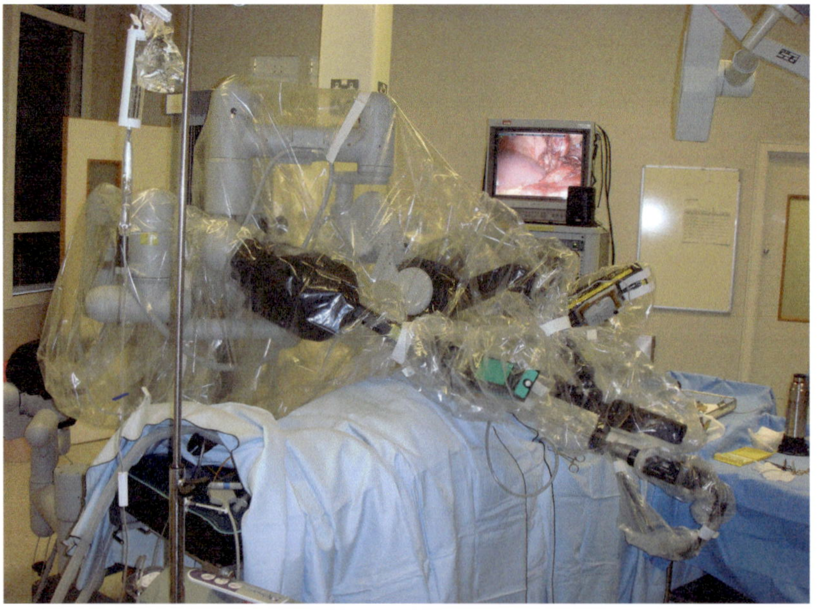

Fig. 7.1 Robotic pyeloplasty performed successfully with one scrub nurse and no medical assistant

entirely upon visual cues in tissue deformation, familiarity with the surgical anatomy and instruments. The robotic arms are powerful, so surgeons must remain careful while manipulating tissues and suturing. It is reassuring that only a small number of robot-related intraoperative and post-operative complications have been reported in the literature [8–11].

Other disadvantages arise from the size of the slave arms and the instruments (Figs. 7.1 and 7.2). The size discrepancy may allow arm and instrument collision outside the patient and potentially restrict anaesthetist and/or assistant access to the patient. The smallest available telescope size is 8 mm. The 5 mm instruments are effective but less versatile than the 8 mm instruments. These disadvantages may become relevant in infants and small children [12]. The slender-sized arms and rotational characteristics of the da Vinci Xi system have addressed some of the above-mentioned drawbacks of the S and Si models.

The capital and maintenance costs of the da Vinci system are significantly higher than conventional endoscopic surgery infrastructure. However, the cost of consumables per procedure can be made comparable to, or lower than, that of disposable endoscopic surgery instruments by reducing the number of robotic instruments used for any given procedure and by the use of reusable ports. In the authors' unit, such measures have been assessed prospectively and have been shown to be beneficial, financially. Furthermore, the increased cost of the robotics may be offset by the improved quality of surgical technique, reduced conversion and complications rates [1, 4, 9, 10, 13], wider application of minimal access surgery and the reduced manpower in the operating room.

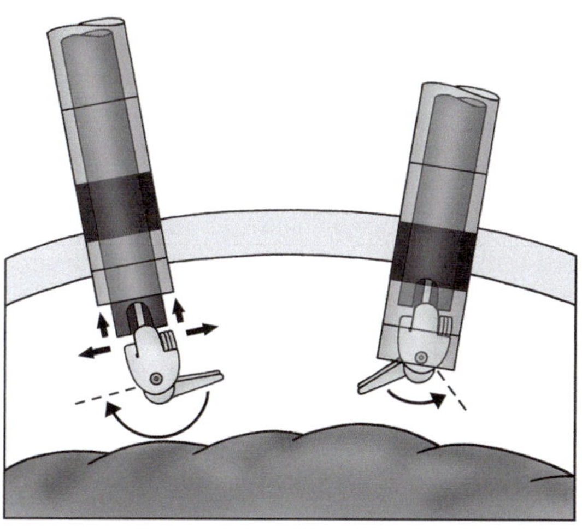

Fig. 7.2 The restricted working space in paediatric robotic surgery. Note the position of the port and its effect on the instrument function

7.3 Training

Current practice in medicine and surgery demands even more than formerly to focus major emphasis on the acquisition of skills. Good surgical management requires appropriate decision-making and competent manipulative skills. The surgeon's ability to perform safe and successful robotic procedures relies heavily on the understanding of general and specific principles of conventional surgery and minimal invasive surgery as well as robotics. A lack of understanding of any of the above principles produces unnecessary difficulties, complications and poor outcome, and expose patients to risks.

Endoscopic surgeons acquire skills of robotics much quicker than surgeons who are naïve to endoscopic surgery. Surgeons exclusively trained in open techniques may find learning robot-assisted surgery less problematic than learning conventional endoscopic surgery [6, 7]. Therefore, prior skills in endoscopic surgery are not a prerequisite to the acquisition of robotic surgery skills. As with all fields of surgical practice, an apprentice can acquire the craft skills of robotics from one or more masters by listening, watching, assisting and being encouraged, assisted and corrected. Hands-on practice on the robotic system, outside and inside the operating rooms, allows for a safer and shorter skills acquisition [14] (Fig. 7.3). Before starting clinical robotics, all surgeons must familiarise themselves with the use of console, slave unit, docking and undocking, emergency undocking, instruments and adjusting to the near-complete loss of tactile feedback during surgery.

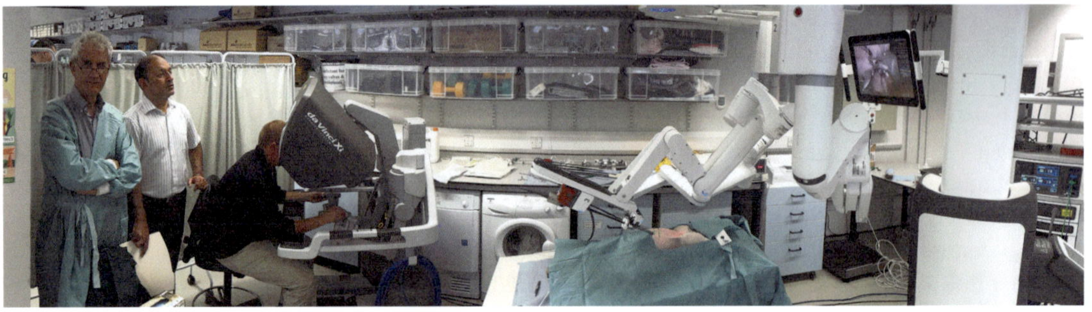

Fig. 7.3 Leeds annual endoscopic and robotic workshop

7.4 Operative Considerations

As with conventional endoscopic surgery in children, preoperative colon preparation is rarely required for abdominal or urological procedures. An informed consent must be obtained in all cases. The patients/guardians must be informed about all risks including potential complications and the possibility of conversion to a manual endoscopic or open technique.

Theatre layout is crucial to the success of any robotic procedure. A dedicated theatre and theatre team improve productivity, speed of surgery and safety. Position of the mobile slave unit must be planned and discussed with the anaesthetic and nursing teams. This is particularly important in multidisciplinary and dedicated paediatric theatres, where a wide range of procedures (thoracic, upper and lower abdominal, left or right sides) are undertaken by one or more teams in different age groups and different sized patients (infants to fully grown adolescents). The position of the S and Si mobile slave units depends on the size of the patient and the types of the procedure to be executed (Table 7.1).

As for conventional manual thoracoscopic and laparoscopic procedures, a slight to moderate head, lateral or foot tilts "before docking" often facilitate access and manipulation. Position of the da Vinci Xi system in both thoracic and abdominal procedures are less complicated compared to S and Si da Vinci system models.

Ready access to the patient's airway and intravenous lines must be ensured at all times. The access for the assistant (if any) and the external position of the accessory conventional endoscopic port/instruments must be planned before the start of the procedure. It is a common mistake to only consider the distance between port sites, instead of the movement arc of the robotic arm and the external part of the conventional port/instrument, as they may clash and make the assistance very difficult.

Table 7.1 The position of the S and Si slave units around the operating table in paediatric robotic surgery

Procedure	Robot slave position
Cervical and thoracic inlet	Head of the table
R/L upper abdominal	R/L shoulder
Posterior mediastinum	Behind semiprone
Anterior mediastinum	In front semisupine or lateral
Transperitoneal renal and adrenal gland	Behind with a slight turn to face the patient's foot in semisupine or semilateral position
Small and large intestine	R/L supine ± slight tilt
R/L lower abdomen and pelvic in older children	R/L of the foot of the table, supine ± slight tilt
Lower abdomen, pelvic and transvesical	Direct foot of the table (infants) or between legs (older), supine

As with conventional endoscopic surgery, all procedures are performed under general anaesthesia with intubation, total muscle relaxation and controlled ventilation. During induction of anaesthesia for a robotic-assisted procedure, gaseous distension of the gastrointestinal tract should be avoided, as even a slight dilatation of the intestines can jeopardise safe and easy access, with a higher risk of complications and increased risks of conversion to open method surgery and complications. This is particularly so in infants and small children, complex procedures, pelvic and retroperitoneal organ surgery and if the procedure is being executed without a surgical assistant or fourth robot slave arm. In the author's experience, inadequate muscle relaxation and/or intestinal tract distension has been the commonest reason for conversion [13]. After induction, nasogastric tube aspiration can improve access in the upper abdomen and minimise the risk of pulmonary aspiration but is less effective in preventing gaseous distension of the intestinal tract. A palpable bladder can usually be adequately emptied by a Credé manoeuvre, and catheterisation is required only in sick patients and complex and prolonged or certain pelvic procedures.

As with the conventional thoracoscopic surgery, endotracheal intubation with or without lung retraction and/or low-pressure insufflation provide adequate access for most hemi-thoracic and mediastinal procedures. Double-lumen intubation and selective bronchial intubation with or without contralateral bronchial occlusion are technically demanding manoeuvres, particularly in small children, and may be required in certain circumstances.

Although the fourth arm of the da Vinci system is easy to operate and may prove helpful in many circumstances, we prefer the use of three robotic arms with or without an accessory conventional endoscopic port and instrument in most paediatric cases, particularly in infants and small children. Reasons for this are listed below.

- Many paediatric procedures can easily be performed using two instruments only.
- The fourth arm takes additional space at and around the operating table and increases the chance of arms and instruments' collision. This is particularly so in small patients.
- An accessory conventional laparoscopic or thoracoscopic port is more versatile for different types and different sized retractors, suction and irrigation devices, special instruments or drains/tubes, sealing devices, staplers, suturing materials, retrievals and specimen bags, in all age groups.

As for conventional endoscopic surgery, it is important to recognise that in children, particularly infants and small children, the surface area for access is limited, The body wall is thin and highly compliant, intercostal spaces are narrow, the liver edge is below the costal margin, the bladder is largely an intra-abdominal structure, viscera and major vessels are closer to the body surface, tissues are delicate, thoracic and abdominal working spaces are small (200–500 mL in infants), and high-pressure insufflation may not be tolerated easily (abdomen 8–12 mmHg, thoracic 4–6 mmHg are usually safe). These characteristics make access and manipulation in paediatric surgery more difficult and complicated when compared with adults. However, the lack of excess visceral fat in infants and small children makes recognition and dissection of structures a relatively easy exercise.

In general, the position and number of access ports are similar to those of equivalent conventional laparoscopic and thoracoscopic procedures [15]. However, it is important to appreciate the following special considerations in robot-assisted surgery:

- Ports, instruments and telescope are usually positioned towards the mobile slave units, though vision and/or instrument function may still be preserved with the instruments at a perpendicular or slightly sideway positions.
- Ports are positioned so that they do not allow collision between the robot slave arms and either the patient's head, ventilation lines, patient's bony landmarks, operating table, assistant, conventional endoscopy ports, deployed instruments or other robot arms.
- The rule of four fingers space between ports is applicable only to large children. In infants and small children, surgeons have to compensate by changing the level at which ports are placed and by being especially careful during robot-assisted surgery.
- Access to the patient (airway, intravenous lines, aspiration and drain) is maintained throughout the procedure.

In children, open technique is the preferred method for the insertion of the primary optical

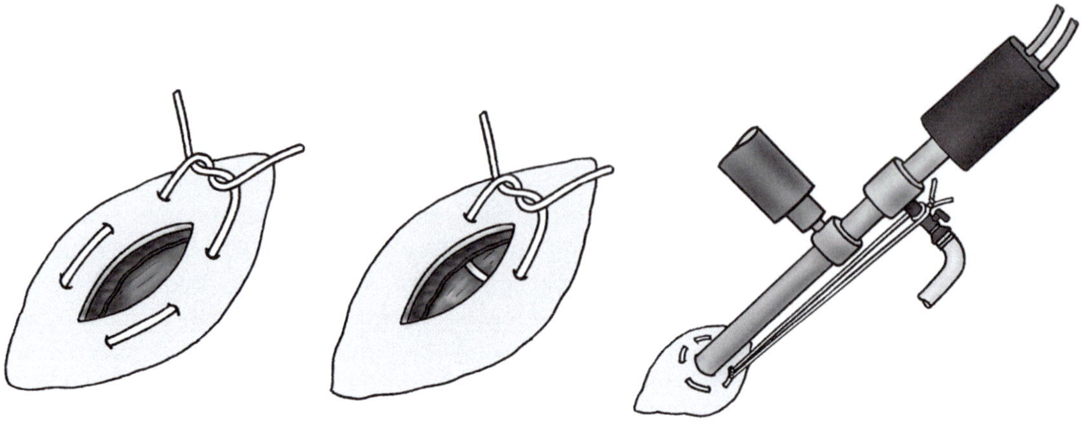

Fig. 7.4 Open technique insertion of the optic primary port

port [15]. A strong purse string or single suture through the fascia and peritoneum with a double throw prevents gas leak around the port. Hitching the suture around the port inlet or insufflation nipple prevents outward displacement of the port during the procedure (Fig. 7.4). The gas flow and insufflation pressure parameters used in robotics are similar to those of conventional manual endoscopic surgery. However, robotic procedures can be executed safely and successfully with lower insufflation (smaller spaces) for the following reasons:

- The fixed ports of the robot act as a lift (anterior abdominal wall only).
- The multijointed instruments allow for a degree of retraction near the operating field.
- The improved dexterity, precision and ergonomics provided by the system.
- The improved camera control and vision.
- The lesser need for instrument changes during any given procedure.

The working space for both 8 and 5 mm instrument functions may be critically reduced if more than 5–10 mm of the port is allowed inside the intra-cavity working space (Fig. 7.2). Once the robot is docked, the arms should be unclutched carefully; one arm at a time, using both hands and the safety and anticipated range of movements for each individual arm and instrument including the telescope, the possibility of internal and external collisions (between arms and instruments, arms and patient, ventilation lines, accessory port, fixed external retractor, assistant) and the required optimal operating view are checked. The position of the robot arms may have to be readjusted before the start of the procedure.

The tissue manipulation, dissection, suturing and the use of energy sources are carried out in a manner similar to that of conventional endoscopic surgery. As described earlier in this chapter, the near-complete loss of tactile feedback must always be remembered during the entire procedure. Care must be taken while loading and unloading instruments, and instruments should only be moved under direct vision, at all times.

Once the procedure is completed, the instruments are removed, arms undocked, and cartwheeled away from the patient. The telescope is held by hand and working ports removed under direct vision, and finally the telescope and the primary port removed. It is essential that the patient is kept fully relaxed while the deeper layers (peritoneum and fascia) of all 8–12 mm (possibly 5 mm in infants) wounds are closed safely. If the patient is not relaxed, wound closure becomes extremely difficult, and the risks of omentum and bowel herniation or being caught in the wound closure increase significantly. As for conventional laparoscopy, layer closure can be difficult in overweight children and adolescents. In such circumstances, a fascial closure device can be used, which has to be deployed while the ports and telescope is still in situ. Wound infiltration with an appropriate local anaesthetic agent may be completed before the skin closure.

Post-operative pain control may be achieved as for conventional manual thoracoscopy and laparoscopy. However, in our experience, less than 20% of patients require one to three doses of Oramorph or iv morphine infusion in the first 8–24 h post-operative period.

7.5 Conclusions

Robotic surgery represents an advance for endoscopic minimal invasive surgery. Application of this technology in children continues to be demonstrated as safe and effective in an increasing variety of procedures and age range. An underappreciated role for this technology is its ability to make a minimally invasive surgical option more available to children who otherwise might undergo an open-technique procedure. Growing numbers of surgeons are reporting low conversion and complication rates and excellent long-term outcomes. Increased surgical precision and dexterity, superior camera control and ergonomics as well as near-normal eye and instrument co-ordination are significant advantages. The system allows for easier and shorter learning curve, reduced manpower in the operating room and possibly shorter operating time.

Compared with conventional endoscopic surgical approach, the costs of equipment, instrument and maintenance are high. The size of the mobile slave unit and instruments and the current single company market monopoly are also a disadvantage.

Robotic surgical technology is here to stay and will continue to evolve to become more advanced, affordable and better suited for our young patients. We anticipate robot-assisted surgery to be an important component in the future of paediatric surgery.

References

1. Najmaldin A. Paediatric robotic surgery: where do we stand. Int J Med Robot Comput Assisted Surg. 2007;3:183–6.
2. Cundy TP, Marcus HJ, Hughes-Hallett A, Najmaldin A, Yang GZ, Darzi A. International attitudes of early adopters to current and future robotic technologies in paediatric surgery. J Pediatr Surg. 2014;49(10):1522–6.
3. Alizai N, Dawrant M, Najmaldin A. Robotic assisted resection choledochal cyst and hepaticojejunostomy in children. Pediatr Surg Int. 2014;30:291–4.
4. McGuinness LA, Rai BP. Robotics in urology. Ann R Coll Surg Engl. 2018;100(Suppl 6):38–44.
5. Cundy TP, Gattas NE, White A, Yang GZ, Darzi A, Najmaldin A. Learning curve evaluation using CUSUM analysis—a clinical example of pediatric robotic assisted laparoscopic pyeloplasty. J Pediatr Surg. 2015;50(8):1368–73.
6. Prassad SM, Manian HS, Soper NJ, et al. The effect of robotic assistance on learning curves for basic laparoscopic skills. Am J Surg. 2002;183:702–7.
7. Yohannes P, Rotariu P, Pinto P, et al. Comparison of robotic versus laparoscopic skills: is there a difference in the learning curve? Urology. 2002;60:39–45.
8. Meehan JJ, Sandler A. Pediatric robotic surgery: a single institutional review of the first 100 consecutive cases. Surg Endosc. 2008;22(1):177–82.
9. Lee RS, Retik AB, Borer JG, Peters CA. Pediatric robotic assisted laparoscopic dismembered pyeloplasty: comparison with a cohort of open surgery. J Urol. 2006;175:683–7.
10. Najmaldin A, Antao B. Early experience of telerobotic surgery in children. Int J Med Robot Comput Assisted Surg. 2007;3:199–202.
11. Cundy TP, Gattas NE, Yang GZ, Darzi A, Najmaldin A. Experience related factors compensate for haptic loss in robotic assisted laparoscopic surgery. J Endourol. 2014;28(5):532–8.
12. Cundy TP, Marcus HJ, Hughes-Hallett A, Mackinnon T, Najmaldin A, Yang GZ, Darzi A. Robotic versus nonrobotic instruments in spatially constrained operating workspaces: a preclinical randomised crossover study. BJU Int. 2015;116(3):415–22.
13. Di Fabrizio D, Cundy TP, Alizai N, Najmaldin A. Conversion rates in paediatric robotic surgery. Best paper presentation at 7th Annual Congress of European Society of Paediatric Endoscopic Surgeons. Wroclaw, Poland. 27–29 Sept 2017.
14. Cundy TP, Mayer EK, Camps JI, Olsen LH, Pelizzo G, Yang GZ, Darzi A, Najmaldin A. Education and training in pediatric robotic assisted minimally invasive surgery: lessons learned from an inaugural multinational workshop. J Robot Surg. 2015;9(1):57–63.
15. Najmaldin A. Chapter 29: Laparoscopy—basic technique. In: Najmaldin A, Rothenberg S, Crabbe D, Beasly S, editors. Operative endoscopy and endoscopic surgery in infants and children. London: Hodder Arnold; 2005.

Training in Pediatric Minimal Access Surgery

8

Aly Shalaby and Amulya K. Saxena

8.1 Introduction

Moulding today's surgeon goes beyond technical skills to build depth of knowledge, professional values and the ability to work in a multidisciplinary environment. Minimal access surgery (MAS) has integrated itself in all aspects of operating which involves comprehensive preoperative skill development. Training therein has moved outside the operating theatre to laboratories with simulators of all guises: real, virtual and combinations thereof. Designing surgical MIS skills training is a challenge. It should be based on acquisition of knowledge and operative skills of progressive complexity. While it is easier to assess a technical skill versus a nontechnical one (e.g. thought processes), objective measures that evaluate MAS skills can be quite complex.

Surgical innovation is fickle. What may be hailed today at the "next big thing" may turn out to be but a blip on the way a few years down the line. Smartphones and augmented reality (AR) have taken the world by storm and are finding themselves in every nook of our daily lives. In a world of evidence-based practice, surgical education is no exception. It is no longer a subjective discipline but a series of objective, validated and quantifiable assessments that aim to curate the well-rounded surgeon of today. Simulation, with all its guises, came to the fore with changes in work-time restrictions, evolving technology, the rising demand for patient safety and the increase in patient expectations. This chapter aims to review the theory behind MIS skill acquisition, the tools available for this purpose with a focus on their application in pediatric surgery.

8.2 Learning Theory

Surgical training has moved on from the traditional apprenticeship model that is based on several years of textbook knowledge combined with workplace training. Traditional learning has now also expanded to encompass virtual learning environments (VLEs) that characterise e-learning. It not only provides supplementary information and support but also allows flexibility in time and place of access—two elements of high importance to surgical trainees balancing on-call duties and learning. In addition, this type of blended learning makes use of a plethora of tools such as box trainers, virtual reality (VR) simulators, inanimate models, cadaveric or explanted tissue and live animal models.

An effective grasp of educational theory is the backbone of improving the teaching of practical skills. Kolb's Learning Style Inventory (LSI) categorises learner types as converging

A. Shalaby · A. K. Saxena (✉)
Department of Pediatric Surgery, Chelsea Children's Hospital, Chelsea and Westminster NHS Foundation Trust, Imperial College London, London, UK
e-mail: amulya.saxena@nhs.net

C. Esposito et al. (eds.), *ESPES Manual of Pediatric Minimally Invasive Surgery*,
https://doi.org/10.1007/978-3-030-00964-9_8

(problem-solving), accommodating (practical involvement), diverging (passive observation) and assimilating (theoretical formulation). Convergence seems to be highest amongst surgeons. It is served well by current training methods involving problem-based discussions, podcasts, blogs and instructional videos.

Two major theories impact on MIS learning. The first is the *Cognitive Load Theory* [1]. It involves three different "loads": *intrinsic*, *exogenous* and *germane* that should come together to provide optimal learning. The *intrinsic* loads are the resources needed for a task, the *exogenous* loads are the resources needed to understand direction and deal with interference, and finally the *germane* load is when the learner has sufficient spare cognitive capacity to reflect on what is being learned. It is important to know that MIS taxes the *germane* load, especially in novices. Stress in peculiar settings, such as trauma or uncontrolled bleeding, decreases the cognitive load.

The second theory is the *Contextual Interference Effect* (CI) [2]. When task parameters are increasingly altered, an impaired performance occurs in the skill acquisition phase. Multiplying the amount of CI, should in theory, improves the subsequent phases of retention and transfer [2]. In an experimental study involving laparoscopic skills, it was found that CI did not provide added benefit and could in fact be detrimental on the retention phase. They recommended that it be tailored to the trainee's level. "Complex variations on training tasks and different camera orientations can be applied later in training, when trainees have attained a higher proficiency level. In this way, trainees are not overly challenged, but flexibility of their skills can still be enhanced" [2].

8.3 Skills, Competence and the Expert

The two major skill areas needed in MIS are visuospatial awareness and fine motor dexterity. Motor skill development is associated with perception, memory, communication skills and managerial processes. As an extension to the Howell model of learning, there is a cognitive phase, integrative phase and an autonomous phase [3].

Skill gain can also be described as three phases: *acquisition*, learning a new skill; *retention*, reproducing same skill several (weeks/months) later; and *transfer*, moving from simulation to theatre. Low variability in learning settings is frequently correlated with poor transfer (third phase of skill gain).

Skill gain reaches a deep learning state by three modes of practice:

(a) **Varied practice** where tasks are done in smaller time slots and alternated more frequently compared to a standard practice where the learner trains on tasks in a sequential order starting from the easiest to the most difficult. Similarly, the *spacing effect* states that dividing training into distinct blocs improves learning.
(b) **Distributed practice** (over weeks) results in improvement and retention of motor skills.
(c) Finally, **deliberate practice** where the learner has an explicit intention and motive to improve (not just time spent operating). Components of deliberate practice are goal-directed training, repetition, reflection and feedback, the latter being the most important.

Competence in surgery is defined as the ability to successfully apply professional, skills, knowledge and attitudes to new situations and familiar tasks. It is evaluated by setting a clear definition, providing up to date documentation complimented with assessments. A behaviourist approach assesses competence using clearly defined set of criteria such as skill sets. A holistic approach assesses competence in context of a wider scope involving other characteristics such as situational awareness. In understanding competence, there are three common educational theories. **Miller's** hierarchical triangle of competence and skills describes a surgeon who "knows", "knows how", "shows how" and finally "does". **Howell's** model on the other hand moves from having unconscious incompetence to conscious competence to unconscious competence. Finally, the **Cambridge** model distinguishes competence (what a trainee is capable of doing) from performance (what actually happens in real life) as other factors affect performance (patient-related factors, colleagues and hospital policy/level of technology).

Defining an expert is a challenging task and has been extensively debated by researchers in medical education. In flying, there are five levels of skill: novice, advanced beginner, competent, proficient and expert. In the medical field, it is not as clear-cut. Economy of movement has been proposed as the best indicator of expert status, and it is a skill level discriminator in simulation. The expert has domain-specific memory skills that tap into long-term memory. Planning and reasoning for alternative courses of action to anticipate adverse events become second nature. Hence some tasks can be done "automatically": primary tasks are done with no obvious intentional effort in addition to capacity to do other simultaneous tasks with relative ease. The expert is capable of recognising his or her own errors and self-correct.

Two types of expert are recognised. The *routine* expert applies learned routines repetitively. New problems are adapted to their learned routines. New learning improves efficiency by modifying aspects of the learned routines. The *adaptive* expert adapts problems to learned routines relying on flexibility, innovation and creativity (as opposed to speed, accuracy and automaticity). This may not particularly be helpful in surgery!

Some authors argue that experts are essentially made despite cultural notions that some doctors are innately geared to be surgeons [4]. In one study looking at training potential, novice subjects ended up clustered into three groups: (a) those with an inborn skill, (b) those who were trainable and (c) those who could not gain competency despite repeated training [5]. Taken at face value, it can suggest that the latter group are untrainable; however a more moderate approach would interpret this group as one which would require additional/alternative training to reach the desired competencies.

8.4 Simulation

Traditionalists will interpret simulation as a static, laboratory-based entity. This may be true to a certain extent in the context of this chapter; however the trainee and the educator reading this should be aware that simulation can offer much more. Simulation's evolved definition is "a spectrum of resources alongside clinical care in order to complement its richness" and "to offer an opportunity to abstract from a complex reality to generalise from the particular aspects and to create suitable conditions for self practice, minimising patient harm".

The need for simulation stemmed from shorter working hours and hospital pressures such as increased theatre utilisation efficiency and medicolegal pressures. Back in 2008 the UK Chief Medical Officer announced that simulation will be of central importance in healthcare education especially for surgery and related craft specialities [6]. It has proven to be an excellent adjunct to surgical education, offering a safe environment where trainees can repeatedly practise a range of clinical skills without endangering patients. It is now central to education and has evolved into a discipline of its own: simulation-based medical education (SBME) is a recognised field. One no longer debates the effectiveness of simulation, rather how to make the best of it.

Simulation should go beyond the operation and incorporate complex reality. This helps to not only hone the technical skills but to bring out the often unseen flaws in the nontechnical skills such as team working. It can be categorised into:

- High fidelity: This includes complex simulation involving all aspects of clinical care and often involves costly mannequins, equipment and simulation labs (laparoscopic simulators).
- Novice-based procedural simulation: Teaches basic skills, is deconstructed and focuses on learning a skill. It is a low-cost and easy way of teaching.

- Patient simulation: Uses real people either actors or chronic patients.
- Hybrid simulation: Combines models with SPs.
- Distributed simulation: Uses low-cost props that are easy to transport to areas beyond the simulation laboratory.
- Sequential simulation: Simulates areas where transition of care might be problematic.

Simulation does not have to involve the entire scenario. It can focus on a certain element and can be therefore broken down into four elements: (a) selection of the desired point to focus on; (b) abstraction, isolating the point from its original setting; (c) representation of that point in another milieu; and (d) intensification, the net result of dismantling the bigger picture and only focusing on one aspect.

8.5 Types of Simulators

Simulators can be classified into virtual (no realistic setting), physical (no virtual setting) and hybrid (combination of virtual and realistic). Another classification according to setup can be box trainers, virtual reality and augmented reality. Box simulators are simple, basic, portable and cheap and allow for basic skills training (Fig. 8.1). Evaluation is done by experienced surgeon or tracking.

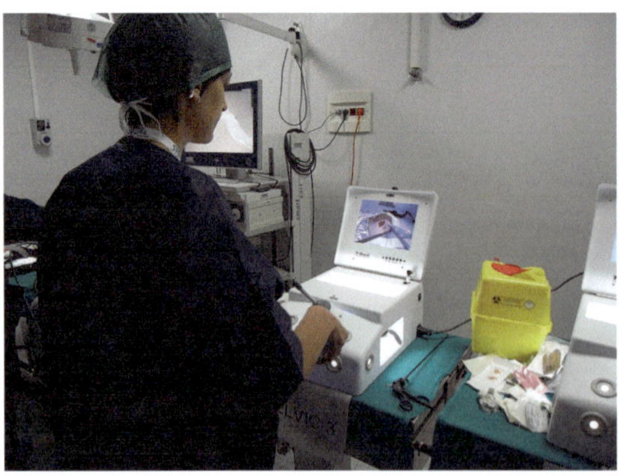

Fig. 8.1 Box trainers with integrated camera and screen to perform procedures in real time on fresh tissue or training objects

Table 8.1 Virtual reality simulators with their characteristics

Device	Manufacturer	Training options
Lap Mentor	Simbionix Ltd. Golan, Israel	Basic/advanced tasks
Sinergia	Sinergia Consortium	Basic tasks
LapSim	Surgical Sciences, Gothenburg, Sweden	Basic/advanced tasks
MIST-VR	Mentice AB, Goteborg, Sweden	Basic tasks
Simendo	SimSurgery AS, Oslo, Norway	Basic/advanced procedures
SEP	SimSurgery AS, Oslo, Norway	Basic/advanced procedures
LapVR	CAE Healthcare, Mainz, Germany	Basic/advanced procedures

Table 8.2 Characteristics of physical simulators for objective measurement of technical skills

Device	Technology	Training evaluation
HUESAD	Optical	Instrument motion
Zebris	Acoustic	Instrument motion
SurgicalSIM LTS	Sensor-based	Physical models with sensors
CELTS	Optical	Instrument motion
ADEPT	Gimbal mechanism	Instrument motion

VR is more complex, is less portable, is more expensive and trains more advanced skills. Evaluation is by forced feedback. VR cons are low realism and poor haptic feedback. AR is most sophisticated, is expensive, trains advanced skills and uses pictures, has better haptic feedback and makes use of actual consumables. Assessment is with complex performance metrics. The commonest simulators currently on the market are summarised in the tables below (Tables 8.1 and 8.2) [7].

AR simulator presently available on the market amongst others includes the more commonly known PROMIS.

8.6 Simulator Assessment

Any simulation or test must be both *reliable* and *valid* in order to give objective feedback on a certain skill or set of skills.

Reliability is how predictable the test is to convey consistent results time after time. It consists of three elements:

- **Inter-rater**: The degree of difference between assessors given to a single trainee (not applicable in VR situations where the data is computer generated)
- **Intra-rater**: The degree of variation when assessing under different conditions and times
- **Test-retest**: The degree of variation when the same individual repeats the test under different conditions and times

Validity means to how true to reality a test is and if it really measures what it sets out to do. Validity has five elements: [8]

- **Face**: subjective but requires the user to measure design, functionality and how close to reality the test is.
- **Content**: assessed by experts but can also be subjective—it aims to determine if the test contains the relevant elements and tasks required for the assessment and its training capacity.
- **Construct**: ability to differentiate between levels of quality (or skill levels).
- **Concurrent**: similarity between two instruments or test that set out to assess the same skill.
- **Predictive**: measures how well the individual will perform the task in a real-life setting.

8.7 MIS Skill Assessment

All the laparoscopic skills such as bimanual dexterity, access and suturing are measured with metrics. There is a huge number of "performance metrics" in the literature such as task duration, number of hand movements and instrument path length (Table 8.3) [9]. The best/most reliable metrics are time, path length, depth perception and motion smoothness. Task difficulty is generally related to poor haptic feedback, loss of depth perception, fulcrum effect, decreased range of motion, amplified tremor, and parallax errors.

Table 8.3 Metrics for objective skill assessment

Efficiency	Force analysis	Tool-tissue forces Torsion
		Force sensitivity
	Motion analysis	Depth perception Tool rotation
		Speed and acceleration Optimal path deviation Energy expenditure
		Angular area Volume
Quality		Task outcomes Errors Manoeuvres' repetitions Manoeuvres' order Idle states

Simple box trainers rely on an "expert" assessor applying a set of predefined scores. Some rely on video assessment. Some tracking systems are rigid and can restrict instrument movement—affecting the trainee's metrics. Performance is better tracked by the VR simulators. Poor haptic feedback and lack of verisimilitude are compensated by combined/hybrid models. Finally, motion analysis attempts to track, quantify and interpret skill level based on the trainee's movements.

8.8 Minimal Access Surgery in Pediatrics

Pediatric surgery is no stranger to MAS procedures, but lack of exposure to index cases can be problematic. In addition, there is a lack of a uniform and structured MIS training program in Europe. The difference in pediatric surgical training in MAS to adults is that the surgeon is exposed to a wide size range of patient in which the procedures have to be performed. This requires adaptation skills in newborns and infants, toddlers, school-age children and teenagers. This size variation has another aspect as procedure in newborns and infants is easier to perform with 3 mm instruments (rather than 5 mm). Besides the instrument size, a large assortment of instruments that are present in 5 and 10 mm options are not available in 3 mm sizes. This unavailability of specialised instruments in smaller sizes has been a major factor in the development of pediatric minimal access surgery as technical step changes have led to procedures goal being achieved using existing instruments of altered surgical steps. Besides this, the small working spaces in newborns offer restricted space for manipulations with risk of injury to organs if instruments during procedures are moved excessively in an uncontrolled fashion. With direct training programs in pediatric surgery where trainees do not have prior exposure to adult minimal access cases, trainees in pediatric surgery are able to perform complete index cases towards the end of their training, however under supervision.

Following a survey in 2013, the European Society of Paediatric Endoscopic Surgeons (ESPES) puts forward such a framework [10]. Its basic four blocks are theoretical, laboratory-based skills, personal logbook and time spent at a dedicated MAS centre (Fig. 8.2). ESPES defines a high-volume centre as one that does at least 200 MAS cases per year [10]. The theoretical block is to include at least a couple of MAS courses. The latter have been shown to complement and enhance learning. The minimum number of cases to reach a high skill level remains still unclear.

The ESPES training takes the Fundamentals of Laparoscopic Surgery (FLS) program to the next level of learning to involve a "step-by-step" teaching that ends in MAS certification (Fig. 8.3) [10].

In children, as in adults, the laboratory-acquired skills remain largely the same:

1. Entry into cavities
2. Suturing and intra- and extracorporeal knot tying
3. Haemostasis
4. Cutting precision
5. Tissue reconstruction

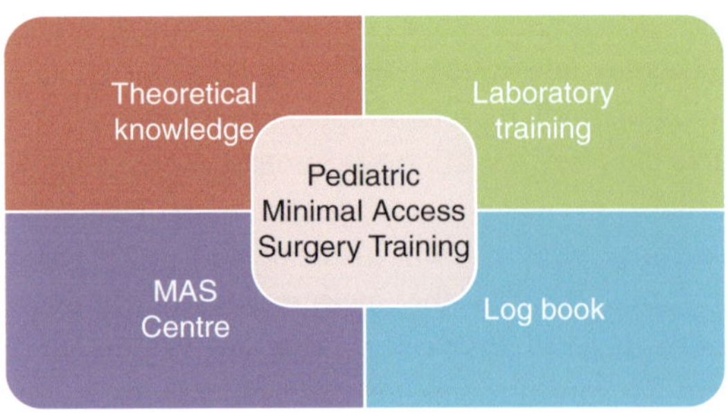

Fig. 8.2 The interrelated areas of pediatric minimal access surgery from the training perspective according to the ESPES 2013 framework

The key skills however identified are "two-handed instrument manipulation, dissection, intra-corporeal suturing and intra- and extracorporeal knot tying".

Static simulation models for pediatric surgery include basic skills and for training on neonatal procedures for pathologies such as oesophageal atresia/trachea-oesophageal fistula, pelvi-ureteric junction obstruction (PUJO), diaphragmatic hernia and duodenal atresia. Advanced courses have been introduced to perform procedures on live tissues in skill labs to mimic real-life scenarios (Fig. 8.4).

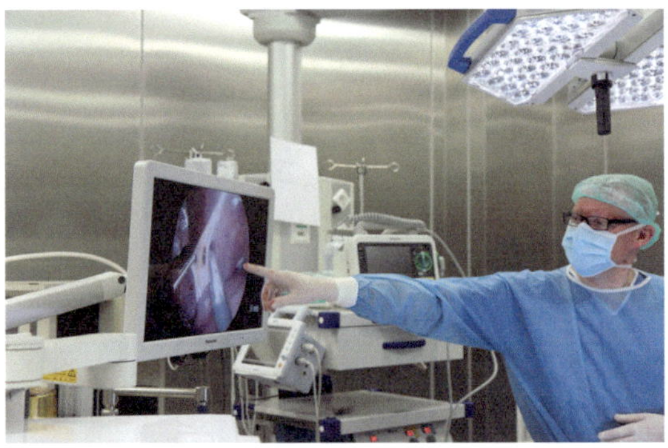

Fig. 8.3 Trainees are guided through various aspects of performing procedures under the guidance of experts who carefully monitor every step of the procedure

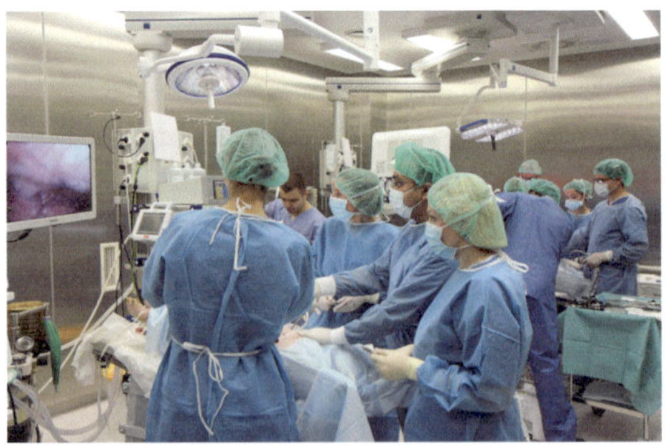

Fig. 8.4 Procedures being performed on live tissue to offer a live model hands-on experience under guidance from experts

The porcine model is the most common used in animal models of pediatric surgery as it allows for complex procedures such as cholecystectomy, splenectomy and nephrectomy but can also be used for hernia repair and varicocelectomy. Rabbits are especially fitting for neonatal procedures owing to their small abdominal and thoracic cavities which mimic those of a neonate.

A learning curve, defined as the time taken for improvement of outcomes, comes hand in hand with MAS. It is characterised by three phases: the start (which differs depending on experience), the incline (skill progression) and the plateau [11]. Learning curves are not just surrogate indicators of skill, but they also affect hospitals and institutions as a whole. A recent systematic review of learning curves in pediatric surgery showed poor representation and measurement thereof. Operative time was the commonest measure in use; however as stand-alone, it is not useful in pediatric surgery where other factors such as co-morbidities and instrument setup can be confounding factors [12]. Ideally, one would use the same performance metrics used in simulation discussed above. Macdonald et al. make a valid statement that attempting to set up such metrics for a routine day case would be prohibitive for most centres [12]. Nevertheless, the authors have put forward a framework that would allow for a standard format of reporting which in turn opens the door for cross-study comparisons (Fig. 8.5) [12].

Whereas some authors were referring to the reporting of novel MAS techniques that might involve multiple surgeons, we believe that maintaining a structured framework per individual would also be good practice.

8.9 Discussion

Technical skills are one of the hallmarks of surgical training compared to other fields of medicine. Educational theory is a complex field, but a good understanding of it influences outcomes. The best most effective surgical curricula will support and train all levels of students to the desired competency level, innate abilities notwithstanding. The answer to a comprehensive program is to use a combination of all the available tools, divided and stratified across the board and tailored to each stage of the surgical training process. An example of development and validation of a laparoscopic colorectal curriculum was published in 2012 [13].

The trainee is an essential component in the learning equation. They must be engaged in training. Surgical trainees count on experiential learning and lament today's lack of contact with trainers and other trainees. However, it must be noted that many factors affect engagement. They can be personal factors such as having well-defined targets/personal development plans (personal interest in MAS, application for a post that involves MAS) or external factors such as work load, free time, simulator placement, protected teaching time and mandatory training sessions/tests. In a systematic review on voluntary participation attitudes of trainees, the biggest reported obstacle was lack of

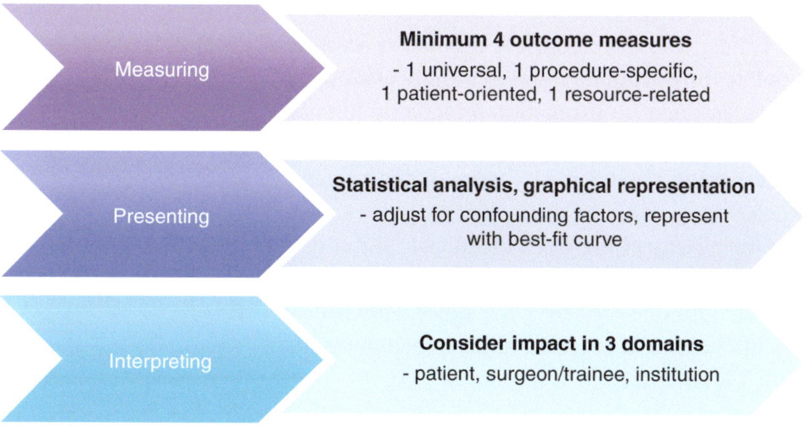

Fig. 8.5 Framework for reporting learning curves in pediatric minimal access surgery

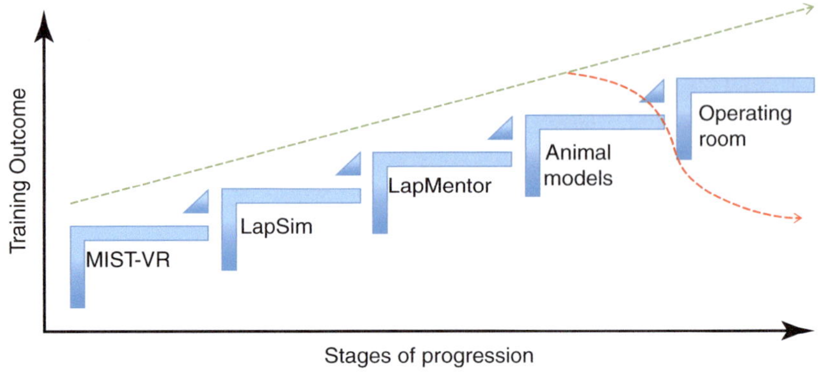

Fig. 8.6 Training outcome improvement (green dotted line) can be best achieved in the following sequential order of skill development. However, if there is a long time lag between any of the animal model and operating room, training outcomes decrease (red dotted line)

free time. Protected teaching time or mandatory participation might be the only way to ensure effectiveness of a training program.

The ideal combination of teaching methods (simulation/reality) that yields maximum training might be difficult to achieve. The relationship between fidelity and training effectiveness is not clear. A hypothetical model (Fig. 8.6) [14] traces such a line where its authors argue that training is best with effective (forced) feedback in simulators but may actually decrease owning to the stresses of real-life operating [15].

In the apprenticeship model of surgical education, there are fewer opportunities for deliberate practice. This is where simulation plays a vital role. It is important to realise that simulators can go beyond the laboratory and skill training in evaluating surgical performance as a whole.

Live models are very realistic, with comparable anatomy, and provide an opportunity to mirror real-life intraoperative complications. They are of course expensive and are restricted by ethical protocols, and they require technical input from anaesthetists.

Trainers often feel that VR simulators are very suitable for teaching. However a study evaluating trainee attitudes to simulation found a preference for live animal models over VR tools. The former were especially favoured by more senior trainees. Respondents deplored the lack of graphic realism and the quality of the forced feedback. Initially it was thought that there was no robust evidence that favours one tool over the other. However a Cochrane review reported slightly better results with VR compared to box training [15].

Regardless of the tools, short bursts/blocks of varied intensity and difficulty over a long period of weeks and months coupled with didactic and operating room experience appear to yield the best results.

Conflict of Interest None.

References

1. Paas F, Renkl A, Sweller J. Cognitive load theory and instructional design: recent developments. Educ Psychol. 2003;38:1–4.
2. Spruit EN, Kleijweg L, Band GPH, Hamming JF. Varied practice in laparoscopy training: beneficial learning stimulation or cognitive overload? Front Psychol. 2016;7:685.
3. Reznick RK, MacRae H. Teaching surgical skills changes in the wind. N Engl J Med. 2008;256:2664–9.
4. Ericsson KA. Deliberate practice and the acquisition and maintenance of expert performance in medicine and related domains. Acad Med. 2004;2004:S70–81.
5. Alvand A, Auplish S, Gill HS, Rees JL. Innate arthroscopic skills in medical students and variation in learning curves. J Bone Joint Surg Am. 2010;93-A:e1151–9.
6. CMO. 150 years of the annual report of the chief medical officer on the state of public health 2008. 2009. http://www.dh.gov.uk/en/Publicationsandstatistics/Publications/AnnualReports/DH_096206. Last accessed 10.05.18.
7. Sanchez-Margallo J, Sanchez-Margallo F, Oropesa I, Gomez E. Systems and technologies for objective evaluation of technical skills in laparoscopic surgery. Minim Invasive Ther Allied Technol. 2014;23:40–51.
8. Gallagher AG, Ritter EM, Satava RM. Fundamental principles of validation, and reliability: rigorous science for the assessment of surgical education and training. Surg Endosc. 2003;17:1525–9.

9. Oropesa I, Lamata P, Sanchez Gonzaled P, Pagador J, et al. Virtual reality simulators for objective evaluation on laparoscopic surgery: current trends and benefits. In: Kim J-J, editor. Virtual reality. IntechOpen; 2011. p. 349–74.
10. Esposito C, Escolino M, Saxena A, Montupet P, Chiarenza F, De Agustin J, Draghici IM, Cerulo M, Sagaon MM, Di Benedetto V, Gamba P, Settimi A, Najmaldin A. European Society of Pediatric Endoscopic Surgeons (ESPES) guidelines for training program in pediatric minimally invasive surgery. Pediatr Surg Int. 2015;31:367–73.
11. Harrysson IJ, Cook J, Sirimanna P, Feldman LS, Darzi A, Aggarwal R. Systematic review of learning curves for minimally invasive abdominal surgery. Ann Surg. 2014;260:37–45.
12. Macdonald A, Haddad M, Clarke S. Learning curves in pediatric minimally invasive surgery: a systematic review of the literature and a framework for reporting. J Laparoendosc Adv Surg Tech A. 2016;26:652–9.
13. Palter VN, Grantcharov TP. Development and validation of a comprehensive curriculum to teach an advanced minimally invasive procedure: a randomized controlled trial. Ann Surg. 2012;256:25–32.
14. Lamata P, Gómez EJ, Bello F, Kneebone RL, Aggarwal R, Lamata F. Conceptual framework for laparoscopic VR simulators. IEEE Comput Graph Appl. 2006;26:69–79.
15. Nagendran M, Gurusamy KS, Aggarwal R, Loizidou M, Davidson BR. Virtual reality training for surgical trainees in laparoscopic surgery. Cochrane Database Syst Rev. 2013;(8):CD006575.

Medicolegal Aspects in Pediatric Minimally Invasive Surgery

9

Isabela Drăghici and Liviu Drăghici

9.1 Introduction

In recent years, a special aspect of medicine called "medicolegal aspects" has emerged and surprisingly developed. In pediatric surgery, this branch is more sensitive because of the patient whose life expectancy must be as close as 100%. No one will ever come to terms with the idea that for a child no matter how sick he is, "nothing can be done."

We wanted to look at this delicate medical side with totally and totally special features, given the age of the patient. How should the problem be asked? How can the doctor or all the medical staff prove that he has done everything he/she has to do about the case? How can a guy who is judged by a forum that is not only a doctor can be blamed, both morally and physically? How can parents accept that the doctor has no fault? How can medical error be quantified? How can you share it on different degrees? Countless questions we will try to find answers to.

I. Drăghici (✉)
University of Medicine and Pharmacy "Carol Davila", Bucharest, Romania

Pediatric Surgery Department, Emergency Hospital for Children "Maria Sklodowska Curie", Bucharest, Romania

L. Drăghici
University of Medicine and Pharmacy "Carol Davila", Bucharest, Romania

9.2 Discussions

The medical profession is considered to be one of the noblest professions in the world. The practice of medicine is capable of rendering noble service to humanity provided due care, sincerity, efficiency, and professional skill are observed by the doctors. However, today, the patient-doctor relationship has almost diminished its fiduciary character and has become more formal and structured. Doctors are no longer regarded as infallible and beyond questioning. Corporatization of healthcare has made it like any other business, and the medical profession is increasingly being guided by the profit motive rather than that of service. On the other hand, a well-publicized malpractice case can ruin the doctor's career and practice. The law, like medicine, is an inexact science. One cannot predict with certainty an outcome of cases many a time. It depends on the particular facts and circumstances of the case and also the personal notions of the judge concerned who is hearing the case. The axiom "you learn from your mistakes" is too little honored in healthcare. The best way to handle medicolegal issues is by preventing them [1].

Several years ago, a completely unknown profession until that time, the patient's rights defender, came into being. He has legal training, but he specializes in medical aspect, he is trained in this respect, and he knows the medical and surgical diseases. Thus, a new concept appeared,

C. Esposito et al. (eds.), *ESPES Manual of Pediatric Minimally Invasive Surgery*,
https://doi.org/10.1007/978-3-030-00964-9_9

malpraxis. This concept is very comprehensive, includes both medical and legal aspects, and involves both the doctor and the patient, as well as his lawyer.

We try to enumerate the preventive measures in safeguarding the doctor against negligence suit.

The potential for medical malpractice claims is one of the most troubling and frustrating situations. The physician is often unknowledgeable and poorly prepared for these events, with little emphasis on this aspect of medicine in either medical school or residency training [2].

Medical profession has its own ethical parameters and code of conduct. However, negligence by doctors has to be determined by judges who are not trained in medical science. They rely on experts' opinion and decide on the basis of basic principles of reasonableness and prudence [1].

The level of negligence depends on the entire context—which includes the place, the time, the individuals involved, and the level of complications. The difference between medical negligence and medical error is well-settled, and the principles are well-founded being clearly laid down in numerous cases by the Supreme Court [1, 3].

There are countless reasons why a patient or, in the case of pediatric surgery, a doctor thinks that he or she has the right to claim a blame or medical negligence in his/her own opinion.

Patients sue because of a feeling that they were not heard, that their needs were not attended to, and that nobody seemed to care, and as a result, a bad outcome resulted due to a mistake or negligence [1, 4].

It is very important that the doctor maintains a better communication with both the patient and his or her patients. A patient (depending on his or her age and degree of understanding) or a patient has the right to be informed about what is happening to the person in question. The physician must have a more open relationship with the parents and the patient. Regardless of the evolution of the case, parents will have much more understanding and respect for their physician if they have developed a professional relationship based on trust. If the doctor keeps a misunderstanding distance with the patient and his/her family and does not create some bridges between the two parties, there will always be a dose of distrust of the family in the that will generate suspicions, perhaps unintelligible.

It is important to let the patient and their caregivers to know that as a treating doctor, their problems are understood [5]. It is a good practice to maintain eye contact while addressing the patient and put a comforting hand on the individual's arm (comforting touch) [1].

Communicate clearly and effectively. Take time to ensure your patient understands their diagnosis, treatment, and medication plans, and then check their understanding by asking them to explain it back. This ensures instructions are properly followed and demonstrates your care toward patient [1, 6].

It is also very important for the doctor to spend a good time with the patient and his/her family, explaining how best to understand all the diagnosis and treatment. The more the doctor spends more time communicating and empathizing with the family, the more the risk of being sued or sued.

The longer the quality time a physician spends with the patient, the less likely will that physician be sued [7].

A big gain in the doctor's favor is the creation and dissection of a set of *clinical guidelines*. These are the fruit of the experience of many specialists and many years of experience and define a kind of "law" in the field of that specialty. They must be strictly observed, and their application should lead to the best result for the given case. Complying with these guides should cover the law with the doctor if he is held accountable for a possible medical fault.

Adherence to clinical guidelines is an effective way to improve quality care and reduce variation in care. Clinical guidelines have been systematically developed nationally and globally to assist clinical decision-making (practice of evidence-based medicine). In medical negligence claims and in court, these guidelines may act as a source of information, provided they are the product of a recognized body and are deemed reliable [8]. They can be seen as normative standards and are used as explicit standards of care at the time of the index clinical event and also to assess the degree to which a questionable practice was in line with accepted standards [9].

Clinical guidelines are also based on specialist literature.

It is very important that everything that happens with the patient is recorded in the observation sheet. The doctor cannot and does not have to rely exclusively on memory, especially when the event took place long before a complaint was filed.

Regardless of the system used, the purpose of documentation, from a legal perspective, is always to accurately and completely record the care given to patients, as well as their response to that care. Documentation has legal credibility when it is contemporaneous, accurate, truthful, and appropriate [10].

Although the ethical obligation of providing the relevant information to patients is not new, the legal concept of informed consent is a development over the past century. "Every human being of adult years and sound mind has a right to determine what shall be done with his own body; and a surgeon who performs an operation without his patient's consent commits an insult for which he is liable in damages" [11].

For laparoscopic or open surgery, the physician needs to obtain informed consent from the patient. Because in pediatric surgery, the patient has not yet reached the age of 18, this consent should be given by one of the parents or, in case of unavailability, by a legal guardian.

Informed consent means that the patient's family specifically consents to the proposed medical procedure. Informed consent is more than just consent. For a patient to give informed consent to a medical procedure, the healthcare provider must inform the patient's family about all of the risks and complications that may reasonably occur during that procedure, however, minor they may be. Furthermore, the treating doctor should mention about alternative treatments available and what happens if no treatment is done. Only after a patient's family is truly informed about the potential risks of a medical procedure can a patient give informed consent to the procedure [1, 12].

A legal duty exists in the patient-doctor relationship and is established when the surgeon undertakes an operation on a patient. The adoption of new technology and surgical techniques will be inevitably associated with a learning curve and a potential for increase in complications [2].

McLean found that despite increased formal training during residency, the nature of injuries leading to malpractice litigation after laparoscopic cholecystectomy changed very little over time with persistence of bile duct (70%), bowel (10%), and vascular (10%) injuries [2, 13, 14]. It is important to note that over 80% of injures were missed and few cases (15%) were converted to open procedures. Other international reviews of malpractice cases in laparoscopic cholecystectomy also stress the importance of (1) early identification of injury and (2) conversion when appropriate [15, 16]. What is also clear is the fact that the introduction of laparoscopic cholecystectomy resulted in an increase of a previously uncommon complication, bile duct injury, but that nearly 25 years of experience has not further reduced this rate much below 1 in 200 cases (0.1–0.5%) [17].

For laparoscopic and robotic operations, explicit mention should be made of injury to blood vessels, bowel, bladder, and other organs, as well as the potential need to convert to an open procedure in some cases [2].

The innumerable advantages of the minimally invasive technique versus the classic technique should be clearly explained to the parents when there is a clear indication for the laparoscopic variant. The indication must not be forced. All absolute or relative contraindications that prevent or complicate the application of the mini-invasive technique should be taken into account. Parents must be fully informed of all these aspects that, when they give their written consent, they will do so in full knowledge of the matter.

It is not necessary to minimize, but to explain in detail all the possible complications, incidents and intraoperative accidents that can occur, as well as the ways to solve them.

Despite the smaller incisions visible to the patients, it should be emphasized that minimally invasive surgery still has major risks and that the underlying risks associated with the operation itself remain essentially unchanged when compared with the corresponding open procedure. The minimally invasive approach does not necessarily equate with minimal risk or complications [2].

Patients should be given the opportunity to convert to open surgery as a way to complete the procedure in a safe manner, not as an abandonment or failure of mini-invasive surgical technique.

The potential need for conversion to open procedure exists for any surgeon in all patients, and this fact should not be viewed as a complication nor as a failure [2].

The parents should not consider the coelioscopic procedure as an "experience" done to their child nor to consider that his non-application for objective reasons represents an inferiority of the surgeon.

Also, pediatric surgeons who do not perform laparoscopic techniques should inform parents about this, as well as the possibility for parents to change their doctor if they opt for a mini-invasive procedure.

In 2017, an international study conducted by Prof. Ciro Esposito (Italy) aimed to assess malpractice in pediatric minimally invasive surgery (MIS) and attitudes, prevention strategies, and mechanisms to support surgeons while they are under investigation. An observational, multicentric, questionnaire-based study was conducted. The survey questionnaire was sent via mail, and it comprised four sections. Twenty-four pediatric surgeons (average age 54.6 years), from 13 different countries, participated in this study. The majority had >15 years of experience in MIS. Three (12.5%) surgeons reported a total of five malpractice claims regarding their MIS activity. The reasons for the claims were a post-operative complication in 3/5 (60%) cases, a delayed/failed diagnosis in 1/5 (20%) cases, and the death of the patient in 1/5 (20%) cases. The claims concluded with the absolution of the surgeon in all cases and monetary compensation to the claimant in two (40%) cases. Eleven (45.8%) surgeons were invited as expert counsels in medicolegal actions. Medicolegal aspects have a minimal impact on the MIS activity of pediatric surgeons. In this series, claims concluded with the absolution of the surgeon in all cases, but they had a negative effect on the surgeon's reputation and finances. A key element in supporting surgeons while they are under investigation is always to choose a surgeon who is an expert in pediatric MIS as legal counsel. A constant update on innovations in pediatric MIS and appropriate professional liability insurance may also play a key role in reducing medicolegal consequences [17].

9.3 Conclusions

We must pay close attention to the forensic aspects of minimally invasive pediatric surgery, especially because of the patient whose life expectancy has to be very high. We have to apply the rules published in the clinical guidelines and to explain to the family all the details of both diagnosis and treatment and also the prognosis of the child's illness.

References

1. Raveesh BN, Nayak RB, Kumbar SF, Raveesh BN. Preventing medico-legal issues in clinical practice. Ann Indian Acad Neurol. 2016;19(Suppl 1):S15–20. https://doi.org/10.4103/0972-2327.192886. PMCID: PMC5109754, PMID: 27891020.
2. Meng MV, Hsieh MH. Medicolegal aspects of minimally invasive urologic surgery. In: Ghavamian R, editor. Complications of laparoscopic and robotic urologic surgery. New York: © Springer Science + Business Media, LLC; 2010. https://doi.org/10.1007/978-1-60761-676-4_24.
3. Panta LS. Supreme Court of India. Kirplani & Ors. 2009. https://indiankanoon.org/doc/1226604/. Last cited on 14 Sept 2016.
4. Oyebode F. Clinical errors and medical negligence. Med Princ Pract. 2013;22:323–33. [PMC free article] [PubMed].
5. Kreimer S. Six ways physicians can prevent patient injury and avoid lawsuits, medical economics. http://www.medicaleconomics.modernmedicine.com. Last updated on 10 Dec 2013; Last cited on 5 Sept 2016.
6. Hagihara A, Tarumi K. Association between physicians' communicative behaviors and judges' deci-

sions in lawsuits on negligent care. Health Policy. 2007;83:213–22. [PubMed].
7. Hickson GB, Federspiel CF, Pichert JW, Miller CS, Gauld-Jaeger J, Bost P. Patient complaints and malpractice risk. JAMA. 2002;287:2951–7. [PubMed].
8. Hurwitz B. How does evidence based guidance influence determinations of medical negligence? BMJ. 2004;329:1024–8. [PMC free article] [PubMed].
9. Davies J. Clinical guidelines as a tool for legal liability. An international perspective. Med Law. 2009;28:603–13. [PubMed].
10. Flynn M. Medical malpractice—medicolegal perspectives: negligence, standard of care. In: Encyclopedia of forensic and legal medicine. 2nd ed. Sydney: Elsevier; 2016. p. 365–9.
11. Chervenak J, LB MC, Chervenak FA. Surgery without consent or miscommunication? A new look at a landmark legal case. Am J Obstet Gynecol. 2015;212(5):586–90.
12. Rubin EB, Bernat JL. Consent issues in neurology. Neurol Clin. 2010;28:459–73.
13. McLean TR. Risk management observations from litigation involving laparoscopic cholecystectomy. Arch Surg. 2006;141:643–8.
14. Kern KA. Malpractice litigation involving laparoscopic cholecystectomy. Arch Surg. 1997;132:392–8.
15. Kienzle HF. Malpractice in laparoscopic cholecystectomy. Results of cases recently considered by the Expert Commission. Zentralbl Chir. 1999;124:535–41.
16. de Reuver PR, Wind J, Cremers JE, et al. Litigation after laparoscopic cholecystectomy: an evaluation of the Dutch arbitration system for medical malpractice. J Am Coll Surg. 2008;206:328–34.
17. Esposito C, Escolino M, Bailez M, Rothenberg S, Davenport M, Saxena A, Caldamone A, Szavay P, Philippe P, Till H, Montupet P, Holcomb Rd GW. Malpractice in paediatric minimally invasive surgery—a current concept: results of an international survey. Med Sci Law. 2017;57(4):197–204.

10 Multimedia Aspects of Pediatric Minimally Invasive Surgery

Modupeola Diyaolu and Todd A. Ponsky

10.1 Introduction

Prior to the twenty-first century, medical professionals, training residents, and medical students were reliant on textbooks, academic or institutional conferences, and medical journals in order to remain up to date on the latest innovations in medicine. As the amount of information to be learned grew, physicians found themselves with a large amount of knowledge to digest with little time to do it. Eventually, as technology advanced, there was a shift to alternate forms of education which incorporated multimedia to enhance the learning experience. This created a chance for physicians to learn in an interactive, engaging, and hands-on manner and allowed them to remain up to date on current surgical technique, technological advances, and surgical education. In addition, by utilizing social media, physicians were able to network across the globe and share relevant resources. In this chapter, different aspects of multimedia will be discussed as it pertains to the education and continued training of practicing physicians.

10.2 Digital Textbooks

With increasing frequency there has been a transition from paper journals to digital, online journals. Some journals are exclusively available online, and this same process is occurring with textbooks [1]. With devices such as Amazon Kindle and iPads, textbooks can now be available in a compact, inexpensive, and efficient manner. Coran's *Pediatric Surgery*, the *Atlas of Pediatric Surgery*, and Aschcraft's *Pediatric Surgery* have online editions of their textbooks available [1, 2]. With functions such as searching for specific topics or keywords, highlighting, note-taking, audio, and videos, digital textbooks have endless benefits for pediatric surgeons who prefer textbooks as one of their main resources. Having a textbook available digitally allows a faster way to access pathophysiology, anatomy, and current surgical technique.

10.3 Video Libraries

For over 10 years, YouTube has been a one-stop website where individuals can find instructions or video clips to almost any topic. It provides a platform that can be reached worldwide in which

M. Diyaolu
Division of Pediatric Surgery, Akron Children's Hospital, Akron, OH, USA

T. A. Ponsky (✉)
Division of Pediatric Surgery, Akron Children's Hospital, Akron, OH, USA

Division of Pediatric Surgery, Cincinnati Children's Hospital Medical Center, Cincinnati, OH, USA
e-mail: TPonsky@akronchildrens.org

C. Esposito et al. (eds.), *ESPES Manual of Pediatric Minimally Invasive Surgery*,
https://doi.org/10.1007/978-3-030-00964-9_10

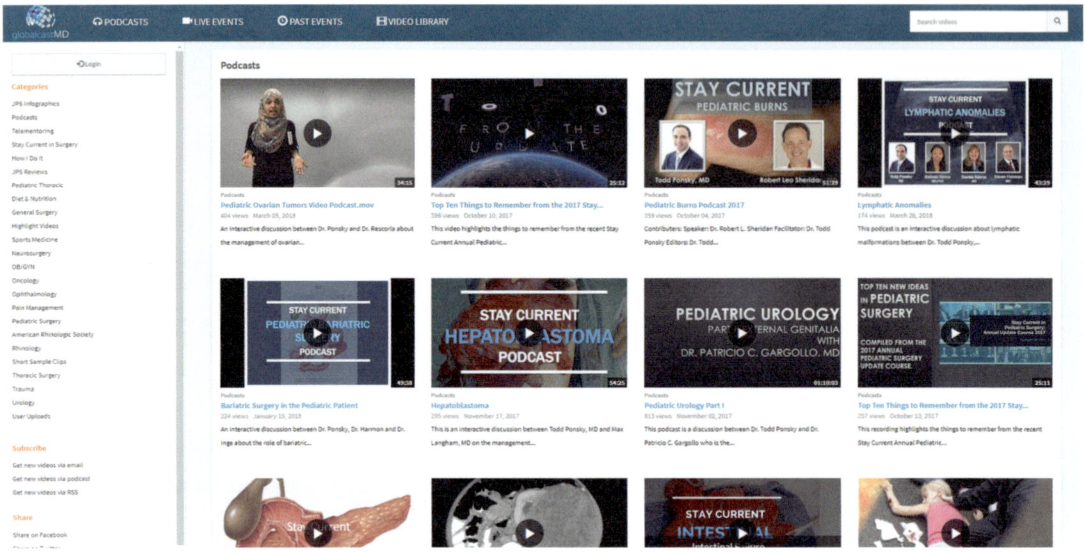

Fig. 10.1 Videos organized by specialty and content

information can be shared and users can create specific channels that cater to particular interests. Individuals within pediatric surgery have created their own versions of video libraries where surgeons can view, learn, and submit videos. For example, the Journal of Laparoendoscopic and Advanced Surgical Techniques has an online video journal called Videoscopy which contains video demonstrations of the latest surgical techniques and technologies. CSurgeries categorizes videos by surgical specialty, association, and vender allowing for an efficient and easy way to find specific surgeries, and Medtube.net offers free e-courses, access to journal articles, and videos of surgical operation.

The authors have developed a video library for pediatric surgeons at the website https://videolibrary.globalcastmd.com. This library contains "How I Do It" surgical technique videos, clips from pediatric surgical conferences, lectures, debates, and pertinent surgery article reviews (Fig. 10.1). This content is free to anyone with the purpose of democratizing pediatric surgical knowledge around the world.

The Hendren Project is another video library that is focused on pediatric surgery. According to their website, The Hendren Project's mission is to "provide sponsor-supported digital resources that enable a global pediatric surgical community to help one another better serve children with complex surgical issues" [3]. They collect and categorize links to high-quality, current research and educational information by expert practicing pediatric surgeons. Some of the content includes conference presentations, content-specific links to major textbooks and journal publications, and links to podcasts and webinars. This project began with videos from Dr. Hardy Hendren's own personal video library.

10.4 Online Resources

The American Pediatric Surgical Association (APSA) has multiple resources for pediatric surgeons to keep up to date and current on literature and education. The Pediatric Surgery Not a Texbook (NaT) is a comprehensive reference for general pediatric surgery that is written by pediatric surgeons [4]. It is updated quarterly and is organized into clinical modules and learning objectives. It also contains high-resolution images, videos, and links to continuing medical education and medical literature. Surgeons are also able to submit feedback, comment on material, and submit interesting cases.

Exam-based Pediatric surgery Educational Reference Tool (ExPERT) is also provided by the APSA. This tool is a continuing medical education program that helps practicing pediatric surgeons review current evidence-based literature and incorporates it into patient care. Members receive two questions weekly to help retain information presented, and there are self-assessments available that cover the core competencies of pediatric surgery. Users are able to create custom courses, but there are also pre-made courses [5].

The Standardized Toolbox for Education for Pediatric Surgery (STEPS) is for pediatric surgeon and senior residents to use for teaching. STEPS was designed by the APSA Education Committee and contains PowerPoint web-based teaching tools organized by modules. Each module starts as a disease-based presentation which is ideal for group interactive learning. They should be used as an adjunct to study [5].

Resources such as UpToDate, AccessSurgery, ClinicalKey, and PubMed are essential to providing current and relevant peer-reviewed journals, review articles, and textbooks [6]. Many institutions provide free access to these websites for employees.

10.5 Social Media

While there are disparities in healthcare, there should not be disparities in knowledge or current advantages in visual technology. Facebook has historically been used for entertainment purposes, but it provides a unique opportunity for physicians to share knowledge. Medical knowledge is exponentially expanding, and the number of pediatric surgery publications is drastically increasing making it very difficult for pediatric surgeons to keep up to date and be aware of the most important publications. It's estimated that by 2020, cumulative knowledge will double every 73 days [4]. Currently, there are 2.5 million studies published each year, and it's becoming increasingly difficult for individuals to know what to read [4]. By using social media, it's possible to highlight critical articles and distribute them to a wider audience. Articles can be summarized in a few key slides, and brief videos can be made that get to the crux of the information. In this form, the information becomes more digestible and easier to assimilate.

The authors have utilized social media to help share the major points and conclusions of the best pediatric surgery articles as they are published. Two social media campaigns were started by the authors, The Journal of Pediatric Surgery and Stay Current in Pediatric Surgery. Given that the social media habits of pediatric surgeons vary widely, multiple channels were used to spread the information such as Facebook, Twitter, YouTube, etc.

The Journal of Pediatric Surgery (JPS) Facebook page was launched in July 2016. Posts include links to newly published Journal of Pediatric Surgery articles, infographics, and video reviews of journal articles. JPS has a YouTube channel that was created in 2016. JPS Reviews contain video reviews of the top articles from the Journal of Pediatric Surgery. To date, the channel has over 160 subscribers. Each video is approximately 2-min long and breaks down journal articles into the essential components, themes, major takeaway points, and possible arguments for or against the article. By subscribing to this channel, notifications can be sent to your smartphone about when new videos are posted keeping up to date on content relatively effortless.

Currently, there are approximately 13,000 followers of the Journal of Pediatric Surgery Facebook Page. There is also a private group of physicians only for surgeons to discuss issues privately. Stay Current in Pediatric Surgery also launched in 2016 and to date has over 1500 members. It aims to provide educational material that's interactive and can be shared with individuals all over the world.

10.6 Mobile Phone Applications

Given that there are multiple styles of learning and limited time for surgeons to read textbooks, the authors designed a mobile application that contains podcast which surgeons can listen to during downtime. Stay Current MD and Stay

Current in Surgery are two free mobile applications by GlobalCast MD which provide podcasts pertaining to medical education. Podcasts are available in a number of different specialties and are led by experts in their respective fields. Unlike most other podcasts which are meant to be listened to from start to finish, these podcasts are reference material. Therefore, the chapters are indexed so the users can choose specifically which subtopic they are curious about and fast forward directly to that spot in the podcast (Fig. 10.2). While some professionals learn by listening, others learn by reading or watching videos. These applications can be used in many different formats to supplement the resources from which pediatric surgeons are reading (Fig. 10.3).

Stay Current in Surgery was released in 2015 and is available for Android and iOS. The new updated version, StayCurrent MD, was released in October 2017 which has a more rich video library consisting of over 700 videos but is only available in iOS at this point in time. Between April 2015 and May 2018, Stay Current in Surgery had over 5700 app units and over 14,000 impressions, while Stay Current MD had 999 app units and 8155 impressions. Currently, there are a total of 29 podcasts for pediatric surgery. There have been over 70,000 podcast listens to date in over 50 countries.

The Stay Current mobile apps have been downloaded in countries such as China, Mexico, and the United Kingdom signaling that the applications have had a very broad reach. Podcasts have the luxury of being readily accessible at any time. Whether you are driving to work or waiting for an appointment, these apps are available for any downtime individuals may have. However, not only surgeons prefer to listen to information. Therefore, each podcast is accompanied by a text manuscript as well. Also, most topics also have associated videos.

10.7 Teleconferencing and Tele-education

Traditionally, physicians would travel to society conferences in order to stay abreast of surgical literature and to get an advanced look into new medical discoveries. While this was a viable option in the past, nowadays the cost of travel as

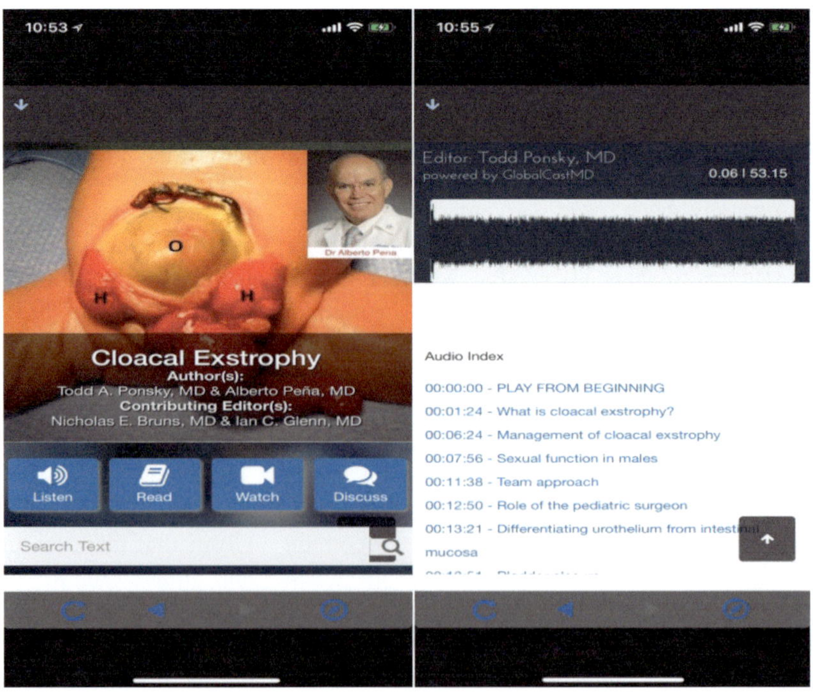

Fig. 10.2 Stay Current in Pediatric Surgery podcast has ability to select which section to listen to of a given chapter

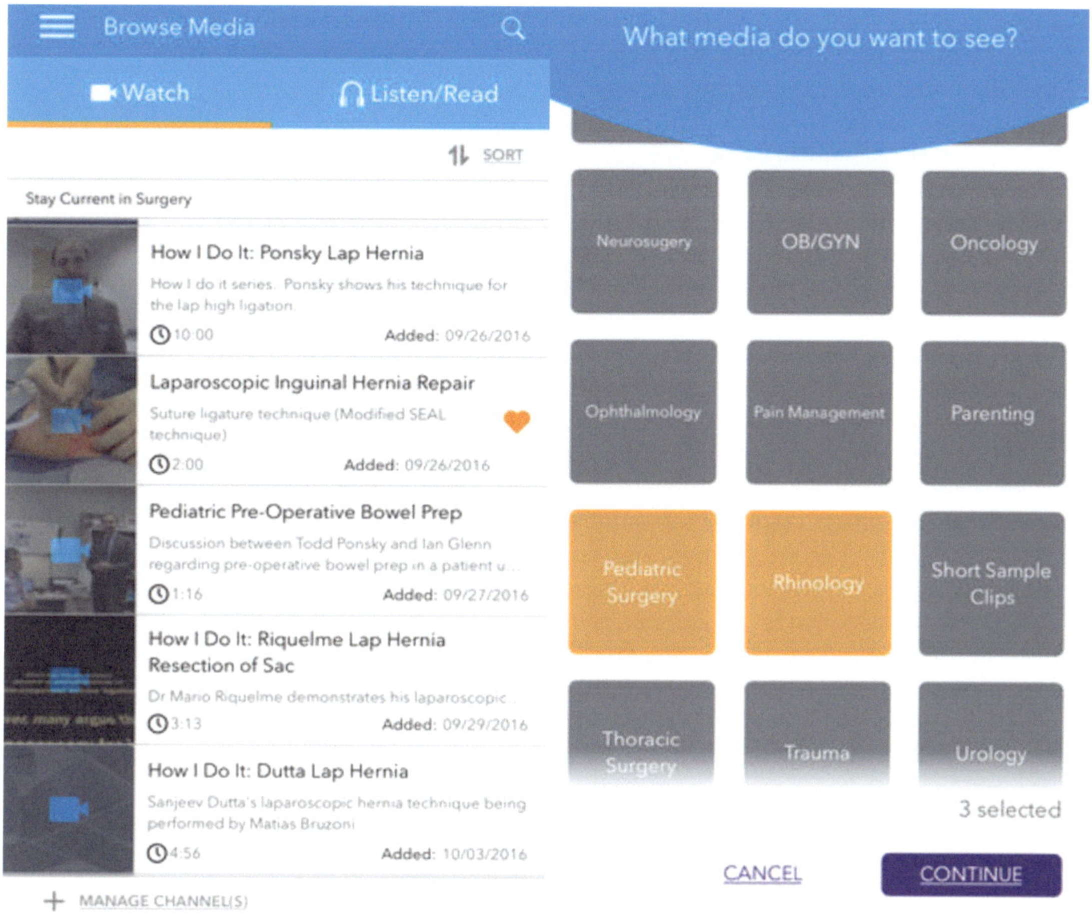

Fig. 10.3 Watch, learn, or read from a variety of different specialties on the Stay Current in Surgery App

well as the time needed to take off from work become barriers to attending conferences. Webinars were a temporary solution to these problems; however, they were akin to being lectured at and were not engaging nor as effective as a live conference. In this day and age of "screen learning," topics must be engaging and stimulating similar to how television and movies operate.

Teleconferencing has been utilized in many different applications such as in multidisciplinary teams like tumor board, inpatient and outpatient consultation, and rural trauma settings. Teleconference allows for practitioners located at different sites to communicate through video and audio. Not only is it relatively inexpensive; individuals find it an acceptable supplement to medical education. From medical students to postgraduates, and across medical fields, teleconferencing has been comparable to having live instruction [6].

In South Africa, at the Division of Paediatric Surgery of University of Cape Town, Dr. Alp Nomanoglu has created a free web weekly conferencing service that also discusses key topics in pediatric surgery via teleconferencing. The hardware uses either ISDN or Internet Protocol (IP), and with increased availability of bandwidth, it's possible to share PowerPoint presentation, operative videos, live web cam images, audio, drawings, instant polls, and drawing boards. Programs such as Adobe Connect®, Web-Ex®, Skype®, and Vidyo® are all tools that can be used to broadcast. As of 2016, approximately 400 sessions have been conducted. A survey conducted revealed that in the past year, 90% of pediatric surgeons had been attending a web meeting, and over 90% of surgeons would be interested in watching surgical videos with experts being able to answer questions immediately [7].

GlobalcastMD is a virtual conference service developed by the authors and provides cutting-edge, live, interactive video conferences on the most pertinent topics in pediatric surgery. These conferences are filmed and broadcast live around the world and are led by experts in the field. The audience is able to participate and interact with the experts by chatting or calling in the phone line with comments or questions. Not only is the audience able to communicate with the presenter and vice versa; they are also able to communicate with each other creating a rich and vibrant dialogue. To keep this content exciting and fast paced, most of these conferences are in the form of case presentations followed by audience polling and then interactive chat and discussions. By holding virtual conferences, you are able to effectively reach a broader audience, bring physicians together making stronger contacts, and keep costs low (Fig. 10.4). These conferences are then available in the video library 1 week after the event. GlobalCastMD events are also archived and discussions can be continued online.

10.8 Telemedicine and Teleconsultation

Telemedicine evolved as a solution for rural or isolated regions to have access to physicians who are more experienced in dealing with complex or challenging medical cases [8–10]. Some formats used are real-time video conferences, mobile or cellular telemedicine, or a combination of both. In 2017, Pandley et al. investigated the use of WhatsApp within the Pediatric Surgery Division of the General Surgery Department at UP Rural Institute of Medical Sciences and Research in India. WhatsApp is a secure messaging, calling, and video calling application that uses Internet connection instead of mobile data. Individuals are able to send pictures, documents, and files through the system. In this study, since a pediatric surgeon was not always in the hospital, a group was created in the app that included radiologists, residents, and consultants. All medical management decisions were made by the pediatric surgeon and were delegating through direct telephone communication. The patient was evaluated by the surgeon the following day. They found that there were no delays in diagnosis or management of patients while using this system [8].

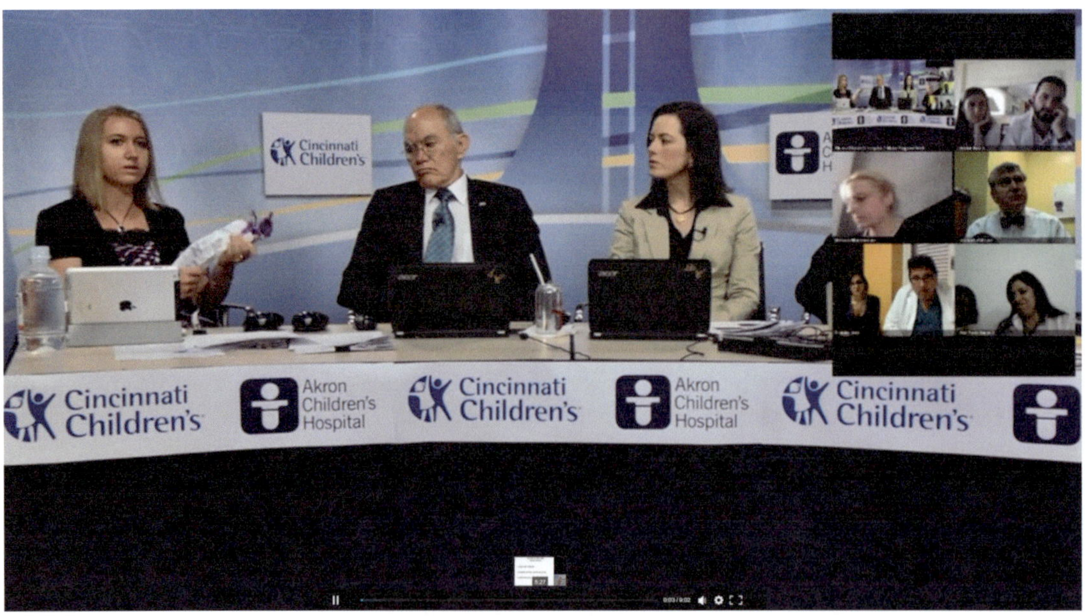

Fig. 10.4 Live discussions with faculty

In the United States, the Medical University of South Carolina designed a pilot program to connect patients in their primary care physician office to subspecialist. Using a software technology, called Jabber, carts composed of a desktop computer, flat screen monitor, and high-definition videoconferencing camera, and patients in rural areas were able to undergo consultations with pediatric surgeons who were located at an academic center [10]. Patients were scheduled during the pediatric surgeon's dedicated clinic time, and a full history was performed as well as a physical exam by a telepresenter (physician, physician extender, or nurse). While telemedicine has the potential to increase access to specialists for patients in rural area, Lesher and Shah noted that physicians need to be specifically licensed to provide telementoring services by the institution which employs them. In addition, the receiving clinic or hospital has to provide credentials to that physician for their services provided. Given how new this technology is, there are no established federal standards. This means that policy is regulated by state laws and medical regulatory commissions. In terms of billing, some states have parity laws that require similar reimbursement rates for professional services provided by telemedicine as an in-person encounter. This is not universal, however, and has the potential to create issues for those providing telemedicine services. Nevertheless, this telemedicine continues to be initiated and used in children's hospitals across the United States.

10.9 Telementoring

As surgical residents, physicians are under the close supervision of an attending. Not only do residents foster a relationship with the attending; they also get consistent and detailed instruction on surgical technique and approach to numerous cases. Once a physician graduates residency, he or she relies on workshops, simulations, animal models, or even in-person proctors to learn new surgical technique. In specialties like pediatric surgery, where some cases are rarely performed, it becomes difficult to become proficient [11–13]. Telementoring has emerged as an excellent resource that provides expert mentoring to physicians. Similar to teleconferencing and telemedicine, telementoring utilizes audiovisual communication to help guide inexperienced physicians through surgical, most often laparoscopic, cases. Mentors are able to see the patient's anatomy, direct where to place instruments and use telestration (drawing on a monitor which both physicians can see), robotic arms, and electrosurgical control to provide visual cues (Fig. 10.5) [6, 11–13].

Ponsky et al. discussed their experiences using the Karl Storz Endoscopy-America, Inc. VisitOR1 telementoring robot to perform a video-assisted left lower lobe resection, placement of temporary gastric stimulator, and laparoscopic inguinal hernia repair between pediatric surgeons at Akron Children's Hospital in Akron, Ohio, and pediatric surgeons, general surgeons, and gastroenterologists at the Rocky Mountain Hospital for Children in Denver, Colorado, and University Hospital Case Medical Center in Cleveland, Ohio [13]. The mentor, an experienced pediatric surgeon who had performed numerous cases, used a laptop that connected directly to the telementoring robot to provide internal and external views of the operation and allowed telestration. The mentees, who had performed 0 or 1 case, sited that the use of the robot was especially helpful with patient setup, trocar placement, and instruction of surgical technique [13]. There are minimal to no adverse effects or complications using telementoring, and it has been shown that it does not increase operative time or complications [11–

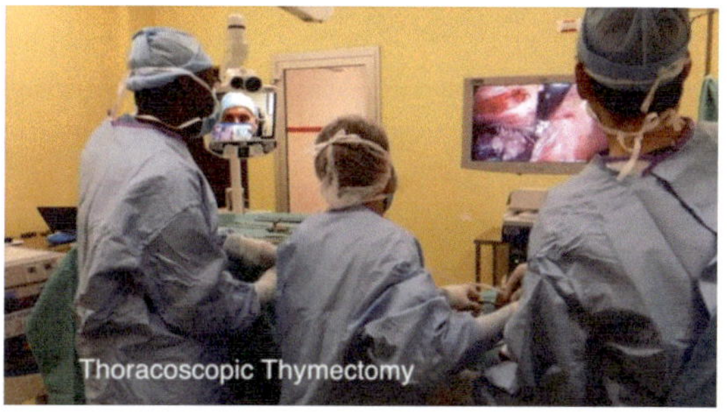

Fig. 10.5 Telementoring from remote location with telementoring robot

13]. Recently, newer, more cost-effective options are becoming available to allow telementoring even between hospitals in developing locations.

Bruns et al. expanded the use of surgical telementoring where pediatric surgeons at Akron Children's Hospital and Rocky Mountain Hospital for Children used telementoring to guide pediatric surgeons in Paris, France, as they performed an interval laparoscopic appendectomy and a thoracoscopic total thymectomy [12]. Similar to the previous study, there was high satisfaction from the telementors and telementees and the use of telestration and laser pointer features on the telementoring robot facilitated the operation. In the case of the appendectomy, the patient had a perforated appendicitis that had been treated with intravenous antibiotics and had developed a pelvic abscess that had been drained, however, had a retained fecalith, prior to the procedure. Telestration was especially beneficial identifying the appendix by pointing out the teniae of the cecum and following it to the base of the appendix. By using the laser pointer and telestration features, the mentor was able to provide tips and tricks to help facilitate the procedure. During the thymectomy, the telementor was able to provide guidance on thoracoscopic technique and helped to identify key anatomic structures.

The use of this technology has obvious advantages in terms of being able to reach and instruct a wide variety of surgeons who in any other circumstances would not have been able to have such a learning experience. With the group of surgeons who would profit the most being rural surgeons, they were surveyed about the possible benefits and applications of surgical telementoring in their practices. The majority of surgeons responded that having surgical telementoring would be useful in their practice and the primary uses would be to learn new techniques or skill sets or help with unexpected intraoperative challenges [14].

Still in its infancy, telementoring is not yet widely known within the patient population. A survey about surgical telementoring was given to patient families in the pediatric surgery and gastroenterology clinic at Akron Children's Hospital after having watched a 1-min video that described telemedicine and surgical telementoring. Out of 129 people, about half would consider telementoring for their child's operation, and 58% would consider it for themselves [15]. The most common objection to surgical telementoring was concern about the operating surgeon's competence. It is suspected that as telementoring becomes commonplace and patients receive more education on the topic that support for this surgical innovation will increase.

Some studies cite the cost of telementoring and the professional relationship between mentor and mentee as some concerns about adopting the practice. The latter is typically resolved with having the mentor and mentee meet or communicate prior to surgery in pretelementoring sessions [11, 13]. In fact, a skill and acquisition model has been created to help practicing physicians learn a new skill. The mentee first undergoes a course or didactic instruction and then observes and assists the export, followed by performing the case with the mentor observing or assisting. Afterward, telementoring is used for cases, which can slowly be escalated from the mentor being in the operating room to the mentor being at a different location. Lastly, via teleproctoring the mentor watches the mentee perform the case (Fig. 10.3). In terms of cost, Akron Children's hospital was able to utilize iPads® (Apple, Cupertino, CA) over a secure connection. The mentor was still able to use the telestrator feature and have a high-definition feed of the operating room camera. Using this solution, they were able to significantly cut down on cost. While obtaining the software, the telementoring robot and the use of equipment can be expensive; this should be weighed against both the acquisition and improvement of surgical skill as well as the traveling cost, time, and expense of flying an expert to an institution for a period of time [13, 14]. In any case, telementoring has proven to be a rapidly evolving field in surgical education.

10.10 Discussion

Within the field of medicine, education does not stop at residency. There are constantly new procedures, surgical techniques, and information that surgeons are required to know in order to continue to practice at a high standard of care. Telemedicine, teleconferencing, and telementoring have allowed surgeons across the world to keep up to date on information within the surgical community. By engaging in interactive virtual conferences, physicians become an active participant in discussions allowing for a more complete experience and assimilation of information.

Social media has also proven to be a powerful resource for not only communicating with peers but also sharing information on a global scale. Between online resources, social media groups and mobile applications like Stay Current MD, physicians are able to tailor the quality and quantity of resources they receive. In addition, with these applications physicians are able to capitalize on their time and focus on relevant and current information within the pediatric surgery field.

References

1. Chung DH, Chen MY. Atlas of pediatric surgical techniques: a volume in the surgical techniques atlas series. 1st ed. Philadelphia: Saunders; 2010.
2. Coran AG, Adzick NS, Krummel TM, Laberge J-M, Shamberger R, Caldamone A. Pediatric surgery. 7th ed. Philadelphia: Saunders; 2012.
3. The Hendron Project. https://www.hendrenproject.org. Accessed 13 May 2018.
4. Glenn IC, Abdulhai S, Ponsky TA. Role of new media for the young pediatric surgeon: fighting exponential knowledge growth with Moore's law. Eur J Pediatr Surg. 2017;27:218–22.
5. The American Pediatric Surgical Association. http://www.eapsa.org/continuing-education/cme-opportunities/. Accessed 13 May 2018.
6. Ponsky TA, Rothenberg SS. Modern, multi-media, advances in surgical information. Semin Pediatr Surg. 2015;24(3):124–9. https://doi.org/10.1053/j.sempedsurg.2015.02.010.
7. Numanoglu A. Using telemedicine to teach paediatric surgery in resource-limited countries. Pediatr Surg Int. 2017;33:471–4.
8. Pandey A, Singh SP, Pandey J, Gupta V, Verma R. Use of WhatsApp in pediatric surgery division of general surgery department: is it worthwhile? J Indian Assoc Pediatr Surg. 2017;22(1):62–3. https://doi.org/10.4103/0971-9261.194632.
9. Martinez R, Rogers AD, Numanoglu A, Rode H. The value of WhatsApp communication in paediatric burn care. Burns. 2018;44(4):947–55. https://doi.org/10.1016/j.burns.2017.11.005.
10. Lesher AP, Shah SR. Telemedicine in the perioperative experience. Semin Pediatr Surg. 2018;27:102–6.
11. Bilgic E, Turkdogan S, Watanabe Y, et al. Effectiveness of telementoring in surgery compared with on-site mentoring: a systematic review. Surg Innov. 2017;24(4):379–85. https://doi.org/10.1177/1553350617708725.
12. Bruns NE, Irtan S, Rothenberg SS, Bogen EM, Kotobi H, Ponsky TA. Trans-Atlantic telementoring with pediatric surgeons: technical considerations and lessons learned. J Laparoendosc Adv Surg Tech A. 2016;26(1):75–8. https://doi.org/10.1089/lap.2015.0131.
13. Ponsky TA, Bobanga ID, Schwachter M, et al. Transcontinental telementoring with pediatric surgeons: proof of concept and technical considerations. J Laparoendosc Adv Surg Tech A. 2014;24(12):892–6. https://doi.org/10.1089/lap.2014.0363.
14. Glenn IC, Bruns NE, Hayek D, Hughes T, Ponsky TA. Rural surgeons would embrace surgical telementoring for help with difficult cases and acquisition of new skills. Surg Endosc Other Interv Tech. 2017;31:1264–8.
15. Abdulhai S, Glenn IC, McNinch NL, Craner D, Chou E, Ponsky TA. Public perception of telemedicine and surgical telementoring in the pediatric population: results of a parental survey. J Laparoendosc Adv Surg Tech A. 2017;28:215–7.

A Short History of the European Society of Paediatric Endoscopic Surgeons (ESPES)

11

Azad Najmaldin, Ciro Esposito, Philippe Montupet, and Henri Steyaert

During the late 1960s, well before their counterparts in adult surgery, Stephen Gans and George Berci anticipated the future of endoscopic surgery (minimal invasive surgery (MIS)) in infants and children would be promising. However, progress in the evolvement of this subspecialty remained slow, partly due to the minimal levels of political and commercial interest this type of surgery attracts in a small speciality like paediatrics. Furthermore, surgery in children encompasses a wide variety of conditions in a wide range of patients of differing age groups and sizes.

With this in mind and sensing safety in numbers, the advantages of a dedicated scientific society brought together many paediatric surgeons from across Europe, who took the initiative to establish their own National Paediatric Endoscopic Surgery groups and societies during the late 1990s. This included Societa Italiana di Videochirurgia Pediatrica (SIVI), Italy; British Association of Paediatric Endoscopic Surgeons (BAPES), the UK; and Groupe d'Etude en Coeliochirurgie Infantile (GECI), French-speaking communities.

At the BAPES fourth Annual Congress in Leeds November 2003, Azad Najmaldin, President, successfully sought permission from the annual general meeting to hold every third BAPES Annual Congresses in a European City outside of the UK. The idea was to create a forum at which European talents, individuals and groups could exchange experiences and develop a collaborative scientific and training relationship. At that meeting, a leading figure of MIS in Europe and one of many BAPES members from outside the UK, Philippe Montupet, volunteered to host the first meeting in Paris the following year. After exchanging countless telephone calls and emails, Azad and Philippe, together with the help and support from BAPES executives and many individuals from all over Europe, arranged a joint meeting between BAPES and GECI in Paris during 24–25 September 2004. This included free paper sessions, hands on laboratory and live operating workshops, as well as a truly pleasurable "Seine" river boat cruise and an annual dinner. The meeting was attended by more than 120 surgeons and trainee surgeons from all over Europe and beyond, as well as leading figures of MIS (Fig. 11.1). BAPES may have lost a sum of 5000 Euros on this occasion, but the Congress certainly succeeded in achieving its scientific and political goals of gathering European paediatric MIS under one roof for the very first time.

A. Najmaldin (✉)
Leeds Teaching Hospitals, Leeds, UK
e-mail: azad.najmaldin@nhs.net

C. Esposito · P. Montupet
Pediatric Surgery Unit, Department of Translational Medical Sciences (DISMET), University of Naples "Federico II", Naples, Italy

CHU Bicetre Paris, Paris, France

H. Steyaert
Department of Pediatric Surgery, Université Libre de Bruxelles (ULB), HUDERF Children's Hospital, Brussels, Belgium

C. Esposito et al. (eds.), *ESPES Manual of Pediatric Minimally Invasive Surgery*,
https://doi.org/10.1007/978-3-030-00964-9_11

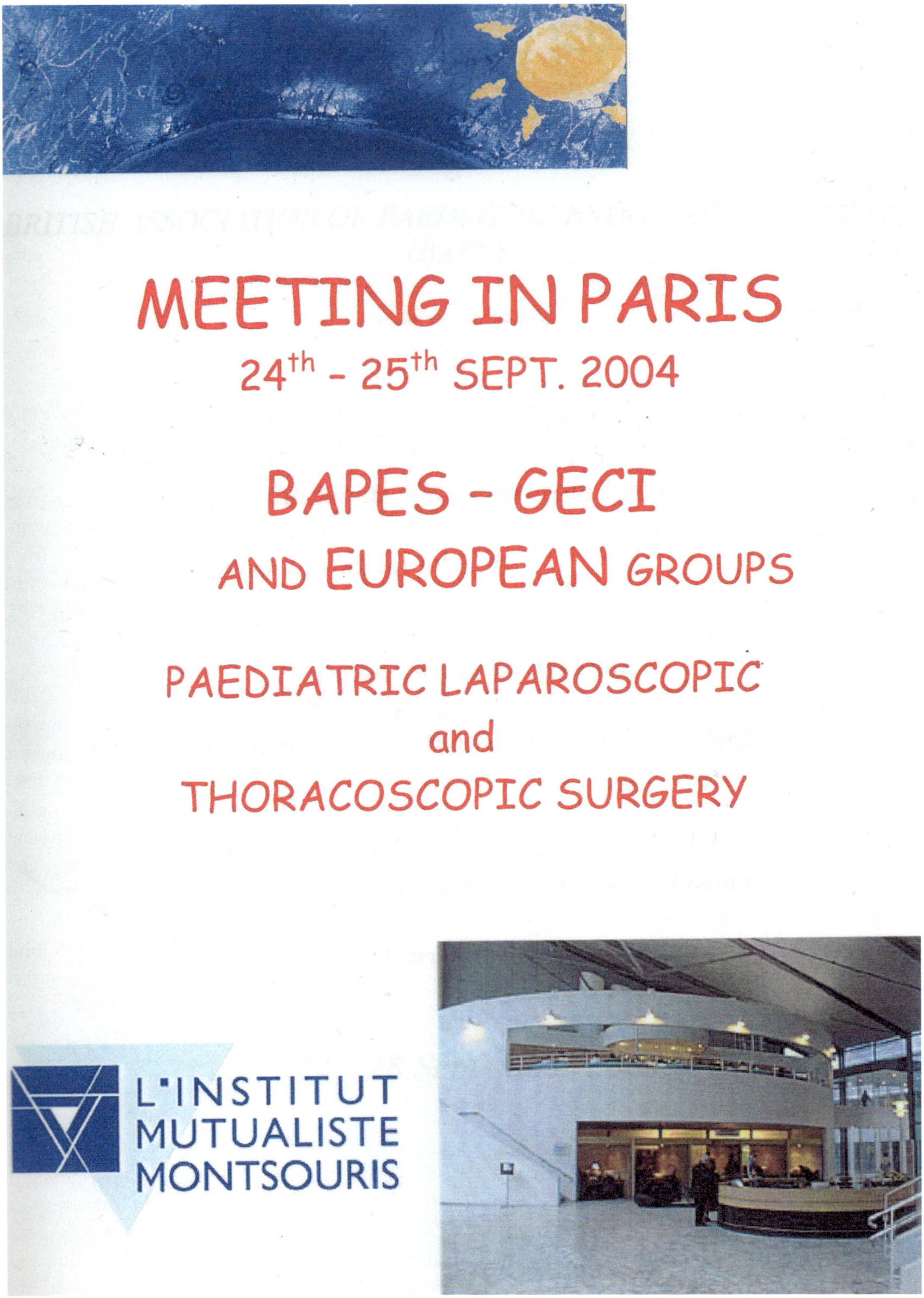

Fig. 11.1 BAPES 1st joint European Congress in Paris, September 2004

Three years later the second European Collaborative Congress and workshop was hosted by Hasan Dogruyol in Istanbul between 7 and 10 Oct 2007 (Fig. 11.2). This joint effort included BAPES, Turkish Association of Paediatric Surgeons and SIVI.

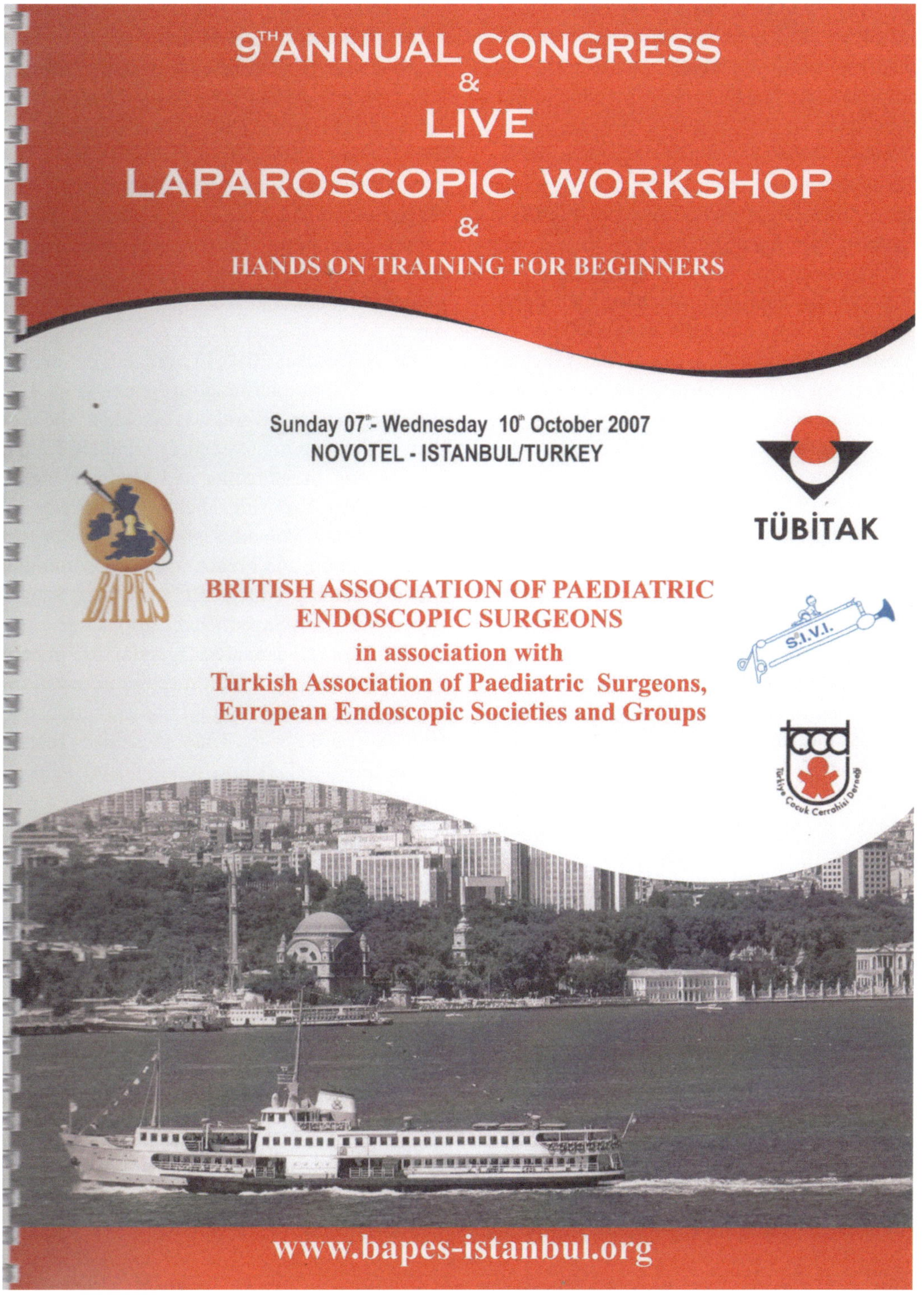

Fig. 11.2 BAPES 2nd Joint European Congress in Istanbul, October 2007

The meeting was attended by more than 200 delegates from Europe and beyond. The workshops were oversubscribed, and the feedbacks from delegates were very positive. On this occasion BAPES shared a small fortune which helped fund future similar efforts. By then plans were already in advanced stages to hold the third European BAPES collaborative meeting in Berne 3 years later.

During IPEG's Annual Congress in Cannes June 2008, Oliver Reinberg and few of his colleagues from GECI invited Azad to address the idea of a pan European society to a French-speaking audience at an informal dinner in a beach restaurant. The political aspects of his reception met little if any enthusiasm; nonetheless the atmosphere stimulated a more than previously serious discussion amongst the French-speaking paediatric endoscopic surgeons.

In July of the same year, once again, Azad took the opportunity and presented his case for a European MIS society to several European small groups and prominent individual surgeons during the British Association of Paediatric Surgeon's Annual Congress in Salamanca, Spain. Whilst many leant their full support and willingness to collaborate, few leading figures refused to support the idea. This was mainly due to the overarching opinion that an independent European paediatric society would inevitably mean there would be less influence for the already functioning non-European or non-paediatric organisations.

By this point, the idea had been widely shared. In early 2010, Azad invited many leading surgeons and representatives of individual national groups and societies to a foundation meeting in Leeds. Whilst the majority agreed to meet, some still refused.

Around the same time, Manuel Lopez, then the President, and Gloria Pelizzo the local organiser of that year's Annual Congress of GECI in Venice invited Azad to address the audience at the Congress. The title of his speech was "The Need for a European Society of minimal invasive surgeons", and the date was 9 October 2010. After months of deliberations, it was agreed to stage the foundation meeting somewhere in or near Venice where GECI's meeting was taking place. Fabio Chiarenza, Ciro Esposito and Luciano Musi volunteered to host the meeting.

At the GECI's meeting, Azad's lecture sparked a great deal of controversy and discussion amongst the delegates, with the clear majority being French-speaking, some Italians and a few other Europeans including British. Many opposed the idea for one reason or another, whilst others remained silent, but few nodded a sign of support. However, GECI's influential figures decided to send several representatives to the planned foundation meeting on the following day.

On 10 October 2010, in a small meeting room in a small suburban hotel in Venice (Fig. 11.3), Azad Najmaldin led and was elected as the chairman of the meeting. Attendees included from the UK, Henrik Steinbrecher and Munther Haddad; Italy, Ciro Esposito, Fabio Chiarenza and Luciano Musi; Poland, Piotr Czanderna; Austria, Amir Haxhida; and French-speaking community, Manuel Lopez, Paul Philippe, Henri Steyaert, Mario Mendoza-Sagaon and Carlos Gine.

With a well-prepared agenda, the meeting attracted hours of heated discussion, often ending in disagreement and a polarised atmosphere from few participants. The topics raised included name, structure, vision, mission and values of the new organisation. Also discussed was the importance of the leadership roles, transparency, research, education and training as well as inclusion of all surgeons from all over Europe and our relationship with other European and international groups and societies. Azad was elected unanimously to lead the group and was given the task of writing the constitution. The group also proposed to plan for the first Congress the following year, jointly with either GECI in Tours or BAPES in London. It was proposed that the second meeting of the "Foundation Group" would take place during the third European BAPES Congress in Berne the following month.

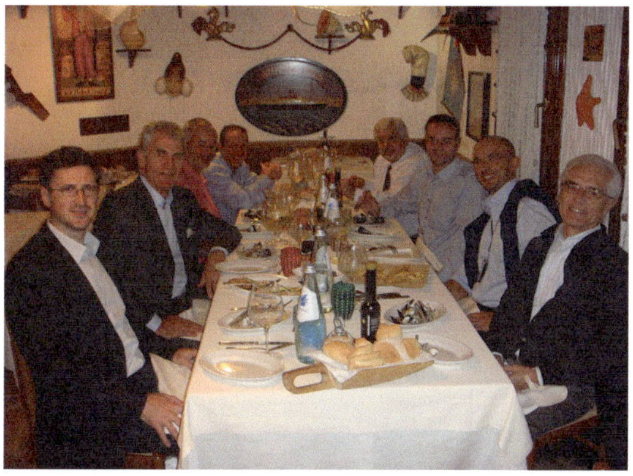

Fig. 11.3 The enthusiasts at the famous dinner on 10 October 2010. From left Amir, Azad, Piotr, Fabio, Munther, Henrik, Ciro, Luciano

Zacharias Zachariou hosted the third Joint BAPES, SIVI, Greek Association of Paediatric Surgeons in Berne on 15–17 Nov 2010 (Fig. 11.4). This again turned out to be a truly successful, inclusive and pleasurable Congress with a full scientific programme, live operating workshop and a fantastic social programme. In between the busy hours of the Congress, official and unofficial discussions relating to the creation of the new European Society took place between the enthusiasts mainly from the UK and Italy led by Azad and Ciro.

The following months, further intensive negotiations driven by Azad led to the foundation of the new society (Fig. 11.5).

- Name: European Society of Paediatric Endoscopic Surgeons (ESPES).
- The first (Inaugural) Congress was planned to be held jointly with BAPES in London.
- ESPES logo was prepared by Ciro.
- Henrick Steinecker on behalf of BAPES agreed to host the "Inaugural Congress" at no cost.
- Ciro and Fabio on behalf of SIVI agreed to underwrite any loses if needed to the tune of 3500 Eu.
- A website was initiated by Ciro first and was later refined and run by Juan de Agustin.
- A bank account was set up by Zacharias in Switzerland.

ESPES Inaugural (First) Congress took place as a joint meeting with BAPES between 2 and 5 November 2011 at Chelsea Football Club, London (Fig. 11.6). The sessions included fantastic key note lectures by eminent speakers, round table discussions with experts, free papers and posters and prizes for the best paper and idea. There were 95 abstract submission, 30% rejected, and the Congress was attended by few hundred delegates from 25 different European and non-European countries.

During the Congress on November 3, the first annual general meeting (assembly) was attended by 51 of 100 members and chaired by Azad. At this meeting aspects of the constitution, structure of the organisation, membership and future relationships were discussed. An executive team was elected for the offices in a friendly and democratic atmosphere. Azad Najmaldin was nominated and elected as the first President. Other executives were nominated and elected including Ciro Esposito Secretary, Amulya Saxena Treasurer, Juan de Augustin Webmaster, Piotr Czauderma Education Officer, Naved Alizai Research and Audit Officer and Fabio Chiarenza Guidelines Executive. The President then nominated special advisors to the society, namely, Philippe Montupet, Munther Hadad, Viladimir Cingel, Mauel Lopez and Zacharias Zachariou.

Within a few months, a comprehensive constitution was written by Azad which was later debated at the second annual meeting in Naples and the subsequent year in Marseille. Soon ESPES became an internationally respected and a major force in the world of Paediatric MIS and new technology. Many have contributed hugely to this success over the years. Some are already identified by name within this short article,

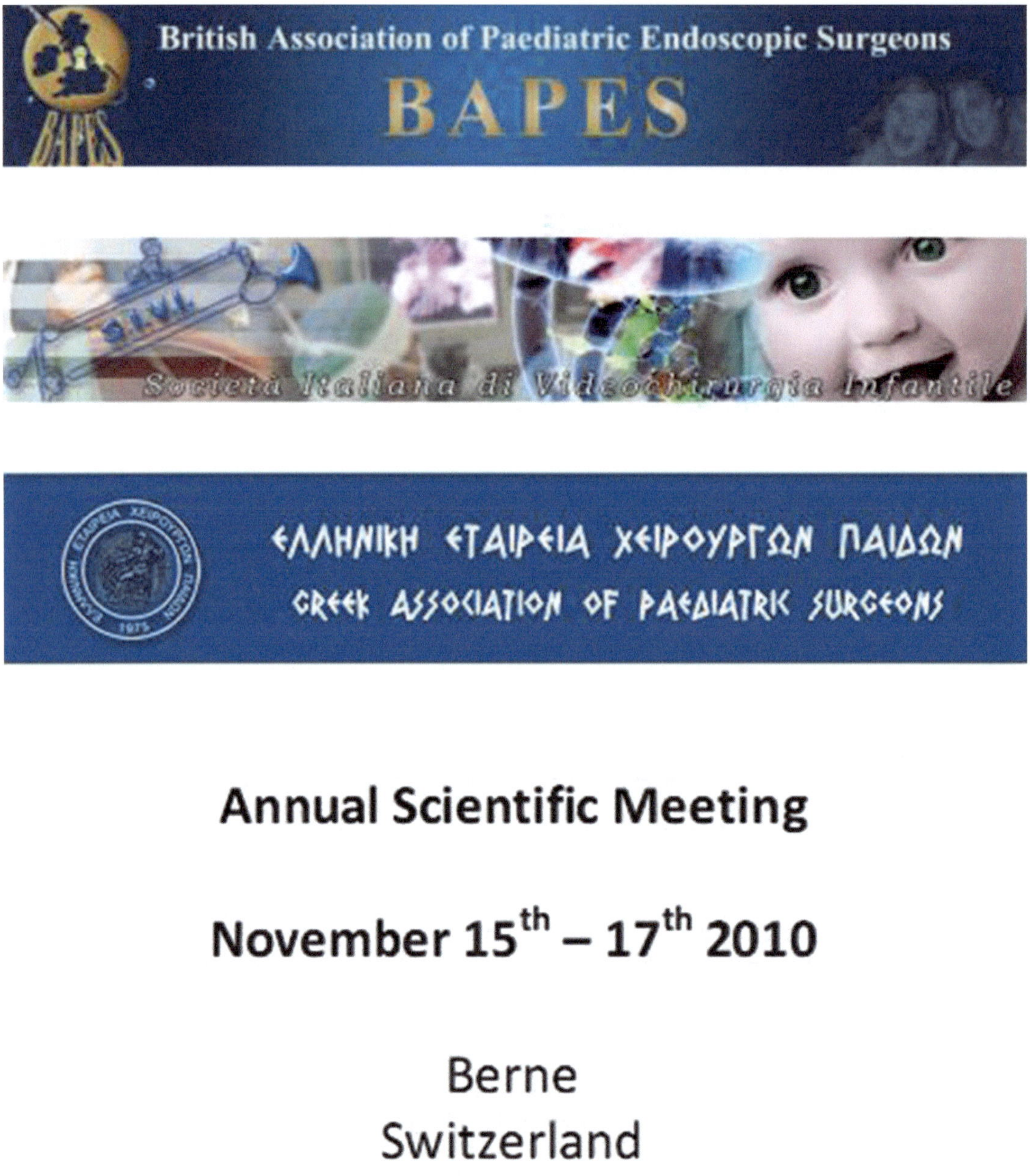

Fig. 11.4 BAPES third joint European Congress in Berne, November 2010

whilst others will undoubtedly have their names included in future communications.

The second ESPES Congress was held in Naples in 2012 (Fig. 11.7). This was a major event during the maturity of the society, setting the momentum for the future of ESPES. Much credit went to the lead local organiser, Ciro. The third Annual Congress was held in Marseille (2013), fourth Bratislava (2014), fifth Bucharest (2015), sixth Madrid (2016) and seventh Wroclaw (2017). The meetings were all equally as successful and well attended, and by 2017 the society's membership exceeded 500 marks. We are now preparing for this year's congress in Brussels which I am confident will be of a high standard.

European Society of Paediatric Endoscopic Surgeons

European Society of Paediatric Endoscopic Surgeons

Founding Members:

Juan de Agustin

Fabio Chiarenza

Vladimir Cingel

Piotr Czauderna

Hasan Dogruyol

Ciro Esposito

Stefan Gfrorer

Carlos Gine

Munther Haddad

Emir Haxhija

Manuel Lopez

Mario Mendozasgaon

Luciano Musi

Azad Najmaldin

Marcel Oancea

Dariusz Patkowski

Amulya Saxena

Hans Skari

Henrik Steinbrecher

Zacharias Zachariou

It is a pleasure to introduce you all to the – *European Society of Paediatric Endoscopic surgeon* **"ESPES", our new society** which promises to be an outstanding scientific and educational organisation for all paediatric surgeons, trainee doctors as well as allied specialists and nurses who may have an interest in paediatric minimal invasive procedures and advances of technology throughout Europe.

Many of you remember our previous pan European collaborative efforts involving BAPES, GECI, SIVI and TAPS, as well as other small groups and individuals from other European countries – first in Paris 2004, then Istanbul 2007 and last Berne 2010. These successful meetings prompted us to think of alternative ways of joining our efforts to deal with the ever-increasing new challenges on the European stage.

In Europe, important matters, such as health care system, patients' rights, employment, education and training, and financing research are becoming increasingly integrated, bringing about a host of new challenges on a regular basis to all and we the paediatric minimal invasive surgeons are not an exception. No single organisation can possibly look after your interest as well as an independent and dedicated society can, one-that is created and led by you.

We are conscious of the fact that you all are busy professionals, and there are more than enough number of societies and meetings about. At the same time, we are aware of too many national and small groups in Europe that are replicating much too much hard work towards the same goal on a regular basis, and this is becoming hard to sustain.

This new society shall involve all Europeans old and young on merit and on a rotational basis. We shall not compete, but instead respect, complement and work closely with all European national, European international and global professional groups and societies which bear similar objectives to ours – ESPES.

Our aims are:

- To foster the development of new technology, endoscopy and minimal invasive techniques across Europe.
- To promote scientific and clinical research.
- To promote and maintain high standards of paediatric minimal invasive therapy across Europe.
- To involve all Europeans at all levels of activities and assist in advancing new and young talents.
- To interact closely with European and international surgical, medical and scientific bodies, and industries.
- To establish an interactive web-platform.
- To organise and support scientific meetings and training courses across Europe at affordable costs.

We already have a constitution in place and a logo, and a website is in the process of being built www.espes.org / www.espes.org.es. The London Inaugural Meeting (joint ESPES/BAPES) was a success. This year's meeting will take place in Naples – September 2012. If any one of you wishes to play an active role or contribute one way or another, please get in touch.

ESPES is yours and waiting your involvements and leadership.

Azad Najmaldin
President

azad.najmaldin@leedsth.nhs.uk parmjit.jajuha@leedsth.nhs.uk msavio@unina.it **www.espes.org**

Fig. 11.5 Letter from Azad Najmaldin to all European Paediatric Surgeons

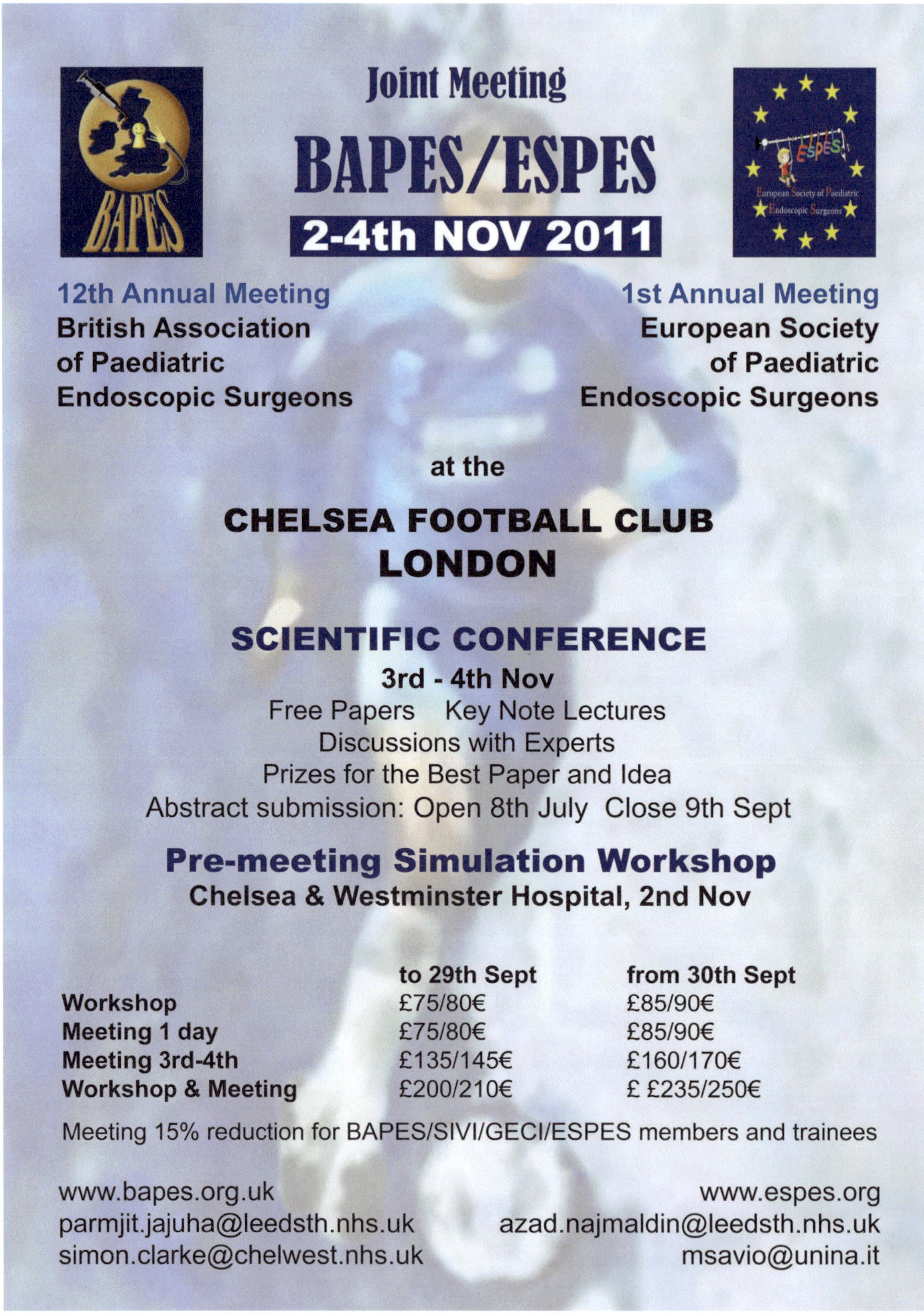

Fig. 11.6 ESPES Inaugural (first) Congress held jointly with BAPES in London, November 2011

During the 2014 Bratislava meeting, the well-known leader of MIS in Europe, Philippe Montupet, became the second President who ushered in many new changes to the life of ESPES (Fig. 11.8). Two years later another well-recognised European leading MIS trainer Ciro Esposito, famously known as Azad's right hand man, was elected President at the Madrid Congress. Current President Henri Steyaert was elected at Wroclaw.

Being a technology-centred organisation, there will always be a future for ESPES. It's current and future success is in the hands of dedicated members, particularly the new generation of paediatric surgeons.

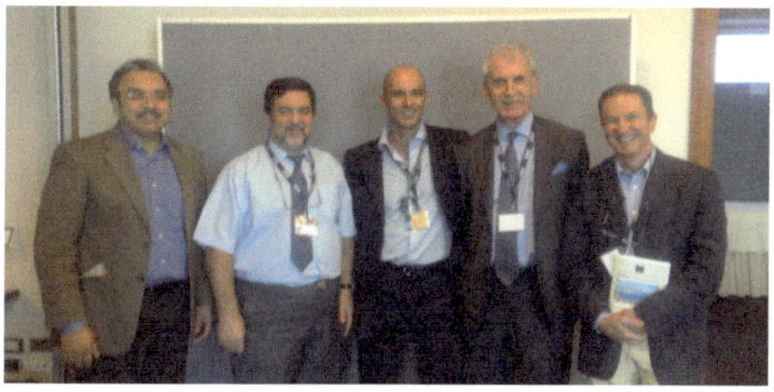

Fig. 11.7 ESPES second Annual Meeting Naples, Italy

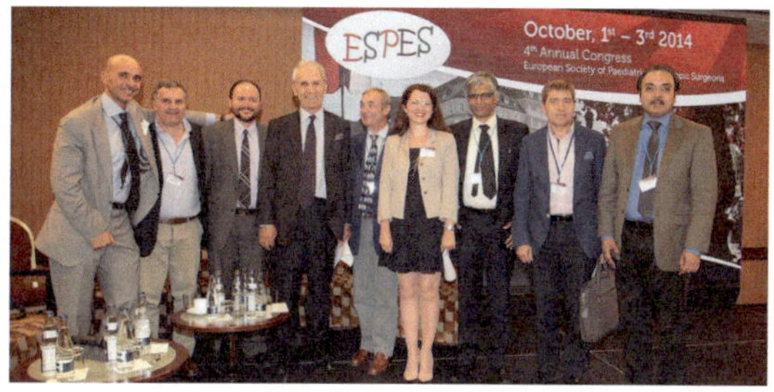

Fig. 11.8 ESPES Executive Board at ESPES Bratislava Annual Meeting

12 Anesthesia in Pediatric Minimally Invasive Surgery

Giuseppe Cortese, Costanza Tognon, Giuseppe Servillo, and Piergiorgio Gamba

12.1 Introduction

Minimally invasive surgery (MIS) may be selected for its speed, efficacy, and security. A minimally invasive approach improves surgical times, reduces the postoperative course, and guarantees a less traumatic recovery for a young patient. The continuing developments in pediatric minimally invasive surgery represent a great challenge for anesthesiologists, who must have the necessary competence to cope with relatively new surgical situations [1]. The pneumoperitoneum produces important changes in cardiovascular and respiratory balance that must be recognized and managed. In addition, pediatric video-assisted thoracoscopic surgery has major physiological derangements that must be understood to correctly perform a procedure; technical skills and familiarity with airway control and single lung ventilation are also required [2]. This chapter focuses on these issues in the pediatric patient, especially in infants and small children whose reactions to thoracic and laparoscopic surgery are unique.

G. Cortese (✉) · G. Servillo
Departments of Nephrology, Urology, General Surgery, Kidney Transplantation, Anesthesia, and Intensive Care, Azienda Ospedaliera, University of Naples "Federico II", Naples, Italy

C. Tognon (✉)
Department of Anesthesia, Azienda Ospedaliera, University of Padua, Padua, Italy

Department of Woman's and Child's Health, Azienda Ospedaliera, University of Padua, Padua, Italy
e-mail: costanza.tognon@aopd.veneto.it

P. Gamba (✉)
Pediatric Surgery, Department of Woman's and Child's Health, Azienda Ospedaliera, University of Padua, Padua, Italy
e-mail: piergiorgio.gamba@unipd.it; piergiorgio.gamba@aopd.veneto.it

12.2 Laparoscopy

12.2.1 Introduction

In recent years, there has been an increasing interest in the use of MIS. Laparoscopic and robotic approaches have become the standard of care for many surgical procedures. MIS offers several potential benefits, including the avoidance of large incisions, less perioperative pain, earlier postoperative mobilization, shorter postoperative ileus, and better cosmetic results. The anesthesiology management of pediatric patients in this operative setting is a new challenge for the anesthesiologist. Any benefits of laparoscopic surgery involve exposing the patient to physiological changes. The changes in normal cardiorespiratory and metabolic physiology represent a potential problem. Minimally invasive surgery does not mean minimally invasive anesthesia.

Laparoscopy requires the formation of a working area in the peritoneal cavity by the insufflation

C. Esposito et al. (eds.), *ESPES Manual of Pediatric Minimally Invasive Surgery*,
https://doi.org/10.1007/978-3-030-00964-9_12

of gas. Insufflated CO_2 is rapidly absorbed across the peritoneum and increases total body CO_2 content, causing changes in many physiological parameters. Insufflation pressure of 4–12 mmHg is typically required for infants [3, 4]. Carbon dioxide is an incombustible and highly soluble gas that can cause excessive absorption, subcutaneous emphysema, intravascular embolization, pneumothorax, and pneumo-mediastinum. Adequate management of surgical access and gas pressure in association with anesthesiology strategies are able to reduce complications.

12.2.2 Physiological Effects of Laparoscopy

12.2.2.1 Respiratory System

The pneumoperitoneum is associated with an abdominal content shove (often in the Trendelenburg position), which determines the cephalad shift of the diaphragm. The total thoracic compliance and functional residual capacity (FRC) decreases and the airway resistance increases (Table 12.1).

A decrease in arterial oxygenation has been reported in adult populations undergoing gynecological surgery [5]. A reduction of FRC and atelectasis may produce a ventilation/perfusion mismatch with hypoxemia [3]. End-tidal CO_2 was reported to increase from a baseline value of 33–42 mmHg during surgery if the ventilator settings were not adjusted [6]. To restore end-tidal CO_2 to baseline levels, an increase of the ventilator rate over 30–60% is necessary [7]. More than 90% of infants required at least one intervention to the ventilator pattern to restore tidal volume and end-tidal CO_2 [8].

Rarely, respiratory changes negatively affect postoperative respiratory functional outcomes. Respiratory acidosis may occur in cases of poor preoperative respiratory function, or residual drugs may depress pulmonary drive.

12.2.2.2 Cardiovascular System

Cardiovascular changes may be caused by the pneumoperitoneum, the absorption of carbon dioxide, and a blood volume shift by positioning.

Several studies have evaluated cardiovascular changes using echocardiography during laparoscopic surgery. The cardiac index decreases by 13% when the intra-abdominal pressure value reaches 12 mmHg [9]. Studies have reported an increase in mean arterial pressure (MAP), vascular resistance (SVR), and central venous pressure (CVP) with a decrease of stroke volume (SV) (Table 12.2).

An increase of intra-abdominal pressure (IAP) induces a neuroendocrine response with the spread of catecholamine and the activation of the angiotensin system. The result is an increase of MAP and SVR [10].

12.2.2.3 Fluid Balance

Plasma renin and aldosterone increase over baseline values; these changes are similar to those in open surgery [11]. Decreased renal plasma flow and glomerular filtration pressure may produce

Table 12.1 Respiratory system changes during laparoscopy

Parameters	Change	Causes
FRC	Decrease	Displacement of diaphragm, positioning
PO_2	Decrease	Atelectasis, preoperative respiratory function, hypoxia-induced vasoconstriction
Lung compliance	Decrease	Elevation of diaphragm, increased intraabdominal pressure
PCO_2	Increase	CO_2 absorption

Table 12.2 Cardiovascular system changes during laparoscopy

Parameter	Changes	Causes
SVR MAP	Increase	Hypercapnia, neuroendocrine response
Cardiac rhythm	Bradyarrhythmia or tachyarrhythmia	Peritoneal stretch, vagal reflex, hypoxia, hypercapnia
Cardiac index	Decrease or stable	Increase in afterload, decrease in venous return Positioning, decrease in cardiac filling

a reduction in urine output. These alterations in healthy patients are well compensated. Permanent renal impairment is not evidenced [12].

12.2.2.4 Temperature

Exposure of the peritoneal cavity to a large volume of cold and non-humidified CO_2 may contribute to the development of hypothermia. The effects of hypothermia on the cardiovascular system and the coagulation pattern remains a possibility during lengthy surgeries, especially in neonates.

12.2.2.5 Intracranial Pressure

Cerebral blood flow and intracranial pressure may be increased [13]. A study of adult patients during laparoscopy has shown that significant changes in cerebral oxygenation are uncommon. Another study detected a similar trend in a pediatric population undergoing laparoscopic surgery [13].

12.2.2.6 Peritoneal Morphology

Carbon dioxide has local and systemic effects. A recent study was designed to evaluate the histopathologic changes on the visceral and peritoneal peritoneum in rats during laparoscopy [14]. CO_2 reacts with peritoneal fluid and reduces peritoneal pH, creating an acidic environment that limits the inflammatory response. The level of intra-abdominal pressure and the type of gas chosen produce different degrees of inflammation. Low pressure and CO_2 cause minor changes in the peritoneum compared with high pressure and air insufflation. An increase in inflammatory cells is represented by eosinophils, mastocytes, and lymphocytes. No clinical modifications are known.

12.2.2.7 Intestinal Function

MIS is associated with faster postoperative rehabilitation compared with open surgery, including a rapid recovery of bowel function, a rapid removal of devices, and rapid mobilization and pain relief [15]. In adult populations, studies have found that when patient-controlled analgesia and a traditional perioperative program are used, a laparoscopic approach to colon surgery promotes earlier restoration of bowel function and more rapid hospital discharge in comparison to laparotomy [7, 12]. Studies of a minimally invasive approach to colon resection have shown that laparoscopy reduces the inflammatory response and the incidence of postoperative wound infection, thus facilitating the recovery process. Preoperative education and optimization of patients' health status, intraoperative attenuation of surgical stress, multimodal analgesia, enforced mobilization, and early oral nutrition, together with revisions to the traditional practice of surgical care, have been applied successfully [12].

12.2.3 Preoperative Assessment and Investigation

Each pediatric patient who undergoes anesthesia is different and requires an individual assessment and management. The spectrum of patients is broad and ranges from healthy children in elective surgery settings to newborns with many systemic diseases in emergency surgery. The principles of management are mostly similar to anesthesia in open surgery.

An anesthesiology evaluation should not be made on day of surgery, but far enough in advance to request for any examinations and allow adequate time for informed consent [10].

A complete physical examination and pathological anamnesis should be carried out to identify contraindications to laparoscopy, particularly heart disease or pulmonary dysfunction. Hydration status, pharmacological therapy, and allergies should be registered. The need for laboratory investigations depends on the general status of the patient. Laboratory examinations are valid for 6 months unless the patient's clinical or pharmacological history changes. The necessary blood tests for a pediatric patient who will undergo anesthesia are specified in Table 12.3. A preoperative electrocardiogram (ECG) is recommended. Routine thoracic radiography is not recommended.

Recommendations for fasting are the same as in adults, with the addition of guidelines

Table 12.3 Recommended blood tests and examinations

Examinations	Conditions
Electrolytes, hematocrit, hemoglobin, transaminase, glucose serum, complete blood count, creatinine, and white blood cell count	Common use (not mandatory)
Coagulation panel (partial thromboplastin time, prothrombin time, INR), platelet count, and blood type	Potential hemorrhagic surgery, anamnesis positive to coagulation problem
Pregnancy test	Female patients of childbearing age
ECG	From birth to 6 months old
Thorax radiography	Risk of broncopulmonary dysplasia (BPD)
ECG and cardiographic examination	Risk of BPD, heart murmur, or obstructive sleep apnea

Table 12.4 Appropriate intake of food and liquids before anesthesia

Ingested material	Minimum fasting period, hours
Clear liquids: Water, fruit juice without pulp, clear tea, black coffee	2
Breast milk	4
Nonhuman milk	6
Light meal (toast and clear liquids)	6

for breast milk and infant formula intake (Table 12.4). In some cases, a bowel preparation is suggested to optimize the working space during laparoscopy [9].

12.2.4 Premedication

The following preparation and setup for anesthesia is recommended. The commonly used acronym SOAPME is useful in planning and to check the ambient conditions before starting any procedure [12]:

- **S** (suction)—size-appropriate suction catheters.
- **O** (oxygen)—adequate O_2 supply and ventilator.
- **A** (airway)—size-appropriate airway equipment (facial masks, laryngoscope blades, endotracheal and rhino-tracheal tubes, stylet, any devices for difficult airway management).
- **P** (pharmacy)—all basic drugs needed to support any phase of anesthesia.
- **M** (monitors)—pulse oximeter, ECG, non-invasive pressure, capnography, and stethoscope are always required; defibrillator periodically checked.
- **E** (equipment)—any special equipment or drugs for a particular case.

Premedication for anesthesia in children presenting for MIS should not be different than that for other types of surgery. The choice depends on the patient's anxiety level and overall physical status. Commonly, midazolam 0.5 mg/Kg orally half an hour before induction is a good choice. Midazolam rectally (0.5 mg/Kg), sublingually (0.3 mg/Kg), or nasally (0.3 mg/Kg) are alternative choices. Atropine or glycopyrrolate may be included in premedication to prevent the reflex bradycardia induced by abdominal insufflation and to dry secretions.

At least one venous catheter must be placed; an additional device is useful in cases where blood loss is expected. It is preferable to position the venous access above the diaphragm, as the pneumoperitoneum may limit the entry of fluid and drugs into the central circulation. Eutectic mixture of local anesthetics (EMLA) should be applied before positioning the intravenous access to reduce pain.

The position of the patient during surgery may be quite extreme; therefore, areas prone to pressure injury should be protected with specific padding (Fig. 12.1).

Each patient must be heated sufficiently (liquids, ambient, devices), remembering that the newborn experiences maximum heat loss from the head and trunk.

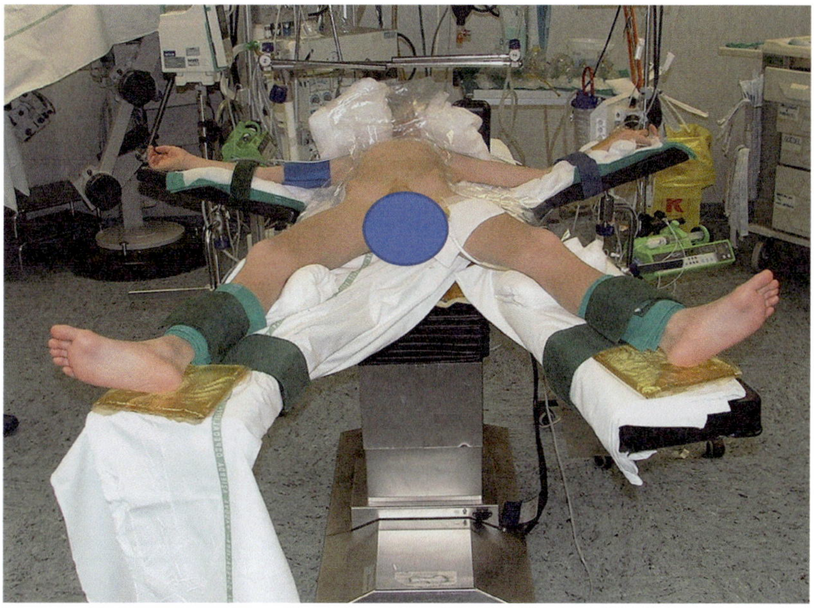

Fig. 12.1 An example of patient position during laparoscopic surgery

12.2.5 Anesthesia

The goals of anesthesia are to provide conditions required for surgery and to rectify the physiological status mutation. General anesthesia with neuromuscular block, intubation, and positive pressure ventilation is the anesthetic strategy. A routine minimum standard of monitoring includes continuous ECG, automated non-invasive blood pressure, pulse oximetry, capnography, and temperature. However, capnography does not consistently reflect $PaCO_2$, especially in infants, because the respiratory rate is usually faster and the arterial to end tidal CO_2 gradient is variable.

Induction may be intravenous or inhalational—the choice depends on the ability of the child to tolerate the placement of an intravenous catheter. Intravenous induction is preferred in older children. Propofol provides rapid induction, reduces intubation-related bronchospasm, and has an antiemetic effect. In cases of inhalational induction, desflurane is not preferred because it may produce coughing, airway irritation, and possible laryngospasm. A protocol of rapid-sequence induction must be considered in children with high risk for regurgitation and pulmonary aspiration. H2-receptor antagonists, such as ranitidine, must be administrated in these patients.

After induction, an orogastric tube should be placed to decompress the stomach, reduce the risk of aspiration, and optimize surgical area visibility. Endotracheal intubation (ETI) is generally preferred to a supraglottic airway (SGA). An appropriately sized endotracheal uncuffed tube should be used in children younger than 8 years of age. However, an uncuffed tube makes positive pressure ventilation and airway safety difficult. Thus, ETI with minimum cuff inflation is preferred [14]. The potential benefits of this practice are better pulmonary protection, improved ventilation in cases with affected pulmonary status, and less gas leakage.

Some authors have reported that the ventilator efficacy of the Proseal laryngeal mask (LMA® (Laryngeal Mask Airway)) is comparable to ventilation through an endotracheal tube [5]. Neuromuscular blockade is required to improve the surgical condition and intubation, using non-depolarizing agents (rocuronium at a dose of 0.6–1.2 mg/Kg). A peripheral nerve stimulator should be used to monitor the degree of blockade.

The maintenance of anesthesia is generally conducted with a balanced technique that includes inhalation gases, intravenous opioids, and neuromuscular agents. The use of nitrous oxide (N_2O) remains controversial because it may cause bowel distension, nausea, and vomiting in the postoperative phase [11].

The major difference in anesthetic management between MIS and open surgery is connected to the cardiopulmonary effect of the pneumoperitoneum. Most cases required controlled ventilation. In younger patients, pressure-controlled ventilation is preferred to reduce the gas leak around the uncuffed tube. In all cases, with the help of modern ventilators, targeted volume is mandatory to prevent lung barotrauma, volume trauma, and depressive effects to the cardiovascular system. The strategy uses a target tidal volume in the range of 6–7 mL/Kg; an increase in the ventilator frequency rate of approximately 30% is required to maintain normocarbia. The ideal ventilation strategy guarantees an optimal arterial oxygen tension, acceptable arterial CO_2, and protective airway pressure.

The requirement for perioperative fluids depends upon preoperative patient status, the patient's age, and the nature and site of intervention. Laparoscopic surgery is associated with less loss of corporeal fluids than open surgery; the goal is usually the maintenance of euvolemic status [7].

12.2.6 Postoperative Pain, Nausea, and Vomiting

Postoperative pain is the result of port insertion in the abdominal wall, irritation of the phrenic nerve, and distention of the peritoneum (Fig. 12.2); its intensity persists for 24 h. The multimodal regimen of local anesthetic infiltration to incision sites, opioids, nonsteroidal anti-inflammatory drugs, and paracetamol reduces the incidence of substantial pain. An example of this approach is the intraoperative administration of intravenous (iv) fentanyl (1–2 y/Kg), iv paracetamol (15 mg/Kg), iv morphine (0.1 mg/Kg), and iv ketorolac (0.5 mg/Kg) [6]. Intravenous or oral paracetamol is the drug of choice to treat postoperative pain. Laparoscopy has been identified as a risk factor for postoperative nausea and vomiting; therefore, routine prophylactic antiemetic therapy should be administrated. Dexamethasone is superior to ondansetron in preventing postoperative nausea after 4–6 h of laparoscopic surgeries. However, both drugs are of equal efficacy in preventing postoperative vomiting up to 24 h after surgery [11].

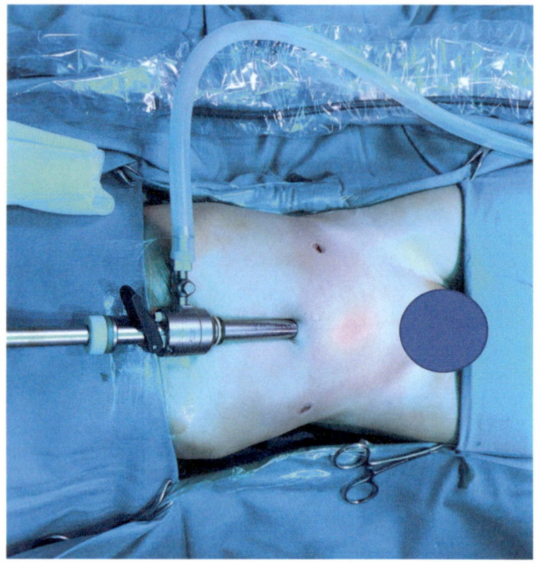

Fig. 12.2 Abdomen view after loss of pneumoperitoneum in the final time of the surgery

12.2.7 Complications

Complications during laparoscopic surgery can be classified into three categories:

1. Effects on hemodynamic and respiratory status (e.g., hypotension, hypoxemia, hypercarbia, gas embolism).
2. Surgical maneuvers related risk (e.g., pneumothorax, vessel lesion, ureter lesion).
3. Patient positioning (e.g., cerebral edema, pressure ulcers, nerve injuries).

The anesthesiologist must prevent and be ready for the quick treatment of potential complications.

It is necessary to control the peak IAP, the grade of stomach deflation, and all changes in respiratory and cardiovascular parameters. In cases of refractory respiratory distress or hemodynamic instability, it may be necessary to convert the intervention to open access. Post-anesthesia recovery usually occurs with no complications, if the patient has no previous compromised physical status. Venous gas embolism is common during laparoscopy, but it is almost always subclinical and does not impair a patient's healthy status. Rarely, carbon dioxide embolism into an artery or large vein may be a potentially fatal complication. Its clinical presentation is characterized by cardiovascular collapse (a sudden drop in end-tidal CO_2, collapse of oxygen saturation, fall in blood pressure, and different arrhythmias) and, depending on the size of the embolus, even death. Life-saving maneuvers include the aspiration of gas through the central vein catheter, placement into Durant's position, and cardiopulmonary resuscitation.

12.2.8 Conclusions

Minimally invasive surgery has advantages in terms of speed, postoperative recovery time, pain control, and patient satisfaction. However, anesthesia associated with the changes brought about by the pneumoperitoneum may cause issues if not properly handled. It is therefore necessary to continue the cooperation and research between surgeons and anesthesiologists to ensure the best standards of care for pediatric patients. In recent years, some laparoscopic surgeries in the adult population have used epidural or spinal anesthesia with excellent results. In the future, it is hoped that MIS anesthesia management achieves international scientific validation, backed by a growing number of randomized controlled trials.

12.3 Thoracoscopy

12.3.1 Introduction

Video-assisted thoracoscopic surgery (VATS) has an ever-increasing number of indications for the pediatric patient. Its minimal invasiveness implies provides known benefits in terms of better cosmetic results, faster recovery, decreased length of hospital stay, and significant reduction of postoperative pain [16, 17]. This surgical choice led anesthesiologists to change their usual anesthetic technique: indeed, a thoracotomy does not always require lung separation and collapse in infants [18]. Moreover, the placement of a peridural catheter is a common choice in our experience and is usually performed before surgery when a thoracotomy is planned, but it is rarely justified in VATS. This approach assures optimal analgesia during and after open surgery with a lower dosage of drugs; in VATS, local anesthetic drugs have a limited role during surgery [19].

One-lung ventilation (OLV), although not mandatory in pediatric thoracic endoscopic surgery [20–22], is very important for the success of VATS and the reduction of the rate of conversion to open surgery because it provides optimal exposure of the surgical field. Many studies have found that non-optimal exposure of the surgical field is a frequent cause of conversion to open surgery [20–23] and that anesthetic management has a big impact on the successful performance of VATS [16, 24]. Moreover, it assures protection from contamination of the healthy, dependent lung. Small children often do not tolerate OLV; in these cases, VATS may be performed with conventional ventilation and insufflation of low-flow, low-pressure carbon dioxide (CO_2) on the operative side, with comparable results [22].

The achievement of reliable separation between the lungs is very different in infants, small children, and adolescents. In the latter, the separate control of airway does not substantially differ from adults; however, difficulties arise in small children whose different airway anatomy and respiratory physiology have to be well understood by anesthesiologists. These aspects are essential to prevent complications and eventually to treat them. In the same way, technical skill with all the available tools is mandatory for airway management. Sharing the planned procedure with the nursing staff and defining their respective roles are recommended for the safe and effective conduct of anesthesia and surgery.

12.3.2 Anatomical Peculiarities of the Airway of Small Children

The small diameter of the infant's airway explains many of the problems that might occur during OLV. The narrow superior airway is the principal factor in the choice of the tracheal intubation technique; this choice affects the quality of lung exclusion and the potential duration and success of thoracic endoscopic surgery. The tracheal and bronchial mucosa might suffer damage during intubation because of the decubitus of the blocker balloon (BB) [16]. A displacement of the tracheal tube or of the BB can occur during a change in the decubitus position or during surgery because the infant's airway is very short. The peripheral airway might close in the dependent lung because the functional residual capacity is closer to the residual volume, and atelectasis ensues. A small lumen is easily obstructed by blood or secretions. Every manipulation of the tracheal tube, airway, and BB is potentially dangerous.

The technical skills required for the management of OLV in infants are of great relevance.

12.3.3 Physiology of OLV and the Lateral Decubitus Position in Infants

In adults and children under normal conditions, respiratory exchanges are optimal if ventilation (V) and perfusion (Q) are well matched. During OLV, the V/Q ratio is increased—that is, the intrapulmonary shunt is increased, with detrimental effects on oxygen exchanges. This effect is due to several factors: diaphragmatic pushing, lung compression by mediastinal structures, abdominal viscera, and rolls placed under the thorax to obtain the correct patient position and better exposure. Moreover, a decrease of residual functional capacity and tidal volume, general anesthesia, surgical maneuvers, and mechanical ventilation are other factors promoting V/Q mismatch.

There is a physiological mechanism that can decrease this negative effect: the hypoxic pulmonary vasoconstriction (HPV). The pulmonary vasoconstriction shifts the blood circulation away from lung areas where the ventilation is poor or absent to the well-ventilated lung. When the lung is collapsed, a large share of the blood is diverted toward the dependent lung, but a small share remains in the non-ventilated lung and is not oxygenated. Although these events occur in adults and children, the lateral decubitus position has negative effects on V/Q mismatch only in children. An adult in the lateral decubitus position does not experience serious difficulties because their rib cage is rigid; the hydrostatic pressure gradient between the lungs and the gravity pressure are higher than in small children. The diversion of the blood circulation from the diseased lung to the healthy, dependent lung is more difficult in children than in adults. Children have soft rib cages and lungs: the dependent hemithorax is compressed by the lateral decubitus position and by the chest rolls placed under the thoracic cage; the lung compliance of the dependent, healthy, ventilated lung decreases and hypoxia ensues [25–27]. These events make small children prone to hypoxia. For this reason, it is essential to maintain the possibility of ventilating both lungs during the whole procedure.

12.3.4 Techniques for OLV in Infants and Small Children

The decreased airway size in infants excludes the choices of double-lumen endobronchial tubes and Univent tubes (Fuji Systems Corp., Tokyo), which are too large for small children. Only two options are possible: selective mainstem intubation and an endobronchial blocker [16, 21–23, 28, 29].

12.3.4.1 Selective Mainstream Intubation

Selective bronchial intubation with a single-lumen tracheal tube is the simplest and least expensive way to achieve OLV in infants. The tube must be a half-size smaller than is suitable for tracheal intubation. The right bronchial insertion is very easy and the auscultation of breath sounds is adequate to control the tube position. The blind left bronchial insertion is more difficult for anatomical reasons; some approaches to solve the problem have been described based on the manipulation of the head and neck [24, 28]. However, in our opinion, blind left bronchus intubation is not advised. Instead, guidance of the tube and the control of its correct position with a fiber-optical bronchoscope (FOB) are recommended. A suitable FOB size for infants is 2.2 mm OD or less.

The tube can be cuffed or uncuffed; a cuffed tube, when compatible, gives a better seal and satisfying lung collapse. In the case of left lung surgery, the placement of the tube in the right main bronchus will cause the exclusion of the upper lobe bronchus, with subsequent atelectasis of the upper right lobe and hypoxia. For this reason, right bronchial intubation is not recommended [30]. The problems occurring with selective bronchial intubation are poor lung isolation and difficulty in quickly re-establishing double-lung ventilation (DLV) if hypoxia should develop during surgery, because tube manipulation under the surgical drapes is very dangerous. Moreover, if main bronchus intubation does not give a completely effective bronchus occlusion, it will be necessary to achieve lung collapse with an intrapleural insufflation of CO_2. CO_2 is absorbed into the blood circulation, and this event can be responsible for the development of hypercapnia and acidosis [16, 24, 30].

12.3.4.2 Bronchial Blocker

In the 1970s a Fogarty embolectomy catheter was used as a bronchial blocker (BB); a 3-Fr Fogarty inserted outside the tracheal tube was considered to be suitable for OLV in infants. However, a low-volume, high-pressure balloon can cause damage to the bronchial mucosa. Moreover, this catheter does not have an internal lumen [23]. A 5-Fr Arndt endobronchial blocker (Cook, Bloomington, IN, USA) represents an improvement in the research for a balloon-tipped catheter that is suitable for infants; it has a high-volume, low-pressure balloon; an internal lumen containing a flexible wire stylet with a loop at its end; and a special adaptor (Arndt Multiport Airway Adapter) with three ports: one of them accommodating the BB, the second one the FOB, and the third one the connector for the ventilation circuit (Figs. 12.3 and 12.4). This adaptor allows the continuation of infant's ventilation during the whole procedure.

The infant trachea does not allow the insertion of a tracheal tube large enough to accommodate the BB and FOB within in; thus, the 5-Fr Arndt blocker is inserted through its port in the adaptor before the tracheal tube, thus remaining outside

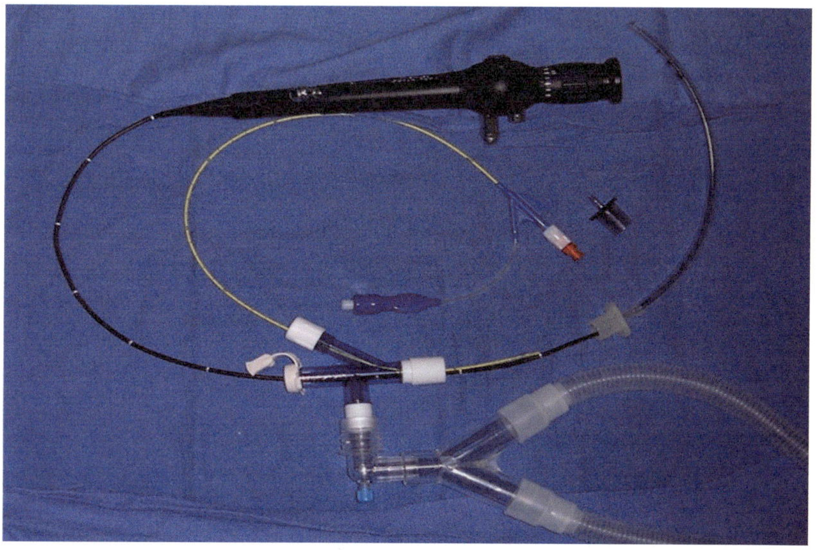

Fig. 12.3 Fiber-optic bronchoscope (FOB) tip inside the Arndt bronchial blocker (BB) loop

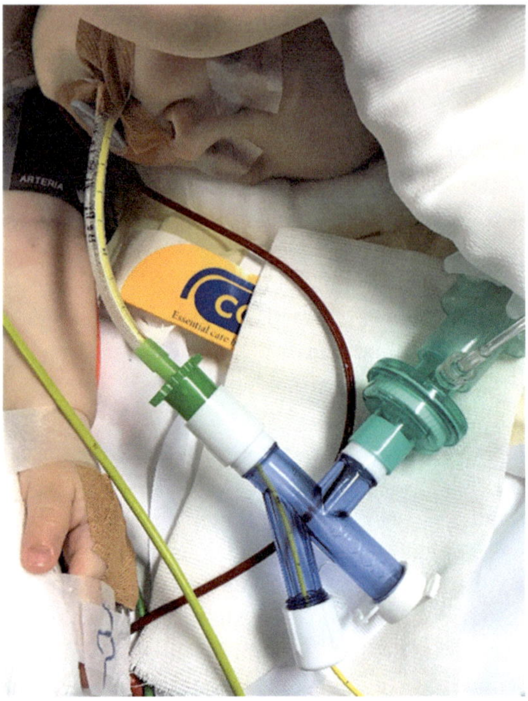

Fig. 12.4 View of the bronchial blocker (BB) inside its dedicated path in the multiport airway adapter

of the tracheal tube. In this way, the extraluminal placement of the blocker leaves more room for ventilation. The FOB is then inserted through its port; the FOB tip must pass through the blocker loop and advance into the mainstem bronchus, which must be blocked. Then, the balloon is slowly inflated under FOB direct vision with small volumes of air, depending on the size of the BB. At this point, the FOB may be removed. Lung auscultation will confirm the silence of breath on the blocked side.

It is suggested to check the correct position of the balloon in the bronchus after turning the child from the supine to lateral position, to exclude the dislodgment of the BB. Some authors suggest placing the BB when the child is already in the lateral position [31]. After checking the correct position and inflation of the BB balloon, the wire guide must be removed to leave the channel available for the lung deflation, aspiration, and oxygen delivery.

The BB allows effective collapse of the diseased lung and isolation of the healthy lung; moreover, it allows for a quick switch from OLV to DLV when necessary. The insertion procedure must be made with extreme care to avoid complications, such as dislodgment of the balloon into the trachea or airway injury.

12.3.5 Techniques for OLV in Children and Adolescents

OLV is faster and easier in children over 6 years of age and usually better tolerated.

The Univent tube (Fuji System Corp.) is a cuffed, single-lumen endotracheal tube made up of two separate channels: the main channel is used for ventilation, whereas the other channel is inside the BB. The BB is movable; by rotating the tube, the BB can be advanced in either right or left bronchus, usually with FOB guidance. The BB is hollow; through its lumen, air can be removed to aid the blocked lung deflation and can be used to insufflate oxygen or suction the operated lung. The advantage of the Univent tube is that the BB is firmly attached to the main endotracheal tube, which means that its displacement is less likely than with other options. The disadvantages are an outer diameter that is very large compared with the inner diameter: an inner lumen of 3.5 mm corresponds to an outer diameter of 7.5–8 mm (the cross-section of this tube is oval). Therefore, this endotracheal tube can be used only in children of 6 years of age or older. Moreover, the BB balloon has low-volume, high-pressure properties, so mucosal injuries can occur.

Currently, Robertshaw tubes (Ruesch, Teleflex Medical Inc.) are the preferred double-lumen endotracheal tubes for older children and adolescents. They are designed to fit a patient's anatomy in both left and right versions. The right version has a side hole for the right upper lobe. However, to avoid the risk of its obstruction, left bronchial tube placement is recommended whenever possible [21]. They do not have a carinal hook. The cuff has high-volume, low pressure properties. The smallest size available is 26 Fr, which can be used for children from 8 years of age. The technique for insertion is the same as in an adult, with an FOB guide for a correct placement. The inner diameter of the 26-Fr size is 3.4 mm, which can accommodate a FOB of 2.2 mm OD. Displacement of double-lumen tubes is less likely compared to BB, and conversion from OLV to DLV can be performed easily.

12.3.6 Preoperative Assessment

The preoperative assessment depends mainly on the patient's age and health status. A pediatric surgery patient may be a newborn with esophageal atresia or congenital diaphragmatic hernia, an infant in very good condition with a congenital cystic adenomatoid malformation, or a child with an oncologic disease either at its onset or after multiple series of chemotherapy and surgical procedures. For a healthy patient, the preoperative evaluation may be based only on an accurate medical history, a physical examination, and a review of tests when required. However, in a seriously ill child, a thorough assessment must also include blood tests and instrumental investigations. Usually, these children have recent tests and many assessments in their medical history; it is not necessary to perform them again if the results are compatible with anesthetic technique, surgery, and OLV and no therapeutic changes have been performed. The availability of blood transfusion has to be assured.

12.3.7 Informed Consent

The anesthesiologist should be very clear and exhaustive in providing information. Although some surgeons might minimize the procedure ("only three small holes"), parents must know that, along with the benefits, there are also some risks, whose frequency and severity must be explained. Minimally invasive surgery does not mean minimal risk [32, 33].

12.3.8 Pre-Anesthesia

Pre-anesthesia is not always necessary, such as when the child goes into the operating room with one parent, as has been our practice for many years. However, many children may benefit from it in particular situations, such as children who have undergone multiple procedures or wth very anxious parents who are unable to reassure their child. Oral midazolam, 0.3–0.5 mg/Kg, is a very common choice. When intravenous anesthetic induction is used and the child does not have venous access already placed, the use of anesthetic EMLA cream can be very helpful.

12.3.9 Anesthetic Technique

Both inhalation and intravenous techniques have been described for the anesthesia of children undergoing VATS. Inhalational agents may inhibit the HPV and be responsible for an intrapulmonary shunt increase and hypoxia; however, a Cochrane database review did not indicate any differences in outcomes between intravenous and inhalational agents [34]. This conclusion has been confirmed by other authors [32, 33].

A large bore intravenous catheter is mandatory because the time necessary to stop bleeding from a large vessel is longer in VATS than in open surgery [33].

Mechanical ventilation for OLV is based on low tidal volume (<10 mL/Kg), respiratory frequency, which is slightly increased in comparison with the usual frequency for the child's age and insufflation of air/oxygen.

The methods available to support respiratory exchanges during OLV and prevent atelectasis and hypoxia are intermittent or continuous positive airway pressure applied to the non-ventilated lung and intermittent insufflations to both lungs. Transient hypoxia occurs frequently during OLV and thoracic surgery; a dislodgement of the tracheal tube or of the BB has to be checked and adjusted. If hypoxia still persists, a higher oxygen fraction is recommended.

Electrocardiography, non-invasive blood pressure, pulse oximetry, end-tidal CO_2 ($EtCO_2$) concentration, inhaled volatile agent concentration, and body temperature are standard monitoring of infants undergoing VATS.

Infants and small children are prone to hypothermia during anesthesia, especially during anesthesia induction and settlement in the right position; it is not clear yet if thoracoscopy is responsible for hypothermia or hyperthermia [24]. In any case, the temperature should be monitored as in all lengthy surgical procedures performed in children and be maintained by warm forced-air devices and warm ventilation gases.

Nitrous oxide (N_2O) is usually used during induction of anesthesia with volatile agents because it increases the speed of induction. However, its interruption is recommended during the maintenance of anesthesia because of its physical property of diffusion into closed spaces full of air. These spaces increase in volume and this effect can be dangerous; the tracheal and bronchial cuff pressure can cause mucosal injuries. The intra-cuff pressure should be checked intermittently when N_2O is used. A safer alternative is the use of saline instead of air to inflate the tube cuffs.

Some authors recommend the placement of an arterial line to control blood gas values [30, 35]. Others think that it is not necessary in healthy children and short (<30 min of OLV) procedure times [32]. Hypercarbia can occur during VATS due to hypoventilation, V/P mismatching, and absorption of CO_2 insufflated into the chest when the seal of the bronchial tube is not reliable [30]. Non-invasive monitoring cannot detect the real amount of the arterial CO_2 value because of the discrepancy existing between $EtCO_2$ and arterial CO_2: $EtCO_2$ underestimates the CO_2 arterial pressure. The difference is due to increased physiologic dead space. Nevertheless, continuous capnography is very helpful for detecting ventilation problems: changes in the $EtCO_2$ waveform occur early when tube or BB displacement and gas exchange problems happen. Moderate hypercarbia can be accepted, provided that oxygen saturation is adequate. When CO_2 is persistently high, acidosis occurs; ventilation must be adjusted by increasing the minute ventilation in the ventilated lung and re-establishing DLV if necessary [29].

12.3.10 Postoperative Pain

Although thoracotomy requires 2–3 days of analgesia, pain resulting from thoracoscopic surgery is of shorter duration and less relevant, probably due to the low invasiveness of the procedure and the reduced need for a chest tube. Pain can be prevented by the preemptive analgesia principle; the injection of a topical anesthetic agent in the port sites is an easy way to prevent and reduce pain. Multimodal analgesia is the best way to achieve excellent results and to reduce the side effects of every single agent. The choice of analgesic drugs depends on the patient's age. Newborns and infants are more susceptible to the collateral effects of opioids, but their pain is usually well controlled by paracetamol. Older children can have a continuous or single-shot paravertebral block or a continuous intrapleural infusion of local anesthetic agents. We place the paravertebral catheter at the end of the surgery but before the camera removal, in order to see every step of the procedure and the correct placement of the catheter (Figs. 12.5 and 12.6), or we place it under ultrasound guidance.

An epidural catheter is advised when VATS has to be converted to open surgery; its placement can be performed at the end of surgery. Several adjuvant drugs can be added to local anesthetic agents, as opioids or alpha-agonist drugs.

Patient-controlled analgesia can be a solution in older children, either as a unique analgesic technique or added to regional anesthesia.

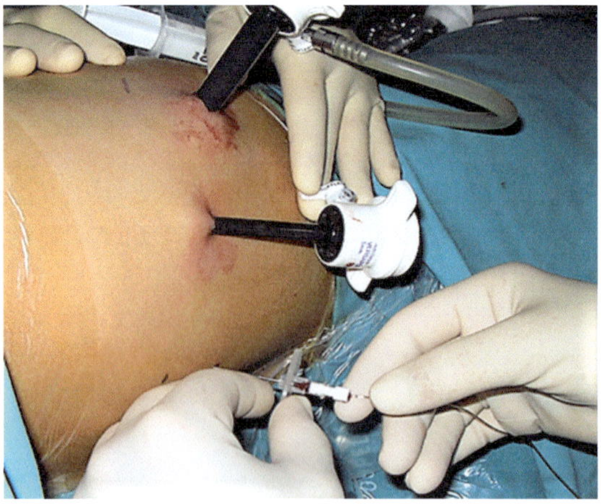

Fig. 12.5 Performance of a paravertebral block under direct view

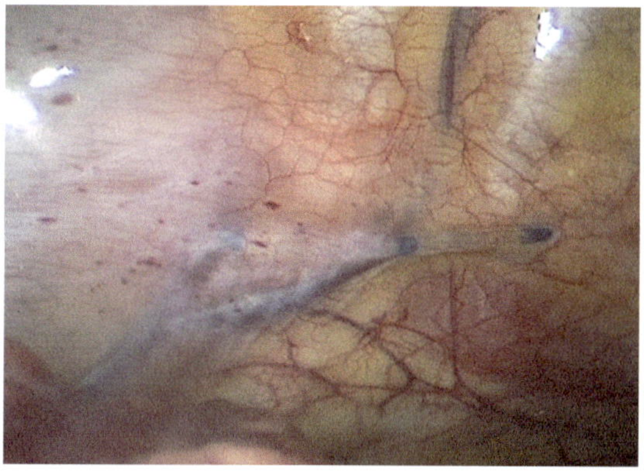

Fig. 12.6 View of the paravertebral catheter

12.3.11 Conclusions

Some items are mandatory for the feasibility and safety of VATS with OLV in children: knowledge of the anatomic and physiologic peculiarities of younger children; an understanding of the respiratory derangement caused by OLV, the lateral decubitus position, and general anesthesia; a familiarity with all available devices; and the importance of a quick conversion to DLV if necessary. Furthermore, coordination of the whole procedure with surgeons and nursing personnel is essential for the successful management of these patients.

Acknowledgments Sincere thanks to Dr. Marta Iannazzone for her important contribution.

I sincerely thank Dr. Franca Giusti who has been and will always be my Mentor in Pediatric Anesthesia and a Teacher of life.

Conflict of interest: The authors have not conflicts of interest to declare.

References

1. De Waal EE, Kalkman CJ. Haemodynamic changes during low-pressure carbon dioxide pneumoperitoneum in young children. Paediatr Anaesth. 2003;13:18–25.
2. Nishio I, Noguchi J, Konishi M, et al. The effects of anesthetic techniques and insufflating gases on ventilation during laparoscopy. Jpn J Anesthesiol. 1993;42:862–6.
3. Kalmar AF, Foubert L, Hendrickx JF, et al. Influence of steep Trendelenburg position and CO2 pneumoperitoneum on cardiovascular, cerebrovascular, and respiratory homeostasis during robotic prostatectomy. Br J Anaesth. 2010;104:433–9.
4. Manner T, Aantaa R, Alanen M. Lung compliance during laparoscopic surgery pediatric patients. Paediatr Anaesth. 1998;8(1):25–9.
5. Pennant JH. Anesthesia for laparoscopy in the pediatric patient. Anesthesiol Clin North America. 2001;19:69–88.
6. Bannister CF, Brosius KK, Wulkan M. The effect of insufflation pressure on pulmonary mechanics in infants during laparoscopic surgical procedures. Pediatr Anaesth. 2003;13(9):785–9.
7. Hatipoglu S, Akbulut S, Hatipoglu F, et al. Effect of laparoscopic abdominal surgery on splanchnic circulation: historical developments. World J Gastroenterol. 2014;20:18165–76.
8. Meininger D, Westphal K, Bremerich DH, et al. Effects of posture and prolonged pneumoperitoneum on hemodynamic parameters during laparoscopy. World J Surg. 2008;32:1400–5.
9. Ortega AE, Peters JH, Incarbone R, et al. A prospective randomized comparison of the metabolic and stress hormonal responses of laparoscopic and open cholecystectomy. J Am Coll Surg. 1996;183:249–56.
10. Joris J, Lamy M. Neuroendocrine changes during pneumo- peritoneum for laparoscopic cholecystectomy. Br J Anaesth. 1993;70(Suppl).
11. Chang DT, Kirsch AJ, Sawczuk IS. Oliguria during laparoscopic surgery. J Endourol. 1994;8:349–52.
12. Rist M, Hemmerling TM, Rauh R, et al. Influence of pneumoperitoneum and patient positioning on preload and splanchnic blood volume in laparoscopic surgery of the lower abdomen. J Clin Anesth. 2001;13:244–9.
13. Cotè CJ, Wilson S. Guidelines for monitoring and management of pediatric patients during and after sedation for diagnostic and therapeutic procedures: an update. Pediatrics. 2006;118(6).
14. Esposito C, Escolino M, Farina A, Cortese G, et al. The role of bowel preparation to optimize working space in laparoscopic inguinal hernia repair in infants. J Pediatr Surg. 2014;49(10):1536–7.
15. Spinelli G, Vargas M, Aprea G, Cortese G, Servillo G. Pediatric anesthesia for minimally invasive surgery in pediatric urology. Transl Pediatr. 2016;5(4):214–21.
16. Lau CT, Leung J, Hui TW, Wong KK. Thoracoscopic operations in children. Hong Kong Med J. 2014;20:234–40.
17. Lau CT, Leung J, Chan IH, Chung PH, Lan LC, et al. Thoracoscopic resection of congenital cystic lung lesions is associated with better post-operative outcomes. Pediatr Surg Int. 2013;29:341–5.
18. Kunisaki SM, Powelson IA, Haydar B, Bowshier BC, Jarboe MD, et al. Thoracoscopic vs open lobectomy in infants and young children with congenital lung malformations. J Am Coll Surg. 2014;218:261–70.
19. Tognon C, Meneghini L, Fascetti Leon F, Gamba PG. The different approaches of single lung ventilation in infants with pulmonary malformation. Int J Pediatr Res. 2018;4:030.

20. Rothenberg SS. First decade's experience with thoracoscopic lobectomy in infants and children. J Pediatr Surg. 2008;43:40–4.
21. Hammer GB. Single-lung ventilation in infants and children. Pediatr Anesth. 2004;14:98–102.
22. Dingemann C, Zoeller C, Bataineh Z, Osthaus A, Suempelmann R, et al. Single- and double-lung ventilation in infants and children undergoing thoracoscopic lung resection. Eur J Pediatr Surg. 2013;23:48–52.
23. Bataineh ZA, Zoeller C, Dingemann C, Osthaus A, Suempelmann R, et al. Our experience with single lung ventilation in thoracoscopic paediatric surgery. Eur J Pediatr Surg. 2012;22:17–20.
24. Oak SN, Parelkar SV, Satishkumar KV, Pathak R, Ramesh BH, et al. Review of video-assisted thoracoscopy in children. J Minim Access Surg. 2009;5:57–62.
25. Byon H-J, Lee J-W, Kim J-K, Kim J-T, Kim YT, et al. Anesthetic management of video-assisted thoracoscopic surgery (VATS) in pediatric patients: the issue of safety in infants and younger children. Korean J Anesthesiol. 2010;59:99–103.
26. Choudhry DK. Single-lung ventilation in pediatric anesthesia. Anesthesiol Clin N Am. 2005;23:693–708.
27. Dimitriou G, Greenough A, Pink L, McGhee A, Hickey A, et al. Effect of posture on oxygen and respiratory muscle strain in infants. Arch Dis Child Fetal Neonatal. 2002;86:147–50.
28. Fabila TS, Menghraj SJ. One lung ventilation strategies for infants and children undergoing video assisted thoracoscopic surgery. Indian J Anaesth. 2013;57:339–44.
29. Tan GM, Tan-Kendrick AP. Bronchial diameters in children—use of the Fogarty catheter for lung isolation in children. Anaesth Intensive Care. 2002;30:615–8.
30. Sutton CJ, Naguib A, Puri S, Sprenker CJ, Camporesi EM. One-lung ventilation in infants and small children: blood gas values. J Anesth. 2012;26:670–4.
31. Hsieh VC, Thompson DR, Haberkern CM. Pediatric endobronchial blockers in infants: a refinement in technique. Pediatr Anaesth. 2015;25:438–9.
32. Fischer GW, Cohen E. An update on anesthesia for thoracoscopic surgery. Curr Opin Anaesthesiol. 2010;23:7–11.
33. Mukhtar AM, Obayah GM, Elmasry A, Dessouky NM. The therapeutic potential of intraoperative hypercapnia during video assisted thoracoscopy in pediatric patients. Anesth Analg. 2008;106:84–8.
34. Cochrane central register of controlled trials, and Cochrane database of systematic reviews. Cochrane Libr. 2013;7.
35. Disma N, Mameli L, Pini-Prato A, Montobbio G. One lung ventilation with Arndt pediatric bronchial blocker for thoracoscopic surgery in children: a unicentric experience. Pediatr Anesth. 2011;21:465–7.

Part II

Chest

Thoracoscopic Lung Biopsy

13

Gloria Pelizzo

13.1 Introduction

Recent advances in endoscopic surgery technology and techniques have dramatically transformed and ameliorated this approach to intrathoracic lesions in the paediatric patient. The anatomy of the thorax with its rigid rib cage and collapsible lung render it ideally suited to endoscopic procedures [1].

The thoracoscopic technique was first described in the early twentieth century and was first applied in children in the mid-1970s [2, 3]. With the advent of minimally invasive surgery over the last few decades, thoracoscopic lung biopsy has become the gold standard and is preferable to the open procedure [4, 5]. This approach is less invasive, minimizes morbidity and visualizes a greater percentage of the lung. Patients have less postoperative pain, a shorter hospital stay and a better cosmetic outcome. Additionally, musculoskeletal sequelae, associated with thoracotomy, can be circumvented [3].

Due to advancements in this surgical technique and perioperative care, thoracoscopic lung biopsy has also become feasible in small infants [3, 5, 6]. Nevertheless, the risk of complications should not be underestimated and should be weighed carefully against the benefits [6].

In this chapter, we describe the indications and contraindications and technical approach to thoracoscopic lung biopsy in children.

13.2 Indications

Lung biopsy for either diffuse or localized processes is a common indication for thoracoscopy [4, 7–9]. Diagnostic thoracoscopic interventions include wedge biopsies of solitary lung lesions, excision and/or biopsy of pulmonary masses, wedge biopsies of diffuse lung parenchymal disease and exploration for trauma.

In Table 13.1, the indications for thoracoscopic lung biopsy in immunocompetent and immunocompromised children are reported.

Table 13.1 Indications for thoracoscopic lung biopsy in children

Indications
Interstitial lung disease in the immunocompromised patient
Diffuse parenchymal lung disease
Pulmonary masses associated with malignancies
Refractory pleural lesion diseases
Pulmonary hydatid cysts larger than 5 cm

G. Pelizzo (✉)
Pediatric Surgery Department, Children's Hospital "G. Di Cristina", ARNAS Civico-Di Cristina-Benfratelli, Palermo, Italy

C. Esposito et al. (eds.), *ESPES Manual of Pediatric Minimally Invasive Surgery*,
https://doi.org/10.1007/978-3-030-00964-9_13

Table 13.2 Absolute and relative contraindications to thoracoscopic lung biopsy in children [8]

Absolute	Relative
• Lack of pleural space due to: – Suspected mesothelioma (where the visceral and parietal surfaces are fused) – Previous pleurodesis – Advanced empyema – Pleural thickening of unknown aetiology	• Inability to tolerate a lateral decubitus position • Unstable cardiovascular or haemodynamic status • Presence of severe, uncorrectable hypoxaemia despite oxygen therapy • Bleeding diathesis • Pulmonary arterial hypertension • Refractory cough • Drug hypersensitivity • Reduced general health status with short suspected survival

13.3 Contraindications

Thoracoscopy is a safe procedure, with only a few absolute and relative contraindications (Table 13.2). An important absolute contraindication is the lack of pleural space resulting from extensive adhesions of the pleural layer, since it is impossible to carry out the procedure if the pleural space has been obliterated [6].

13.4 Preoperative Preparation

A full patient workup should be made to determine general anaesthesia tolerance [3]. Besides a detailed history, a thorough physical examination is a vital component of a pre-thoracoscopic evaluation. The patient's respiratory status must be evaluated, at a minimum, with blood gas analysis and, if necessary, with pulmonary function tests.

The history of the patient may provide important information on possible risk factors [3]. The history should include knowledge of previous drug therapies, in particular anticoagulant treatment, which may be an absolute or relative contraindication to the intervention. Additionally, systemic immunosuppressive treatment, especially corticosteroids, could induce delayed closure of biopsy sites of the lung.

An ECG should be obtained to exclude a recent myocardial infarction or significant arrhythmia. The clinical laboratory should include coagulation parameters, serum electrolytes, serum creatinine, glucose, liver function studies and a complete blood count as well as a blood group typing [6]. Before undergoing thoracoscopic biopsy, it is recommended that patients undergo chest radiography (preferably anteroposterior and lateral views) and a CT or MRI of the chest. The chest x-ray and CT or MRI findings help to localize the lesion and to determine optional patient positioning for the operation [3, 5–7].

All patients and their parents must sign a specifically formulated informed consent before the procedure.

13.5 Positioning

Lung biopsy is usually performed with the patient in the lateral decubitus position. Posterior pleural biopsies are performed with the patient almost prone, and anterior lesions are performed with the patient almost supine. Thus, positioning takes advantage of gravity to allow the lung to fall away from the lesion when the lung is collapsed [3, 6]. For anterior mediastinal masses, a modified supine position is helpful. This position allows gravity to keep the lung out of the operative field.

An axillary point of entry is standard in most cases: entry in the midaxillary line at the level of the fourth or fifth intercostal space allows the best and most complete thoracic cavity inspection [6]. The working trocars are inserted in triangular fashion depending on the biopsy site selected. The biopsy locations are selected according to the visual appearance of the lung. One to four biopsies of at least 1 cm^3 lung tissue each are taken [6] often including pieces of different lobes.

13.6 Instrumentation

Standard equipment to safely perform the thoracoscopic procedure [8] include:

- Thoracoscope.
- High-resolution video monitor.
- 2–4 intercostal access ports
- Endoscopic stapling devices.
- Endoscopic scissors.
- Endoscopic forceps.
- Endoscopic bags.
- Endoscopic dissector.

In Fig. 13.1, the standard paediatric thoracoscopic instruments are illustrated.

Besides affording larger biopsy sizes, thoracoscopic instruments facilitate the extraction of biopsies from very dense lesions. The rigid instruments are also more suitable when it is necessary to control haemorrhage after biopsy [6].

In children, 5 and 10 mm Hopkins rod-lens telescopes are used. In small infants, a 3.5 mm or the new 14-gauge endoscopic telescope may be useful. Short trocars without valves are specifically designed for this procedure [3], and standard hand instruments used in laparoscopy (10, 5 mm/3 mm) may be used. The theatre set-up and operative technique also depend upon the procedure being performed [3].

13.7 Technique

The consecutive steps in thoracoscopic lung biopsy are described in Table 13.3.

Paediatric anaesthesia remains a vital component of the general success in thoracoscopic

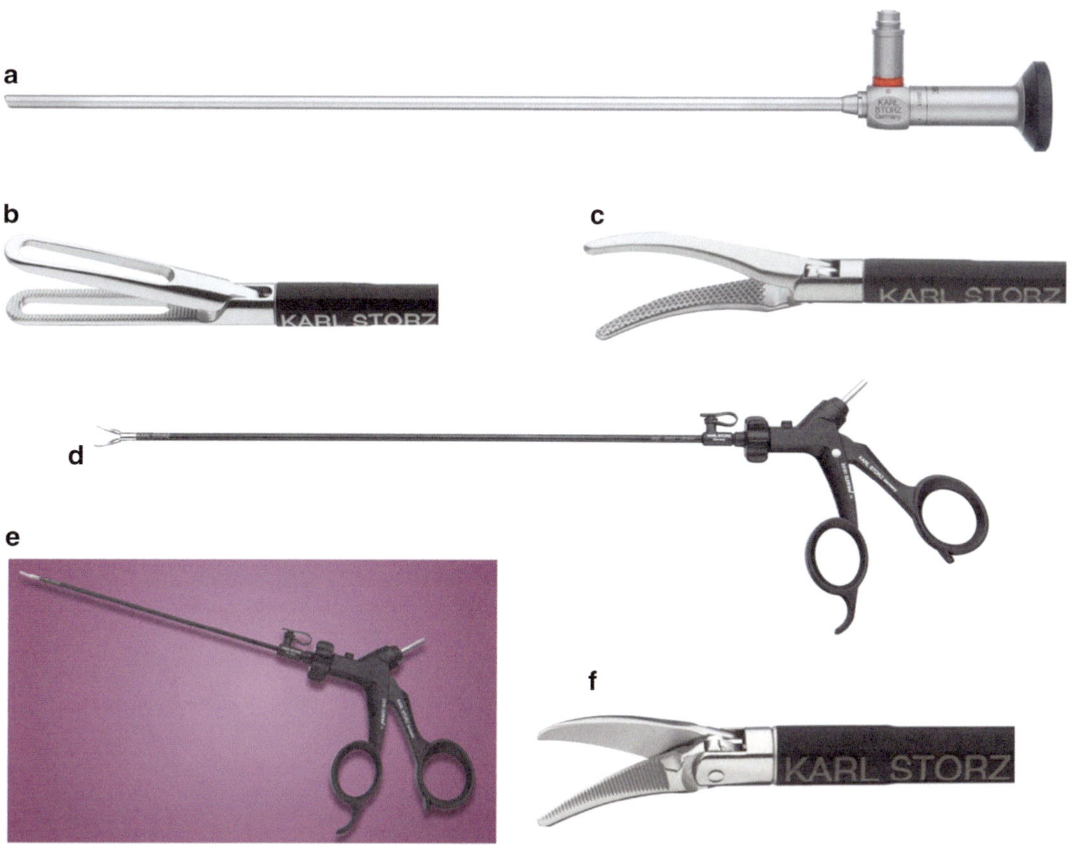

Fig. 13.1 Paediatric thoracoscopic instruments: (**a**) optic, (**b**) fenestrated forceps, (**c**, **d**) grasping forceps, (**e**, **f**) scissors (courtesy of KARL STORZ Endoscopia S.r.l.)

procedures. All biopsies are performed under general anaesthesia using a single-lumen endotracheal tube for conventional double-lung ventilation. Patients are placed in the lateral decubitus position, and a 5 or 10 mm trocar is placed in the pleural space below the tip of the scapula on the middle axillary line, usually at the fourth interspace.

CO_2 insufflation is started with maximal pressures of 3–5 mm of Hg in order to obtain an adequate space within to work. Use of CO_2 insufflation creates a pneumothorax and further collapses the ipsilateral lung and elevates the ipsilateral diaphragm [3, 5]. Single lung ventilation is useful in infants and children, but dual lumen tubes are difficult to place in small children [3]. Instead, the patient may undergo selective contralateral lung ventilation using ipsilateral bronchial blockers or Fogarty balloon catheters.

Table 13.3 Steps in thoracoscopic lung biopsy

Consecutive steps in thoracoscopic lung biopsy
– Preparation of the patient (information, fasting status, skin shaving)
– Radiographic review and patient positioning
– Induction of anaesthesia (selective contralateral lung ventilation)
– Patient positioning
– Choice of entry site/trocar positioning
– Induction of pneumothorax (insufflation of additional air/CO_2 into the pleural cavity if necessary)
– Inspection of the thoracic cavity using a thoracoscope
– Video and photographic recording
– Obtaining biopsy samples
– Control of bleeding
– Placement of thoracic drainage tubes
– Surveillance during recovery

The bioptic procedure is started by choosing the best site for paramount observation of the thoracic cavity. The suitable site for the biopsy is usually selected from the chest high-resolution computerized tomography scan (HRCT) and intraoperative macroscopic findings.

The working trocars are positioned according to the lesion of interest and ease of instrumental access. Each trocar site should be far enough away from the other to avoid the crossing of instruments, and all trocar sites must be located within the same 180° arc to avoid mirror imaging [8]. Trocars have to be placed far enough from the lesion to allow surgical manipulation and observation [8]. When considering these rules, the trocars are usually placed on three neighbouring corners of the lozenge with the target lesion on the remaining one. In most procedures, two to four access sites are necessary.

Biopsy instruments include Endoloop ligature (Fig. 13.2, Panel a), endostapler (Fig. 13.2, Panel b) and scissors (Fig. 13.2, Panel c) and are usually chosen by the performing surgeon [5]. Biopsies are removed through the largest trocar using atraumatic forceps. In smaller children (<15 kg) three 3–5 mm ports are used. In larger children, placement of a 12 mm port is recommended for the use of endoscopic staplers. Smaller children can be biopsied with biopsy forceps or after placement of Endoloops surrounding the tissue [9] and/or may be secured by sutures.

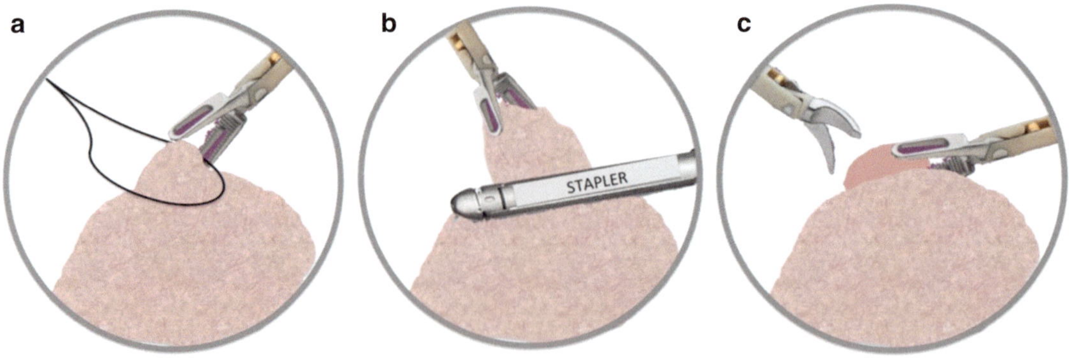

Fig. 13.2 Biopsy instruments: Endoloop ligature (Panel **a**), endostapler (Panel **b**), scissors (Panel **c**)

The 12 mm port for the stapler is placed as caudally as possible to allow the jaws to open properly. The specimen is excised with scissors or staples and removed through the largest trocar using atraumatic forceps. Bleeding and air leakage from the transected lung are controlled with absorbable sutures thoracoscopically placed.

Bleeding can also be controlled with cautery, laser or ultrasonic shears. However, re-expansion of the lung frequently controls bleeding. Placement of a drainage tube at the end of the procedure is recommended and is often based on the extent of ventilatory support the patient will require [5, 6].

13.8 Postoperative Care

In the postoperative period, the patient is kept in a normal decubitus position. As for all conscious sedation protocols, patients should refrain from eating and drinking 6–8 h after the procedure. The analgesic requirement (paracetamol every 6 h) is generally limited to the first 24 postoperative hours. All patients are discharged on the first or at a maximum on the second postoperative day.

13.9 Complications

The incidence of complications associated with thoracoscopic biopsies is considered to be acceptable. As reported in Table 13.4, potential complications can occur before, during or after the procedure [6].

The most serious complication during the procedure is bleeding. The main site of bleeding usually occurs at the intercostal vessels and lung parenchyma. According to various authors, it may occur in 8–12% of cases [10, 11]. Side effects can happen with any procedure. The most common side effect from a thoracoscopy is fever. The most common complication after biopsy is air leakage. An air leak lasting more than 7 days occurs in less than 5% of cases [10, 11]. Infectious complications, such as empyema, lung inflammation and postsurgical wound infections, occur with an incidence similar to that for other thoracoscopic procedure [12].

Table 13.4 Potential complications of the thoracoscopic bioptic approach [8]

Before the procedure
– Air embolism, subcutaneous emphysema and pain during pneumothorax induction
– Shortness of breath after pneumothorax induction
– Hypersensitivity reaction to local anaesthetic
During the procedure
– Pain
– Hypoxaemia
– Hypoventilation
– Cardiac arrhythmias
– Hypotension
– Haemorrhage
– Injury to the lung or other organs
After the procedure
– Pain
– Postoperative fever
– Wound infection
– Hypotension
– Empyema
– Subcutaneous emphysema
– Persisting pneumothorax
– Prolonged air leakage

13.10 Remarks

As reported by Fortman et al. [7], the diagnostic accuracy of thoracoscopic lung biopsies in children with suspected interstitial lung disease is high (98%). Thoracoscopic biopsy is also considered an effective diagnostic procedure for lung masses in immunocompetent and immunocompromised children [13, 14], and histopathologic results help define disease-specific treatment in the majority of cases. The morbidity rates of the procedure are low, and patients may benefit from avoiding thoracotomy [5].

13.11 Tips and Troubleshooting

The drawbacks of the thoracoscopic procedure compared with the open approach are well recognized. The thoracoscopic approach greatly reduces the surgeon's ability to use tactile feedback. The second disadvantage is that the images essentially lack three-dimensional information in spite of their high-quality resolution. The size of operative view is also restricted. Therefore, surgeons are required to be very familiar with the three-dimensional sensation of the phantom images and possess detailed knowledge of the topographical anatomy in the thorax as well as the possibility of anatomical variations [8].

Pulmonary nodules deeper than 1 cm under the visceral pleura may be difficult to identify by thoracoscopy. Ipsilateral lung collapse may help or alternatively a finger can be introduced through one of the port site openings for direct tactile perception. Other options available in such cases are stereotactic needle localization, preoperative localization utilizing CT guidance, preoperative tattooing with methylene blue or India ink and intraoperative ultrasonography [15].

In case a malignancy is suspected, it is important to deliver the specimen into a bag, to avoid port site seeding [4]. Concerning the biopsy technique, the Endoloop technique is considered a safe, effective technique in small paediatric patients. It avoids problems with the limited size of the chest cavity in patients less than 10 kg and avoids the introduction of large incisions in a small child [9].

13.12 Conclusion

Children with interstitial lung disease and isolated lesions associated with tumours frequently require thoracoscopic lung biopsies. The miniaturization of instruments and improved visualization with smaller scopes have enabled the successful performance of thoracoscopic lung biopsy in infants of almost any size, with a low complication rate. The significant benefits of thoracoscopic biopsy over conventional thoracotomy and the improved diagnostic yield over a transbronchial or percutaneous biopsy allow for earlier and more accurate diagnosis and treatment in infants and children with lung parenchymal disease.

References

1. Łochowski MP, Kozak J. Video-assisted thoracic surgery complications. Wideochir Inne Tech Maloinwazyjne. 2014;9(4):495–500.
2. Rodgers BM. Pediatric thoracoscopy: where have we come and what have we learned? Ann Thorac Surg. 1993;56(3):704–7.
3. Shah R, Reddy AS, Dhende NP. Video assisted thoracic surgery in children. J Minim Access Surg. 2007;3(4):161–7.
4. Landreneau RJ, Mack MJ, Hazelrigg SR, et al. Video-assisted thoracic surgery: basic technical concepts and intercostal approach strategies. Ann Thorac Surg. 1992;54(4):800–7.
5. Fortmann C, Schwerk N, Wetzke M, Schukfeh N, Ure BM, Dingemann J. Diagnostic accuracy and therapeutic relevance of thoracoscopic lung biopsies in children. Pediatr Pulmonol. 2018;53(7):948–53.
6. Loddenkemper R, Lee P, Noppen M, Mathur PN. Medical thoracoscopy/pleuroscopy: step by step. Breathe. 2011;8(2):157–67.
7. Fuger M, Clair MP, El Ayoun Ibrahim N, L'Excellent S, Nizery L, O'Neill C, Tabone L, Truffinet O, Yakovleff C, de Blic J. Chronic interstitial lung disease in children: diagnostic approach and management. Arch Pediatr. 2016;23(5):525–31.
8. Asamura H. Thoracoscopic procedures for intrathoracic diseases: the present status. Respirology. 1999;4(1):9–17.
9. Ponsky TA, Rothenberg SS. Thoracoscopic lung biopsy in infants and children with endoloops allows smaller trocar sites and discreet biopsies. J Laparoendosc Adv Surg Tech A. 2008;18(1):120–2.
10. Jancovici R, Lang-Lazdunski L, Pons F, et al. Complication of video-assisted thoracic surgery. Ann Thorac Surg. 1996;61(2):553–7.
11. Kaiser LR, Bavaria JE. Complication of thoracoscopy. Ann Thorac Surg. 1993;56(3):796–8.
12. Imperatori A, Rotolo N, Gatti M, Nardecchia E, De Monte L, Conti V, Dominioni L. Peri-operative complications of video-assisted thoracoscopic surgery. Int J Surg. 2008;6(suppl 1):S78–81.
13. Daniel TM, Kern JA, Tribble CG, Kron IL, Spotnitz WB, Rodgers BM. Thoracoscopic surgery for diseases of the lung and pleura. Effectiveness, changing indications, and limitations. Ann Surg. 1993;217(5):566–74.
14. Tsao K, St Peter SD, Sharp SW, Nair A, Andrews WS, Sharp RJ, Snyder CL, Ostlie DJ, Holcomb GW. Current application of thoracoscopy in children. J Laparoendosc Adv Surg Tech A. 2008;18(1):131–5.
15. Piolanti M, Coppola F, Papa S, Pilotti V, Mattioli S, Gavelli G. Ultrasonographic localization of occult pulmonary nodules during video-assisted thoracic surgery. Eur Radiol. 2003;13(10):2358–64.

Management of Pleural Empyema 14

Anna-May Long and Alex C. H. Lee

14.1 Introduction

Pleural infection in children most commonly occurs after pneumonia, though may complicate trauma or surgery. Following parenchymal lung infection, exudative effusion solidifies over time due to the deposition of fibrin causing encasement of the lung, affecting expansion and trapping pockets of infected fluid preventing resolution [1].

Small effusions will settle with antibiotics alone but larger ones require intervention. Pleural drainage may be sufficient before organisation has occurred, but for those that have become loculated, various management strategies have been described [2–5]. The least invasive of these is the instillation of intrapleural fibrinolytic therapy through a narrow bore chest drain inserted via a *Seldinger* technique [6]. Urokinase and tissue plasminogen activator (tPA) are the most widely used fibrinolytic agents with high levels of success and excellent safety profiles [5–10]. These agents may not be available in all settings, and where they are not, thoracoscopic drainage of the fibrinous coagulum and pyogenic material by video-assisted thoracoscopic surgery (VATS) is a reasonable option, comparing favourably with more aggressive management [4]. After a peak in the usage of VATS in the past decade, its use has declined and in many countries has been supplanted by the use of chest drainage and intrapleural fibrinolysis [11].

For all children with complicated parapneumonic effusion, a multidisciplinary approach with paediatric respiratory medicine, physiotherapy and clinical microbiology alongside surgical care is essential. The use of a standardised clinical care pathway has streamlined the care of these children [7].

14.2 Preoperative Preparation

Following plain radiograph, thoracic ultrasound is used to confirm the diagnosis of parapneumonic effusion and allow assessment of size, inflation of the underlying lung and the level of organisation. This allows preoperative marking of the ideal drain placement site. CT scan should be reserved for those with suspicion or underlying parenchymal abscess formation or lung necrosis [3, 4].

A.-M. Long
Department of Paediatric Surgery, Addenbrooke's Hospital, Cambridge University Hospitals NHS Foundation Trust, Cambridge, UK
e-mail: Anna-May.Long@addenbrookes.nhs.uk

A. C. H. Lee (✉)
Department of Paediatric Surgery, Oxford Children's Hospital, Oxford University Hospitals NHS Foundation Trust, Oxford, UK
e-mail: alex.lee@paediatrics.ox.ac.uk

C. Esposito et al. (eds.), *ESPES Manual of Pediatric Minimally Invasive Surgery*,
https://doi.org/10.1007/978-3-030-00964-9_14

Appropriate broad spectrum antibiotic cover should be administered according to local protocols.

14.3 Chest Drain Insertion

Chest drain insertion can be performed safely under local anaesthesia and sedation where facilities and expertise are available. Otherwise it is done in the operating theatre under general anaesthesia. The patient is positioned supine with the arm folded up behind the child's head. A narrow bore (e.g. 8–9Fr) 'pigtail' chest drain inserted via a *Seldinger* technique is associated with less postoperative discomfort and leak than a larger drain inserted using open technique [6, 7].

Ultrasound guidance during insertion is a useful adjunct to confirm the diagnosis, but this is not essential, particularly if the child has been previously marked during a diagnostic scan. Local anaesthetic instillation at the drain site prior to placement will alleviate postoperative discomfort.

The fifth intercostal space, mid-axilliary line is the most common site for drain placement, although this may depend on the distribution of the effusion.

The effusion should be drained to a maximum of 20 mL/kg in the first instance, to prevent rebound pulmonary oedema. Samples of fluid should be sent for cell count, culture and sensitivity as well as PCR assay for *Streptococcus pneumoniae*. A check chest radiograph soon after insertion should confirm an adequate position and lung re-expansion.

14.3.1 Intrapleural Fibrinolytic Therapy

The first dose of intrapleural fibrinolytic can be administered immediately and the drain clamped for 4 h [7]. A commonly utilised protocol for fibrinolytic therapy involves the administration of a total of six doses of intra-pleural urokinase at 12 h intervals [6, 8]. The doses used are: 40,000 IU in 40 mls of saline for children above 12 months of age and 10,000 units in 10 mls for saline for those under a year. The fibrinolytic is left in the chest for four hours and then the drain unclamped. Children are encouraged to mobilise, particularly when the fibrinolytic is in the chest, to facilitate its distribution. Drains are removed after the 6th dose if the child's condition warrants this.

14.4 VATS

14.4.1 Positioning

The child is placed in the lateral position with the affected side upward. The arm is supported on a pillow or with an arm rest as for a thoracotomy. A roll may be placed under the chest in order to maximally spread the ribs. The surgeon stands at the child's back facing the screen.

The assistant should stand at the surgeon's side to avoid paradoxical movements which may occur when the surgeon and assistant stand on either side of the bed. This is particularly so when the two monitors are placed at either sides of the table and when the endoscope is pointing towards the viewer. This may, however, be unavoidable in smaller children due to limited external space.

14.4.2 Instrumentation

An operating endoscope, where available, provides an effective means of undertaking thoracoscopic debridement through a single port using a suction/irrigation system and blunt (Johann) bowel grasping forceps for dissection and removing the fibrinous peel.

If this is not available, a two-port technique is usually used. Port site placement will depend on the location of the empyema, but commonly a 5 mm 30° endoscope is placed anterior to the mid-axilliary line in the sixth intercostal space. A 3–5 mm working port, depending on size of the child, is placed on the dominant-hand side of the camera port. For older children, a 10 mm port may be useful to facilitate removal of debris, although the width of the rib space may limit this. Optics and instruments may be swapped between ports. If indicated, further third port may be needed to ensure the full thoracic cavity can be inspected and reached.

Special energy devices are usually not required. A sputum trap, placed in the suction circuit, may be used to retrieve samples of fluid.

14.4.3 Technique

Single lung ventilation may be preferred by the surgical and anaesthetic team although this is not essential and may not be tolerated. Total general anaesthetic time should not be significantly prolonged to achieve single-lung ventilation. If used, this can be achieved via a dual lumen tube or bronchial blocker.

Local anaesthetic instillation at the port sites prior to placement will alleviate postoperative discomfort. Alternatively an intercostal block in the relevant rib spaces may be performed at the end of the procedure.

After camera port placement, insufflation should be limited to 4–6 mmHg of CO_2 to disrupt pleural adhesions and to cause lung collapse. Initial dissection to create the working space may begin with gentle broad sweeps of the endoscope especially infero-posteriorly. Once the pleural operative space is established, secondary working port(s) to the right and/or left of the central port is (are) used for suction/irrigation and instrumentation.

A fresh sample of the pleural fluid should be collected for laboratory analysis (see chest drain insertion). The aims are: (i) to further break down any fluid-filled loculations within the pleural cavity, (ii) to remove "peel" or rind as much as possible from the surface of the visceral pleura facilitating lung expansion, (iii) to free the lung from the parietal pleura while avoiding bleeding or damage to the viscera including the phrenic nerve. Blunt grasping forceps are preferred to avoid inadvertent injury. A damp swab may be used externally to remove the peel from the grasping forceps.

Once the pleural fluid has been drained and most of the fibrinous peel is removed, the pleural space is irrigated with warm saline and subsequently suctioned.

A chest drain is left in the anterior port site, guided thoracoscopically and secured externally. Instruments and ports are removed under vision. Lung expansion is enabled by letting out the insufflated CO_2, releasing the ipsilateral airway occlusion if this has been used for double-lung ventilation and a few positive pressure breaths from the anaesthetist. The trocar sites are closed in layers and the chest drain attached to an underwater sealed bottle.

14.4.4 Postoperative Care

A chest radiograph is obtained in recovery or soon after returning to the ward to check the drain position and lung re-expansion. A period of low negative suction may be required to facilitate lung expansion, otherwise drainage using an underwater seal should be sufficient. Chest radiographs are taken to monitor progress. The drain is removed once it is confirmed that the lung has fully expanded, the drainage is physiological, the child has improved clinically and there is no suspicion of residual pleural collection. If the latter is confirmed, intrapleural fibrinolytics may additionally be of use. Antibiotic duration will be guided by the child's condition according to local protocol. Adequate analgesia is important, and usually intravenous opiates are used in the first 24–48 h. Clinic follow up appointments with chest radiographs are arranged to confirm complete resolution.

14.5 Results

The outcomes of intervention for paediatric empyema will vary according to the age, comorbidity, microbiological aetiology and extent of parenchymal lung disease in affected children.

Although a lower mortality is expected in children than adults, a large database study from the USA demonstrated a case fatality among 14,936 with this condition of 3.2% (2003–2008) [12]. In the *Alder Hey Children's Hospital* series (2006–2012), mortality was 0.4% among 239 children [7] and death was associated with significant co-morbidities. In this series 21% of all children were admitted to a high dependency or intensive care unit. Children infected with Group A *Streptococcus* as a causative agent had more severe ilness with 58% requiring HDU or ICU admissions.

Consent for minimally invasive intervention should include the need for re-intervention which varies between published series with most suggesting a rate of 15–20% among all-comers [7, 12]. Re-intervention approaches include the insertion of a larger bore chest drain, VATS or thoracotomy, the latter may be necessary in children with necrotising disease and bronchopleural fistula [4, 7].

Both mechanical and chemical debridement with fibrinolytics have a low rate of complications and have demonstrated similar outcomes in clinical trials. Median post-procedural length of hospital stay is similar among those treated with VATS or fibrinolysis and is 6–10 days in published series [4, 7, 13].

14.6 Tips and Tricks

Attachment of a "three-way tap" to the chest drain allows drainage and easy access for instillation of fibrinolytics. A sturdy fixation such as a "drain-fix" dressing helps to prevent dislodgement and does not involve suture removal on the ward.

The suction/irrigation device may be used to suction fluid as well as to perform blunt dissection.

Short length endoscopic instruments are preferable and may be inserted directly a stab incision without a trocar. Handheld instruments, e.g. large haemostat clips or sponge holding forceps, can be used to insert directly under thoracoscopic vision to peel the pleural rind though the pleural space may be limited (due to the non-collapsed lung).

14.7 Discussion

A few randomised controlled trials have compared VATS to thoracostomy drainage in children with complicated parapneumonic effusion [5, 8, 10, 13, 14]. The evidence from these was assessed and synthesised in a recent Cochrane review [5]. No difference was found in the included studies in mortality, length of hospital stay or procedural complications. The quality of the evidence was found to be low and particularly lacking concerning the use of fibrinolytics. A few randomised controlled trials and several large observational studies have, however, shown these to be safe, and they appear as effective as VATS [7–10, 12–15].

Chemical debridement is a more cost-effective approach than VATS due to a shorter operative time [4, 10, 13]. For this reason, where the preparations are available, fibrinolytic therapy is recommended as a primary management strategy over VATS. This approach has been endorsed both by the American Paediatric Surgical Association Outcomes and Clinical Trials Committee [4] and the British Thoracic Society [3] and is gaining popularity [11].

Some children will inevitably fail this treatment course, and VATS may be an appropriate second-line therapy [4] although, where failure is due to necrotizing disease or bronchopleural fistula open surgery may be preferable, particularly in the presence of physiological instability [4, 7].

References

1. Hamm H, Light RW. Parapneumonic effusion and empyema. Eur Respir J. 1997;10(5):1150–6.
2. Cremonesini D, Thomson A. How should we manage empyema: antibiotics alone, fibrinolytics, or primary video-assisted thoracoscopic surgery (VATS)? Semin Respir Crit Care Med. 2007;28:322–32.
3. Balfour-Lynn IM, Abrahamson E, Cohen G, Hartley J, King S, Parikh D, et al. BTS guidelines for the management of pleural infection in children. Thorax. 2005;60(suppl 1):i1–21.
4. Islam S, Calkins CM, Goldin AB, Chen C, Downard CD, Huang EY, et al. APSA Outcomes and Clinical Trials Committee, 2011-2012. The diagnosis and management of empyema in children: a comprehensive review from the APSA Outcomes and Clinical Trials Committee. J Pediatr Surg. 2012;47:2101–10.

5. Redden MD, Chin TY, van Driel ML. Surgical versus non-surgical management for pleural empyema. Cochrane Database Syst Rev. 2017;(3).
6. Thomson AH, Hull J, Kumar MR, Wallis C, Balfour Lynn IM. Randomised trial of intrapleural urokinase in the treatment of childhood empyema. Thorax. 2002;57:343–7.
7. Long AM, Smith-Williams J, Mayell S, Couriel J, Jones MO, Losty PD. 'Less may be best'—pediatric parapneumonic effusion and empyema management: lessons from a UK center. J Pediatr Surg. 2016;51:588–91.
8. Sonnappa S, Cohen G, Owens CM, van Doorn C, Cairns J, Stanojevic S, et al. Comparison of urokinase and video-assisted thoracoscopic surgery for treatment of childhood empyema. Am J Respir Crit Care Med. 2006;174:221–7.
9. Gasior AC, Knott EM, Sharp SW, Ostlie DJ, Holcomb GW III, St Peter SD. Experience with an evidence-based protocol using fibrinolysis as first line treatment for empyema in children. J Pediatr Surg. 2013;48:1312–5.
10. St Peter SD, Tsao K, Spilde TL, Keckler SJ, Harrison C, Jackson MA, Sharp SW, et al. Thoracoscopic decortication vs tube thoracostomy with fibrinolysis for empyema in children: a prospective, randomized trial. J Pediatr Surg. 2009;44:106–11.
11. Dorman RM, Vali K, Rothstein DH. Trends in treatment of infectious parapneumonic effusions in U.S. children's hospitals. 2004–2014. J Pediatr Surg. 2016;51:885–90.
12. Goldin AB, Parimi C, LaRiviere C, Garrison MM, Larison CL, Sawin RS. Outcomes associated with type of intervention and timing in complex pediatric empyema. Am J Surg. 2012;203:665–73.
13. Marhuenda C, Barceló C, Fuentes I, Guillén G, Cano I, López M, et al. Urokinase versus VATS for treatment of empyema: a randomized multicenter clinical trial. Pediatrics. 2014;134:e1301–7.
14. Cobanoglu U, Sayir F, Bilici S, Melek M. Comparison of the methods of fibrinolysis by tube thoracostomy and thoracoscopic decortication in children with stage II and III empyema: a prospective randomized study. Pediatr Rep. 2011;3:e29.
15. Griffith D, Boal M, Rogers T. Evolution of practice in the management of parapneumonic effusion and empyema in children. J Pediatr Surg. 2018;53:644–6.

Thoracoscopic Lobectomy

15

Steven Rothenberg

15.1 Introduction

There are numerous indications requiring pulmonary lobe resections in infants and children. The majority are for the broad spectrum of bronchopulmonary malformations that present in early infancy and childhood. These include bronchogenic cysts, bronchopulmonary sequestrations (BPS), congenital pulmonary airway malformation (CPAM), and congenital lobar emphysema (CLE) [1]. These lesions may be detected by prenatal ultrasound, present as acute respiratory distress in the newborn period, or may remain undiagnosed and asymptomatic until later in life. The other major indications include chronic infection resulting in bronchiectasis and malignancy. Treatment may vary somewhat depending on the time of diagnosis and the presentation, but in most cases complete lobar resection is the desired therapy. Minimally invasive techniques now allow these procedures to be done with much less pain and morbidity and avoid the long-term consequence of a thoracotomy in an infant or small child.

However, thoracoscopic lobectomy can be one of the most technically demanding procedures performed by a pediatric surgeon. The ability to first correctly identify vital structures to both the affected lobe and those going to areas needing to be preserved, and then safely secure the large pulmonary vessels, and a general lack of adequate lung case volume for most pediatric surgical trainees make these procedures even more difficult to adopt. In order to address these issues, we have developed a standardized approach to perform thoracoscopic lobectomy and applied these techniques in training fellows and junior staff.

15.2 Positioning

The procedure should be performed with the patient in a lateral decubitus position with the affected side up. In most cases with single lung ventilation, obtained by mainstem intubation of the contralateral side. In larger patients a double lumen endotracheal tube or bronchial blocker can be used. In cases where single lung ventilation cannot be achieved, CO_2 insufflation alone can used. The surgeon and assistant stand at the patient's front. In smaller children the patient should be placed near the edge of the table, so the handle of the instruments are not obstructed by the table.

S. Rothenberg (✉)
Rocky Mountain Hospital for Children,
Denver, CO, USA
e-mail: steven.rothenberg@hcahealthcare.com

C. Esposito et al. (eds.), *ESPES Manual of Pediatric Minimally Invasive Surgery*,
https://doi.org/10.1007/978-3-030-00964-9_15

15.3 Instrumentation

Three valved ports, ranging from 3 to 5 mm, are used. In the majority of cases, a bipolar vessel-sealing device is used to manage the pulmonary vessels. In most cases, a 3 mm vessel sealer (JustRight Surgical, Louisville, CO) is employed; in patients over 15 kg, a Maryland 5 mm LigaSure is used. These devises are also used to seal and divide the lung parenchyma in cases of an incomplete fissure. The vessels are managed by obtaining adequate length of the vessel to create two seals approximately 3–5 mm apart and then dividing the vessel between them (Fig. 15.1). In larger patients (generally those over 15–20 kg), a 5 or 12 mm endoscopic stapler can be used to secure some or all of the major pulmonary vessels. If these are not available, clips for smaller bronchi or division and suture ligature can be used.

15.4 Technique

The room is set up to facilitate an anterior approach. The surgeon and assistant are at the patient's front with the monitor at the patient's back (Fig. 15.1). First the chest is insufflated with CO_2 using a Veress needle to help collapse the lung and avoid injury of the parenchyma with a trocar. Three trocars are used in almost all cases. The first port is placed in the mid- to anterior axillary line in the fifth or sixth interspace to determine the position of the major fissure and evaluate the lung parenchyma. Position of the fissure should dictate the placement of the other ports. The working ports are placed in the anterior axillary line above and below the camera port (Fig. 15.2).

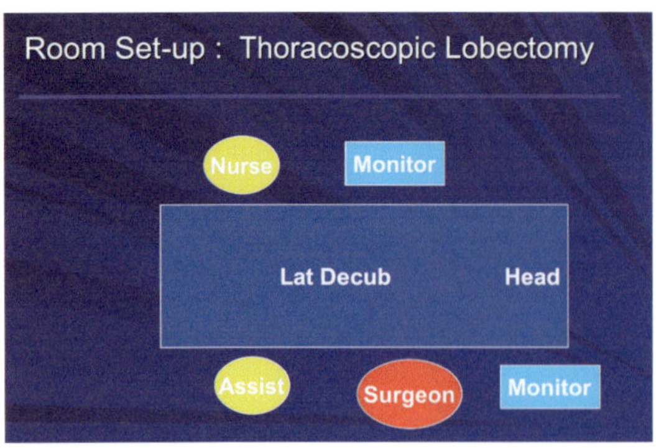

Fig. 15.1 Appropriate room setup for thoracoscopic lung resection

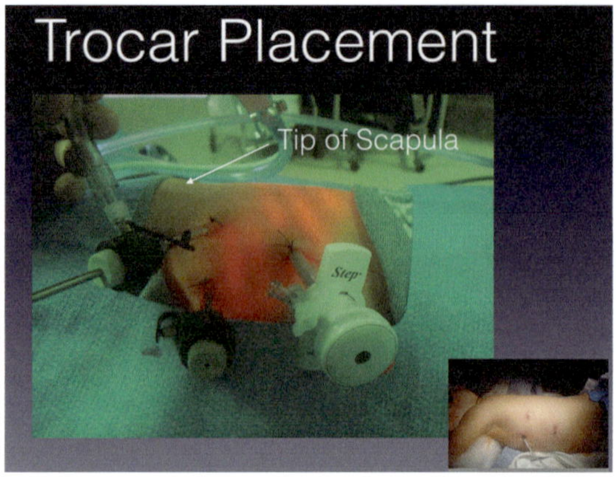

Fig. 15.2 Trocar placement for LLL. 4 mm camera port, left hand 3 mm port, and right hand 5 mm port for endoscopic stapler

For a lower lobe, the inferior pulmonary ligament is taken first until the inferior pulmonary vein (PV) is exposed. During this portion care is taken to look for a systemic vessel arising from the thoracic aorta or up through the diaphragm. The major fissure is then examined and if necessary completed using tissue sealing. This is done in an almost finger fracture technique until the pulmonary artery is seen transversing the fissure. The branches of pulmonary artery to the lower lobe are then sealed and divided, often at the segmental level. If necessary dissection can be carried out into the parenchyma of the lower lobe to obtain adequate length of the segmental branches for safe sealing and division. After this the bronchus to the lower lobe is visualized lying directly under the divide arterial trunk. It is mobilized and divided with the endoscopic stapler (Fig. 15.3). In many cases it is beneficial to take the superior segmental bronchus first and then the trunk to the basal segments. This exposes the inferior pulmonary vein trunk which can be easily divided with the 5 mm stapler (Fig. 15.4). If not available, the vessel should be followed proximally toward the parenchyma where it branches,

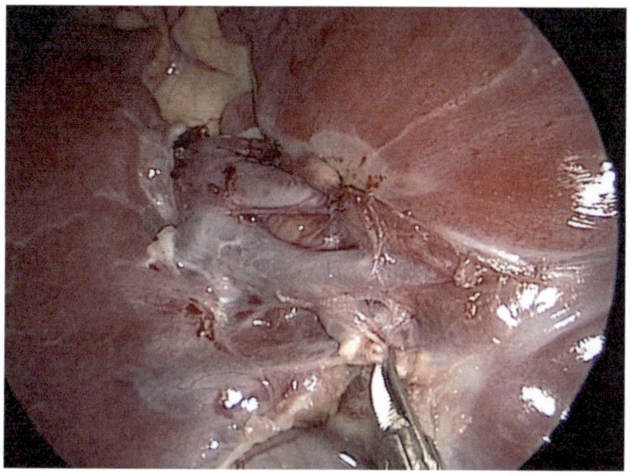

Fig. 15.3 Proximal and distal seals on anterior basal branch of pulmonary artery with scissors dividing vessel between the two seals

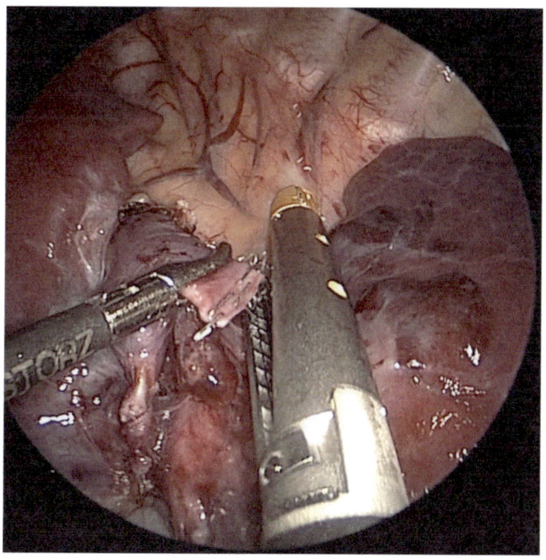

Fig. 15.4 Dividing main pulmonary artery to LLL with 5 mm stapler. The 3 mm Maryland keeps proximal vascular control until it is clear that the staple line is secure

and the smaller branches can be sealed and divided as already described. If there are large space-occupying cysts, these are "collapsed or popped" first using the vessel sealer. The cystic areas of the lung are grasped and energy applied (Fig. 15.5). This causes the cyst to decompress and collapse, creating more intrathoracic space and improving the surgeon's ability to manipulate the lung and identify important structures. The specimen is then removed in a piecemeal fashion through a slightly dilated 5 mm trocar

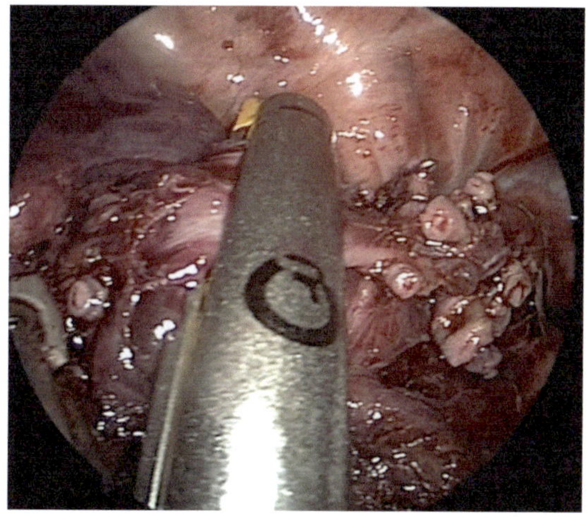

Fig. 15.5 Taking bronchus to RUL with 5 mm stapler

site. A chest tube is left in all cases of lobar resection.

15.5 Postoperative Care

The patient is managed on the ward with IV narcotics for the first night. The CT is kept to 10–15 mmH_2O suction. If there is no air leak, it is placed to H_2O seal, and an X-ray is obtained in 2 h. If there is no pneumothorax, the CT is removed. Most patients are discharged on the second postoperative day.

15.6 Results

Over the last 25 years, 499 of 502 procedures were completed thoracoscopically. Operative times ranged from 35 to 240 min (avg. 115 min). Average operative time when a trainee was the primary surgeon was 160 min (N = 83) and 95 min when the senior surgeon was performing the procedure. There were 109 upper, 33 middle, and 260 lower lobe resections. There were four intraoperative complications (1.1%) requiring conversion to an open thoracotomy. Three of these were secondary to bleeding, and one was to repair a compromised bronchus to an upper lobe following a lower lobectomy. Only one of these, a bleeding vessel to a pulmonary sequestration, occurred in the last 15 years of the study period. The postoperative complication rate was 3.3%, and three patients (0.8%) required re-exploration for a prolonged air leak. In two cases a small accessory bronchus was found and sutured closed. In the third, no leak was identified, and the patient had no air leak postoperatively. Hospital stay (LOS) ranged from 1 to 16 days with a mean of 3.2 days. In patients <5 kg and < 3 months of age, the average operative time was 78 min, and LOS was 1.8 days. The postoperative complication rate was 2.6% and LOS 2.1 days.

15.7 Tips and Tricks

Use vessel sealing as the primary mode of vessel division.

Collapse all large cystic spaces.

Dissect into the lung parenchyma to gain greater vessel and bronchus length.

15.8 Discussion

Thoracoscopic lobectomy in children for congenital cystic lung disease is now an accepted and well-described technique [2–6]. Most authors agree on the relative merits of a thoracoscopic approach including less pain, shorter hospital stay, and decreased long-term morbidity, including chest wall deformity, shoulder girdle weakness, and scoliosis [7]. Despite this general consensus, the adoption of this technique and surgeon comfort with the approach remains relatively low primarily because of the procedure is technically demanding and because most surgeons see a low volume of cases which results in a decreased familiarity with pulmonary anatomy. Using a thoracoscopic approach further compounds this, as the surgeon can no longer put their hand in the chest cavity to palpate the structures and identify the anatomy. Therefore, standardization of technique and approach is critical.

One of the most difficult aspects of these cases is when the fissure is incomplete and the pulmonary vessels are not readily visible. We have found that using the tissue sealing technology to dissect and divide the parenchyma of an incomplete fissure is the safest way to approach this. The fissure is approached layer by layer until the pulmonary artery is visualized (Fig. 15.4). In our experience using the vessel sealer results in limited bleeding and air leak as compared to other methods.

The second issue has been standardizing an anterior approach. During an open thoracotomy, the surgeon is generally positioned at the patients back. For thoracoscopic lobectomies the surgeon and assistant are positioned at the patient's front. This is especially important in smaller patients, as there is more room from the chest wall to the mediastinum, where the pulmonary vessels arise.

The anatomic relationships for each lobe using this anterior approach are critical. The three-dimensional relationships of the vessels and bronchi to each lobe, which cannot always be seen in the two-dimensional view of the scope, are critical in understanding and comfort with the anatomy.

The third major issue is standardizing the management of the pulmonary vessels. Early in our experience we learned that thoracoscopic suture ligation of each individual vessel was difficult and time-consuming. The small working space, difficulty in achieving traction and counter-traction to obtain adequate vessel length while suturing, and the technical demands of tying a secure knot made this process laborious. We did not favor endoscopic clips for most vessels because of the risk of dislodging them during the extensive tissue manipulation necessary during a lobectomy. Therefore, we adopted vessel sealing as a way to safely manage the pulmonary vessels [8]. The initial 5 mm sealing device used could manage a vessel up to 7 mm in diameter and was an adequate tissue dissector. The 3 mm sealing device now available can seal vessels up to 5 mm and works well as a dissector especially in the smaller chest cavities of infants. It is more than adequate for most pulmonary vessels in children under 10 kg and for segmental branches in larger children. A key to using vessel-sealing technology effectively is to make proximal and distal seals on the vessel approximately 3–5 mm

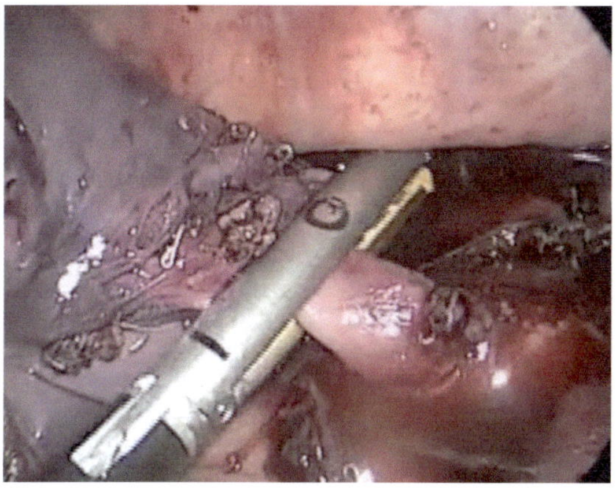

Fig. 15.6 Taking the inferior pulmonary vein to the RLL with the 5 mm stapler. Care is taken to insure there is an adequate stump length in case there are any issues

apart. Using scissors, a partial cut is made to determine that the seals are secure and that there is no bleeding once the lumen is entered. Once the vessel is partially divided and no bleeding is seen, the vessel can be completely divided (Fig. 15.6). If there appears to be some bleeding, there is an opportunity to reseal the vessel before the vessel retracts and control is lost. Because of the relatively large nature of the pulmonary vessels, and the limited space in the chest cavity, it takes very little blood to obscure the operative field and force conversion to an open thoracotomy. For this reason we have avoided any energy devises which seal and divide the vessel in one step, because if the seal fails the ability to salvage the situation is minimal.

For bronchus management we initially cut and then suture the bronchus using PDS suture in smaller patients. This can be time-consuming and technically demanding. We discovered that in most patients less than 10 kg, the lobar or segmental bronchus could be occluded using 5 mm endoscopic clips. If the lobar bronchus is too large, then distal dissection allows for a segmental bronchus to be taken. This decreases the size of the remaining main trunk. For example, the superior segment bronchus in a lower lobectomy can be occluded separately, and then the trunk to the basal segments can be taken with a second clip. In larger patients we used the 12 mm endoscopic linear staplers. However, because of the variations in anatomy and the close proximity of the bronchus to the other lobes, extreme care must be taken to avoid compromising the other bronchi. Therefore, if there is any question, the bronchus to the target lobe should be divided sharply and sutured close. There is now new 5 mm stapling technology which better fits in the chest cavity of infants and children and should eliminate the use of clips and larger staplers in these smaller patients.

The timing of surgery remains somewhat controversial, but there is little evidence to suggest that delayed resection improves outcome. We favor earlier resection of prenatally diagnosed lesions before they become infected or the patients become symptomatic. We have previously documented our experience with infants under 10 kg and showed that these procedures had shorter operative times, lower complication rates, and shorter hospital stays [9]. In older infants, there can be significant adenopathy and inflammation in the fissures and around the pulmonary artery making identification and safe division of these vessels much more difficult. These procedures are technically easier in infants at or near 5 kg despite the smaller working space as evidenced by the shorter operative times in this group as compared to older patients. The length of stay in this group is also shorter. Lastly for those who argue for conservative nonoperative management of these lesions in asymptomatic patients, despite the high incidence of infection, we had two cases of unsuspected pulmonary blastoma [10, 11]. We feel the risk of recurrent infection and possible malignancy outweigh the risks of intervention if a thoracoscopic approach is used in an institution with a large experience in these procedures.

References

1. Rothenberg SS, Cromblehome TM. Congenital lung malformations. In: Ziegler M, Azizkhan R, Weber T, Von Allmen D, editors. Operative pediatric surgery. 2nd ed. New York: McGraw Hill; 2014.
2. Rothenberg SS. First decades experience with thoracoscopic lobectomy in infants and children. J Pediatr Surg. 2008;43:40–5.

3. Cano I, Anton-Pacheco JL, Garcia A, Rothenberg S. Video-assisted 322 thoracoscopic lobectomy in infants. Eur J Cardiothorac Surg. 2006;29:997–1000.
4. Diamond IR, Herrera P, Langer JC, Kim PC. Thoracoscopic versus open resection of congenital lung lesions: a case matched study. J Pediatr Surg. 2007;42:1057–61.
5. Vu LT, Farmer DL, Nobuhara KK, Miniati D, Lee H. J Pediatr Surg. 2008;43:35–9.
6. Albanese CT, Sydorak RM, Tsao K, et al. Thoracoscopic lobectomy of prenatally diagnosed lung lesions. J Pediatr Surg. 2003;38:553–5.
7. Lawal TA, Gosemann JH, Kuebler JF, Gluer S, Urer BM. Thoracoscopy versus thoracotomy improves mid-term musculoskeletal status and cosmesis in infants and children. Ann Thorac Surg. 2009;87:224–8.
8. Yoshida K, Toishi M, Eguchi T, Saito G, Shiina T, Kondo R, Amano J. Feasibility of using a vessel sealing system in a human pulmonary lobectomy: a retrospective comparison of this procedure with or without a vessel sealing system. Ann Thorac Cardiovasc Surg. 2014;20(5):353–8.
9. Rothenberg SS, Kuenzler K, Middlesworth W, Kay S, Yoder S, Shipman K, Rodriguez R, Stolar C. Thoracoscopic lobectomy in infants <10 kg with prenatally diagnosed cystic lung disease. J Laproendosc Adv Surg Technol. 2011;21(2):181–4.
10. Fingeret A, Garcia A, Borczuk AC, Rothenberg SS, Aspelund G. Thoracoscopic lobectomy for type 1 pleuropulmonary blastoma in an infant. Pediatr Surg Int. 2013;30:239–42.
11. Rothenberg SS, Middlesworth WE, et al. Two decades of experience with thoracoscopic lobectomy in infants and children: standardizing techniques for advanced thoracoscopic surgery. J Laproendosc Adv Surg Technol A. 2015;25(5):423–8.

Thorascoscopic Management of Pulmonary Sequestration

16

Henri Steyaert

16.1 Introduction

Extralobar sequestration is a part of a lung, separated from the normal lung, with a separate pleura, and attached to the mediastinum by only its feeding systemic vessels (Fig. 16.1).

Intralobar sequestration is a part of a lung separated from the normal bronchial tree, included in a normal lobe, and also attached by feeding systemic vessels. Differentiation between congenital cystic adenomatoid malformations (CCAM) and intralobar sequestration is not always easy and not accurate anymore since those lesions may be mixed ones. The term congenital pulmonary adenomatoid malformations (CPAM) has to be used for these lesions nowadays [1].

In this chapter we will only discuss management of extralobar sequestration. Bronchogenic cysts and esophageal duplication are treated by the same way and technique [2]. For intralobar sequestration a lobectomy is mostly mandatory and will be discussed in another chapter.

More and more sequestrations are diagnosed prenatally. Debate about the ideal age of resection is still ongoing and depends mainly on surgeon's experience [3]. In the majority of the cases, for anesthesiologic reasons, surgery is scheduled after 3–6 months of age.

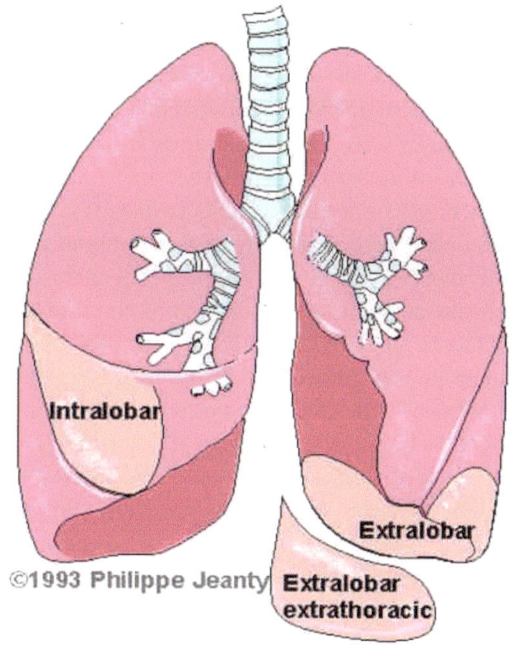

Fig. 16.1 Types of sequestrations

H. Steyaert (✉)
Department of Pediatric Surgery, Université Libre de Bruxelles (ULB), HUDERF Children's Hospital, Brussels, Belgium
e-mail: henri.steyaert@huderf.be

C. Esposito et al. (eds.), *ESPES Manual of Pediatric Minimally Invasive Surgery*,
https://doi.org/10.1007/978-3-030-00964-9_16

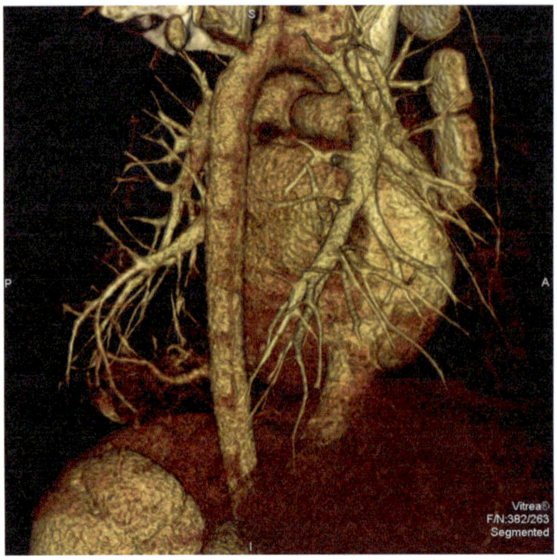

Fig. 16.2 3D reconstruction—vascular supply of an extralobar sequestration

16.2 Preoperative Preparation

Diagnosis is mostly confirmed with the help of an MRI (or CT scan) just before surgery. 3D reconstruction is more and more used and may be helpful in cases were the sequestration is fixed to the lobe or intralobar [4] (Fig. 16.2).

A single intravenous line is sufficient in most cases along with pulse oximetry and blood pressure monitoring. A single preoperative dose of cephalosporin is given depending on hospital protocols. A nasogastric tube is mostly placed due to the lateral decubitus position of the patient.

Whenever possible, single-lung ventilation is obtained because it will give the surgeon time and space in order to do a proper dissection of the feeding vessels, ligate, and cut them. Surgery without single-lung ventilation is possible but needs a perfect collaboration between the anesthesiologist and the surgeon. Indeed, hypercapnia is quickly increasing during thoracoscopy, much more than during laparoscopy.

16.3 Positioning

Because the lesion is mostly posterior, the patient is positioned in a modified prone position (affected side elevated 30–45°). This position allows the lung to fall down anteriorly. An axillary role is always placed.

As for all minimal invasive surgeries, surgeon and assistant stand in line with the organ to be operated and the video screen. In this case the surgeon and assistant stand ventrally. Little children must be placed anteriorly close to the border of the table (not in the middle) in order to increase mobility of the instruments. Main monitor is placed posteriorly in line with surgeon's eyes. The monitor has to be placed low enough helping to avoid neck pain. Accessory monitors may eventually be placed in front of the anesthesiologist and/or the scrub nurse who stands toward the patient's back.

16.4 Instrumentation

Like for the vast majority of the minimal invasive surgeries in children, the preferred scope is a 5 mm 30° one. A 3 mm one can be used, but the advantage is not really important because specimen removal is mostly conducted through enlargement of the scope orifice.

In order to deal with vessels, energy applying system such as thermofusion may be interesting. Clip appliers are also useful. An aspiration/lavage system is, of course, mandatory before the beginning of the operation. A curved, fine dissection device is the most important instrument in order to facilitate dissection of the vessels. 3 mm instruments may be used in babies. In that case ligation of the vessels is mandatory.

16.5 Technique

An open technique is mostly used. Three ports are normally needed. The one for the scope is placed on the anterior axillary line in between the fifth to seventh intercostal spaces. The two operating trocars are placed on the midaxillary line, above and under the first trocar. After a little skin incision, a forceps is pushed into the thorax followed by a first blunt trocar. After insufflation under low pressure and low flow (maximum of 4 mmHg), the two other trocars are inserted. A Veress needle may be used first in order to help collapsing the ipsilateral lung, but we don't use it.

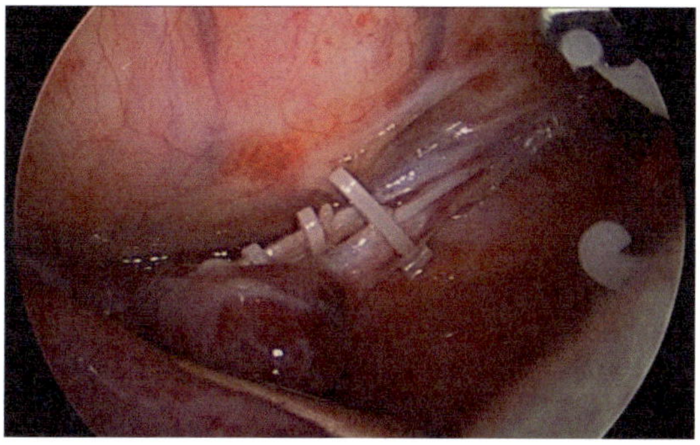

Fig. 16.3 Clipping of the systemic vessels before division

First step of the operation consists in pushing gently on the lung in order to collapse it. Time must be taken to wait for equilibration of the parameters in particular if the lung is not excluded. Once the anesthesiologist is happy, exploration of the posterior part of the thorax may begin in order to find the lesion mostly situated close to the diaphragm. Second step is to identify the systemic artery that may reach from under the diaphragm. Gentle dissection around the vessel with a thin dissector is done after opening of the pleura with the help of the monopolar hook. The vessel can be ligated either using sutures, clips, or the thermofusion device (Fig. 16.3). Instrument sealing and dividing at the same time must be avoided. Once the vessels divided (there could be more than 1 artery) dissection of the sequestration may be conducted easily using the hook or thermofusion. Thermofusion is mandatory in case the sequestration is fixed to the lower lobe. In such case the limit between normal and sequestered tissue is better seen when the lung is insufflated. Help of the anesthesiologist is important at that time, in particular if the lung was excluded. Once the specimen is freed, it may be extracted through an enlargement of a trocar site. An endobag is mostly not necessary.

16.6 Postoperative Care

No drain is needed in most of the cases [5]. The child may drink and eat immediately. Discharge is scheduled on the first day after the operation in the majority of the cases. No X-ray is mandatory except particular cases.

16.7 Tips and Tricks

- Don't forget to put the little children anteriorly close to the border of the table.
- Pulmonary exclusion facilitates dissection but needs expertise in babies and takes time.
- When cutting the arterial vessel, it's safe to have a forceps on the stump in order to control eventual bleeding. Indeed vessel may retract under the diaphragm.
- In case of sequestration fixed to the lower lobe, insufflation and exsufflation of the lobe may help to determine the limit of the resection.
- In case of drainage, the use of a Redon with repeated extraction of the thoracic air in the recovery room may be used. Once there is no air anymore in the Redon, it may be taken out (mostly in the recovery room).

16.8 Discussion

Extrapulmonary sequestration is a well-known disease more and more diagnosed prenatally. Alternative treatments are described even prenatally such as laser obliteration of the systemic vessels. After birth, a radiologic treatment is also described but not widely used [6–8].

Sequestration may become symptomatic due to infection of the excluded lung, the reason why most authors suggest an elective removal soon after birth. The ideal age for operation depends on anesthesiologic and surgeon's habits and is mostly scheduled after 6 months of age. Operation is mostly easy and fast in experienced hands. Main danger is bleeding of the systemic vessels. Care must be taken during dissection and ligation.

Cancer is not a real concern in extralobar sequestration [9]. That's why some authors suggest to wait [10, 11]. But eventual infection of the tissue may complicate dissection, and follow-up needs probably repeated sonographies and/or MRI increasing the costs. Sequestration becomes sometimes symptomatic late in adulthood, so needed follow-up is very long [12].

In case of operation, there is no indication any more for a thoracotomy that increases hospital stay and may lead to scoliosis and other thoracic deformations [13–15]. Referral to a center with knowledge in thoracoscopic anesthesia and surgery is mandatory.

References

1. Pelizzo G, Costanzo F, Andreatta E, Calcaterra V. Congenital pulmonary airway malformations: from prenatal diagnosis to postnatal outcome. Minerva Pediatr. 2016;68(4):299–311.
2. Rothenberg SS. Thoracoscopic management of esophageal duplications, bronchogenic cysts, and extralobar sequestration. In: Endoscopic surgery in infants and children. Berlin: Springer; 2008. p. 131–5.
3. Jesch NK, Leonhardt J, Sumpelmann R, Gluer S, Nustede R, Ure BM. Thoracoscopic resection of intra- and extralobar pulmonary sequestration in the first 3 months of life. J Pediatr Surg. 2005;40(9):1404–6.
4. Saeed A, Kazmierski M, Khan A, McShane D, Gomez A, Aslam A. Congenital lung lesions: preoperative three-dimensional reconstructed CT scan as the definitive investigation and surgical management. Eur J Pediatr Surg. 2013;23(1):53–6.
5. Ponsky TA, Rothenberg SS, Tsao K, Ostlie DJ, St Peter SD, Holcomb GW III. Thoracoscopy in children: is a chest tube necessary? J Laparoendosc Adv Surg Tech A. 2009;19(Suppl 1):S23–5.
6. Cho MJ, Kim DY, Kim SC, Kim KS, Kim EA, Lee BS. Embolization versus surgical resection of pulmonary sequestration: clinical experiences with a thoracoscopic approach. J Pediatr Surg. 2012;47(12):2228–33.
7. KH L, Sung KB, Yoon HK, Ko GY, Yoon CH, Goo HW, Kim EA, Kim KS, Pi SY. Transcatheter arterial embolization of pulmonary sequestration in neonates: long-term follow-up results. J Vasc Interv Radiol. 2003;14(3):363–7.
8. SJ A, Kim EY, Kim JH, Byun SS, Kim HS, Choi HY, Sun YH. Successful endovascular treatment of bilateral intralobar pulmonary sequestration with a bridging isthmus in a child. Pediatr Pulmonol. 2014;49(6):E126–9.
9. Feinberg A, Hall NJ, Williams GM, Schultz KA, Miniati D, Hill DA, Dehner LP, Messinger YH, Langer JC. Can congenital pulmonary airway malformation be distinguished from type I pleuropulmonary blastoma based on clinical and radiological features? J Pediatr Surg. 2016;51(1):33–7.
10. Brown SC, De Laat M, Proesmans M, De Boeck K, Van Raemdonck D, Louw J, Heying R, Cools B, Eyskens B, Gewillig M. Treatment strategies for pulmonary sequestration in childhood: resection, embolization, observation? Acta Cardiol. 2012;67(6):629–34.
11. Stanton M. The argument for a non-operative approach to asymptomatic lung lesions. Semin Pediatr Surg. 2015;24(4):183–6.
12. Kestenholz PB, Schneiter D, Hillinger S, Lardinois D. Thoracoscopic treatment of pulmonary sequestration. Eur J Cardiothorac Surg. 2006;29(5):815–8.
13. Patrick DA, Rothenberg SS. Thoracoscopic resection of mediastinal masses in infants and children: an evolution of technique and results. J Pediatr Surg. 2001;36:1165–7.
14. de Lagausie P, Bonnard A, Berrebi D, Petit P, Dorgeret S, Guys JM. Video-assisted thoracoscopic surgery for pulmonary sequestration in children. Ann Thorac Surg. 2005;80(4):1266–9.
15. Adams S, Jobson M, Sangnawakij P, Heetun A, Thaventhiran A, Johal N, Böhning D, Stanton MP. Does thoracoscopy have advantages over open surgery for asymptomatic congenital lung malformations? An analysis of 1626 resections. J Pediatr Surg. 2017;52(2):247–51.

17 Thoracoscopic Management of the Mediastinal Masses

Arnaud Bonnard and Liza Ali

17.1 Introduction

The mediastinum is the most common location of chest masses in the pediatric population. They are representing a variety of pathology in children. Causes are mostly related to the location of the mass either in the anterior, middle, or posterior mediastinum. Mainly, mediastinal masses are represented by tumor or congenital malformation. Although the mediastinum is located right in the middle, the surgical approach is most of the time coming from the right or the left side depending of the location of the mass. Vascular anomalies such as double aortic arch, in the middle mediastinum, won't be treated here although the surgical approach is also thoracoscopic. Anterior approach, just above the manubrium is well developed in adult surgery but needs to be extended to the children for some indication. At last, for the anterior diaphragmatic hernia, which is one of the causes for anterior and inferior mediastinal mass, laparoscopy is most likely to be used to repair the hernia and close the diaphragm.

Due to the size of the mass, an associated open approach might be necessary to remove the tumor. Otherwise, if the mass can be crushed, doing this using an endobag is highly recommended.

17.2 Thoracoscopic Approach

17.2.1 General Consideration

A perfect collaboration is necessary between the anesthesiologist and the surgeon. The patient should be paralyzed to avoid the diaphragmatic incursion into the chest. Single lung ventilation is not necessary. Indeed, insufflation with CO_2 at 5 mmHg allows in most of the cases to perform the procedure. A positive expiratory pressure (PEP) should be avoided so the lung can be deflated easily. In addition, higher frequency ventilation with small volume can be used to obtain a good CO_2 clearance.

17.2.2 Generality and Operating Room Setup

Three or four port can be used depending of the surgical procedure. The room setup is mostly depending on the mass you have to remove or the procedure you have to perform.

Indeed, for a mass placed in the posterior mediastinum, it is better to place the patient in

A. Bonnard (✉) · L. Ali
Department of General Pediatric Surgery and Urology, Robert Debre Children University Hospital, APHP, Paris, France
e-mail: arnaud.bonnard@aphp.fr

C. Esposito et al. (eds.), *ESPES Manual of Pediatric Minimally Invasive Surgery*,
https://doi.org/10.1007/978-3-030-00964-9_17

70° lateral decubitus, almost in prone position, with the surgeon in front of the patient and the screen back to the patient, in line with the operator. Scrub nurse is usually placed in front of the operator and the assistant either on his right or left side (Fig. 17.1).

For a mass placed in the anterior mediastinum, the patient is better positioned on strict lateral decubitus or slightly at 100° to make the lung fall down and have a direct vision of the anterior mediastinum. The surgeon is then placed on the patient's back and the screen in front of the patient (Fig. 17.2).

Table 17.1 is showing the operating setup related to the indications. Bronchogenic cyst can be operated in the same approach than a mediastinal posterior lesion.

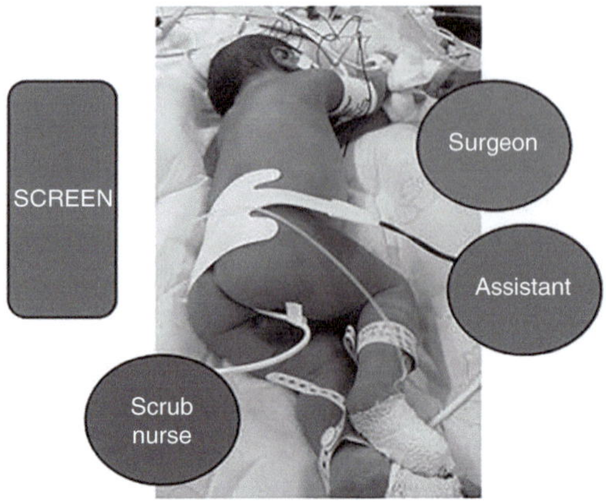

Fig. 17.1 Room setup for a right thoracoscopy and surgery of the posterior mediastinum

17.2.3 Port Placement

Usually, three ports are necessary. A fourth extra port can be placed to push away the lung. It has to be placed most of the time at the base of the chest, not too close from the operative port.

The first port for the camera is usually placed at the tip of the scapula, a few millimeters below. Once the lesion is visualized down or up to the chest, the operative ports are placed respecting a good triangulation. Some operators prefer to place the camera port slightly below and anterior to the tip of the scapula. This way, the scope can push the lung away down allowing to get a larger operative field.

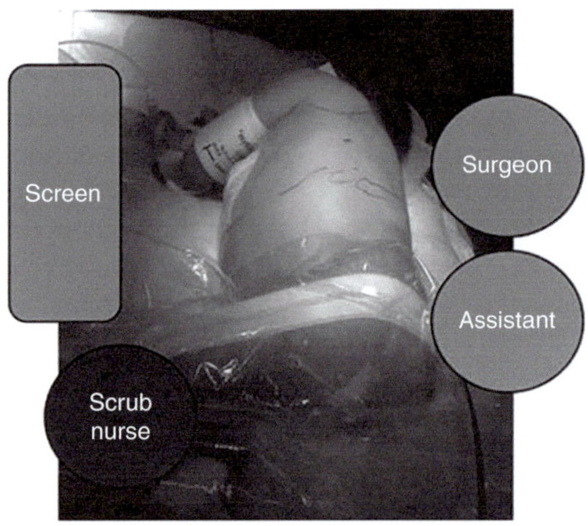

Fig. 17.2 Room setup for a left thoracoscopy and surgery for the anterior mediastinum

Table 17.1 Pathology related to the mediastinum part and room setup

Mediastinum	Anterior	Middle	Posterior
Superior	Thyroid (rare)	Lymph nodes	Neuroblastoma, ganglioneuroma, esophageal duplication
Middle	Thymoma, lymphoma, teratoma	Lymph nodes, bronchogenic cyst	Neuroblastoma, ganglioneuroma, esophageal duplication
Inferior	Pleuro-pericardial cyst, anterior larrey diaphragmatic hernia	Bronchogenic cyst, hiatal hernia	Neuroblastoma, ganglioneuroma, esophageal duplication
	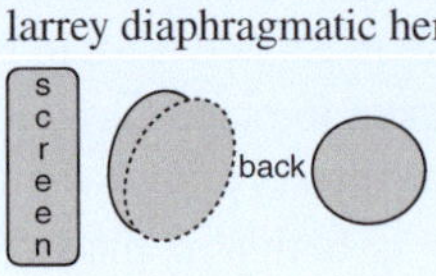		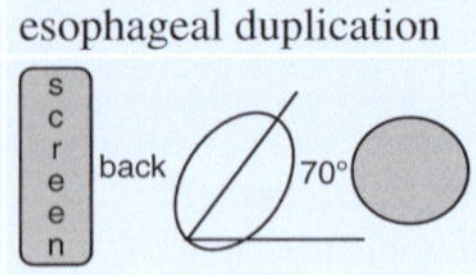

17.2.4 Port and Instrument Size Camera Angle

Ideally, a 5 mm diameter should be used for the camera with a 30° scope which can help to get a better visualization. Three millimeters instruments is the better option, especially if the patient is a small baby. For those who have an access to the 3 mm JustRight™ Vessel Sealing System (JustRight Surgical, Louisville, USA), this makes the surgery safer to perform. Otherwise, hook cautery can be used. Five millimeters instrument can be also an option for children and older. Sometimes, a stapler is necessary, but a 12 mm port have to be introduced which is quite impossible if the surgery is done on a small baby, and this could be avoided.

17.3 Indications

The most frequent indication of the thoracoscopic approach for a mediastinal mass in children is cystic lesion, either a bronchogenic cyst or an esophageal duplication cyst, a thymus lesion (thymoma), or neuroblastoma.

17.3.1 Esophageal Duplication and Bronchogenic Cyst

Foregut duplication cyst are most likely diagnosed now prenatally. Once the diagnosis has been done, parents are seen in prenatal counselling to explain what could be the postnatal management. Surgical removal of the cyst can be easily performed within the 3 months of age. The diagnosis of cyst is made sometimes from an incidental finding on chest radiograph or due to respiratory compromise due to mass effect or infection. Thoracoscopic resection has been reported as a safe and effective method to remove this kind of cyst [1]. Moreover, a study comparing thoracoscopy versus thoracotomy demonstrated an operating time and anesthesia time not different between the two groups. However, the thoracoscopy group had significantly fewer chest tube days (1.6 vs. 3.3 days) and a shorter hospital stay (2.6 vs. 6.6 days) [2].

A nasogastric tube is inserted to make the procedure safer and recognize any esophageal perforation during the dissection. Operating room setting and position of the patient has been described already, and the cyst will be operated through a right thoracoscopic approach, the operator in front of the patient, and the screen in his back (approach of the posterior mediastinum). The cyst can be placed at different level of the esophagus, either at the thoracic inlet or above the diaphragm. Most of the time, it is located in the second third of the esophagus (Fig. 17.3). The bronchogenic cyst is surrounding the trachea or the main bronchus or even the carina, which make sometimes his excision difficult and at risk for tracheal or bronchus injury (Fig. 17.4).

Resection must be performed staying as close as possible from the cyst to avoid any surrounding tissue injuries. Sometimes, in case of duplication cyst, the lesion and the esophagus are sharing a common muscular wall which needs to be opened if we want a complete resection. This situation is at high risk of mucosal injury. At the end of the procedure, the operator can ask the anesthesiologist to pull up the nasogastric tube and put it at the same level of the resection. Pushing some air in, and using some saline, bubbles will be in favor of a mucosal hole which needs to be perfectly identified and

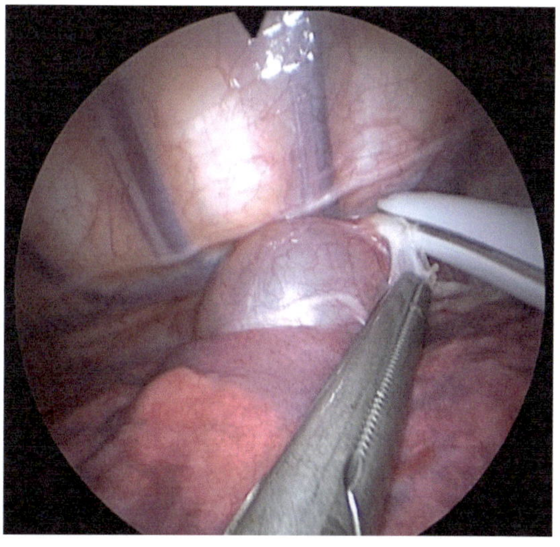

Fig. 17.3 Duplication cyst of the esophagus

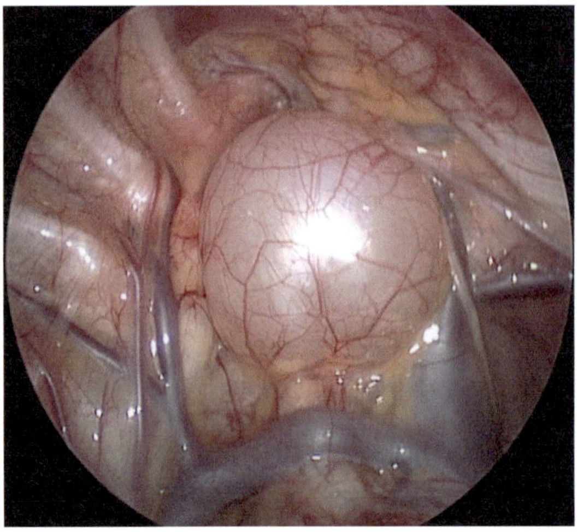

Fig. 17.4 Bronchogenic cyst in the superior part of the chest

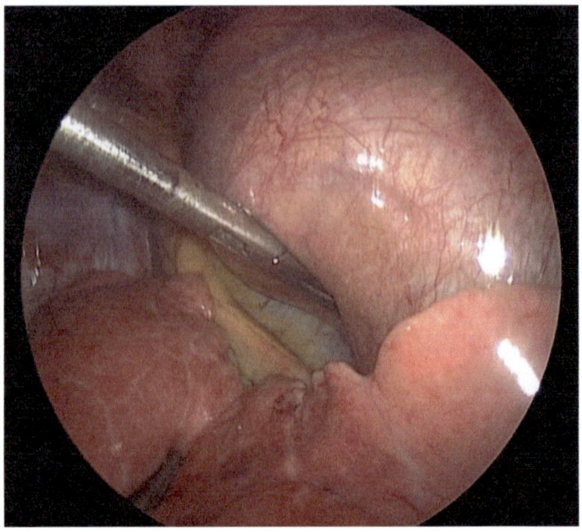

Fig. 17.5 Huge thymoma—dissection done through a left thoracoscopic approach

sutured. The muscular layer would be closed over to avoid development of a mucosal diverticulum.

17.3.2 Thymoma

Myasthenia gravis (MG) is an autoimmune chronic disorder affecting postsynaptic acetylcholine receptors causing progressing weakness and fatigue of voluntary striated muscles. Children with MG account for 11–24% of all cases [3–5]. Medical treatment of myasthenic children is based on anticholinesterase drugs, corticosteroids, and other immunosuppressive medications [4, 6]. Since the early reports by Blalock suggesting that removal of the thymus led to clinical improvement in patients with MG, thymectomy has played an important role in the management of MG [7]. Complete radical thymectomy is believed necessary to maximize surgical results [8–10]. Standard open techniques include total or partial sternotomy, the transcervical approach, and the "maximal" thymectomy combining the trans-sternal and transcervical approaches. The trans-sternal approach is aggressive with a postoperative morbidity as high as 33% [8]. The transcervical approach is implicated as a cause of incomplete thymectomy due to the poor exposure of the anterior mediastinum. Thus, the thoracoscopic approach offering a perfect vision of the anatomy and the entire part of the thymus should be the preferable approach now [11] (Fig. 17.5). The actual indications for thymectomy are early, generalized, and moderate to severe disease stabilized by medication and resistant ocular disease.

The patient is placed on right lateral side for a left thoracoscopy. The operator is on the patient's back and the screen in front of the patient. The dissection is usually starting by the thymus inferior left horn since it's the first structure visualized. The dissection is done immediately under the sternum taking care about the internal mammal vessel. All the vessels can be perfectly identified due to the magnification especially those coming from the top of the thymus and the vein coming into the brachiocephalic venous trunk. They can be controlled either by knotting or using any device such as harmonic scalpel or a thermofusion device.

17.3.3 Neuroblastoma

Neuroblastoma is a good indication of thoracoscopic approach. Indeed, the posterior mediastinum, especially in his superior part, is quite difficult to access through an open approach. Thus, the thoracoscopic approach is offering a good vision of the tumor and the surrounding tissues. The other advantages is that some neurogenic tumor can be crushed into an endobag which is not possible for other kind of tumor such as teratoma. Pathology is showing either neuroblastoma or ganglioneuroma or even ganglioneuroblastoma. Advantages such as less blood loss has been also reported with this approach [12].

As described previously, the approach of the posterior mediastinum is done with the operator in front of the patient and the screen on the back. The patient is placed slightly in prone position to push down away the lung.

In his dominant localization, the upper part of the chest, the camera is introduced as usual at the tip of the scapula. A 30° camera angle is better to use. The operating ports are introduced following the rules of mini-invasive surgery with a good triangulation. It means that, depending of the localization of the tumor, the ports can be inserted either on the same camera port posterior axillary line or one port posteriorly and the other anteriorly (Fig. 17.6).

Thermofusion, LigaSure™ (Medtronic, Minneapolis, USA), or HARMONIC® scalpel (Ethicon, Issy-Les-Moulineaux, France) [13] are helping to the resection taking care to not injure the adjacent structures such as the subclavian artery, the superior vena cava, the pneumogastric nerve, or even the stellar ganglion or the laryngeal nerve. Parents should be aware about all these complications and especially the risk of vocal cord paresis or Horner syndrome [14]. In this localization, the tumor can go into the intervertebral foramen, but the complete resection is optional, and residual disease can be left in place. Once the complete dissection has been done, an endobag have to be used to pull out the specimen. A 5 mm or a 10 mm might be necessary. The use of the posterior incision is preferable avoiding a more visible scare.

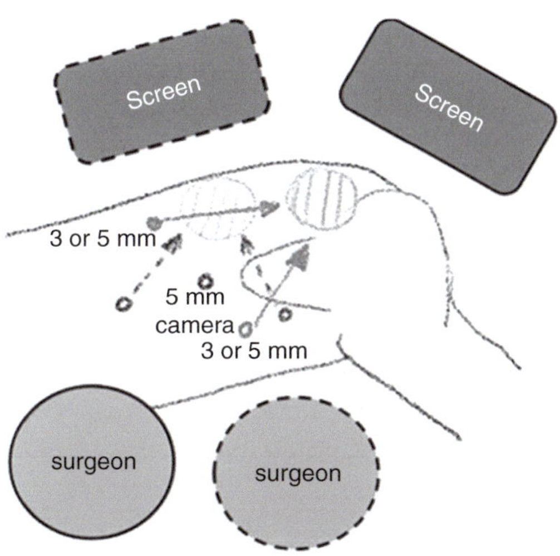

Fig. 17.6 Room setup in relation with the place of the neuroblastoma

17.4 Conclusion

Thoracoscopic approach for a mediastinal mass should be the preferred approach and even the gold standard. Indeed, the possible adverse effect of a thoracotomy on a chest ingrowth is something that should be avoided as often as possible. In some selected cases, such as duplication cyst or bronchogenic cyst, this surgery could be done on a day-case surgery basis.

References

1. Hirose S, Clifton MS, Bratton B, Harrison MR, Farmer DL, Nobuhara KK, Lee H. Thoracoscopic resection of foregut duplication cysts. J Laparoendosc Adv Surg Technol A. 2006;16(5):526–9.
2. Bratu I, Laberge JM, Flageole H, Bouchard S. Foregut duplications: is there an advantage to thoracoscopic resection? J Pediatr Surg. 2005;40(1):138–41.
3. Lakhoo K, De Fonseca J, Rodda J, et al. Thymectomy in black children with juvenile myasthenia gravis. Pediatr Surg Int. 1997;12:113–5.
4. Morita MA, Gabbai AA, Oliveira ASB, et al. Myasthenia gravis in children. Analysis of 18 patients. Arq Neuropsiquiatr. 2001;59:681–5.
5. Youssef S. Thymectomy for myasthenia gravis in children. J Pediatr Surg. 1983;18:537–41.
6. Roberts PF, Venuta F, Rendina E, et al. Thymectomy in the treatment of ocular myasthenia gravis. J Thorac Cardiovasc Surg. 2001;122:562–8.
7. Blalock A, Mason MF, Morgan HJ, Riven SS. Myasthenia gravis and tumors of the thymic region: report of a case in which the tumor was removed. Ann Surg. 1939;110:544–61.
8. Jaretzki A III. Thymectomy for myasthenia gravis: analysis of the controversies regarding technique and results. Neurology. 1997;48:S52–63.

9. Pompeo E, Nofroni I, Lavicoli N, et al. Thoracoscopic completion thymectomy in refractory nonthymomatous myasthenia. Ann Thorac Surg. 2000;70:918–23.
10. Ruckert JC, Walter M, Müller JM. Pulmonary function after thoracoscopic thymectomy versus median sternotomy for myasthenia gravis. Ann Thorac Surg. 2000;70:1656–61.
11. Seguier-Lipszyc E, Bonnard A, Evrard P, Garel C, De Ribier A, Aigrain Y, de Lagausie P. Left thoracoscopic thymectomy in children. Surg Endosc. 2005;19:140–2.
12. Dingemann C, Ure B, Dingemann J. Thoracoscopic procedures in pediatric surgery: what is the evidence?Eur. J Pediatr Surg. 2014;24(1):14–9.
13. Short SS, Naik-Mathuria BJ, Hunter CJ, Papillon S, Stein JE. Use of the harmonic blade scalpel as a novel technique for thoracoscopic resection of pediatric paraspinal masses in children. J Laparoendosc Adv Surg Technol A. 2014;24(4):274–9.
14. Fraga JC, Rothenberg S, Kiely E, Pierro A. Video-assisted thoracic surgery resection for pediatric mediastinal neurogenic tumors. J Pediatr Surg. 2012;47(7):1349–53.

18 Primary Focal Hyperhidrosis: Surgical Management

Pablo Laje

18.1 Introduction

Primary focal hyperhidrosis (PH) is a condition in which the sweat glands of certain areas of the body produce more sweat than what would be expected at any given circumstance for adequate thermoregulation. The condition generally affects the soles, the axillae, and the palms, bringing deleterious consequences from psychological, functional, and social perspectives. The actual prevalence of the condition is unknown, mostly due to underreporting, but it has been estimated to be between 2 and 4% in the general Caucasian population. The etiology of PH is largely unknown, although the frequently positive family history suggests a genetic component [1, 2]. Why it affects only certain areas of the body and why each patient has a different combination of areas affected remain a complete mystery. PH affects males and females, tends to begin in early childhood, and is more prevalent in the Asian population than in the Caucasian population. The excessive sweating occurs regardless of the temperature of the environment, tends to worsen in stressful situations, and in general does not occur during sleep.

P. Laje (✉)
Division of General, Fetal and Thoracic Surgery, Children's Hospital of Philadelphia, Philadelphia, PA, USA
e-mail: laje@email.chop.edu

Patients with certain generalized conditions can have excessive sweating in their entire body, in sharp contrast with PH. Hyperthyroidism, systemic hypertension, lymphoma, and chronic infections are among those conditions, and the excessive sweating, named *secondary* hyperhidrosis, is just a sign of an underlying disease. Secondary hyperhidrosis must be completely ruled out before starting treatment for PH.

Typically, patients with PH have involvement of their palms, and/or the soles, and/or the axillae. The excessive sweating of the palms interferes with all manual tasks. Handling papers, using touchscreens, driving, and playing certain sports (among many other activities) become difficult and often impossible. Needless to say, the social aspect of daily life becomes significantly impaired as well.

18.2 Physiology of the Sweat Glands

The human body has two main types of sweat glands: (1) the *eccrine* glands, which are located throughout the entire body (with a few exceptions), concentrated mostly on the palms, soles, and face, and which have a thermoregulatory function through the production of odorless sweat, and (2) the *apocrine* glands, located exclusively in the axillae, areolas, and perineum, which are inactive before puberty and produce a

C. Esposito et al. (eds.), *ESPES Manual of Pediatric Minimally Invasive Surgery*,
https://doi.org/10.1007/978-3-030-00964-9_18

thicker secretion which initially is odorless but generates a characteristic odor when it mixes with bacterial debris. The ducts of the apocrine glands typically open into the distal ends of hair follicles, whereas the ducts of the eccrine glands open directly on the surface of the skin.

The eccrine glands are the ones involved in the pathophysiology of PH. Their function is controlled by a number of local and systemic mechanisms. The direct application of heat on areas with eccrine glands triggers a locally mediated sweating response. Most importantly, the eccrine sweat glands receive sympathetic innervation in response to changes in the core body temperature and in stressful situations. The sympathetic innervation of the sweat glands is mediated mainly by the thermoregulatory center of the hypothalamus. The preganglionic cholinergic fibers originate from the thoracolumbar region of the spinal cord and synapse with the postganglionic neuron via nicotinic acetylcholine receptors, as in the entire sympathetic system. But the postganglionic fibers, which exit the spinal cord and travel along the paravertebral sympathetic chain, stimulate the sweat glands releasing acetylcholine, which is a remarkable exception, since all other postganglionic neurons in the sympathetic system release norepinephrine. The acetylcholine stimulates the eccrine sweat glands via muscarinic receptors.

18.3 Medical Management

There are several forms of medical therapy for patients with palmar PH. All these forms are ongoing treatments, require a long-term commitment, and are by no means a cure.

- *Topical antiperspirants*: They are the easiest form of therapy [3]. These products consist of highly concentrated aluminum chloride (up to 30%) that is applied daily on the palms, usually at night, and acts by physically blocking the outlet of the sweat glands. This is generally the first line of therapy, but the results are actually quite variable. A common side effect and a reason why the treatment is frequently abandoned is skin irritation.
- *Botulinum toxin*: It works by blocking the release of acetylcholine by the postganglionic neurons, which prevents the stimulation of the eccrine glands. The toxin has to be injected directly in the dermis of the skin of the affected areas. The procedure is painful and causes swelling and inflammation of the area for 2–3 days. The toxin wears off relatively quickly, so it has to be injected every 3–6 months. It is not a common treatment in the pediatric population, and furthermore, the use of botulinum toxin for hyperhidrosis in pediatrics is not approved by the Food and Drug Administration [4].
- *Iontophoresis:* It is a form of therapy in which the hands are submerged into a pan that contains tap water to which an electrical current is applied. The hands need to be submerged for 20–30 min, once or twice per day, for several days. The sweating decreases for a few days, and when it returns, the patient needs to repeat the treatment. The mechanism of action of this form of therapy is unknown. It is not a very common therapy, particularly in pediatrics, because it requires a significant time commitment and causes a number of unpleasant side effects (tingling, numbing, and skin changes). The compliance with this form of therapy is generally low [5]. There are published series in the pediatric population, but the follow-up time is short [6, 7].
- *Oral anticholinergic agents:* These agents work by blocking the muscarinic receptors in the cells of the sweat glands, preventing them from being activated by the acetylcholine released by the postganglionic neuron. The most commonly used agents are glycopyrrolate and oxybutynin. They are quite effective, but due to their systemic absorption, they are associated to the whole range of side effects that all anti-muscarinic agent have: dizziness, dry mouth, blurred vision, urinary retention, and tachycardia, among others. Additionally, the long-term consumption of anticholinergic agents has been associated

with a high incidence of cognitive impairment and dementia [8, 9].

– *Other treatments:* There is a variety of other options that include liposuction of the axillary region, thermal ablation of the sweat glands of the axillary region, ultrasound ablation of sweat glands, topical application of traditional medicine compounds, topical application of anticholinergic gel, oral calcium-channel blockers, oral clonidine, and laser application, among others, but generally the effectiveness of those forms of therapy is very limited, and most of them are not approved to be used in children.

18.4 Preoperative Evaluation

For patients with palmar PH who do not respond, do not tolerate, or do not want to try medical therapies, a thoracoscopic bilateral sympathectomy (TBS) is a feasible option. It is recommended, however, that patients try topical antiperspirants before committing to surgery due to their minimal side effects, because even though the likelihood is low, if the topical antiperspirants provide adequate relief, the operation can be avoided.

In order to undergo a TBS, patients must fulfill the following criteria:

- Secondary hyperhidrosis must be ruled out. This is done through a comprehensive history and physical exam. No laboratory tests are necessary for typical cases, but cases that are questionable must be evaluated by a pediatrician who should rule out hyperthyroidism, hypertension, and all other common forms of secondary hyperhidrosis.
- Patients must have a normal cardiac physical exam and a normal electrocardiogram. Patients with any type of arrhythmia or severe baseline bradycardia may not undergo TBS (life-threatening bradycardia has been reported after TBS, requiring lifelong pacing) [10].
- All pediatric patients must be evaluated by a pediatric psychologist to make sure that they understand the implications of the procedure and do not have unrealistic expectations for after the procedure. Teenagers in particular tend to withdraw from social activities due to their hyperhidrosis and may erroneously expect that all aspects of their social life will improve after the operation. If patients are not deemed good candidates due to any psychologic concerns, the TBS should not be done.
- It is imperative that both, patient and parents, are in agreement with the plan of undergoing a TBS, have read the available literature, and have been informed thoroughly about all the potential benefits, complications, and side effects of the operation. Patients must complete a quality-of-life questionnaire as an objective tool to evaluate the postoperative outcomes.

18.5 Surgical Technique

– *Anesthesia*: The operation is done under general anesthesia, with a double-lumen endotracheal tube that will allow the sequential deflation of each lung. For smaller patients who cannot accommodate a double-lumen endotracheal tube, the lungs need to be collapsed with the CO_2 pneumothorax. Patients do not need an arterial catheter but must have an active blood type and screen sample, and blood needs to be readily available. A central venous catheter is not needed.

– *Positioning*: Patients are positioned in supine decubitus with the arms extended exposing the axillary regions and the arms flexed. The elbows and wrists must be carefully padded and not hyperextended (Fig. 18.1). The anterior aspect of the neck, the axillary regions, and the anterior chest to the level of the xyphoid process are prepared and included in the surgical field.

– *Trocars*: A 3-mm trocar and a 5-mm trocar are inserted 1 in. apart in the axillary region at the level of the third or fourth intercostal space. The 3-mm trocar is placed anteriorly (Fig. 18.2).

– *Instruments*: A 5-mm, 30-degree scope and a 3-mm monopolar hook are the only instruments needed. A 3-mm suction cannula must

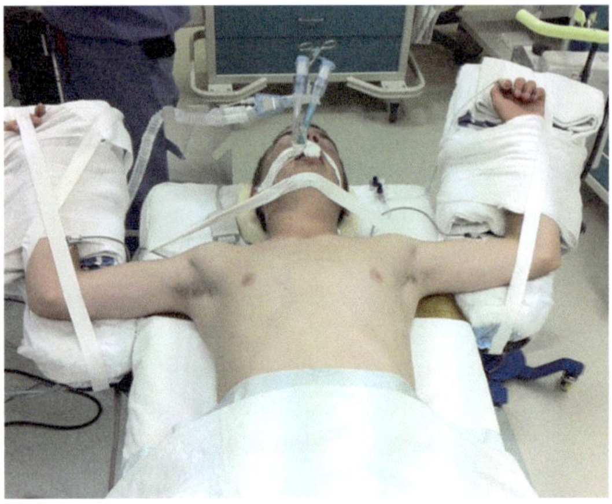

Fig. 18.1 Patient positioning for a thoracoscopic bilateral sympathectomy. Ideally patients are intubated with a double-lumen endotracheal tube

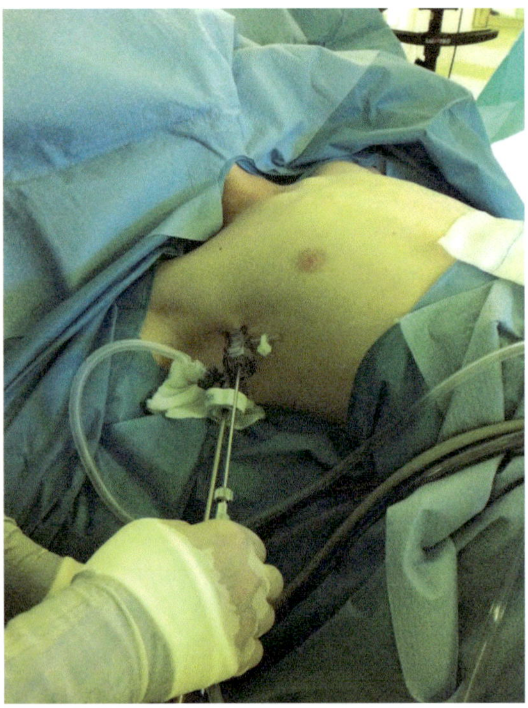

Fig. 18.2 Trocar placement. The trocars are placed high within the axillary region along a skinfold. The 3-mm trocar is anterior to the 5-mm trocar

be ready to use *on* the operating table, as well as an open thoracotomy instrument tray. We typically start on the right side, disconnecting the right lung from the ventilator circuit and insufflating the thorax with CO_2 at very low pressure: 2–4 mmHg. Once the right side is completed, we re-expand the right lung and repeat the procedure on the left side.

– *Procedure*: The exact type of intervention to be done on the sympathetic chain is a matter of constant debate in the literature, and oftentimes, articles contradict each other. The sympathetic chain can be clipped (a potentially reversible technique), severed (sympathotomy), or partially removed (sympathectomy), and the level at which to intervene is also a matter of debate [11–13]. As a rule, the higher the intervention (closer to T2), the higher the efficacy but the higher the incidence of compensatory sweating. In our hyperhidrosis center at the Children's Hospital of Philadelphia, we performed a bilateral T3 sympathotomy with monopolar cautery in all cases [14]. The head of the third rib is identified by fluoroscopy prior to the cauterization (Fig. 18.3). The parietal pleura covering the sympathetic chain is incised with cautery, and the chain is carefully severed without excessive pulling, to avoid damage to the stellate ganglion (Fig. 18.4). Once the chain is divided, the cut ends are pushed apart as far as possible, and the third rib is cauterized for a length of 2–3 in. to burn potential nerve branches that

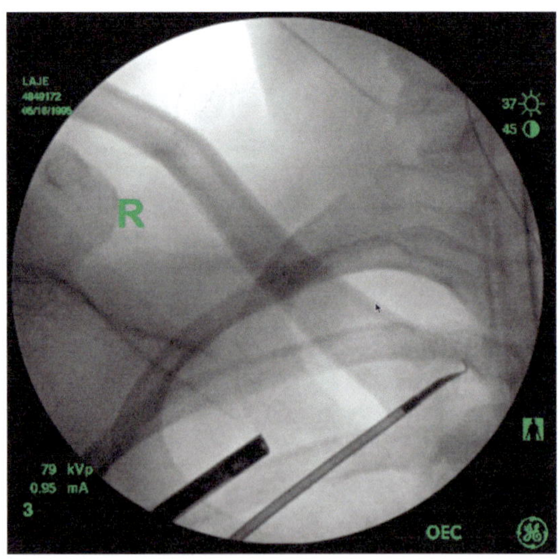

Fig. 18.3 Identification of T3 by fluoroscopy prior to the intervention

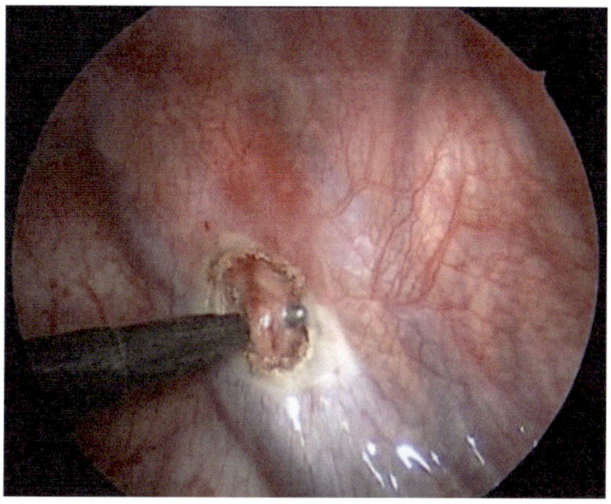

Fig. 18.4 Monopolar hook cautery is used to divide the sympathetic chain (strictly a sympathotomy) without excessive traction

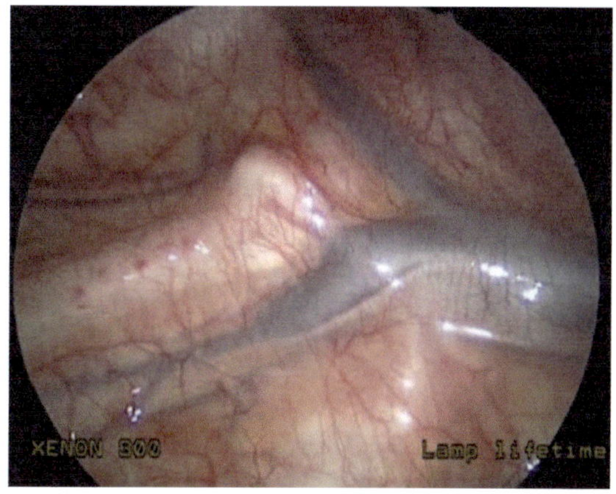

Fig. 18.5 Branches of the azygous vein covering the sympathetic chain

may exit and reenter the chain above and below the transection point. Once this is complete, we remove the instruments and ports and evacuate the pneumothorax with a red rubber catheter under water seal. If there has been no injury to the lung, no chest tube is necessary.

– *Potential intraoperative challenges*: If the patient has adhesions of the lung to the chest wall covering the paravertebral space, which is common in adults, a third port may be needed to dissect them and expose the sympathetic chain. If the sympathetic chain is covered by branches of the azygous vein, these need to be dissected and cauterized very carefully because delayed bleeding can occur (Fig. 18.5).

18.6 Potential Complications and Side Effects

The potential complications of the TBS are of two types: (1) those related to any thoracoscopic procedure (hemothorax, pneumothorax, subcutaneous emphysema, and postoperative infections, among others) and (2) those inherent to the intervention on the sympathetic chain. Within the second category, the most common one is transient bradycardia. It tends to occur right after the first or the second chain is transected and is generally self-limiting, but intraoperative atropine or other anticholinergic agents may be needed. Also within the second category is Horner's syndrome, temporary or permanent, which results from direct or indirect damage to the stellate ganglion by excessive stretching of the sympathetic chain or by thermal damage. The manipulation of the sympathetic chain must be extremely gentle.

Compensatory sweating (CS) is a potential side effect of the operation but, interestingly, can also occur during medical treatments of hyperhidrosis [15]. The pathophysiologic mechanism of CS is unknown, and there is no reliable way to predict what patient will develop it and how severe it will be. A thoracoscopic temporary sympathetic nerve block with local anesthetics is sometimes used in adults as an attempt to predict the development of CS, but the reliability is low because the anesthetic wears off within 1 week and at least 50% of the cases of CS start several weeks after the operation. This technique should not be used in children. The incidence of CS after TBS varies greatly in the literature because it is not well defined and patients don't always report it. In general, teenagers have a much lower incidence of CS than adults [16]. Prior to undergoing a TBS, the surgeon must clearly discuss with the patient and the parents the potential risk of CS.

18.7 Postoperative Care and Follow-up

After the operation is completed, patients are admitted for overnight observation in the regular surgical unit (intensive care is not needed). Adult patients can potentially be discharged the same day of the operation. After the operation, patients are seen in the hospital 1–2 weeks postoperatively, and in our program, we follow up in the long term by phone and email at 1 month, 6 months, 1 year, and yearly thereafter. At all the follow-up time points, the patients complete the quality-of-life questionnaire.

18.8 Results

The results of the TBS in terms of permanently curing the excessive sweating of the palms are extremely high (above 95% across the literature), and the recurrence rate is remarkably low. Improvement of the sweating of the soles, if concomitantly present, occurs in 30–50% of the patients who undergo TBS for palmar hyperhidrosis.

18.9 Conclusions

For children with focal palmar PH, the TBS is a remarkably effective and safe therapeutic option. While it carries an intrinsic risk of compensatory sweating, it provides a cure in the vast majority of cases without any of the lifelong side effects and complications of all forms of medical therapy. The operation, however, needs to be done by experienced pediatric surgeons in multidisciplinary centers.

References

1. Yamashita N, Tamada Y, Kawada MJ, et al. Analysis of family history of palmoplantar hyperhidrosis in Japan. Dermatology. 2009;36:628–31.
2. Ro KM, Cantor RM, Lange KL, et al. Palmar hyperhidrosis: evidence of genetic transmission. J Vasc Surg. 2002;35:382–6.
3. Gordon JR, Hill SE. Update on pediatric hyperhidrosis. Dermatol Ther. 2013;26:452–61.
4. Bohaty BR, Hebert AA. Special considerations for children with hyperhidrosis. Dermatol Clin. 2014;32:477–84.
5. Özcan D, Güleç AT. Compliance with tap water iontophoresis in patients with palmoplantar hyperhidrosis. J Cutan Med Surg. 2014;18:109–13.
6. Dagash H, McCaffrey S, Mellor K, et al. Tap water iontophoresis in the treatment of pediatric hyperhidrosis. J Pediatr Surg. 2017;52:309–12.
7. Dogruk Kacar S, Ozuguz P, Eroglu S, et al. Treatment of primary hyperhidrosis with tap water iontophoresis in paediatric patients: a retrospective analysis. Cutan Ocul Toxicol. 2014;33:313–6.
8. Gray SL, Anderson ML, Dublin S, et al. Cumulative use of strong anticholinergics and incident dementia: a prospective cohort study. JAMA Intern Med. 2015;175:401e7.
9. Cooper CS. Fat, demented and stupid: an unrecognized legacy of pediatric urology? J Pediatr Urol. 2017;13:341–4.
10. Lai CL, Chen WJ, Liu YB, et al. Bradycardia and permanent pacing after bilateral thoracoscopic T2-sympathectomy for primary hyperhidrosis. Pacing Clin Electrophysiol. 2001;24:524–5.
11. Zhang W, Wei Y, Jiang H, et al. T3 versus T4 thoracoscopic sympathectomy for palmar hyperhidrosis: a meta-analysis and systematic review. J Surg Res. 2017;218:124–31.
12. Gunn TM, Davis DM, Speicher JE, et al. Expanded level of sympathetic chain removal does not increase the incidence or severity of compensatory hyperhidrosis after endoscopic thoracic sympathectomy. J Thorac Cardiovasc Surg. 2014;148:2673–6.
13. Lee SS, Lee YU, Lee JH, et al. Comparison of the long-term results of R3 and R4 sympathicotomy for palmar hyperhidrosis. Kor J Thorac Cardiovasc Surg. 2017;50:197–201.
14. Laje P, Rhodes K, Magee L, et al. Thoracoscopic bilateral T3 sympathectomy for primary focal hyperhidrosis in children. J Pediatr Surg. 2017;52:313–6.
15. Baumgartner FJ, Bertin S, Konecny J. Superiority of thoracoscopic sympathectomy over medical management for the palmoplantar subset of severe hyperhidrosis. Ann Vasc Surg. 2009;23:1–7.
16. Bell D, Jedynak J, Bell R. Predictors of outcome following endoscopic thoracic sympathectomy. ANZ J Surg. 2014;84:68–72.

19 Thoracoscopic Treatment of Chylothorax

Lucas E. Matthyssens

19.1 Introduction

Chyle or lymph is a milky, noninflammatory, alkaline, bacteriostatic bodily fluid composed of electrolytes, proteins, glucose, abundant lymphocytes, and fat (chylomicrons derived from alimentary fatty acids) [1]. Chylomicrons are collected in the lacteals and transported by a network of lymphatic vessels in the small bowel wall, connecting to the cisterna chyli (CC), which lies in front of the first lumbar vertebral bodies, between the abdominal aorta and the inferior caval vein. The CC ascends via the aortic hiatus into the chest to continue as the thoracic duct (TD). The distal TD lies extrapleurally in the posterior right mediastinum between the aorta and azygos vein, running dorsal from the esophagus. At the sixth to fourth thoracic vertebral body, the TD crosses the vertebral column to the left, entering the superior mediastinum between the aortic arch and the subclavian artery. At the thoracic inlet, the proximal TD arches above the clavicle, passing anterior to the subclavian artery to terminate into the circulation at the level of the confluence of the left subclavian and jugular veins [1].

L. E. Matthyssens (✉)
Department of Paediatric Surgery/Gastrointestinal Surgery (GIHK)—2K12C, Princess Elisabeth Children's Hospital, Ghent University Hospital, Ghent, Belgium
e-mail: lucas.matthyssens@uzgent.be

Many anatomic variations exist, however, in all portions of the TD [1] and can be explained by its embryology: during development, the TD first grows as two symmetrical tubes, with numerous points of fusion between the two tubes that can partly develop or disappear. The lower right part and the upper left part normally remain and become connected, to form a single TD [2], but, e.g., duplication of the caudal TD is described in 38.7% of people [3].

19.2 Chylothorax: Definition, Diagnosis, and Classification

Chylothorax (CTX) can be defined as the accumulation of chylous fluid in the pleural space. It is a rare condition and the exact incidence in children is unknown [1]. Paediatric CTX (pCTX) is congenital or acquired and may have several causes, according to the age of the child and the mechanism; see Table 19.1. In neonates, congenital or spontaneous CTX is mostly idiopathic, but genetic predispositions have been described. The most common cause of CTX in childhood is trauma, specifically surgical treatment of congenital (cardio)thoracic disorders [4]. After congenital cardiac surgery, CTX is reported in 1 to 6.6% [5–8], with a higher risk at a younger age, in the presence of genetic syndromes (Down, Noonan, Turner), with increased procedure complexity and after cavopulmonary anastomosis

C. Esposito et al. (eds.), *ESPES Manual of Pediatric Minimally Invasive Surgery*,
https://doi.org/10.1007/978-3-030-00964-9_19

Table 19.1 Causes of chylothorax in children

A. *Congenital (mostly presenting as prenatal hydrops fetalis or neonatal CTX):*
– Congenital lymphatic malformations and aplasia, hypoplasia or obstruction of the TD, Gorham-Stout disease
– Genetic predispositions: Down syndrome, Noonan syndrome, Turner syndrome, Yellow nail syndrome, etc.
– Idiopathic
B. *Acquired:*
– Trauma to the TD or its tributaries: surgical (congenital cardiac, congenital diaphragmatic hernia, vascular ring, esophageal, scoliosis surgery, neck dissection, or lymphadenectomy), central venous catheterization, blunt or penetrating, or birth trauma
– High central venous pressure: single ventricle palliation surgery (Fontan, Glenn), thrombosis of the superior caval vein
– Tumor: mediastinal, neurogenic, lymphoma, teratoma, Wilms, ovarian, sarcoma
– Infection: granulomatous (tuberculosis, histoplasmosis), staphylococcal discitis
– Other: sarcoidosis, Henoch-Schönlein purpura

CTX chylothorax; *TD* thoracic duct

procedures (Fontan, Glenn) with elevated superior vena cava pressure [5]. After congenital diaphragmatic hernia repair, CTX has been reported in 4.6–27%, probably associated to prenatal diagnosis, patch repair, and the need for ECMO treatment [8–10].

pCTX should be suspected in a child when X-ray or ultrasound of the chest shows pleural effusion, especially after a thoracic operation [11] (Figs. 19.1 and 19.2). The diagnosis of CTX is based upon laboratory analysis of pleural fluid [12, 13]; see Table 19.2.

At present, there is no specific classification for the reporting of pCTX. To better define the severity of pCTX and to allow for better comparison between treatment study outcomes, a novel classification system for pCTX is proposed, based upon two recent complication classifications [14, 15] and taking into account different pediatric management algorithms [1, 5, 6, 16]. The novel pCTX classification system (see Table 19.3) is easy to use and classifies pCTX in three grades with two severity levels. The consequences of prolonged/persisting CTX in children may be serious: dehydration by fluid loss, malnu-

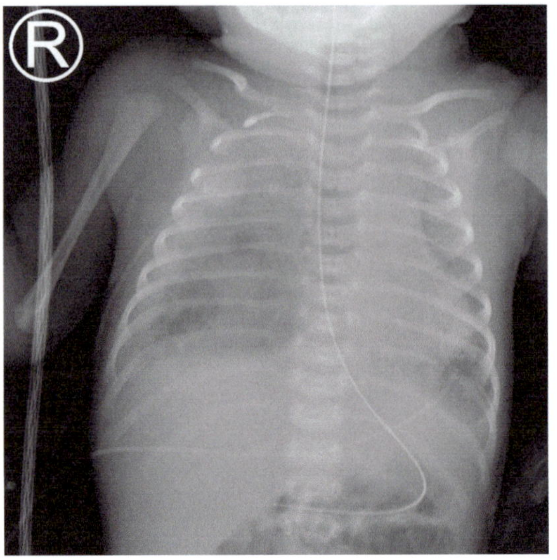

Fig. 19.1 Chest X-ray of a right-sided pleural effusion in a neonate

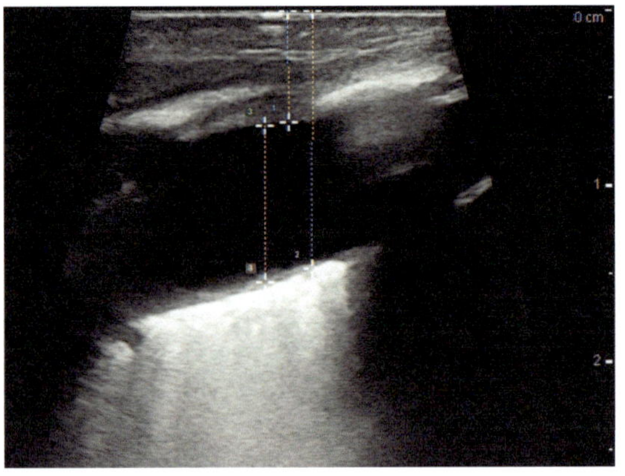

Fig. 19.2 Diagnosis of pleural effusion by thoracic ultrasound in the same neonate as Fig. 19.1

Table 19.2 Diagnostic criteria of chylothorax, at biochemical and microscopic analysis of pleural fluid (see also [12, 13])

Main criteria:
– Triglyceride concentration in the fluid: >110 mg/dL (1.2 mmol/L)
– White cell count >1000 cells/μL with a significant lymphocyte fraction (>80%)
Additional criteria:
– Triglyceride/cholesterol ratio >1
– Presence of chylomicrons at microscopy
– Sterile culture

Table 19.3 Proposal for classification of chylothorax in infants and children (based upon [1, 5, 6, 14–16])

Paediatric Chylothorax (pCTX) grade
pCTX Grade I: Treatment by thoracocentesis/drainage and dietary modifications (enteral MCT-diet) with/without medication[a]
pCTX Grade II: Treatment by thoracocentesis/drainage and Nil Per OS (NPO), total parenteral nutrition (TPN) with/without medication[a]
pCTX Grade III: Treatment by thoracocentesis/ drainage and surgical (or interventional-radiological) therapy
Severity level:
A: Drain output, <100 mL per year of age per day (infants, <10 mL/kg/day)
B: Drain output, ≥100 mL per year of age per day (infants, ≥10 mL/kg/day)
For example, a chylothorax in a 2-year-old child with drain(s) initially producing 300 mL per day and successfully treated by initiating TPN with octreotide = chylothorax grade IIB

MCT medium chain triglycerides; *kg* kilogram; *mL* milliliter; *TPN* total parenteral nutrition; *with/without* with or without
[a]Somatostatin, octreotide, etilefrine, and others

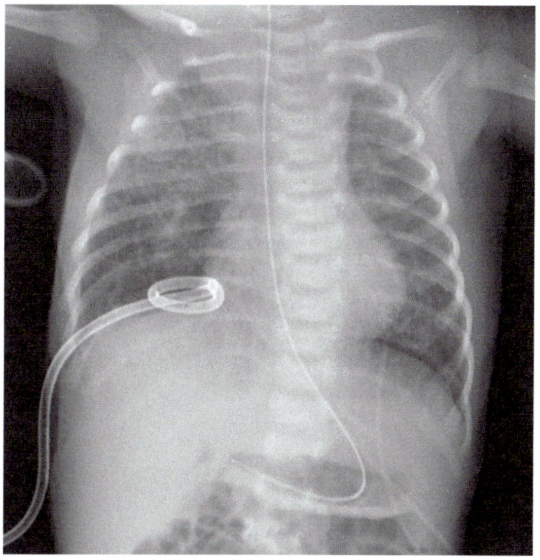

Fig. 19.3 Chest X-ray after the placement of a thoracic drain on the right side, same neonate as Figs. 19.1 and 19.2

trition, and immunosuppression due to loss of lymphocytes, lipids, and proteins (protein C, protein S, antithrombin III, etc.) may predispose the young patient to infections, delayed healing, thrombosis, weight loss, failure to thrive, and longer hospital stay with increased need for suppletion of fluids, albumin, fresh frozen plasma, intravenous immunoglobulins, and a potential increased risk for inhospital mortality [7, 8].

19.3 Management and Indications for Surgery

There is at present no overall evidence-based consensus regarding the best management of CTX in children. Authors from several institutions have reported different algorithms based on physician experience and preference [1, 5, 6, 16]. Treatment starts by repeated thoracocentesis/thoracic drainage (Fig. 19.3) and generally a conservative therapy by step-up approach going from dietary changes (starting enteral feeding with medium chain triglyceride (MCT) diet) (pCTX grade 1) to nil per os (NPO) and total parenteral nutrition (TPN) (pCTX grade II), with or without the addition of drug treatment (somatostatin, octreotide, etilefrine, others) and adjuvant, supportive measures. Depending on age and cause, approximately 71–87% of children will be treated conservatively [5, 12, 13, 16, 17]. The remaining 13–29% will need more invasive, surgical treatment [7].

The ideal timing of surgical treatment for pCTX remains however controversial. Surgical treatment is generally recommended in pediatric patients if:

- Chylous drainage exceeds 100 mL per year of age daily or more than 50 mL/kg/day for more than 7 days [4, 10].
- Conservative treatment is not successful with chylous drainage of more than 10 mL/kg/day after 3–4 weeks of treatment [6, 10, 12, 13, 17].
- Earlier in case of nutritional or cardiorespiratory complications [10, 18].

The goals of surgical therapy for CTX are twofold: to drain the chyle from the pleural space to relieve effects of compression and to stop the leak of chyle with its resulting fluid, electrolyte, nutritional, and immunologic losses [19].

Different surgical options are available for the treatment of persisting CTX:

- Closure of the leak or TD.
- Pleurodesis (mechanical or chemical).
- Placement of a pleuroperitoneal shunt.

Especially in postoperative CTX patients, where a localized leak can be expected, is TD ligation a very effective intervention, with high success rate and relatively low morbidity [19].

In case of congenital/spontaneous CTX, treatment by pleurodesis is more recommended [20–23]. Both techniques can be performed by thoracoscopy and will be discussed in detail below.

19.4 Why (Not) Thoracoscopy?

Thoracoscopy is now the treatment approach of choice for CTX, also in children: it is safe and attractive as it reduces surgical trauma while enhancing visualization of intrathoracic structures by magnification, which is especially useful in small children and for identification of the TD and leaks [19, 24]. Compared to thoracotomy, thoracoscopy offers easy manageability, low morbidity [11], a low rate of complications, and potentially better cost-effectiveness [17, 25], but single-lung ventilation is needed. Extensive pleural adhesions can be an unforeseen problem and may force conversion to an open procedure [19, 24]. In case of problems or contraindications to obtain single-lung ventilation, a mini-thoracotomy of 4–5 cm with one additional 5-mm trocar for the scope may offer a good alternative [16].

19.5 Locating the Leak?

In postoperative CTX, the location of the leak is mostly clear. If not, lymphangiography (direct or intranodal), lymphangio-magnetic resonance imaging (MRI), or computed tomography (CT)-lymphangiography may be performed. Lymphoscintigraphy or multidetector-row CT may also identify the location of chylous leak. Most authors do however not recommend preoperative localization by diagnostic lymphangiography in postoperative CTX before thoracoscopic exploration. In the rare cases of CTX recurrence after thoracoscopic treatment, lymphangiography may be useful to indicate whether the leak follows an alternate route or if there is intent to embolize the TD [26].

19.6 Preoperative Preparation of the Patient

Apart from the routine fasting regime, 3–4 h preoperatively, the patient is given 200 mL lipids (cream) per os or by nasogastric tube to enhance visualization of the thoracic duct [4]. If necessary, this can be repeated intraoperatively.

19.7 Positioning

Under general anesthesia, the child is ventilated by elective left main stem bronchus intubation (controlled by fiber-optic bronchoscopy), to obtain total collapse of the right lung. Prophylactic intravenous antibiotics (cefazolin) are adequately administered, and a large-bore nasogastric tube (Ch 12–16, depending on the size of the patient) is introduced into the esophagus to facilitate intraoperative identification. The child is then positioned in left lateral decubitus and in 30–45°/near total prone position with axillary roll and protective paddings [22]. As for most thoracoscopic procedures, the operating surgeon stands in front of the patient (facing the ventral side of the patient) with the first assistant (camera-person) beside him. The operating nurse stands opposite them at the foot-side of the operating table, to easily pass the instruments. The insufflator column with first monitor/screen is positioned in front of the operating surgeon and assistant. An additional monitor/screen for the operating nurse is placed behind the operating surgeon (Fig. 19.4).

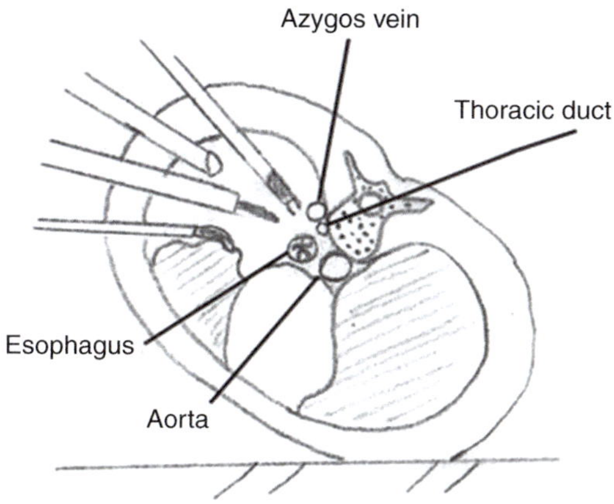

Fig. 19.4 Schematic position of the patient and operative instruments during thoracoscopy [27]

19.8 Operative Technique

19.8.1 Thoracoscopic Thoracic Duct Ligation

After cutaneous disinfection with chlorhexidine digluconate 0.5% in alcohol 70% and sterile draping of the right chest, a 5-mm incision is made in the direction of the skin creases near the distal point of the scapula (posterior axillary line) at the 6th–seventh intercostal space. After blunt dissection by curved hemostat forceps onto the pleura, a 5-mm trocar with blunt tip is introduced into the pleural cavity. Introduction of a 5-mm 30-degrees laparoscope with camera confirms correct intrapleural position by direct vision. The 5-mm trocar is temporarily fixed to the skin with a 4–0 stitch, and a pneumothorax is created by gentle insufflation of carbon dioxide (CO_2) at a maximum pressure of 4 mmHg (torr) and a flow of 1 L/min, aiding at total collapse of the right lung. Two 3-mm working trocars are then introduced by stab incisions under direct thoracoscopic control: one at the midaxillary line in the fifth intercostal space and one at anterior axillary line in the 7th–eighth intercostal space. If later on clips are to be used, a 3-mm trocar will be changed for a 5-mm trocar. Treatment starts with the evacuation of chyle by suction and irrigation with warm physiological serum. Adhesiolysis is gently performed where necessary. The azygos vein and aorta are identified, and the parietal pleura between the azygos vein and spine is opened with electrocoagulation, which is also used for the division of the inferior pulmonary ligament [4, 22, 25]. The mediastinal pleura is incised just above the diaphragm to expose and identify the esophagus. By blunt dissection, the esophagus is mobilized away from the spine and retracted anteriorly [19]. After identification of the pale, tubular TD (if necessary helped by intraoperative administration of extra cream or olive oil via the nasogastric tube), active leakage of chylous fluid may be observed. The leak in the TD is then controlled by placing at least two transfixing sutures (polypropylene 4–0) (or endoscopic clips), first above/proximal and then distal on the TD, just above the diaphragm [4]. Fibrin glue can be sprayed over the mediastinal region, especially if the exact site of injury cannot be identified or if fibrosis of the tissues near the duct makes dissection difficult [11, 19, 22]. In case of doubt on the exact identification of the TD, supradiaphragmatic mass ligature is preferable, by placing several sutures in the soft tissue of the area between the aorta and azygos vein, covered thereafter with fibrin glue [3]. At the end of the procedure, a silicone chest tube (mostly 15Fr, but depending on the size of the patient) is left in place, exteriorized by one of the trocar openings, fixed to the skin with a braided 3–0 stitch, and connected to a conventional thoracic drainage reservoir with water seal system. Insufflation is stopped, trocars are removed under direct vision, hemostasis is checked, and while the right lung is gently recruited by the anesthesiologist, the incisions are closed in layers where appropriate with polyglactin 4–0 or 5–0 intracutaneous sutures, covered by Steri-Strips or glue (Fig. 19.5).

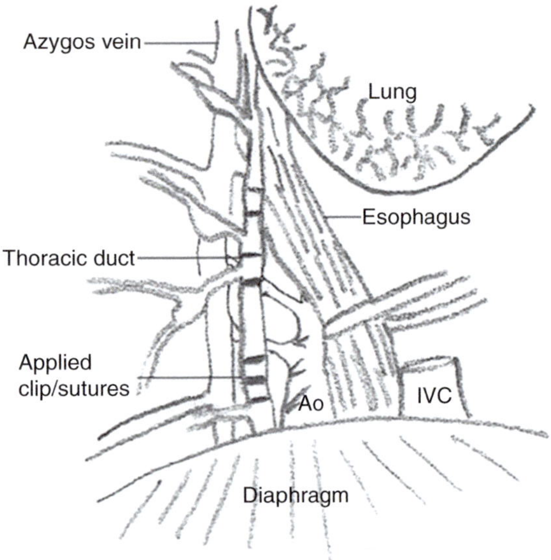

Fig. 19.5 Schematic intraoperative view on the thoracic duct and its anatomical relations during thoracoscopy [27]

19.8.2 Thoracoscopic Pleurodesis

Obliteration of the pleural space either chemically (by instillation of talc, fibrin glue, povidone-iodine, OK-432, or other sclerosing agents) or mechanically (by pleural abrasion) is another surgical option to the management of CTX that can also be performed thoracoscopically in children [17, 28]. Pleurodesis (PD) can be performed primarily as a stand-alone procedure [21] or concomitant after TD or mass ligation [16, 20, 22, 29]. PD can also be performed as a second-line procedure, in rare cases of CTX recurrence after TD ligation [17]. Mechanical PD by pleural abrasion is preferable, especially in neonates and small infants as severe adverse effects have been reported after chemical PD with povidone-iodine [21]. Thoracoscopic abrasion is performed by scratching the parietal, mediastinal, and diaphragmatic pleura with the raw surface of an instrument or tissue, and a cut piece of tip cleaner is very useful for this [21]. Care must be taken not to injure the phrenic or other nerves. PD by pleurectomy is not really recommended in case of CTX, as damage to subcostal lymph vessels may actually worsen the CTX [11].

19.9 Postoperative Care

After the operation, the patient is kept nil per os with TPN administered intravenously until the thoracic drain volume shows a decrease below 10 mL/kg/day. At this moment, enteral feeding by MCT-diet is gently restarted. When further volume decrease is seen, TPN can be weaned stepwise. The chest drain can be removed if enteral feeding is restarted and drainage volume drops below 2 mL/kg/day. The MCT-diet is continued for 4 weeks after removal of the chest drain.

19.10 Results

Success of the procedure can be defined as cessation of chylous drainage (< 2 mL/kg/day) within 14 days after the surgical intervention [7]. Surgical TD ligation has a success rate of up to 90% in children refractory to medical therapy [7, 16]. Review of the literature on thoracoscopic treatment of pCTX (Table 19.4) shows many case reports and small case series but very good results with a contemporary success rate between 86 and 100% [4, 9, 16, 17, 20–25, 28–33].

19.11 Tips and Tricks

- CTX may present at the right or left side or bilateral. Thoracoscopic exploration and TD ligation are possible from both sides. The procedure is preferably performed on the side of the effusion or in the right hemithorax if bilateral [16].
- Pledgetted sutures can be used to reinforce TD ligation [16].
- The use of tissue-sealing technology to seal and/or divide the TD has been described in pediatric thoracoscopic CTX treatment with success [22, 30].

Table 19.4 Reported patients and outcomes of thoracoscopic treatment of chylothorax in children in the literature

Author (year)	Ref	n CTX	Cause	**n VATS**	Age[a]	Weight[b]	Type	Success	%
Graham (1994)	[25]	6	SCVT,I/C	**6**	1	nc	PD, 1 PPC + FG	6	100
Burke (1995)	[24]	2	PCS	**2**	4.6	16.5	TDL	0	0
Stringel (2000)	[4]	1	PCS	**1**	4	nc	TDC + ML	1	100
Takahashi (2001)	[31]	1	PCS	**1**	0.08	2.5	TDC? (ns)	1	100
Watanabe (2005)	[32]	1	I/C	**1**	0.16	1.7	TDL? (ns)	1	100
Achildi (2006)	[29]	1	Spont.	**1**	2	13	TDL + FG + PD	1	100
Khelif (2007)	[30]	6	PCS	**2**	4.5	nc	TDS	2	100
Soto-Martinez (2009)	[17]	1	Traum.	**1**	2	nc	ML	1	100
Cleveland (2009)	[20]	23	PCS, I/C, O	**1**	0.08	3.5	ML	1	100
Komuro (2010)	[9]	1	CDHL	**1**	0.08	2.5	TDL + FG	1	100
Le Nué (2010)	[21]	10	I/C	**3**	0.08	nc	PD	3	100
Pego-Fernandes (2011)	[16]	64	PCS	**14**	2.3	nc	TDL, 4TDL + PD	12	86
Kumar (2013)	[33]	1	Spont.	**1**	1.7	12	TDC	1	100
Noda (2013)	[28]	1	GSD	**1**	15	nc	ML + FG + PD x2	1	100
Slater (2015)	[22]	21	PCS, I/C, O	**21**	nc	nc	TDS + FG + PD	19	90
Clark (2015)	[23]	14	I/C	**6**	0.08	2.7	PPC + FG + PD	6	100

CDHL left congenital diaphragmatic hernia repair; *CTX* chylothorax; *FG* fibrin glue; *GSD* Gorham-Stout disease; *I/C* idiopathic/congenital chylothorax; *ML* mass ligation; *nc* not communicated; *n CTX* number of patients with CTX; *ns* not specified; *n VATS* number of CTX patients treated by thoracoscopic intervention; *O* other causes; *PCS* post cardiac surgery; *PD* pleurodesis; *PPC* parietal pleural clipping; *SCVT* superior caval vein thrombosis; *spont.* Spontaneous CTX; *success* resolution of CTX after the surgical intervention; *TDC* thoracic duct clipping; *TDL* thoracic duct ligation; *TDS* thoracic duct sealing; *traum.* traumatic

[a]Age of the patient: mean age in years (0.08 = first month of life)

[b]Weight of the patient: mean weight in kilograms

– Mass ligation in the fatty tissue between the azygos vein, aorta, esophagus, and spine may also be performed after TD ligation as there may be anatomical variations including accessory ducts [16].

19.12 Discussion

Forty-eight years after the first successful TD ligation by Lampson in 1946, Graham et al. reported on the successful thoracoscopic diagnosis and treatment of a 15-month-old child with spontaneous CTX [25]: thoracoscopy revealed a rent in the posteroinferior pleura, multiple clips were applied to the pleural defect, and the area was covered with fibrin glue. The chest tube was removed on postoperative day 3, and the child was discharged the following day [25]. At present, there are no evidence-based data available favoring one specific surgical method for the minimal invasive treatment of CTX in children. Reported case series are small, causes and clinical presentations vary, and different surgical treatment options are available. It seems however logical to approach this rather rare problem by a minimal invasive and patient-tailored approach:

First, the minimal invasive approach by thoracoscopy is safe and effective, offering augmented visualization and avoiding the morbidity of thoracotomy. Second, the type and timing of surgical treatment need to be adapted to the individual patient, based upon age, history, and clinical presentation: neonates with congenital CTX and especially high-output CTX (exceeding 50 mL/kg/day) will certainly benefit from mechanical pleurodesis, with or without TD (or mass) ligation (with or without fibrin glue) [20–23, 29]. Children with traumatic/postoperative CTX caused by a leak are likely treatable by thoracoscopic TD ligation. If the TD cannot be identified at thoracoscopic exploration, supradiaphragmatic mass ligature, with or without fibrin glue instillation, may be the best alternative [3, 19]. The timing of surgical treatment should also be adapted to the individual patient, and correct classification may be of help: in order to prevent further chylous losses and clinical deterioration, patients with severe, high-output pCTX (pCTX severity level "B," Table 19.3) may benefit from earlier surgical treatment. Finally, every patient may have a different anatomy of the TD due to frequent embryological variations. As technology evolves fast, novel techniques are on their way to better delineate lymphatic anatomy preoperatively by MR-TD-ography or 3D imaging [2, 34], and also intraoperative guidance by near-infrared fluorescence lymphography (NIRFL) with indocyanine green (ICG) is promising [35].

References

1. Tutor JD. Chylothorax in infants and children. Pediatrics. 2014;133:722–33.
2. Oguma J, Ozawa S, Kazuno A, et al. Clinical significance of new magnetic resonance thoracic ductography before thoracoscopic esophagectomy for esophageal cancer. World J Surg. 2018;42:1779–86.
3. Patterson GA, Todd TRJ, Delarue NC, Ilves R, Pearson FG, Cooper JD. Supradiaphragmatic ligation of the thoracic duct in intractable chylous fistula. Ann Thorac Surg. 1981;32(1):44–9.
4. Stringel G, Teixeira JA. Thoracoscopic ligation of the thoracic duct. Journal of the Society of Laparoendoscopic Surgeons. 2000;4:239–42.
5. Chan EH, Russell JL, Williams WG, Van Arsdell GS, Coles JG, McCrindle BW. Postoperative chylothorax after cardiothoracic surgery in children. Ann Thorac Surg. 2005;80:1864–71.
6. Panthongviriyakul C, Bines JE. Post-operative chylothorax in children: an evidence-based management algorithm. J Pediatr Child Health. 2008; 44:716–21.
7. Nath DS, Savla J, Khemani RG, Nussbaum DP, Greene CL, Wells WJ. Thoracic duct ligation for persistent chylothorax after pediatric cardiothoracic surgery. Ann Thorac Surg. 2009;88:246–52.
8. Levy SM, Lally PA, Lally KP, Tsao K, Congenital Diaphragmatic Hernia Study Group. The impact of chylothorax on neonates with repaired congenital diaphragmatic hernia. J Pediatr Surg. 2013;48(4):724–9.
9. Komuro H, Kudou S, Matsubara M, Hoshino N. Thoracoscopic treatment of chylothorax after patch repair of congenital diaphragmatic hernia. J Pediatr Surg. 2010;45:1748–50.
10. Zavala A, Campos JM, Riutort C, Skorin I, Godoy L, Faunes M, Kattan J. Chylothorax in congenital diaphragmatic hernia. Pediatr Surg Int. 2010;26: 919–22.
11. Fahimi H, Casselman FP, Mariani MA, van Boven WJ, Knaepen PJ, van Swieten HA. Current management of postoperative chylothorax. Ann Thorac Surg. 2001;71:448–51.
12. Büttiker V, Fanconi S, Burger R. Chylothorax in children: guidelines for diagnosis and management. Chest. 1999;116(3):682–7.
13. Beghetti M, La Scala G, Belli D, Bugmann P, Kalangos A, Le Coultre C. Etiology and management of pediatric chylothorax. J Pediatr. 2000;136(5):653–8.
14. Low DE, Alderson D, Cecconello I, et al. International consensus on standardisation of data collection for complications associated with esophagectomy. Ann Surg. 2015;262:286–94.
15. Besselink MG, Bengt van Rijjsen L, Bassi C, et al. Definition and classification of chyle leak after pancreatic operation: a consensus statement by the ISGPS. Surgery. 2017;161(2):365–72.
16. Pego-Fernandes PM, Nascimbem MB, Ranzani OT, Shimoda MS, Monteiro R, Jatene FB. Video-assisted thoracoscopy as an option in the surgical treatment of chylothorax after cardiac surgery in children. J Bras Pneumol. 2011;37(1):28–35.
17. Soto-Martinez ME, Clifford V, Clamette T, Ranganathan S, Massie RJ. Spontaneous chylothorax in a 2-year-old child. Med J Aust. 2009;190(5): 262–4.
18. Selle JG, Snyder WH, Schreiber JT. Chylothorax: indications for surgery. Ann Surg. 1973;177(2): 245–9.
19. Wurnig PN, Hollaus PH, Ohtsuka T, Flege JB, Wolf RK. Thoracoscopic direct clipping of the thoracic duct for chylopericardium and chylothorax. Ann Thorac Surg. 2000;70:1662–5.
20. Cleveland K, Zook D, Harvey K, Woods RK. Massive chylothorax in small babies. J Pediatr Surg. 2009;44:546–50.
21. Le Nué R, Molinaro F, Gomes-Ferreira C, Scheib-Brolly C, Escande B, Kühn P, Lacreuse I, Favre R, Becmeur F. Surgical management of congenital chylothorax in children. Eur J Pediatr Surg. 2010;20:307–11.
22. Slater BJ, Rothenberg SS. Thoracoscopic thoracic duct ligation for congenital and acquired disease. J Laparoendosc Adv Surg Tech A. 2015;25(7):605–7.
23. Clark ME, Woo RK, Johnson SM. Thoracoscopic pleural clipping for the management of congenital chylothorax. Pediatr Surg Int. 2015;31(12):1133–7.

24. Burke RP, Wernovsky G, van der Velde M, Hansen D, Castaneda AR. Video-assisted thoracoscopic surgery for congenital heart disease. J Thorac Cardiovasc Surg. 1995;109(3):499–508.
25. Graham DD, McGahren ED, Tribble CG, Daniel TM, Rodgers BM. Use of video-assisted thoracic surgery in the treatment of chylothorax. Ann Thorac Surg. 1994;57(6):1507–12.
26. Reisenauer JS, Puig CA, Reisenauer CJ, Allen MS, Bendel E, Cassivi SD, Nichols FC, Shen RK, Wigle DA, Blackmon SH. Treatment of postsurgical chylothorax. Ann Thorac Surg. 2018;105(1):254–62.
27. Misthos P, Kanakis MA, Lioulias AG. Chylothorax complicating thoracic surgery: conservative or early surgical management? Updates Surg. 2012;64:5–11.
28. Noda M, Endo C, Hoshikawa Y, Ishibashi N, Suzuki T, Okada Y, Kondo T. Successful management of intractable chylothorax in Gorham–Stout disease by awake thoracoscopic surgery. Gen Thorac Cardiovasc Surg. 2013;61(6):356–8.
29. Achildi O, Smith BP, Grewal H. Thoracoscopic ligation of the thoracic duct in a child with spontaneous chylothorax. J Laparoendosc Adv Surg Tech A. 2006;16(5):546–9.
30. Khelif K, Maassarani F, Dassonville M, De Laet MH. Thoracoscopic thoracic duct sealing with LigaSure in two children with refractory postoperative chylothorax. J Laparoendosc Adv Surg Tech A. 2007;17(1):137–9.
31. Takahashi M, Kurokawa Y, Toyama H, Hasegawa R, Hashimoto Y. The successful management of thoracoscopic thoracic duct ligation in a compromised infant with targeted lobar deflation. Anesth Analg. 2001;93:96–7.
32. Watanabe K, Miyamoto Y, Kinouchi K, Kagawa K, Kitamura S. Anaesthetic management of a 1.7-kg premature infant undergoing thoracoscopic thoracic duct ligation. Masui. 2005;54(10):1165–7.
33. Kumar A, Bin Asaf B, Chugh K, Talwar N. Thoracoscopic ligation of thoracic duct for spontaneous chylothorax. Indian Pediatr. 2013;50:796–8.
34. Nakano T, Okamoto H, Maruyama S, Ohuchi N. Three-dimensional imaging of a thoracic duct cyst before thoracoscopic surgery. Eur J Cardiothorac Surg. 2014;45(3):585.
35. Shirotsuki R, Uchida H, Tanaka Y, Shirota C, Yokota K, Murase N, Hinoki A, Oshima K, Chiba K, Sumida W, Hayakawa M, Tainaka T. Novel thoracoscopic navigation surgery for neonatal chylothorax using indocyanine-green fluorescent lymphography. J Pediatr Surg. 2018;53(6):1246–9.

20 Thoracoscopic Congenital Diaphragmatic Hernia (CDH) Repair

Holger Till and Ahmed El Haddad

20.1 Introduction

Since the introduction of thoracoscopic repair for congenital diaphragmatic hernia (CDH) by Van der Zee and Bax in 1995 [1], this approach has always been one of the most challenging in neonatal MIS. For more than two decades, technology improved and made it increasingly feasible, but surgical complications like recurrence rate never reached open standards. It seemed that minimal invasive surgery (MIS) of CDH had a performance problem [2]. Furthermore observations of intraoperative hypercapnia and severe acidosis raised medical concerns [3]. Thus today, unlike other neonatal MIS procedures, CDH repair has not yet reached the status of a "gold standard" for the complete spectrum of patients [4]. Instead the academic discussion has identified key points of success calling for a "smart" selection of neonates and specialized teams. The following chapter will deal with such details to improve overall success rate in this very delicate group of patients.

H. Till (✉) · A. El Haddad
Department of Paediatric and Adolescent Surgery, Medical University of Graz, Graz, Austria
e-mail: holger.till@medunigraz.at

20.2 Preoperative Preparation

Neonates with CDH present a spectrum of perinatal pathophysiology, especially pulmonary hypoplasia associated with decreased oxygenation as well as pulmonary vascular hypertension causing impaired pulmonary circulation. When it comes to timing of surgery, any repair should take these comorbidities into consideration. The CDH EURO Consortium recommends surgery [5] once the following criteria have been met:

- Mean arterial blood pressure has reached normal values for gestation.
- Preductal saturation levels of 85–95% SaO_2 on fractional inspired oxygen below 50%.
- Lactate below 3 mm/L.
- Urine output more than 2 mL/kg/h.

Besides timing of surgery, "smart" preoperative selection of neonates seems advisable especially to improve outcome of thoracoscopic procedures. Putnam [6] published for the CDHSG a query from 2007 to 2015 and concluded that larger defects (types C and D) were associated with higher recurrence rates. Costerus [7] recommended avoiding neonates with "liver up." We will discuss such details later again, but it seems worth mentioning at this point for optimal preoperative preparation.

Since thoracoscopic repair of neonatal CDH requires a well-trained and well-educated team,

C. Esposito et al. (eds.), *ESPES Manual of Pediatric Minimally Invasive Surgery*,
https://doi.org/10.1007/978-3-030-00964-9_20

all of these preoperative considerations should be discussed within the team ahead of any operation to avoid intraoperative disagreement and impaired performance.

20.3 Positioning

The patient is placed in an almost prone position (Fig. 20.1) with the affected side slightly up and the arm raised above over the head. Especially in neonatal CDH repair, the baby could be placed across the table if the surgeons prefer to work over the head (Fig. 20.2). As for all MIS procedures, the room should be set with ergonomic precision with the surgeon, the patient, and the monitor arranged in a straight line.

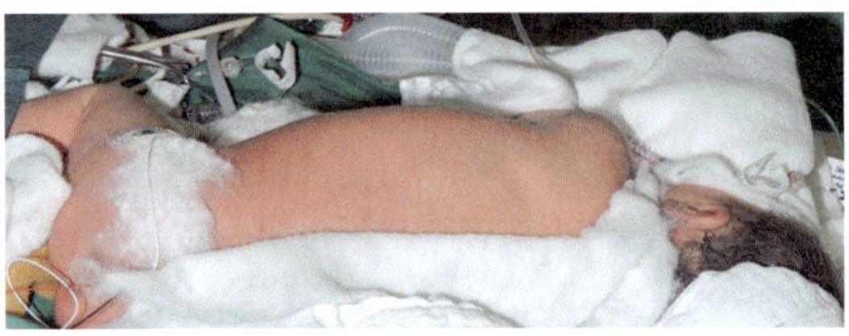

Fig. 20.1 Newborn with CDH placed lateral or almost prone with the affected side slightly up

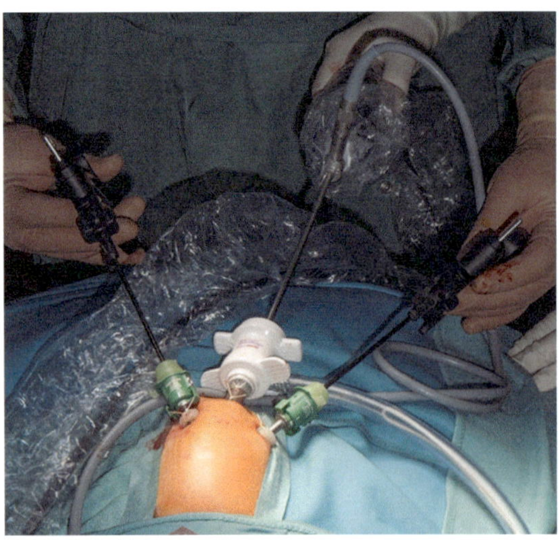

Fig. 20.2 The surgeon stands at the head of the newborn with CDH, the camera man on his left. Triangulation of the ports (5 mm expandable optic port, 3 mm working ports, RoTaLock™). Ports positions: camera port at the tip of scapula, right and left working ports in the axillary lines creating an ergonomic triangle

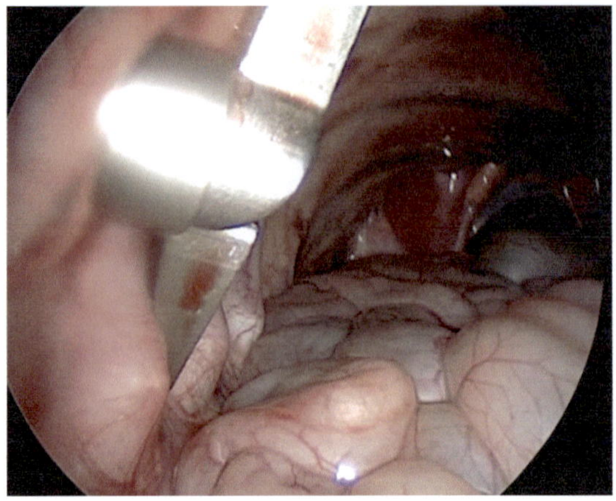

Fig. 20.3 "Early" view down toward the CDH with most of the intestine still in the thorax. Note the RoTaLock™ port anchored and using hardly any space within the neonatal thoracic cavity

20.4 Instrumentation

Basically a regular neonatal MIS set including 3 or 3.5 mm short instruments, hook cautery, needle holder, and knot pusher (in case of extracorporeal knotting) seems sufficient. Any kind or brand of adequate (short) ports seems fine; however there are some special ports available, which require hardly any space within the thoracic cavity and anchor fine at the same time (e.g., RoTaLock) (Fig. 20.3). Similarly any kind of sutures that the surgeon uses for open repair is fine for MIS as well (just follow you standards); however care must be taken about the shape and size of the needle. It must pass through the port without too much bending and should match the limited space inside the small thoracic cavity. We prefer 3/0 or 4/0 Ethibond on a RB-1 needle. Finally, if patch repair is required, it seems advisable to test which material passes through the trocars before surgery.

Finally, if additional pathologies like an extrapulmonary sequestration are expected, the instrumentations must be extended to allow for careful resection, i.e., sutures, clips, and specimen bag.

20.5 Technique

The first port is placed just at the tip of the scapula usually in the mid-axillary line of the fourth or fifth intercostal space (better not too low). We prefer an open introduction without using the Veress needle. The intrathoracic position is carefully checked with the scope, and gentle insufflation of CO_2 (0.1 L/min and a maximal pressure of 3–5 mmHg) is started. If desaturations are noted at this time, the team is prepared to carefully observe, whether equilibration occurs without major acidosis. In case of doubt, CO_2 insufflation may even be stopped for a while and started later. Usually the baby adapts to this situation after 5–10 min. Thereafter two working ports are introduced under vision in the anterior and posterior axillary line of the fourth or fifth intercostal space aiming for an ergonomic triangle with the tip pointing down to the diaphragm (Fig. 20.2).

Once the ports are in place, the procedure continues by gentle reduction of the intestinal organs. Gentle reduction means pushing loops of bowel with open or closed atraumatic graspers down toward the diaphragm (Fig. 20.4). Gradually the thoracic cavity empties, the size of the defect becomes more apparent, but major challenges, i.e., the spleen and the stomach, are still to come. At this point continuous CO_2 insufflation may not be necessary anymore.

Reduction of the spleen requires special attention. It should never be grasped, because this will inevitably damage the capsule and cause bleeding. Sometimes it nicely follows the stomach being reduced (which may be grasped gently). Especially in small defects, it may be advisable to hold the anterior leaf of the diaphragm and "open the door" into the abdominal cavity. In most cases pushing the spleen with the shaft of a blunt grasper placed completely across the spleen allows atraumatic reduction. Once the spleen is in the abdomen, it usually "occludes" the defect avoiding reherniation.

The paradigm that resection of a hernia sac is not necessary has changed. Instead it is believed that it should be incised circumferentially (scissor, electrocautery) close to all diaphragmatic leaves allowing for direct scarring of the muscle. Thereafter, just like in classical open approach, the posterior rim of the diaphragm should be mobilized to reduce as much tension as possible. This concludes the reduction phase. If an additional pathology like an extrapulmonary sequestration covering the CDH is present, it should be dealt with simultaneously. Please note that the aberrant abdominal vessel may pass directly through the hernia sac of the CDH and should be handled with care. Finally the size of the defect can be assessed completely (Fig. 20.5).

The reconstruction of the diaphragm usually starts at the medial portion of the defect. In larger left-sided defects, care must be taken not to include the esophagus into the first stitch. Step by step the diaphragm is approximated, and every time the surgeon should critically assess, whether

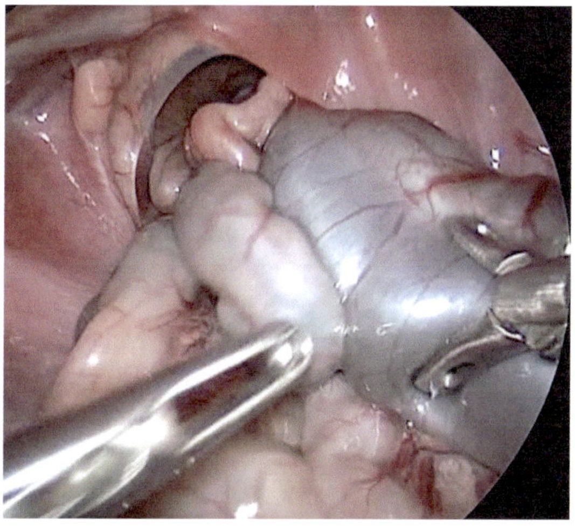

Fig. 20.4 Gentle reduction of the content with open or closed instrument toward the defect

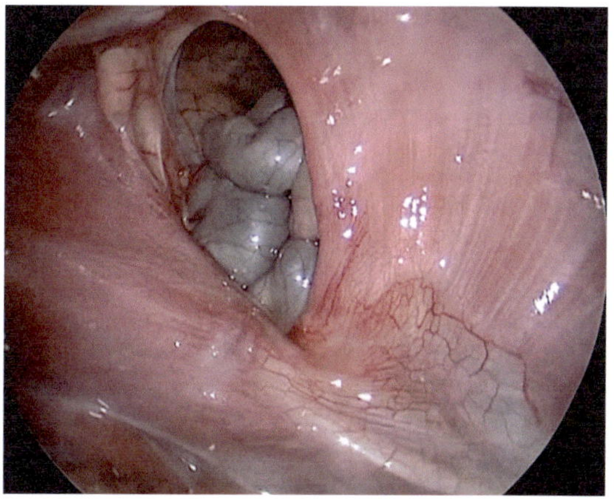

Fig. 20.5 Assessment of the CDH after complete reduction

any tension has been created. Most experts agree today that only a tension-free reconstruction avoids later recurrence. In any case of doubt either a patch repair should be started or according to Costerus [7] recommendation, conversion to open surgery may improve outcome.

Closing the posterolateral portion of the defect remains demanding. In some cases it may be advisable to start with this challenge. Since the space is rather limited, transcutaneous stitches around the rib and into the corner of each diaphragmatic leave may make this step rather easy. We recommend identifying the optimal position of such stitches by pushing from the outside. Then a stab incision is made into the skin, and the (straightened) needle is passed into the thoracic cavity. The needle is grasped from the inside, stitched through both diaphragmatic leaves, and passed to the outside on the other side of the same rib. The same skin incision can be pushed over the tip of the needle, and the knot can be buried underneath. Further interrupted stitches finally close the defect (Fig. 20.6).

If a patch repair is required (Fig. 20.7), it follows the basic principles of open surgery. The only challenge remains how to measure the adequate size (including some redundancy) and pass it inside. Most patch materials can be rolled and passed through the 5 mm optical port after removal of the cap. Then the scope is reintroduced pushing the patch completely inside. With great care the patch is unrolled, positioned, and sutured to the diaphragmatic leaves as well as around the rib(s) (Fig. 20.7).

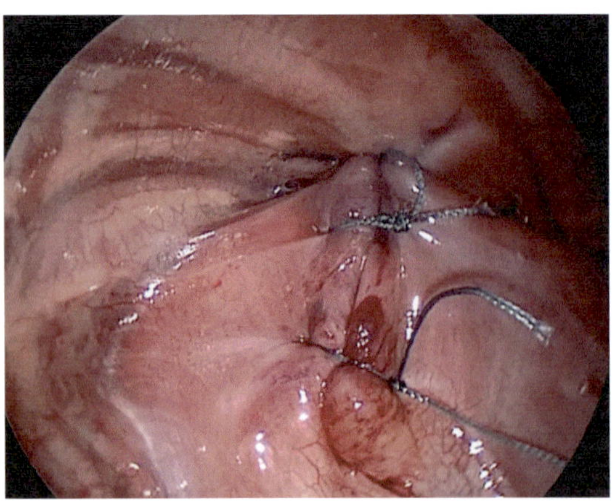

Fig. 20.6 Same patient as Figs. 20.4 and 20.5 after complete and tension-free closure of the CDH

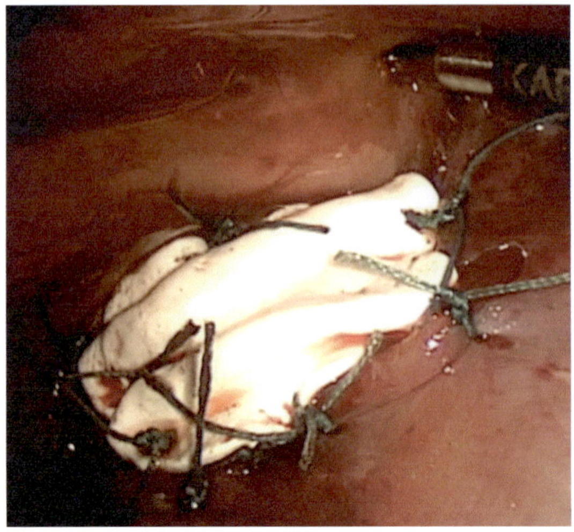

Fig. 20.7 Larger defects may be closed by GORE-TEX® patching for a tension-free repair

At the end of the procedure, suction and irrigation may be necessary to clean the thoracic cavity, but most surgeons would not leave a thoracic drain as it may cause overstretching of the pulmonary parenchyma.

20.6 Postoperative Care

The patient is brought back to the ICU or neonatal ward, and standard care is usually started immediately.

20.7 Results

Over the last decades, numerous reports with variable level of evidence have been published. As mentioned in the introduction, present results of thoracoscopic CDH repair in neonates do not show a general benefit over open surgery. Instead intraoperative complications like hypercapnia, acidosis, or decreased cerebral oxygenation must be observed as much as long-term recurrences. However experts in the field have identified that "smart patient selection" may improve outcome.

Finally note that potential benefits of MIS such as early recovery, less pain, or more rapid extubation may not be as relevant for neonates with CDH if they require prolonged treatment in an ICU anyhow [3].

20.8 Tips and Tricks

- Team training and mutual understanding of intraoperative challenges (hypercapnia, acidosis) seem essential.
- Select your patient's right: careful with liver up and type C or D defects.
- Avoid any tension on the reconstruction.
- Transcutaneous corner stitches, especially around the ribs, add stability.
- Patches should be as redundant as possible.

20.9 Discussion

Despite all technical developments and individual surgical training, MIS repair of neonatal CDH remains a challenge and requires careful considerations and patient selection.

First CDH represents a spectrum of postnatal pulmonary hypoplasia and vascular hypertension. As in open surgery, guidelines should be respected, when to operate. Moreover it seems obvious that extensive CO_2 insufflation during surgery in patients that already suffer from hypercapnia must carefully be observed. Bishay and others raised a special concern about significant intraoperative hypercapnia and severe acidosis [8]. Even impaired cerebral oxygenation observed by near-infrared spectroscopy (NIRS) must be encountered. Consequently most experts in pediatric endosurgery today recommend gentle insufflation and "no gas" after the reduction. Additionally cerebral oxygenation should be monitored intraoperatively by NIRS.

To improve long-term outcome, adequate patient selection seems essential. Lacher et al. [9] performed a survey among IPEG members about the contraindications for thoracoscopic CDH repair. Participants said *no* to patients on ECMO (78%), after ECMO (42%), liver in the chest (32%), and right-sided hernia (15%). Of course this list has not been validated by major studies yet, but it seems "good to know" as an individual guide especially in centers with few cases per year.

Putnam [6] clearly identified two key predictors for failure of the repair when analyzing data from the CDHSG registry from 2007 to 2015: in 3984 patients he found that (1) large defect sizes (type C, odds ratio (OR) 4.3; type D, OR 7.1) and (2) MIS (OR 3.2) were independent predictors of recurrence.

Costerus [7] developed a critical selection process after comparing the Rotterdam data of open versus thoracoscopic neonatal CDH repair. This selection process included all factors mentioned above like hemodynamic stability, liver down, size of defect, but also the surgeon's technical ability and choice. In their hands such a selection process showed its efficacy, because outcome of open versus thoracoscopic CDH repair was almost identical after adequate selection.

Of course surgical risks have to be balanced against benefits for the patient. Avoiding a laparotomy wound is obviously a lifelong benefit over three stab incisions in the axillary lines. However some potential benefits of MIS like less pain or earlier recovery may not be as relevant for neonates with CDH staying in the ICU for a certain period of time anyway [3]. However Putnam [4] confirmed that MIS approached was associated with a decreased length of hospital stay (LOS) and lower incidence of small bowel obstructions (SBO).

In summary thoracoscopic repair of CDH in newborns is certainly technically feasible but requires education about the medical challenges and individual training of surgical skills. Critical preoperative patient selection seems mandatory to minimize long-term morbidity. Critical intraoperative observation of potential "biological" problems like decreased cerebral oxygenation or prolonged acidosis should be standardized. Critical reconstruction avoiding tension on the primary reconstruction or patch repair will certainly decrease recurrence rates. Finally late presenters are obviously perfect candidates for thoracoscopic repair of CDH.

References

1. van der Zee DC, Bax NM. Laparoscopic repair of congenital diaphragmatic hernia in a 6-month-old child. Surg Endosc. 1995;9(9):1001–3.
2. Tsao K, Lally PA, Lally KP, Congenital Diaphragmatic Hernia Study Group. Minimally invasive repair of congenital diaphragmatic hernia. J Pediatr Surg. 2011;46(6):1158–64.
3. Fujishiro J, Ishimaru T, Sugiyama M, Arai M, Suzuki K, Kawashima H, et al. Minimally invasive surgery for diaphragmatic diseases in neonates and infants. Surg Today. 2016;46(7):757–63.
4. Putnam LR, Tsao K, Lally KP, Blakely ML, Jancelewicz T, Lally PA, et al. Minimally invasive vs open congenital diaphragmatic hernia repair: is there a superior approach? J Am Coll Surg. 2017b;224(4):416–22.
5. Snoek KG, Reiss IK, Greenough A, Capolupo I, Urlesberger B, Wessel L, et al. Standardized postnatal management of infants with congenital diaphragmatic hernia in Europe: the CDH EURO Consortium Consensus—2015 update. Neonatology. 2016;110(1):66–74.
6. Putnam LR, Gupta V, Tsao K, Davis CF, Lally PA, Lally KP, et al. Factors associated with early recurrence after congenital diaphragmatic hernia repair. J Pediatr Surg. 2017a;52(6):928–32.
7. Costerus S, Zahn K, van de Ven K, Vlot J, Wessel L, Wijnen R. Thoracoscopic versus open repair of CDH in cardiovascular stable neonates. Surg Endosc. 2016;30(7):2818–24.
8. Bishay M, Giacomello L, Retrosi G, Thyoka M, Garriboli M, Brierley J, et al. Hypercapnia and acidosis during open and thoracoscopic repair of congenital diaphragmatic hernia and esophageal atresia: results of a pilot randomized controlled trial. Ann Surg. 2013;258(6):895–900.
9. Lacher M, St Peter SD, Laje P, Harmon CM, Ure B, Kuebler JF. Thoracoscopic CDH repair—a survey on opinion and experience among IPEG members. J Laparoendosc Adv Surg Technol A. 2015;25(11):954–7.

Thoracoscopic Repair of Esophageal Atresia and/or Tracheoesophageal Fistula

21

Dariusz Patkowski

21.1 Introduction

The thoracoscopic repair of esophageal atresia (EA) and/or tracheoesophageal fistula (TEF) is one of the most challenging endoscopic procedures. The first reported thoracoscopic repair of pure esophageal atresia (EA) was in 1999 followed by the next year report of first case of EA/TEF, both done by S. Rothenberg [1, 2]. The experience with a novel technique is growing systematically however only in a few centers is regarded as a standard procedure. The citied advantages of a novel procedure are an excellent visibility of anatomic structures and a potential decreased morbidity due to avoidance of the open thoracotomy consequences. The results are at least comparable to open technique [3]. However, according to IPEG 2013 survey, only half of the responders were using thoracoscopic approach [4].

The primary aim of this chapter is to provide the practical information about thoracoscopic repair of EA/TEF. Author's personal experience is more than 160 cases operated by thoracoscopic approach for different types of EA/TEF malformations [5].

D. Patkowski (✉)
Pediatric Surgery and Urology Department, Wroclaw Medical University, Wroclaw, Poland
e-mail: dariusz.patkowski@umed.wroc.pl

21.2 Preoperative Preparation

The preoperative assessment follows the same principle as for open repair that include X-ray examination, cardiac echo, and abdominal ultrasound. More than 50% of patients with EA/TEF have additional malformations that should be diagnosed before starting the operation. The X-ray examination in a vertical position including the chest and the abdomen with a small amount of contrast in the upper pouch of the esophagus is carried out. The examination done by experienced team carries a low risk of contrast aspiration into the respiratory tract. However, some recommend not to use the contrast as air in the upper pouch should be enough to delineate it.

Patients are usually operated within 24 h after arriving to the hospital in the morning or afternoon session. Almost in each case with distal fistula the primary or delay esophageal anastomosis is possible.

Just before starting the surgery, the rigid bronchoscopy is performed as a routine procedure to look for trachea and larynx malformations and a fistula position. Any signs of tracheomalacia suggest possible postoperative respiratory problems. Knowing the fistula position helps with the distal pouch localization during the operative procedure and usually corresponds to the distance between pouches. If the fistula is located at the level of carina, it is found at the surgery directly under the azygos vein, and the distance between

C. Esposito et al. (eds.), *ESPES Manual of Pediatric Minimally Invasive Surgery*,
https://doi.org/10.1007/978-3-030-00964-9_21

pouches is greater. If the fistula enters the trachea on its posterior wall, the dissection should start above the azygos vein, and both pouches should be in proximity. The preoperative bronchoscopy is extremely important for cases regarded as a pure EA. It is not rare to discover undiagnosed proximal fistula.

My personal experience suggests that newborns with the weight above 1500 g are good candidates for thoracoscopic repair. The only principal contraindication is surgeon's lack of experience in newborn endoscopic surgery. For cases below 1500 g, unstable babies mainly with respiratory insufficiency due to the distal fistula or if any problems with anesthesia occur, only thoracoscopic closure of the distal fistula as the first-stage operation should be considered followed later by a final thoracoscopic repair.

21.3 Positioning

The proper patient's position is crucial. At the beginning, a lateral position was used; however, with the growing experience, a complete prone position turned out to be the most suitable. It ensures a good exposure of posterior mediastinum by lung collapse with gravitation and the insufflation pressure aid. I found that it is even not necessary to elevate the right side as it was being done earlier. It is important to put a newborn at the table border—it ensures a full extent of free instruments movement (Fig. 21.1).

The surgeon is standing on the left side of the table, and camera assistant is sitting to the surgeon's left hand on the same side. The video equipment is located in front of the surgeon on

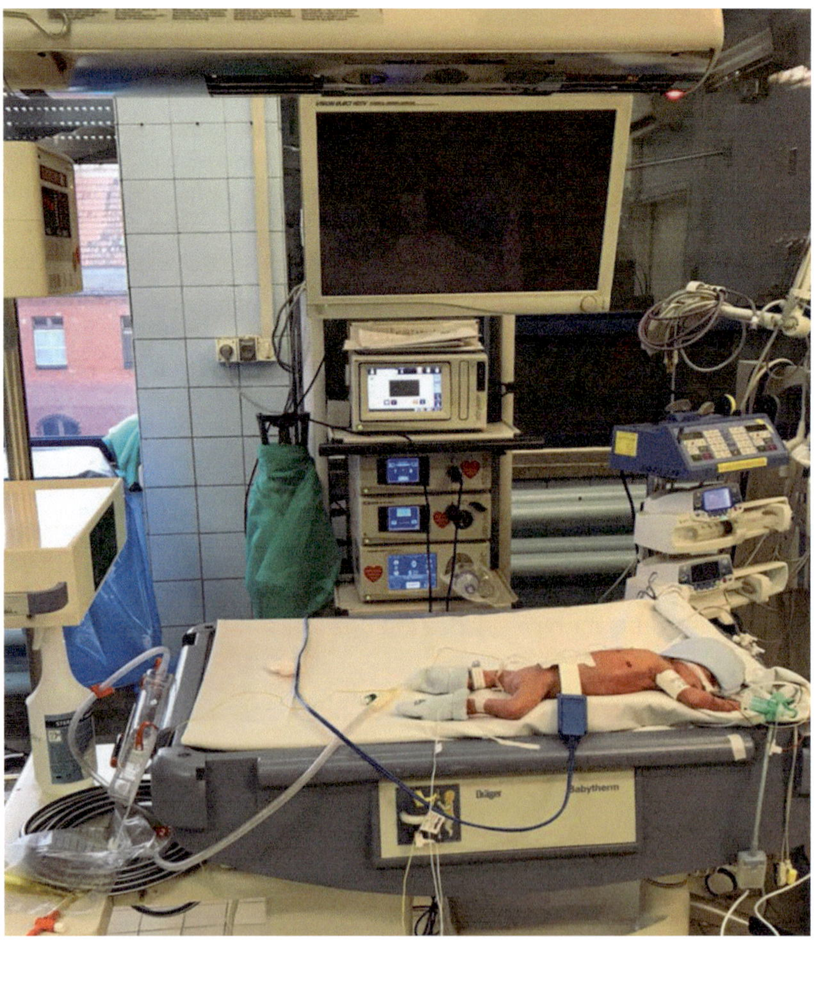

Fig. 21.1 Patient's position on operating table and TV monitor setup

Table 21.1 Suggested instruments set for thoracoscopic EA/TEF repair

	Instrument	Diameter	Number of items
1.	Maryland dissector	3–3.5 mm	1
2.	Fenestrated grasper	3–3.5 mm	1
3.	Babcock-type grasper	3–3.5 mm	1
4.	Metzenbaum scissors	3–3.5 mm	1
5.	Hook scissors	3–3.5 mm	1
6.	Needle holder	3–3.5 mm	1
7.	Hook electrode	3–3.5 mm	1
8.	Trocar	5 mm	1–2
9.	Trocar	3.5 mm	2
10.	Clip applier—optional	5 mm	1
11.	Scope 30° short	4–5 mm	1

the opposite side of operative table, and the scrub nurse is standing on the same side left to the video screen.

21.4 Instrumentation

The optimal equipment for EA/TEF repair consists of 3.0–3.5 mm instruments preferably not longer than 25 cm listed in Table 21.1. The best view comes from 4–5 mm short telescope with 25–30 degrees connected to HD camera. The 5 mm optical trocar and two 3–3.5 mm working trocars are needed. The trocars should be fixed to the skin with sutures as they easily move up and down during the procedure. Short trocars are more suitable. Depending on what way the fistula is going to be closed, it may be necessary to have a 5 mm clip applier and one 5 mm trocar to accommodate it. The clip applier is also needed for long-gap stage repair. Electrocautery is needed seldomly—hook electrode is enough. It is essential to have insufflated CO_2 heated.

21.5 Technique

The first 5 mm cannula for a video camera is inserted using the open technique 1–2 cm below the inferior scapula angle in the posterior axillary line. With 5–6 mmHg insufflation pressure, the lung on operated side will collapse within a few minutes after starting the procedure. After pneumothorax with heated CO_2 insufflation is established, two additional ports are inserted under the camera control: 3.5 mm near the paravertebral line at the same level as the first one and 3.5 or 5 mm (if a clip applier is going to be used) in posterior axillary line through the third or fourth intercostal space. With such trocars, positioning both the scope and auxiliary working instrument retracts partially the lung preventing it from coming into the posterior mediastinal view. There is no need for an extra trocar and a lung retractor. The right thoracoscopy is done even for the diagnosed right aortic arch cases; however, left approach is also advocated.

The azygos vein serves as an anatomical landmark demarcating TEF location and is never divided what will be discussed later. The mediastinal pleura is opened by blunt dissection below or above the azygos vein depending on preoperative bronchoscopy. Staying within anatomical borders, blunt dissection gives excellent tissue separation with almost no bleeding. The lower part of the esophagus is mobilized close to the trachea only on a very short distance. However, it is not a mistake to dissect the lower esophagus down to the diaphragm level if it is required. The TEF is being dissected completely around at the connection with the trachea and then occluded with 5 mm titanic clips or with a suture ligature close to the trachea. The upper part of the esophagus is localized with the aid of nasogastric tube placed through the mouth by an anesthesiologist—tube movement helps to distinguish upper pouch in operating area. Then it is mobilized circumferentially mainly by blunt dissection. There is usually firm and fibrous adhesion to the posterior tracheal wall that should be dissected or cut with care to avoid opening the trachea. After sufficient mobilization, the proximal esophageal pouch is opened with scissors and the TEF cut below the ligation suture. The 6–8 Fr nasogastric tube is passed through both parts of the esophagus into the stomach. The esophageal anastomosis is created above the azygos vein over the tube by placing 6–8 interrupted sutures of 4–0 or 5–0 absorbable braided suture including all layers starting from posterior wall (Fig. 21.2).

After placing the first suture, it is easy to rotate the anastomosis around the tube using cut suture ends to have a good exposure. All knots are tied intracorporeally using the sliding (slip) knot. The sliding knot, that I am using every time, is very helpful as it lets to approximate both esophageal ends even under the considerably tension. If the anastomosis was uneventful, there is no need for pleural drainage. The skin wounds are closed with single sutures.

21.5.1 The Long-Gap EA

There are different definitions of long-gap EA; however, to avoid any confusions, it should be reserved only for EA without distal fistula. Long-gap EA is always a challenge for a surgeon, and it is hardly ever possible to make primary esophageal anastomosis during the first days of life. The thoracoscopy is the only method to precisely define the gap between esophageal pouches. Having such a case, the author is using stage repair with internal traction technique. The same principles of thoracoscopic approach as described earlier are used at the beginning of the procedure. Usually the distal pouch is found directly above the diaphragm level. It is mobilized circumferentially in a full extent down even below the diaphragm. In the same way, the upper pouch is dissected. If there is an upper fistula, the pouch mostly ends highly in the chest inlet and looks small and hypotrophic; in other case, it is longer, distended with a thick wall. It is extremely difficult to suture the upper fistula located highly at or above thoracic inlet. Placing the clips across is the best way to close it and then to divide it between clips. Having both pouches, fully mobilized internal traction suture between them is placed. It goes through the tips of both esophageal ends taking a good bite of tissue. To prevent any leakage and tissue disruption, two clips are placed across the tips of both esophageal pouches taking the threads into the clips—they are not tightened at that moment. In this way, the traction force is dispersed along the clips instead of tissue puncture spot, and one can use the greater traction force. Two sliding (slip) knots are created, and both esophageal ends are approached step by step. It is surgeon's experience how much traction force to use. Usually there is no need for chest drainage (Fig. 21.3).

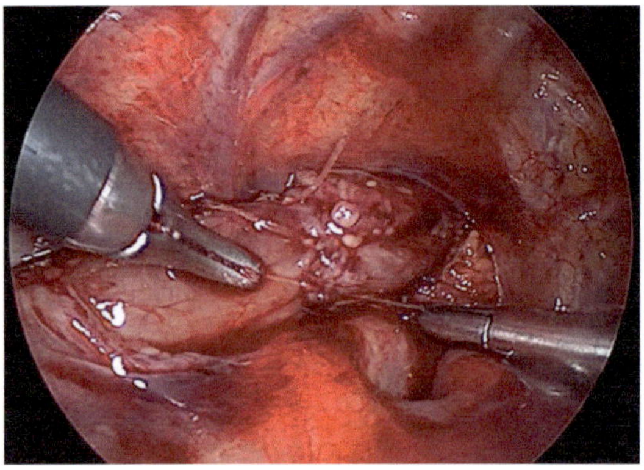

Fig. 21.2 The final esophageal anastomosis above the azygos vein

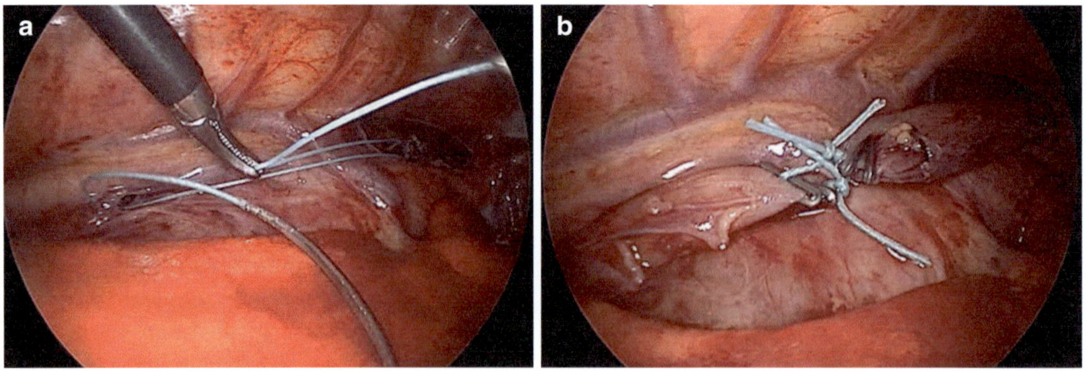

Fig. 21.3 Internal traction technique: (**a**) Before starting the traction. (**b**) Esophageal end approximation with the internal traction

The next stage procedure is scheduled 5 days later. The trocars are placed using the previous skin incisions. Usually only very soft adhesions are found at the mediastinum around the pouches and the traction suture. They are dissected easily. If both pouches overcome each other, the anastomosis is possible; in other case, the previously created sliding (slip) knots are used to get them closer. Using the described technique, the anastomosis is possible in majority of cases in two stages; sometimes, the third one is needed. One author's case had final anastomosis at sixth thoracoscopy. If the surgical treatment is started within first days after birth, it is not necessary to create a gastrostomy that seems to be one of advantage.

21.5.2 The Isolated Congenital Tracheoesophageal Fistula (H-Type)

The H-type fistula is mostly repaired by right neck incision above the clavicle. The thoracoscopy may be considered as alternative approach for the cases with fistula located at the entrance to the chest or below. It is a good idea to put the guidewire through the fistula at the preoperative bronchoscopy to help its identification. One can use a nylon thread instead and take the esophageal end out for traction. The thoracoscopic approach for H-type fistula is almost similar to EA/TEF repair. The main difference is difficult intracorporal suturing of the fistula located high in the entrance to the chest. If this is a case, the fistula can be closed with clips and divided between them.

21.6 Postoperative Care

The postoperative care during the first days is provided by neonatal intensive care unit (NICU). Most patients represent a wide spectrum of problems related not only to performed operation but also to associated malformations, prematurity, and arising complications. Patient remains intubated for at least 24 h. Direct extubation after operation should be avoided. The eventual reintubation is always danger for esophageal anastomosis and the tracheal fistula closure site. If in surgeon's opinion there is considerable anastomotic tension, especially for long-gap EA, then prolonged muscle paralysis is maintained even up to 5 days. The oral secretion is removed by suction only as needed. The enteral feeding starts in small amounts through nasogastric tube on the second postoperative day. There is no need to keep pleural drainage until the contrast examination, so it is removed as early as possible. The contrast study/imaging is done on 5th–sixth postoperative day. If there is no leakage, oral feeding starts, and if tolerated, the nasogastric tube is removed. The antacid prophylaxis is continued for at least 3 months. In case of any leakage, a good and efficient drainage is enough. Usually the leakage stops within a few days on conservative management. There is no routine anastomosis dilatation as long as any clinical manifestations of stenosis arise.

21.7 Results

The first thoracoscopic repair of EA with TEF was done by the author in 2005 [5]. Since then, he was personally involved in more than 160 cases (EA, EA/TEF, isolated, or recurrent TEF) operated in different centers around the world. The presented results are referred to cases operated at the Pediatric Surgery and Urology Department, Wroclaw, Medical University, Poland, with my personal involvement (Tables 21.2, 21.3, and 21.4).

Table 21.2 Patients operated at Ped. Surg. and Urol. Dept. in Wroclaw (author's personal involvement)

No of cases of EA/TEF	113
Type I	6
Type II	9
Type III	91
Type IV	1
Type V (H-type TEF)	6

Table 21.3 Results for EA and TEF type III and IV Ped. Surg. and Urol. Dept. in Wroclaw (author's personal involvement)

Weight	av. 2397 g (min. 900 g, max. 4700)
Operating time	av. 1:47 (min. 0:55, max. 4:05)
Conversion	0
Accidental tracheal opening	2/92 (2.2%)
Anastomotic leakage 6/92	(6.5%)
Stenosis 19/87	(21.8%)
Recurrent TEF	1/87 (1.15%)
Death[a]	5/92 (5.4%)

[a]Not directly related to the surgical procedure

Table 21.4 Results for long-gap EA with internal traction staged repair at Ped. Surg. and Urol. Dept. in Wroclaw (author's personal involvement)

No of cases	15
2 stages	7 (46.7%)
3 stages	4 (26.7%)
5 stages	1 (6.7%)
6 stages	1 (6.7%)
Not completed (death)	1 (6.7)
Final Collis-Nissen open repair	1 (6.7)

21.8 Tips and Tricks

1. There is no need for one lung ventilation; the bilateral lung conventional mechanical one is always used.
2. I am against using Replogle tube. Both preoperatively and postoperatively, the suction of oral secretion is only on demand. In my opinion, Replogle tube with continuous suction may cause mucosa dryness and subsequent irritation and local infection.
3. The azygos vein was never divided in my experience with thoracoscopic approach. Leaving intact vein may improve vascularity of surrounding tissues and in majority of cases will separate the fistula site closure from esophageal anastomosis line decreasing the risk for recurrent fistula formation with native tissue between them.

21.9 Discussion

Many studies showed that even complex endoscopic procedures in newborns and neonates are possible to perform. The results of surgery for esophageal atresia have always been the signs of progress in pediatric surgery. The same we can say about thoracoscopic EA/TEF repair. In a recent review of the literature and meta-analysis of five retrospective comparative studies, there was no difference with regard to complication rate, anastomotic leak, or anastomotic stricture between the thoracoscopic and open approaches for EA/TEF. The review also showed an earlier time to extubation, first oral feeding, and shorter hospital stay after thoracoscopic repair. The only disadvantage was longer operating time; however, it seems to be directly related to surgeon's learning curve [6–9]. Looking to my personal experience, it usually takes no more than 75–90 min to complete a case.

Considering the indication for thoracoscopic EA/TEF repair, main three criterions are discussed: patient's weight, patient's general condition, and type of the defect. To author's opinion, generally speaking, each case of EA/TEF considered for surgical approach is also suitable for thoracoscopic approach. Some surgeons advocate the 2500 g as the lower limit for endoscopic repair; others put the limit to 1500 g [10]. With author's experience, it was possible to successfully repair cases weighting 1000 g, but it was really challenging. In such a case, it is reasonable only to close the fistula with thoracoscopic approach and to perform the final anastomosis after gaining more weight. The same treatment is recommended for patients in poor general condition and severe respiratory insufficiency.

One of the main cited advantages of thoracoscopic approach is avoiding thoracotomy that influenced chest development and natural mechanism of chest wall movement. The thoracotomy morbidity is well known and may result in scoliosis and shoulder girdle weakness later in the life [11, 12]. Using only limited small skin incisions to introduce three trocars minimizes considerably the risk for the chest wall trauma.

The growing surgical scar created at the newborn period is well known. Thoracoscopy gives the excellent cosmetic result as the scars are almost invisible with time [13]. Even with the staged repairs, the same incisions are used for next procedures (Fig. 21.4).

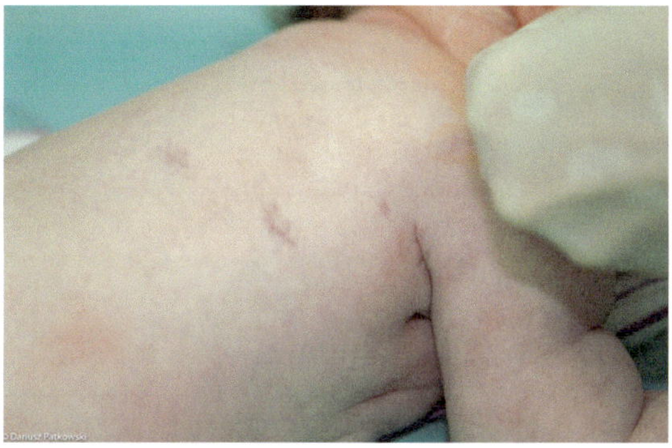

Fig. 21.4 Scars after six thoracoscopic procedures

Another important advantage is mediastinal visualization and mediastinal exposure. The thoracoscopy gives not only a direct view to mediastinal anatomy but also offers great magnification and precise anatomic details view especially with modern HD and 4 K screens. It almost gives the impression of working like under microscope. All the crucial steps of repair including fistula dissection and ligation, pouches, mobilization, and anastomosis are well seen for the entire team not only for operating surgeon that was a rule in open approach. The upper pouch may be dissected delicately from the membranaceous tracheal wall high into the thoracic outlet and neck with constant camera view control. This step was usually done blindly with open approach.

The fistula closure with a clip is the fastest method [13]. It is simple and effective especially in severely unstable patients when closure of fistula is the only procedure planned to do. However, there is a risk of clip migration. Sometimes the clips disappear on X-ray pictures taken later. It happened to one author's patient that his mother brought the clip he had coughed up 3 years after the procedure.

The main challenge and difficulty of thoracoscopic EA/TEF repair is meticulous endoscopic suturing in a small space that forms the basis of success. The lack of experience in making perfect endoscopic knot is a main contraindication to the thoracoscopic approach. In author's opinion, the most practical is a sliding knot. It allows to bring suturing tissues together with precise tension control. Using multiple sliding (slip) knots allow to overcome the tissue tension at anastomosis by distributing the tension between sutures when gradually tightening.

The main discussed disadvantage of thoracoscopic approach is the use of CO_2 for insufflation that may lead to hypercapnia, acidosis, and decreased cerebral perfusion that were reported by the team from Great Ormond Street in London [14]. Looking into their results, one can notice high insufflation pressure and long operative time. Other reports didn't confirm such a problem [15, 16].

The long-gap EA is the most challenging case for surgeon. The thoracoscopy for long-gap EA offers delay anastomosis or staged repairs with different forms of traction for final anastomosis of both esophageal ends. S. Rothenberg advocates initial gastrostomy after birth and waiting for spontaneous esophageal ends growth, delay thoracoscopic anastomosis at the age of 4–8 weeks depending on patients size, overall condition, and failure to show any improvement in gap length [17]. The different protocol is used by D. van der Zee without gastrostomy, and repeated every 3–4 days thoracoscopic oesophageal ends mobilization and external passive traction followed by delay anastomosis [18]. At our department, we developed the described earlier in this chapter "internal traction" technique that works well for all long-gap cases. In my personal opinion, the thoracoscopy will completely change the way we use to manage these cases.

In conclusion the thoracoscopy technique for EA/TEF repair is demanding, difficult, and requiring great experience however should be considered as the procedure of choice. That is the main reason why patients with EA/TEF should be managed only in specialized centers to provide the best available quality of treatment.

References

1. Lobe TE, Rothenberg S, Waldschmidt J, et al. Thoracoscopic repair of esophageal atresia in an infant: a surgical first. Pediatr Endosurg Innov Tech. 1999;3:141–8.
2. Rothenberg SS. Thoracoscopic repair of a tracheoesophageal fistula in a newborn infant. Pediatr Endosurg Innov Tech. 2000;4:289–94.
3. Holcomb GW, Rothenberg SS, Bax KMA, et al. Thoracoscopic repair of esophageal atresia and tracheoesophageal fistula a multi-institutional analysis. Ann Surg. 2005;3:119–26.
4. Lal D, Miyano G, Juang D, et al. Current patterns of practice and technique in the repair of esophageal atre-

sia and tracheoesophage-al fistula: an IPEG survey. J Laparoendosc Adv Surg Technol A. 2013;23:635–8.
5. Patkowski D, Rysiakiewicz K, Jaworski W, et al. Thoracoscopic repair of tracheoesophageal fistula and esophageal atresia. J Laparoendosc Adv Surg Technol A. 2009;19(Suppl 1):S19–22.
6. Lugo B, Malhotra A, Guner Y, et al. Thoracoscopic versus open repair of tracheoesophageal fistula and esophageal atresia. J Laparoendosc Adv Surg Technol A. 2008;18(5):753–6.
7. Borruto FA, Impellizzeri P, Montalto AS, et al. Thoracoscopy versus thoracotomy for esophageal atresia and tracheoesophageal fistula repair: review of the literature and metaanalysis. Eur J Pediatr Surg. 2012;22(6):415–9.
8. Davenport M, Rothenberg SS, Crabbe DC, et al. The great debate: open or thoracoscopic repair for oesophageal atresia or diaphragmatic hernia. J Pediatr Surg. 2015;50:240–6.
9. Yang Y-F, Dong R, Zheng C, et al. Outcomes of thoracoscopy versus thoracotomy for esophageal atresia with tracheoesophageal fistula repair: a PRISMA-compliant systematic review and meta-analysis. Medicine. 2016;95(30):e4428.
10. Dingemann C, Zoeller C, Ure B. Thoracoscopic repair of oesophageal atresia: results of a selective approach. Eur J Pediatr Surg. 2013;23:14–8.
11. Cherup LL, Sieweres RD, Futrell JW. Breast and pectoral muscle maldevelopment after anterolateral and posterolateral thoracotomies in children. Ann Thorac Surg. 1986;41:492–7.
12. Lawal TA, Gosemann JH, Kuebler JF, et al. Thoracoscopy versus thoracotomy improves midterm musculoskeletal status and cosmesis in infants and children. Ann Thorac Surg. 2009;87:224–8.
13. Rothenberg SS. Thoracoscopic repair of esophageal atresia and tracheo-esophageal fistula in neonates: evolution of a technique. J Laparoendosc Adv Surg Technol A. 2012;22(2):195–9.
14. Bishay M, Giacomello L, Retrosi G, et al. Decreased cerebral oxygen saturation during thoracoscopic repair of congenital diaphragmatic hernia and esophageal atresia in infants. J Pediatr Surg. 2011;46:47–51.
15. Tytgat SH, van Herwaarden MY, Stolwijk LJ, et al. Neonatal brain oxygenation during thoracoscopic correction of esophageal atresia. Surg Endosc. 2016;30:2811–7.
16. Stolwijk LJ, van der Zee DC, Tytgat S, et al. Brain oxygenation during thoracoscopic repair of long gap esophageal atresia. World J Surg. 2017;41(5):1384–92.
17. Rothenberg SS, Flake AW. Experience with thoracoscopic repair of long gap esophageal atresia in neonates. J Laparoendosc Adv Surg Technol A. 2015;25(11):932–5.
18. van der Zee DC, Gallo G, Tytgat SH. Thoracoscopic traction technique in long gap esophageal atresia: entering a new era. Surg Endosc. 2015;29(11):3324–30.

Part III

Abdomen

22 Laparoscopic Management of Congenital Morgagni Hernia (CMH)

M. L. Metzelder

22.1 Introduction

Congenital Morgagni hernia (CMH) is a very rare defect of the anterior diaphragm with retrosternal herniation of abdominal content [1–3]. CMH represents less than 5% of all congenital diaphragmatic hernias [1, 4], and males are predominantly affected [3]. In reports with data available for the defect size, intraoperatively, measured size varies from 3 to 11 cm in maximal dimension, respectively, 4 × 7 cm [4, 5].

In larger patient series, it was reported that the defect concerns in about 90% the right anterior part of the diaphragm, whereas the left side is only in 2% affected. Eight % of the defects were bilateral [1]. In contrast, in other reports, so-called midline defects were added with an occurrence of 50% leading to less right- and left-sided defects but same number of bilateral defects [3]. The hernia content is mostly the colon, followed by the liver, the small intestine, omentum majus, and the stomach, depending on the size of the defect [4–6]. Moreover, associated anomalies are mostly cardiac anomalies (30%), followed by chromosomal anomalies (25%) and to a lesser extend intestinal malrotation and other very rare entities like Cantrell Pentalogy [1, 7]. A possible explanation for the higher incidence of CMH in M. Down patients could be the more hypotonic muscle development that could also lead to a higher recurrence rate in this patient group [1].

Several authors reported that about 50–80% of their CMH patients were asymptomatic, and CMH was found by chest X-ray (Fig. 22.1), by other imaging (computed tomography, barium enema, and others), or during surgery in the upper abdomen for other reasons [1, 2]. Other authors reported contrary on a higher incidence of symptomatic CMH patients as the majority of their patients with CMG were investigated for respiratory problems [4, 6]. To this regard, the underlying risk for a severe onset of intestinal obstruction or even bowel strangulation is evident also, and was reported, too [8].

Several techniques for laparoscopic CMH repair were described including a primary closure in an interrupted or running suture technique as well as the use of several types of patches [2, 5, 6].

22.2 Preoperative Preparation

Underlying associated anomalies with CMH, exemplarily cardiac anomalies need precise preoperative cardiac evaluation including a preoperative echocardiogram.

The extend of the defect and the planned use of a patch might lead of a perioperative application of i.v. antibiotics [5]. However, in most

M. L. Metzelder (✉)
Department of Pediatric Surgery, Medical University of Vienna, Vienna, Austria
e-mail: martin.metzelder@meduniwien.ac.at

C. Esposito et al. (eds.), *ESPES Manual of Pediatric Minimally Invasive Surgery*,
https://doi.org/10.1007/978-3-030-00964-9_22

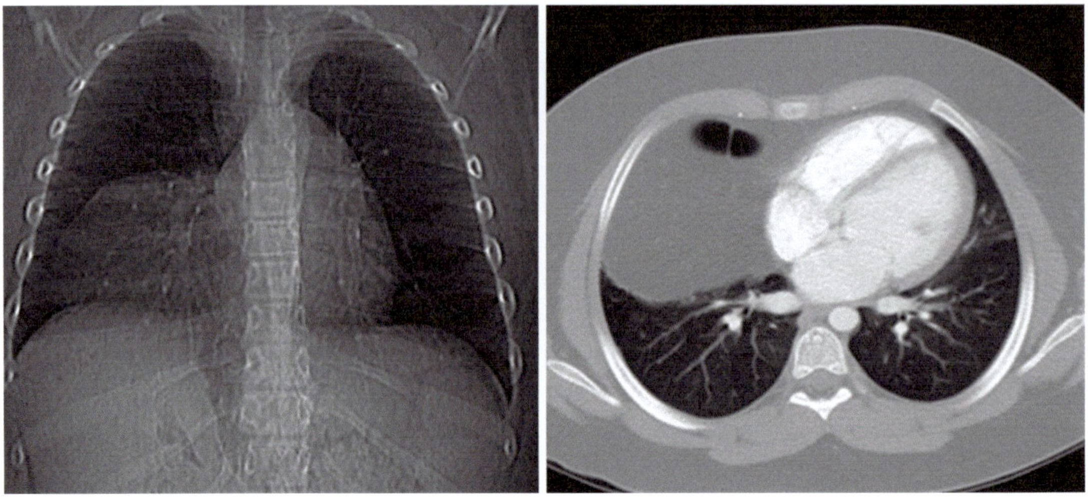

Fig. 22.1 Chest X-ray and CT scan indicating a huge right-sided Morgagni hernia in a 14-year-old female

cases, especially for asymptomatic patients with CMH, there is no need for a special preoperative preparation.

22.2.1 Patient Position

The patient is placed in a supine position. Small infants should be placed in a reverse frog position, whereas older children in a spread leg position. The surgeon stands at the end of the operating table or in older children between the patient's legs. Two monitors should be placed, one above the patient's head and the second in front of the surgeon's camera assistant.

22.3 Instrumentation

In general, a 30° 5 mm optic can be used in our experience irrespective of the age of the patient, whereas a 10 mm optic might be required in obese patients. In addition, a standard pediatric set of endoscopic instruments for laparoscopic surgery is sufficient. Again, depending on patient's size, either 3 or 5 mm trocars and endoscopic graspers and needle holders are required. We use monopolar hook cautery (3–5 mm) or other sealing devices (5 mm) to handle with the falciform ligament and for the resection of the hernia sac. To overcome tension during the intracorporal tying maneuver, we prefer the application of a Goretex® patch to achieve a tension-free repair.

22.4 Surgical Technique

In general, we use a three-trocar technique for a laparoscopic hernia repair of a CMH. At our institution, we prefer an open umbilical approach for the insertion of the 5 mm optic trocar, irrespective the age of the patient and to prevent from intraabdominal injury. Other techniques preferred by others include the insertion of a Veress needle or the use of an umbilical STEP® trocar [5]. Under videoscopic guidance (30° optic) and following application of a limited CO_2 pneumoperitoneum (6–8 mmHg small infants; 8–10 mmHg older children), two 3–5 mm working trocars are placed in the upper right and upper left abdomen with ergonomic angulation (80–0°) shown at Fig. 22.2. The content of the hernia should be pushed back with atraumatic endoscopic graspers (Fig. 22.3). The next step is to incise the falciform ligament with an endoscopic sealing device (Fig. 22.3) for a better exposure of the hernia defect. By surgeon's preference, a hernia sac can be excised by hook cautery or any other sealing device but also left in situ, especially if it is adherent to the pleura or pericardium [2, 5]. In case of leaving the hernia sac in place, it can be plicated and included into the stiches to reduce

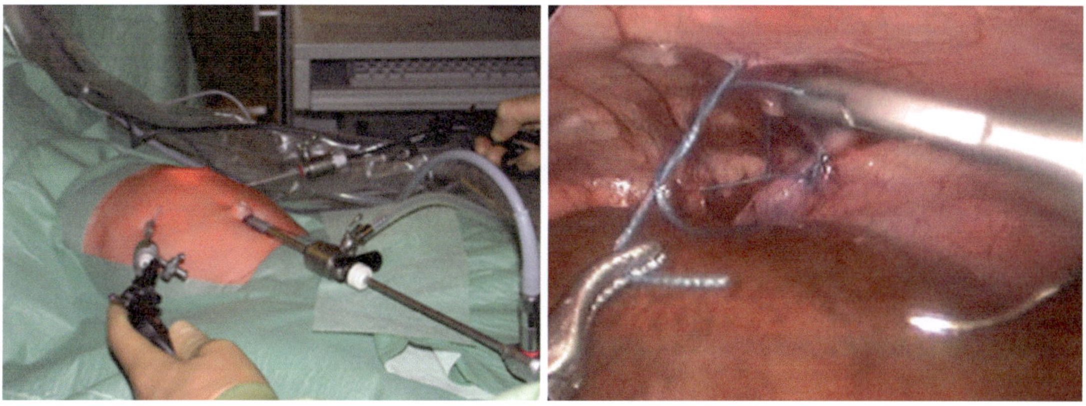

Fig. 22.2 Ergonomic triangulation of camera optic and instruments and intraabdominal laparoscopic view

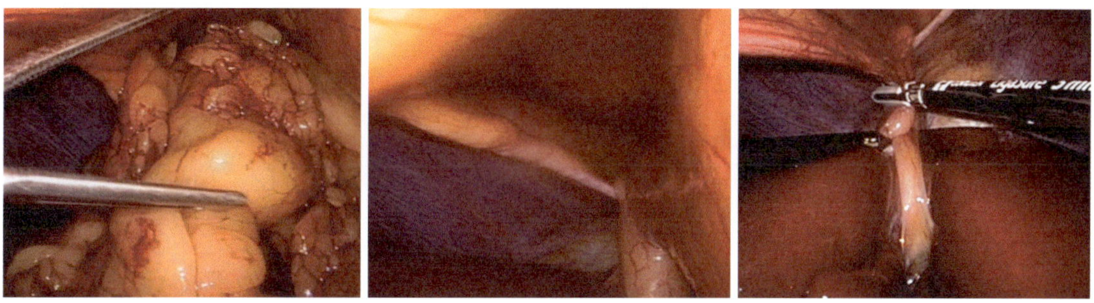

Fig. 22.3 Laparoscopic view during Morgagni hernia repair: reduction of herniated omentum majus; inspection of right-sided part of retrosternal hernia; dissection of falciform ligament

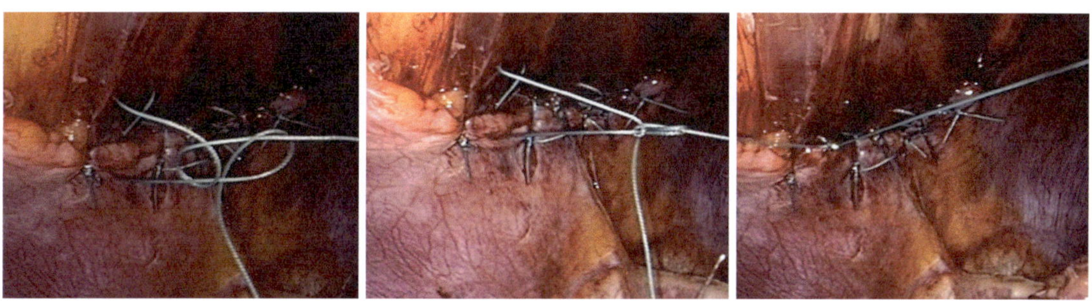

Fig. 22.4 Laparoscopic view: intracorporal technique of a slipping knot to facilitate tying the knot

a residual formation in the thoracic cavity and to obtain a stronger closure. To further reduce the incidence of recurrence, some authors [2] recommend to cauterize the edges of the CMH into scar tissue. High acceptance exists to use a patch for a tension-free hernia closure [2, 6]. To verify and to overcome tension, a transparietal/transabdominal stich to suspend the diaphragm to the abdominal wall is helpful [2]. In addition, transabdominal sutures should be applied, if there is no anterior rim of the diaphragm, and interrupted stitches are subsequently tied in the subcutaneous tissue by separate small skin incisions [2, 9]. We prefer non-resorbable interrupted sutures 3.0 or 2.0 with intraabdominal knotting in the slipping-knot technique in case of primary closure (Figs. 22.4 and 22.5). However, depending on the surgeons skills, intracorporal as well a

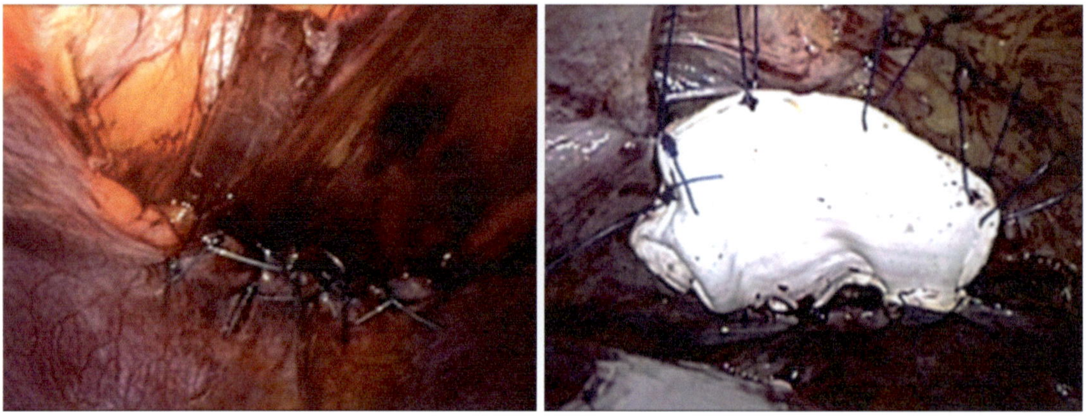

Fig. 22.5 Laparoscopic view of Morgagni hernia repair: example of direct closure with interrupted sutures and example using a Goretex® patch

extracorporal knotting is in use, and in combination of both techniques [4], as suturing parallel to the anterior abdominal wall can be demanding. If a patch is needed, it should be rolled around an endoscopic grasper to facilitate the insertion via the trocar or even trocarless into the abdomen. An example of an intraoperative view of one of our patients who underwent a patch repair is shown at Fig. 22.5. To this regard, the patch should overlap the defect edges for about 1 cm [5]. We like others [6] find that the need for a patch does not add much technical difficulty to the operation. At the end of the procedure and after leaving the pneumoperitoneum, the nasogastric tube as well as the trocars can be removed under videoscopic guidance, followed by skin closure.

22.5 Postoperative Care

Exclusive patients without severe associated anomalies can be treated with fast track surgery concepts by starting eating and drinking postoperative at the day of operation and can be discharged at the first postoperative day [6].

22.6 Results

Whether the laparoscopic closure of a CMH is easy or demanding depends on the age of the patient, the size and location of the defect, and the type of underlying associated disease. However, in experienced centers, the reported average length of the operation was about 60 min, and the overall complication rate was very low and less than 3% [2]. The need of a demanding assisting device like extracorporal membrane circulation is extremely rare [3].

In contrast to several patient series without any conversion of the laparoscopic procedure [2, 5, 6], Garriboli et al. reported on 2 conversions (17%) out of 12, due to one case with severe adhesions and another with severe scoliosis [4].

In several published series with more than 15 patients, the reported recurrence rate was below 3% [2, 5, 6] but tended to be higher in patients with associated anomalies like Down syndrome [1]. The report from Dutta et al. on their patients with patch repair and no case of recurrence underlines the use of a patch if there is any sign of tension [5].This is further underlined by a report from Garriboli et al. who found a high number of recurrence in four out of five of their patients who all underwent primary repair of CMH without a patch as well as without hernia sac resection.

Nonetheless, a recent multicenter surveys found a low recurrence rate irrespective of a primary or a patch repair [2], and thus, it remains of most importance not to underestimate tension during primary CMH repair.

With regard to postoperative patient monitoring, there is no evidence for a recommended follow-up for CMH patients after surgery, and thus, it should be adapted to the individual patient and the underlying disease. Clinical controls after 1 week, 1 and 3 months, and after 1 year with a chest X-ray to detect recurrence were recommended [2, 4]. This algorithm seems to be suitable as published data indicate that recurrence after primary repair occurs within the first year postoperatively [4].

22.7 Tips and Tricks

A simple rule stated by Laituri et al. is to attempt an intracorporal tie with minimal insufflation pressure. If there is too much tension to tie it down, then a patch should be placed for a tension-free repair [6].

22.8 Discussion

Congenital Morgagni hernia (CMH) is a very rare entity. Some authors reported that the majority of patients with CMH is asymptomatic [2], others about 50% [3], while some found the majority of their patients with CMH associated unspecific respiratory symptoms [6]. However, as also asymptomatic patients may beat a risk to experience intestinal obstruction or even a strangulated colon requiring immediate surgery [8], most surgeons opt for surgery, if a CMH is incidentally diagnosed [1, 2, 6].

With the advent of minimally invasive pediatric surgery, anecdotal reports and several retrospective studies confirmed the safety of the laparoscopic repair [10–12] with excellent outcome and some superior aspects compared to the conventional open repair [1, 6, 9].

There are still some other issues that need to be addressed. Whether to resect the hernia sac or not should be an individual decision, as injuries of the pleura or pericardium may occur [2, 5]. To this regard, a partial resection or to include part of the hernia sac into the suture line is an option, too [5]. Nonetheless, in the majority of the published series with exception of the study from Garriboli et al. [4], there is no higher incidence of recurrence of a CMH, irrespective of a resected or non-resected hernia sac [2].

As the majority of authors agrees to use a patch in case of too much tension during the repair, there is no evidence whether to apply an absorbable [6] or a non-absorbable patch [2]. To this regard, the current literature revealed no differences and a similar outcome and very low incidence of infections, as well as the same rate of recurrence without other patch-related morbidity [2]. Nonetheless, in case of a recurrent CMH, after initial laparoscopic primary repair, subsequent laparoscopic patch repair is feasible with an excellent outcome [4]. Concerning suture material, there is consensus to use non-absorbable instead of absorbable sutures in an interrupted fashion [2].

With regard to the advantage of earlier feed, less analgesia, shorter hospital stay, and better cosmesis by using the laparoscopic approach compared to the open repair, we like others [2, 6] recommend to apply the laparoscopic repair to children with CMH at institution familiar with minimally invasive surgical techniques.

References

1. Al-Salem AH, Zamakhshary M, Al Mohaidly M, et al. Congenital Morgagni's hernia: a national multicenter study. J Pediatr Surg. 2014;49:503–7.
2. Esposito C, Escolino M, Varlet F, et al. Technical standardization of laparoscopic repair of Morgagni diaphragmatic hernia in children: results of a multicentric survey on 43 patients. Surg Endosc. 2017;31:3320–5.
3. Golden J, Barry WE, Jang G, et al. Pediatric Morgagni diaphragmatic hernia: a descriptive study. Pediatr Surg Int. 2017;33:771–5.
4. Garriboli M, Bishay M, Kiely EM, et al. Recurrence rate of Morgagni diaphragmatic hernia following laparoscopic repair. Pediatr Surg Int. 2013;29:185–9.
5. Dutta S, Albanese CT. Use of a prosthetic patch for laparoscopic repair of Morgagni diaphragmatic hernia in children. J Laparosendosc Adv Surg Tech A. 2007;17:391–4.
6. Laituri CA, Garey CJ, Ostlie DJ, et al. Morgagni hernia repair in children: comparison of laparoscopic and open results. J Laparoendosc Adv Surg Tech A. 2011;21:89–91.
7. Cigdem MK, Onen A, Okur H, et al. Associated malformation in Morgagni hernia. Pediatr Surg Int. 2007;23:1101–3.
8. Vaos G, Skondras C. Colonic necrosis because of strangulated recurrent Morgagni's hernia in a child with Down's syndrome. J Pediatr Surg. 2006;41:589–91.

9. Azzie G, Maoate K, Beasley S, et al. A simple technique of laparoscopic full-thickness anterior abdominal wall repair of retrosternal (Morgagni) hernias. J Pediatr Surg. 2003;38:768–70.
10. Huntington TR. Laparoscopic transabdominal preperitoneal repair of Morgagni. J Laparoendosc Surg. 1996;6:131–3.
11. Orita M, Okino M, Yamashita K, et al. Laparoscopic repair of a diaphragmatic hernia through the foramen of Morgagni. Surg Endosc. 1997;11:668–70.
12. Bortul M, Calligaris L, Gheller P. Laparoscopic repair of a Morgagnilarrey hernia. J Laparoendosc Adv Surg Tech A. 1998;8:309–13.

Laparoscopic Treatment of Esophageal Achalasia

23

Giovanna Riccipetitoni, Francesca Destro, Claudio Vella, Luciano Maestri, and Tiziana Russo

23.1 Introduction

Esophageal achalasia is a primary motility disorder that is thought to be due to a dysfunction of the enteric nervous system [1]. It is characterized by loss of ganglion cells with degeneration of inhibitory myenteric plexus that innervates the esophageal body and the region of the lower esophageal sphincter (LOS) of unknown origin. It is hypothesized that decreased nitric-oxide synthase leads to a neuronal excitatory/inhibitory imbalance with esophageal aperistalsis, incomplete LOS relaxation in response to swallowing, and increased LOS resting pressures.

The condition is exceedingly rare in the pediatric population with 0.11–0.18/10,000 children observed/year in the UK and a male preponderance [2]. Less than 5% of cases are reported under 15 years of age (mean patient age at diagnosis is 10.9 years) [3, 4].

Achalasia is frequently described in association with trisomy 21, congenital hypoventilation syndrome, glucocorticoid insufficiency, eosinophilic esophagitis, familial dysautonomia, Chagas disease, and AAA syndrome (achalasia, alacrima, and ACTH insensitivity).

Dysphagia (progressive, from solids to liquids) and weight loss are the most common manifestations, followed by regurgitation, aspiration pneumonia, retrosternal chest pain, and respiratory symptoms (younger children).

The diagnosis is easily suspected performing an esophagram with barium that demonstrates a dilated esophagus with "bird's-beak" like tapering of the distal esophagus. The manometry study is important (elevated resting LES pressure, absent or low amplitude peristalsis, or non-relaxing LES upon swallowing), but its interpretation might be challenging (difficulties are reported from 27.6 to 34.5%) [5]. The upper endoscopy is useful to exclude eosinophilic esophagitis and other secondary causes of achalasia.

Medical treatment with Nifedipine (calcium channel blocker) or botulin toxin (BT) has no or limited effect: Hurwitz reported an 83% response rate among children receiving BT, lengthen 4.2 months, with more than 50% of those responders requiring additional procedures [6].

Pneumatic dilatation (PD), with a recommended balloon of 30–35 mm, has an overall success rate ranging from 65 to 80% [7–9]. A Cochrane review of adults demonstrated that PD is superior to BT in symptom remission at 6 and 12 months. Long-term remission of PD is reported to be 40% at 5 years and 36% at 10 years

G. Riccipetitoni (✉) · F. Destro · C. Vella
L. Maestri · T. Russo
Pediatric Surgery Unit, Departement of Paediatric Surgery, Buzzi Children's Hospital, Milan, Italy
e-mail: giovanna.riccipetitoni@asst-fbf-sacco.it; Francesca.destro@asst-fbf-sacco.it; Claudio.vella@asst-fbf-sacco.it; Luciano.maestri@asst-fbf-sacco.it; Tiziana.russo@asst-fbf-sacco.it

C. Esposito et al. (eds.), *ESPES Manual of Pediatric Minimally Invasive Surgery*,
https://doi.org/10.1007/978-3-030-00964-9_23

[10]. Although significant short-term efficacy of PD has been reported, long-term efficacy data in children are lacking.

The treatment of choice remains the surgical correction with the extramucosal longitudinal modified Heller cardiomiotomy (the double myotomy proposed by Heller was modified into a procedure that provides for the anterior cut alone) [11]. An anterior fundoplication has to be performed in order to avoid the onset of gastroesophageal reflux, to protect the esophageal mucosa and to maintain the myotomy open. Laparoscopy is associated with lower recurrence rate because the myotomy can be easily extended also on the gastric side (complete distal myotomy), and it allows the simultaneous anti-reflux procedure. A recent meta-analysis demonstrated remission and relapse rates of 77.8% and 35.7%, respectively, for PD compared with 95% and 5.1%, respectively, for laparoscopic myotomy [12].

23.2 Preoperative Preparation

All patients and their parents have to sign a specifically formulated informed consent before the procedure. Three days before surgery, the patient reduces food intakes and the day before surgery adopts a liquid diet in order to avoid the presence of food in the esophagus. Patients receive antibiotic prophylaxis (cefazolina i.v.) and PPI therapy. The procedure is performed under general anesthesia.

23.3 Positioning

The patient is placed in supine, reverse Trendelenburg position with legs opened or in frog position for younger children (Fig. 23.1). The first surgeon stays between the patient's legs and the assistant on his left (Fig. 23.2). A third surgeon is opposite to the assistant. The scrub nurse is between the first and the third surgeon. The laparoscopy tower with monitors is placed at the head of the child, in front of the surgeon. Three or four trocars are used: 5 or 10 mm in the umbilicus (lens), 3–5 mm operative trocars in left and right hypochondrium, and an additional fourth trocar below the subcostal margin for liver retractor.

23.4 Instrumentation

The set of instruments is the following: 30° 5 or 10 mm lens (3D lenses require 10 mm trocar), atraumatic dissectors, Joanne graspers ($n = 2$), hook (protected and not too long instruments to simplify maneuvering and reducing the risk of injuries), peanuts, high-frequency devices (e.g.,

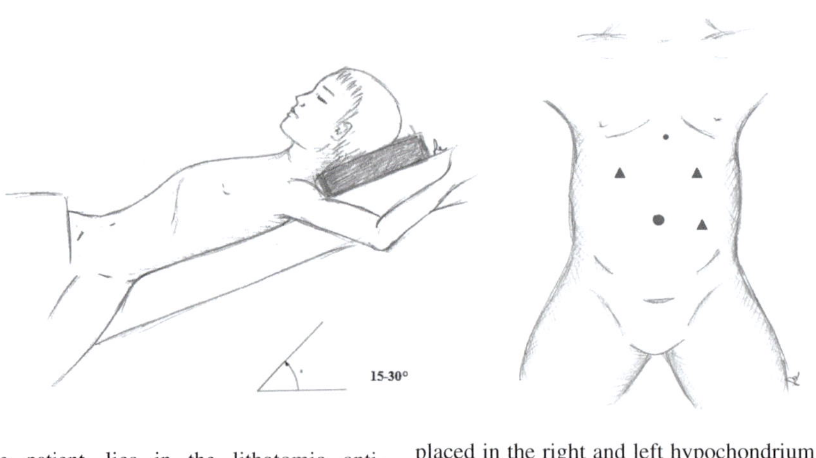

Fig. 23.1 The patient lies in the lithotomic anti-Trendelenburg supine position. The optic is inserted in the umbilicus (circle on the right figure); operative trocars are placed in the right and left hypochondrium or on the left paraumbilical line (triangles on the right figure); and hepatic retractor is in the epigastrium (small circle)

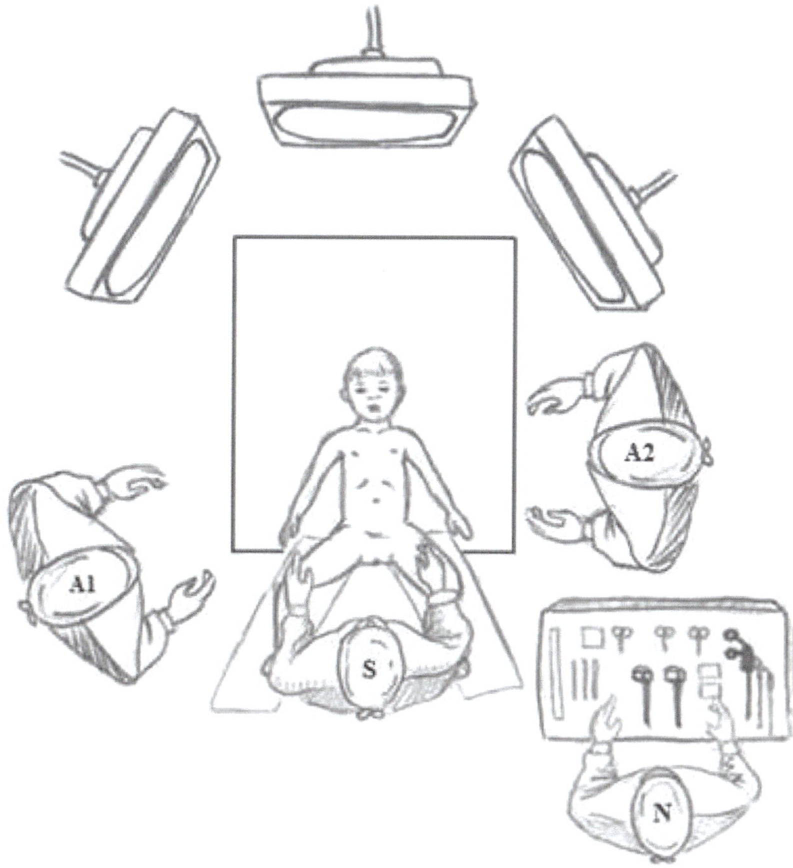

Fig. 23.2 Team position (*S* surgeon; *A1* assistant 1; *A2* assistant 2; *N* scrub nurse)

Ligasure™), 3 or 5 mm needleholders, scissor, Ethibond 2/0 sutures, and gastroscope. In addition, a standard set of instruments for traditional open surgery should be available.

23.5 Technique

At the beginning of the surgical procedure, an endoscopic evaluation can be performed to remove any retained food (if present), but care should be taken not to overextend the stomach complicating the operation. The first umbilical trocar is inserted with open technique, the pneumoperitoneum is created with controlled pressure and flow, and the remaining trocars are placed under direct vision. The esophagogastric junction is exposed after the retraction of the left hepatic lobe and the opening of the lesser omentum (Fig. 23.3). Exercising a downward traction of the stomach, the edge of the diaphragmatic crura appears as a "white line"; the phrenoesophageal junction is divided freeing the

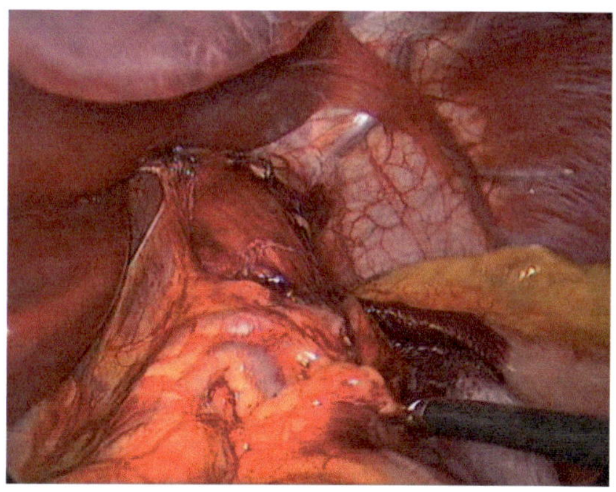

Fig. 23.3 Exposure of the anterior esophageal surface with liver retraction and lesser omentum opening

anterior esophageal surface. The anterior vagal nerve branch is identified on the left side of the esophagus and preserved.

An anterior incision is performed in the esophageal wall far from the anterior vagal nerve and slightly at the right side of the esophagus, including the muscular layers up to the mucosa. The exact site of the incision can be marked with the hook. A blunt dissector is used to separate the longitudinal muscle layers until the mucosa herniates through the window (Figs. 23.4b and 23.5b). The window can be widened using a monopolar hook or two graspers (Fig. 23.5a). The myotomy should be extended proximally until the point of the mediastinum where the anterior vagal branch crosses the anterior esophageal wall from the left to the right side (that is the point where the esophagus dilates). It is very important to limit the upper dissection to the thoracoabdominal junction without extending deeply in the thorax. Distally the myotomy ends on the great gastric curve where transversal muscular fibers become vertical (2 cm from the esophagogastric junction). Both longitudinal and circular esophageal muscles are cut letting the mucosa to herniate. The overall length of the myotomy is almost 6–8 cm. Muscular bleedings at the margins of the myotomy are usually self-limited and therefore should not be treated with electrocautery. At the end of the procedure, the insufflations of air through the nasogastric tube

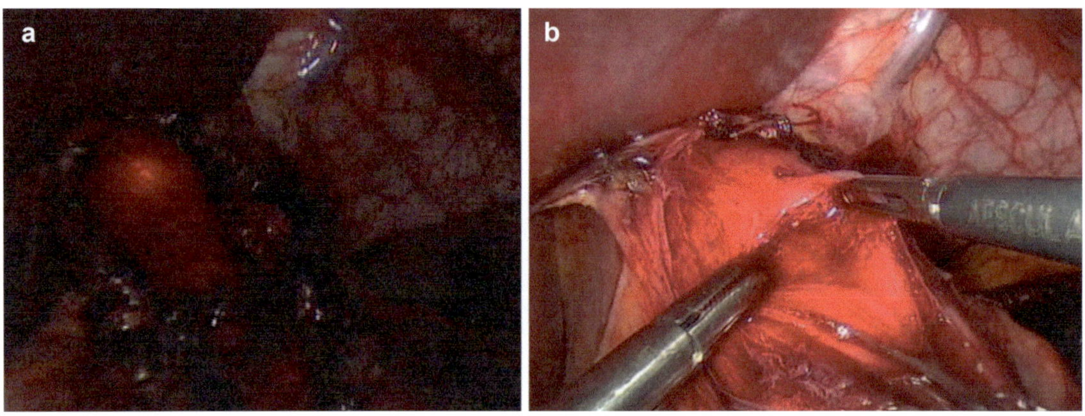

Fig. 23.4 The gastroscopy is performed during surgery (**a**), and the myotomy is spread with two blunt graspers (**b**)

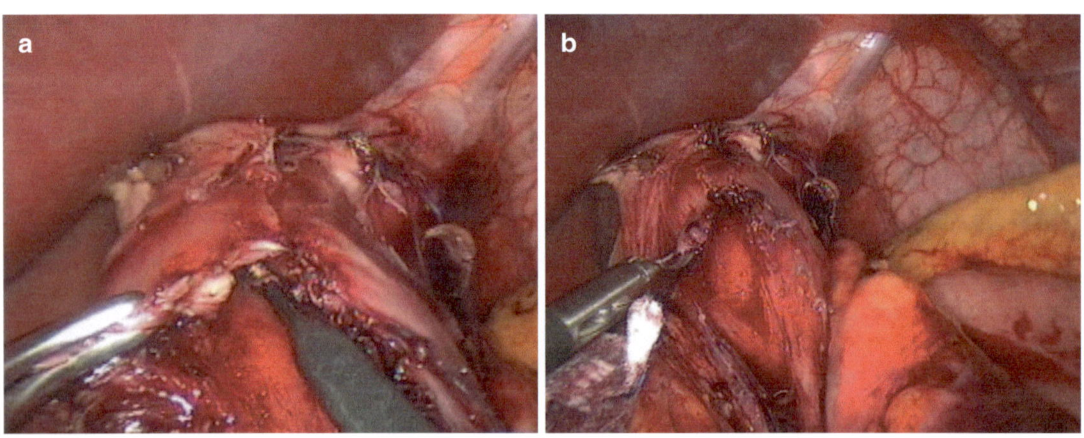

Fig. 23.5 The monopolar hook is used to widen the window (**a**) until the mucosa herniated (**b**)

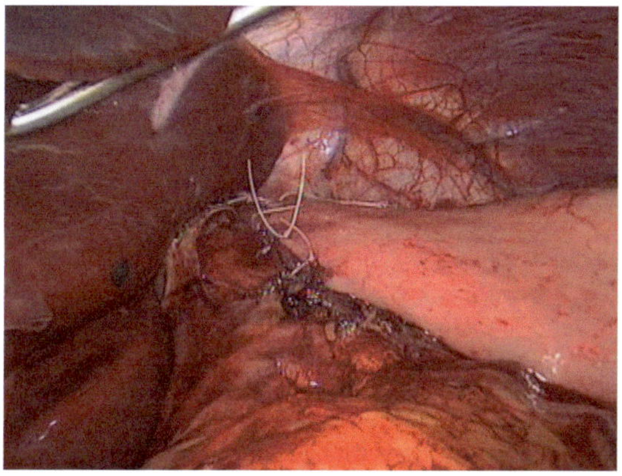

Fig. 23.6 A Dor fundoplication is performed at the end of the procedure

are used to check the tightness of the mucosa and the complete incision of the muscle fibers, prior to the execution of the Dor fundoplication (180° anterior fundoplication the anterior gastric fundus is fixated to the anterior esophageal muscle layers with three stitches) (Fig. 23.6).

23.6 Postoperative Care

After surgery, patients are relieved of symptoms, and they can feed properly after 48 h starting with mildly fluid diet for the first 3–4 weeks. The nasogastric tube, inserted during surgery, is removed after 24–48 h.

23.7 Results

The average length of surgery is about 100 min (range 85–155). We did not report intraoperative neither postoperative complications in our series of a 10-year period. Median hospital stay was 4 days.

Follow-up is performed by clinical evaluation at our outpatient clinic: PPI therapy is administered for 30 days, and contrast X-ray is performed after 1 month.

The average time to return to full daily activities was 7 days, and all patients were highly satisfied of the postoperative outcome and cosmetic results.

23.8 Tips and Tricks

The endoscopic evaluation performed during surgery avoids preoperative gastric overdistension and permits to evaluate the esophageal clearance and the appearance of the mucosa and to facilitate the identification of the esophagogastric junction (Fig. 23.4a).

The identification of the anterior vagal nerve at the beginning of the procedure is important for its preservation.

An excessive mobilization of the esophagus should be avoided, as well as a long myotomy over the esophageal and gastric sides that predispose to gastroesophageal reflux and complications.

The myotomy can be performed with monopolar diathermy, but this approach exposes to deeper thermal damage with delayed perforation.

A mucosal leak can be repaired with absorbable suture.

23.9 Discussion

The aim of surgery is to obtain long-term symptom palliation minimizing GERD that commonly occurs after treatment. Laparoscopic Heller myotomy (LHM) + Dor fundoplication seems the most definitive and successful treatment, and it is considered the gold standard first-line approach. However, in 2015, a systematic review identified two articles in favor of LHM, one for PD and one for both concluding that there is lack of data to determine the ideal treatment [11].

Advantages: the laparoscopic approach is superior to the open approach for the well-recognized benefits including minimal pain, better cosmesis, shorter hospital stay, and faster return to normal activity for the child and parents.

Complications: the most fearful surgical complication of surgical management of achalasia is esophageal perforation. Frequent causes of surgical failure are GERD and recurrent dysphagia. For these reasons, a partial fundoplication (Dor; Toupet) is commonly used to prevent GERD following Heller myotomy [12]. In a randomized controlled trial, Rebecchi determined that laparoscopic Dor fundoplication after a LHM was associated to lower recurrence rate of dysphagia than those after a Nissen procedure, but there is not a significant difference when the anterior fundoplication is compared to the posterior one [13]. There is some controversy as to whether an anti-reflux procedure should be performed in children at the time of LHM. Corda et al. concluded that an anti-reflux procedure is not required after a LHM for the prevention of GERD [14]. Other studies have shown benefits, and in many authors' practice, LHM and partial fundoplication are performed together.

Another proposed option is limited LHM without anti-reflux procedure. Valadez founded a significant decrease in the LOS resting pressure 6 months after limited LHM showing that the procedure is an effective treatment for achalasia. On the other hand, GER was observed in 68.3% of patients, and 21.6% were clinically symptomatic [12].

An evolving endosurgical therapeutic modality is POEM (peroral endoscopic myotomy). The technique includes a submucosal saline injection and the incision of submucosa 2 cm above LOS. The myotomy extends 2–3 cm distally to the gastroesophageal junction. At the end of the procedure, the mucosa is sutured. Among the proposed variants, the myotomy that is started at 2 o'clock is associated with less GER and that at 5 o'clock with less dysphagia.

POEM seems to be effective and with similar outcomes as LHM [15]. However the incidence of complications is high: GER (10.9%), pneumothorax (55%), pneumomediastinum (29%), and pleural effusion (48%).

References

1. Pachl MJ, Rex D, Decoppi P, Cross K, Kiely EM, Drake D, Pierro A, Curry JI. Paediatric laparoscopic Heller's cardiomyotomy: a single centre series. J Pediatr Surg. 2014;49(2):289–92.
2. Marlais M, Fishman JR, Fell JM, Haddad MJ, Rawat DJ. UK incidence of achalasia: an 11-year national epidemiological study. Arch Dis Child. 2011;96(2):192–4.
3. O'Neill OM, Johnston BT, Coleman HG. Achalasia: a review of clinical diagnosis, epidemiology, treatment and outcomes. World J Gastroenterol. 2013;19(35):5806–12.
4. Pacilli M, Davenport M. Results of laparoscopic Heller's myotomy for achalasia in children: a systematic review of the literature. J Laparoendosc Adv Surg Technol A. 2017;27(1):82–90.
5. Morera C, Nurko S. Heterogeneity of lower esophageal sphincter function in children with achalasia. J Pediatr Gastroenterol Nutr. 2012;54(1):34–40.
6. Hurwitz M, Bahar RJ, Ament ME, Tolia V, Molleston J, Reinstein LJ, Walton JM, Erhart N, Wasserman D, Justinich C, Vargas J. Evaluation of the use of botulinum toxin in children with achalasia. J Pediatr Gastroenterol Nutr. 2000;30(5):509–14.
7. Pastor AC, Mills J, Marcon MA, Himidan S, Kim PC. A single center 26-year experience with treatment of esophageal achalasia: is there an optimal method? J Pediatr Surg. 2009;44(7):1349–54.
8. Berquist WE, Byrne WJ, Ament ME, Fonkalsrud EW, Euler AR. Achalasia: diagnosis, management, and clinical course in 16 children. Pediatrics. 1983;71(5):798–805.
9. Nakayama DK, Shorter NA, Boyle JT, Watkins JB, O'Neill JA Jr. Pneumatic dilatation and operative treatment of achalasia in children. J Pediatr Surg. 1987;22(7):619–22.
10. Eckardt VF, Gockel I, Bernhard G. Pneumatic dilation for achalasia: late results of a prospective follow up investigation. Gut. 2004;53(5):629–33.
11. Sharp NE, St Peter SD. Treatment of idiopathic achalasia in the pediatric population: a systematic review. Eur J Pediatr Surg. 2016;26(2):143–9.
12. Zurita Macías Valadez LC, Pescarus R, Hsieh T, Wasserman L, Apriasz I, Hong D, Gmora S, Cadeddu M, Anvari M. Laparoscopic limited Heller myotomy without anti-reflux procedure does not induce significant long-term gastroesophageal reflux. Surg Endosc. 2015;29(6):1462–8.
13. Rebecchi F, Allaix ME, Schlottmann F, Patti MG, Morino M. Laparoscopic Heller myotomy and fundoplication: what is the evidence? Am Surg. 2018;84(4):481–8.
14. Corda L, Pacilli M, Clarke S, Fell JM, Rawat D, Haddad M. Laparoscopic oesophageal cardiomyotomy without fundoplication in children with achalasia: a 10-year experience: a retrospective review of the results of laparoscopic oesophageal cardiomyotomy without an anti-reflux procedure in children with achalasia. Surg Endosc. 2010;24(1):40–4.
15. Talukdar R, Inoue H, Nageshwar Reddy D. Efficacy of peroral endoscopic myotomy (POEM) in the treatment of achalasia: a systematic review and meta-analysis. Surg Endosc. 2015;29(11):3030–46.

24 Antireflux Surgery for Gastroesophageal Reflux Disease (GERD)

Ciro Esposito, Maria Escolino, Fulvia Del Conte, Alessandra Farina, Giuseppe Cortese, Marta Iannazzone, Agnese Roberti, and Philippe Montupet

24.1 Introduction

Gastroesophageal reflux disease (GERD) is a functional disorder that occurs when refluxed gastric contents produce symptoms or tissue damage [1]. Indications for an antireflux procedure in a child are GERD associated with hiatal hernia, failure of medical therapy for GERD, dependence on aggressive or prolonged medical therapy, respiratory symptoms, or high risk to develop GERD after EA repair or following placement of a feeding gastrostomy for nutritional support [2–7].

The first laparoscopic antireflux procedure was performed 25 years ago in 1993 by Georgeson and Lobe [8].

In children, the problem of the management of GERD is more complicated than in adults [1, 9–11]. In fact, almost 30–50% of the indications for surgery in children are represented by children with neurological impairment (NIC), whose management is extremely difficult and represents a true challenge for the surgeon [4].

C. Esposito (✉) · M. Escolino · F. Del Conte
A. Farina · G. Cortese · M. Iannazzone · A. Roberti
Pediatric Surgery Unit, Department of Translational Medical Sciences (DISMET), "Federico II" University of Naples, Naples, Italy
e-mail: ciroespo@unina.it

P. Montupet
CHU Bicetre, Paris, France

In fact, in terms of results, while the management of neurologically normal children can be considered comparable to that of adults with a success rate of 90–95% [2, 9, 11–14], as for the results in NIC they are difficult to analyze because NIC present always GERD, feeding problems, and malnutrition [4, 15].

In this chapter, we will speak only of the laparoscopic management of GERD in neurological normal children.

Laparoscopic antireflux surgery in pediatric patients has shown benefits to patients in reduced hospital stay and improved cosmesis, and this procedure is considered highly effective if performed by expert hands with low morbidity and mortality [13].

Several techniques are available for the surgical treatment of pathologic reflux in children; however, analyzing the international literature, it seems that laparoscopic Nissen and Toupet antireflux procedures remain the standard of care for correction of GERD [2, 8, 11].

24.2 Preoperative Preparation

Before starting the procedure, the parents have to sign a specifically formulated informed consent. The procedure is performed in general anesthesia. A nasogastric tube is placed for gastric decompression after induction of anesthesia and removed at the end of procedure.

C. Esposito et al. (eds.), *ESPES Manual of Pediatric Minimally Invasive Surgery*,
https://doi.org/10.1007/978-3-030-00964-9_24

The bladder is emptied using the Credé maneuver in smaller children. A Foley catheter may be placed in patients where a lengthy procedure is anticipated, such as a redo procedure.

All access sites are injected with bupivacaine with epinephrine to provide for postoperative pain control and assist with cutaneous hemostasis.

24.3 Positioning

Infants and small children are positioned frog-legged at the foot of the operative table and secured with adhesive tape. Larger children and teenagers are positioned in dorsal lithotomy with the legs in stirrups. The operating surgeon stands between the patient's legs. The table is then placed in reversed Trendelenburg. The monitor is position at the head of the patients (Fig. 24.1).

24.4 Instrumentation

Selection of instruments and trocar size is also dependent on the size of the child. In general, for infants and children less than 10 kg, we use 3 mm instruments of 18–20 cm length, and for children over 10 kg standard length 3 or 5 mm instruments are appropriate. A 30-degree angled scope is preferentially used as it greatly enhances the surgeon's ability to view the area of the hiatus,

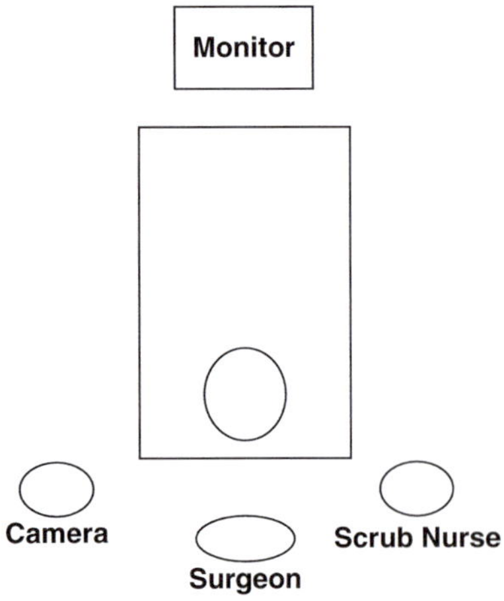

Fig. 24.1 Team position

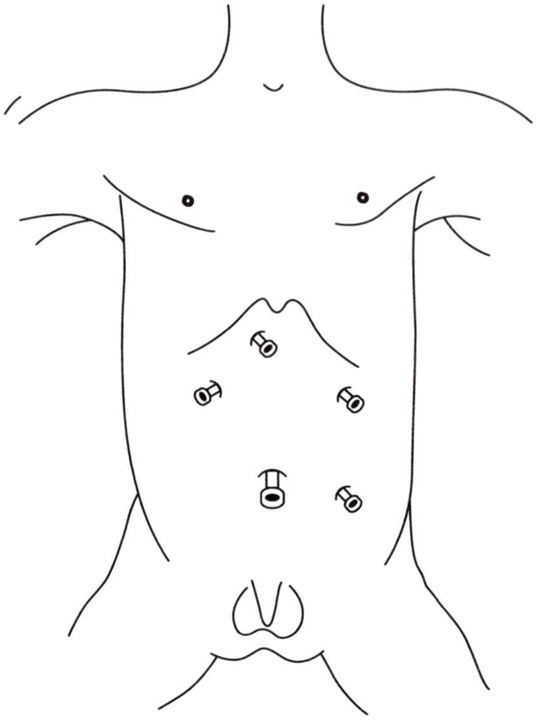

Fig. 24.2 Trocar position for a laparoscopic antireflux procedure

upper short gastric vessels and the retroesophageal space. It also limits instrument dueling as it allows the surgeon to place the telescope above the shafts of the right and left working ports and enabling the surgeon to look down on his working tips. The other instruments to adopt are a needle holder, a hook, a liver retractor, a couple of atraumatic forceps, and a pair of scissors. In general, we prefer to use 5 trocars: an umbilical trocar for the optic, 2 operative trocars, 1 trocar for liver retractor, and 1 trocar to move the umbilical tape placed around the GE junction (Fig. 24.2).

24.5 Technique

After positioning the umbilical trocar in open access, the abdomen is insufflated to a pressure of 8–12 mmHg according to the age of the patient, and four additional 3–5 mm trocars are placed.

The gastrohepatic ligament and the peritoneal reflection overlying the anterior esophagus are divided using monopolar hook or scissors with electrocautery. The crura of the diaphragm is exposed. An umbilical tape is placed around the esophagus to facilitate the dissection of the gastroesophageal junction. This dissection is accomplished with both blunt and sharp dissection. The anterior and posterior vagus nerves are identified and left lying along the esophagus. The hepatic branches of the vagus nerve are carefully preserved.

The crura is approximated using one to three interrupted 2-0 non-absorbable sutures. The fundus is then back around the back of the esophagus, and 3 to 4 interrupted non-absorbable

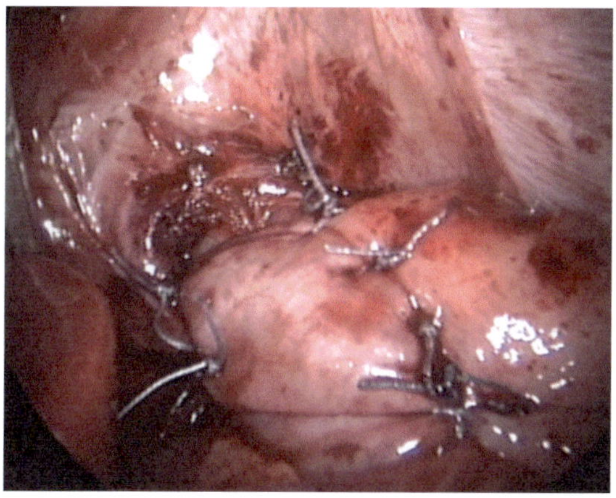

Fig. 24.3 We perform a 360° Nissen fundoplication positioning 3–4 separated stitches between the two sides of the stomach

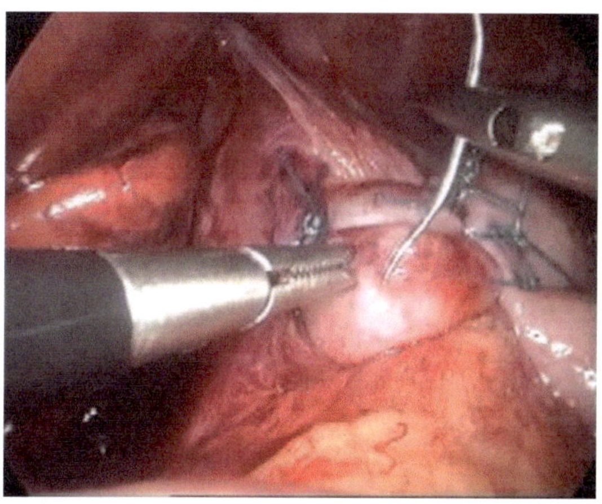

Fig. 24.4 After creating a Nissen valve, we position two separated stitches between the valve and the right crura to stabilize the wrap

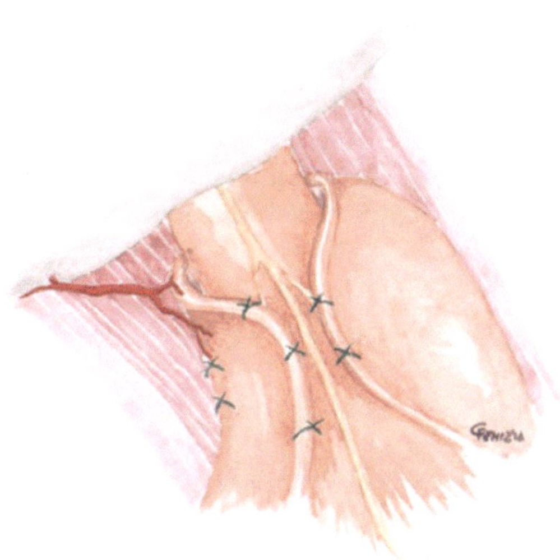

Fig. 24.5 To perform a 270° Toupet valve, we position 5–6 separated stitches to fix the valve onto the anterior part of the esophagus and two separated stitches between the valve and the right crura to stabilize the wrap

sutures are used to create a 360-degree fundoplication according to Nissen (Fig. 24.3). These sutures are placed through the left side of the fundus, the esophagus, and the right side of the fundus. Then we prefer to stabilize the wrap positioning to stitches between the wrap and the right crura (Fig. 24.4). At the end all port sites 5 mm are closed with separated stitches; in case of 3-mm trocars, we prefer to close them using sterile trips. The nasogastric tube is left in place until the following morning.

Toupet antireflux procedures involve wrapping the fundus posterior to the esophagus leaving free the anterior part of the esophagus. Three to four stitches are placed for each side between the stomach and esophagus, and then the wrap is fixed to the right crura with two separated stitches (Fig. 24.5).

24.6 Postoperative Care

Patients start feeding on liquids the morning of postoperative day 1. When patients have tolerated liquids, they are advanced to a "no solid" or semiliquid diet. Patients and their parents are educated by the pediatric surgical team's dietician about the "semiliquid" diet that they must follow for about 4 weeks following the operation.

Pain is controlled using intravenous analgesics for the first 24 h. Hospital stay is 2–3 days.

Patients are seen in follow-up about 1 week, 4 weeks, 6 months, and 1 year after surgery.

Then the controls are performed every year for the first 5 years after surgery.

We performed only clinical controls; instrumental exams are performed only in case of recurrence of symptoms.

24.7 Results

There are no randomized controlled trials of open versus laparoscopic fundoplication in children; however, there are some large retrospective series which form the basis of this review [7, 9].

The complication rates of these large series are very few. The conversion rate ranged from 0.9 to 3.3%, with most occurring in the first 30 operations. The intraoperative complication rates ranged from 2.6 to 5.1% and postoperative complication rates from 3.4 to 7.3%. Intraoperative complications included esophageal and gastric perforations and pneumothorax during hiatal dissection. Postoperative complications include dysphagia, gastroparesis, pneumonia, and recurrent GERD requiring reoperation. The rate of recurrent GERD in these series ranged from 2 to 5%.

The majority of complications occur in small series and in patients of less than 1 year of age.

24.8 Tips and Tricks

After 25 years of experience of antireflux surgery, we think that a key point above all at the beginning of the experience is that you have to use a 5-port technique: the first port for the optic and the second and third port for operative instruments. The fourth trocar is necessary for the liver retractor, and 5th trocar for the traction of the GE junction, with the experience you can switch to a 4-trocar technique.

Key points of the technique are the posterior closure of the crura with one or two standard stitches or with a figure of 8 stitch, to use non-resorbable suture to perform the procedure, and the need to fix the valve to the right crura to stabilize the wrap avoid its torsion and its migration.

As for the valve calibration, we prefer to use only a small nasogastric tube. Additionally, the use of 30° optic is crucial to create a posterior window and to well identify the vagus nerve.

24.9 Discussion

Laparoscopic antireflux procedures were first described in pediatric patients 25 years ago in 1993 [1, 8]. The recurrence rate of GERD in children undergoing open antireflux procedures is well known.

The largest experience reported from Fonkalsrud of over 7400 patients found a recurrence rate of 7.1% [13]. Several studies reported that the laparoscopic antireflux procedure has a lower recurrence rate varying from 2 to 5% [2, 8, 9].

Laparoscopic antireflux surgery has become the gold standard, and two techniques, namely, the Nissen and Toupet, have proven their effectiveness [2, 8, 9, 11]. The results are certainly dependent on the specific training, the surgeon, and on his antireflux experience.

In particular, the dissection phase consisting in the isolation of the esophagus and in the closure of the crura is similar for both procedures.

The critical steps of the procedure are to abdominalize 3–4 cm of the esophagus, to close posteriorly the crura with 1 or 2 stitches, to perform the antireflux mechanism, and then to fix the valve to the right pillar to avoid torsion of the valve and to avoid migration of the valve in the thorax.

As for the choice of procedure to adopt between Nissen and Toupet, it's a surgeon choice [2, 8, 9, 11].

There is no doubt that Nissen procedure is the most popular procedure performed worldwide in adult and also in pediatric patients [8, 9, 15].

There are several studies published in the international literature that show that both procedures give similar long-term results if performed by expert hands [2, 9, 11, 12].

Probably Toupet 270° antireflux procedure is preferred in patients with esophageal dysmotility and in patients with a bad esophageal peristalsis as the patients operated for esophageal atresia [10, 11].

Our chapter is focused only on the treatment of GERD in neurologically normal patients.

In this category of patients, antireflux procedures give excellent long-term results in more than 95% of patients [2, 12, 14]. The results of antireflux procedures in nerurologically impaired children (NIC) are completely different [4, 15], because NIC have a lot of problems, as failure to thrive, tetraparesis and in the majority of cases antireflux procedure alone is not efficient to solve their problems [5], but this category of patients will be treated in another chapter.

Laparoscopic antireflux procedures compared to the open technique have the advantages of a lower complication rate, quicker recovery period, and a lower failure rate than open fundoplication [8, 9, 13]. The learning curve is significant because of the advanced laparoscopic skills required, but once these skills are mastered, the procedure can be performed quickly and effectively.

As for technical details in laparoscopy, we never divide the short gastrics, as happened in open surgery.

Concerning the complications, laparoscopic antireflux surgery requires considerable training.

All techniques demand a precise dissection. In general, intraoperative complications in expert hands are near 0; sometimes dissection can be difficult in case of hiatal hernia or in case of an important esophagitis [6, 7].

Regarding the hiatoplasty, the crura has to be closed posteriorly using one or two separate stitches; in extremely rare cases it is necessary to use a patch in order to reinforce the crura.

As for the postoperative controls, at the beginning of laparoscopic surgery 25 years ago, the patients were followed periodically with instrumental controls as Ph-impedenzometry, barium swallow, manometry, and endoscopy, now after 25 years of experience with this surgery, we performed only clinical controls for 5 years after surgery, and instrumental controls are scheduled only in case of symptoms.

As for the learning curve that is about of 10–15 procedures, it's mandatory to start the experience with a mentor on your side expert in laparoscopic antireflux procedures.

In conclusion, laparoscopic antireflux procedures give excellent results in children with GERD if performed by expert hands. Nissen and Toupet antireflux procedures seem to give similar results [2, 13].

These techniques after 25 years of experience are standardized, and surgeons have to know step by step the procedure. A good preoperative work-up and a correct indication for surgery are important.

Complication rate is very low, and in general, postoperative controls consist only in the clinical exam.

References

1. Esposito C, Montupet P, Rothenberg S, editors. The gastroesophageal reflux in infants and children. Berlin: Springer; 2004.
2. Esposito C, Montupet P, van der Zee D, Settimi A, Paye-Jaouen A, Centonze A, Bax NK. Long-term outcome of laparoscopic Nissen, Toupet, and Thal antireflux procedures for neurologically normal children with gastroesophageal reflux disease. Surg Endosc. 2006;20(6):855–8.
3. Rothemberg SS, Bratton D, Larsen G. Laparoscopic fundoplication to enhance pulmonary function in children with severe reactive airway disease and gastroesophageal reflux disease. Surg Endosc. 1997;11:1088–90.
4. Esposito C, Van Der Zee DC, Settimi A, Doldo P, Staiano A, Bax NM. Risks and benefits of surgical management of gastroesophageal reflux in neurologically impaired children. Surg Endosc. 2003;5:708–10.
5. Esposito C, Settimi A, Capano G, Ascione G, Centonze A. Laparoscopic assisted jejunostomy: an effective procedure for the treatment of neurologically impaired children with feeding problems and GER. Surg Endosc. 2005;4:501–4.
6. Sydorak RM, Albanese CT. Laparoscopic antireflux procedures in children: evaluating the evidence. Semin Laparosc Surg. 2002;9:133–8.
7. Esposito C, Montupet P, Amici G, Desruelle P. Complications of laparoscopic antireflux surgery in childhood. Surg Endosc. 2000;14:622–4.
8. Lobe TE, Schropp KP, Lunsford K. Laparoscopic Nissen fundoplication in childhood. J Pediatr Surg. 1993;28:358–61.

9. Rothenberg SS. Experience with 220 consecutive laparoscopic Nissen fundoplications in infants and children. J Pediatr Surg. 1998;33:274–8.
10. Bensoussan AL, Yasbeck S, Carceller-Blanchard A. Results and complications of Toupet's partial posterior wrap: 10 years experience. J Pediatr Surg. 1994;29:1215–7.
11. Montupet P, Mendoza-Sagaon M, De Dreuzy O, et al. Laparoscopic Toupet fundoplication in children. Pediatr Endosurg Innov Technol. 2001;5:305–8.
12. Esposito C, Saxena A, Irtan S, Till H, Escolino M. Laparoscopic Nissen fundoplication: an excellent treatment of gerd-related respiratory symptoms in children-results of a multicentric study. J Laparoendosc Adv Surg Tech A. 2018;28(8):1023–8. https://doi.org/10.1089/lap.2017.0631.
13. Esposito C, Roberti A, Turrà F, Escolino M, Cerulo M, Settimi A, Farina A, Vecchio P, Di Mezza A. Management of gastroesophageal reflux disease in pediatric patients: a literature review. Pediatr Health Med Ther. 2015;23(6):1–8.
14. Esposito C, De Luca C, Alicchio F, Giurin I, Miele E, Staiano AM, Settimi A. Long-term outcome of laparoscopic Nissen procedure in pediatric patients with gastroesophageal reflux disease measured using the modified QPSG Roma III European Society for Pediatric Gastroenterology Hepatology and Nutrition's questionnaire. J Laparoendosc Adv Surg Tech A. 2012;22(9):937–40.
15. Knatten CK, Kvello M, Fyhn TJ, Edwin B, Schistad O, Aabakken L, Pripp AH, Kjosbakken H, Emblem R, Bjørnland K. Nissen fundoplication in children with and without neurological impairment: a prospective cohort study. J Pediatr Surg. 2016;51(7):1115–21.

MIS Gastrostomy

25

Alberto Sgrò, Rossella Arnoldi, Carlo Gemme, Germana Casaccia, Enrico Felici, and Alessio Pini Prato

25.1 Introduction

Placement of gastrostomy for long-term enteral feeding and therapeutic purposes is fundamental in management of several issues in children including neurologic or metabolic diseases, intestinal failure, oesophageal obstruction and others. In 1980, Gauderer et al. [1] introduced the concept of percutaneous endoscopic gastrostomy (PEG) which reached a wide application due to its minimal invasiveness and low cost. However, it may result not applicable to small children or to those carrying anatomical features which may increase the risk of complication during or after PEG procedure.

A. Sgrò · R. Arnoldi · G. Casaccia
Pediatric Surgery Unit, Alessandria's Children Hospital, Alessandria, Italy

C. Gemme
Endoscopy Unita, AON SS Antonio e Biagio e Cesare Arrigo, Alessandria, Italy

E. Felici
Pediatric Unit, Alessandria Children Hospital, Alessandria, Italy

A. Pini Prato (✉)
Pediatric Surgery Unit, Alessandria's Children Hospital, Alessandria, Italy

The Children Hospital, AON SS Antonio e Biagio e Cesare Arrigo, Alessandria, Italy
e-mail: apini@ospedale.al.it

In the past, the most common and safest method was the open Stamm procedure [2]. More recently, minimally invasive surgery allowed to fashion a safe gastrostomy with the advantages of the PEG technique. Laparoscopic gastrostomy (LAP) and laparoscopic-assisted PEG (LAPEG) have been reported and gained popularity as valid alternatives to the classic open Stamm procedure [3, 4]. Stamm technique itself has been reported as feasible with a minimally invasive approach [5].

25.2 Preoperative Preparation

All patients and parents should undergo informed consent before the procedure. Regardless of the chosen procedure for gastrostomy fashioning, preoperative enema may be useful to deflate the colon, allow a better laparoscopic view and reduce the risk of perforation. All gastrostomy techniques lead to stomach opening. Due to this reason, i.v. antibiotic prophylaxis (cefazolin) should be administered 30 min before the procedure. General anaesthesia is induced. In case of PEG technique, only sedation and local anaesthesia may be considered and discussed with anaesthesiologist on the base of patient's characteristics.

C. Esposito et al. (eds.), *ESPES Manual of Pediatric Minimally Invasive Surgery*,
https://doi.org/10.1007/978-3-030-00964-9_25

25.3 Patient Positioning

Patient lies in supine position for all gastrostomy procedures. Mild reverse-Trendelenburg position may be used to achieve a better visualization during laparoscopic procedures and to reduce the risk of colon interposition between the stomach and the abdominal wall.

25.3.1 PEG

Endoscopy monitor should be placed on the left side of the patient. The endoscopist (either paediatric surgeon or gastroenterologist) is on the right side of the patient at the level of the head. The operator performing the percutaneous manoeuvre should stay at the level of the abdomen, the side based on patient's size and age. Both involved operators should have direct view both of the endoscopic screen and the abdomen. Scrub nurse should stay on one side of the patient or just at the bottom of the field.

25.3.2 Laparoscopic-Assisted PEG

The surgeon is on the right side of the patient. The endoscopist is on the right side at the head level. Endoscopy and main laparoscopic monitors are on the left side of the patient. A second laparoscopic monitor is positioned behind the surgeon. Scrub nurse is on the left side in front of the surgeon.

25.3.3 Laparoscopic Gastrostomy and Laparoscopic Stamm Gastrostomy

The surgeon is on the right side of the patient. Main monitor is on the upper left side, secondary on the upper right. Assistant is on the left side in front of the surgeon. Scrub nurse is on the left side. The possibility for the surgeon to stay in between the legs and for the assistant to stay on the same side of the surgeon represents valid alternatives.

25.4 Surgical Technique

25.4.1 PEG

Gastroscopy is performed using a paediatric endoscope. Adult instrument can be used depending on patient's weight and clinical characteristics. Gastric cavity needs to be fully inflated and distended to obtain the contact with abdominal wall and adequate tension for the following percutaneous puncture. The site for gastrostomy on abdominal wall is identified by transillumination which plays a fundamental role for safety of the procedure. If transillumination can't be obtained, percutaneous procedure should not be performed due to risk of organ (especially colon and liver) perforation. On abdominal wall, gastrostomy should be placed on upper left quadrant at least 2 cm away from rib cage. In gastric cavity, the preferred position for tube insertion is on the anterior wall of the antrum, even if the gastric body is acceptable when it is the only option to obtain a valid transillumination. Correspondence between transillumination and gastrostomy sites can be confirmed by finger pressure on the epigastrium being endoscopically visible from inside the gastric cavity. Once the site of gastrostomy and transillumination is identified, a small skin incision on the site needs to be done. Through that incision, a large bore needle is inserted inside the stomach under endoscopic visualization. In the "pull" technique [1], a string is inserted in the stomach through the needle, then grasped with endoscopic forceps (or a loop) and pulled out through the oesophagus and the mouth. The string is fixed to the external end of the feeding tube which is, then, pulled through the mouth, the oesophagus and the stomach to reach the final positioning of the bumper.

When transit of the bumper along the oesophagus is not considered to be feasible or safe (i.e.

strictures, mucosal fragility, etc.), PEG variation can be used. While endoscopic procedure and site identification through transillumination are similar, tube insertion is different. In the "push" technique with introducer [6], after site identification, the stomach is fixed to the abdominal wall by insertion of three T-fasteners under endoscopic view. Subsequently , a guidewire is inserted in the stomach through a needle, and a indirect Seldinger technique is used to insert an introducer (similar to a peel-away device for percutaneous central venous catheter placement) and, finally, the gastrostomy tube with inflating balloon fixation.

In both "push" and "pull" techniques, the correct positioning and free rotation of the tube should be endoscopically confirmed as the last step of the procedure.

If the PEG kit with a stiff bumper is used, tube replacement will require a second endoscopic procedure under anaesthesia about 10–12 weeks after first surgery. Under endoscopic visualization, the bumper is grasped with an endoscopic forceps or loop. The tube is externally cut at the skin level, and a new gastrostomy tube with balloon is positioned under direct view. The bumper is then extracted through the oesophagus and the mouth together with the endoscope.

25.4.2 Laparoscopic-Assisted PEG

LAPEG [7] is used when no transillumination can be obtained or when PEG is not considered to be safe enough due to patient characteristics (i.e. previous abdominal surgery). A 5 mm port and camera are positioned in the upper right quadrant. Camera may be positioned through the umbilicus, but there is a risk of worse visualization during stomach insufflation. One or two additional 5 mm ports are inserted to gain access for instruments. The stomach is visualized, and causes for failed transillumination are identified. If needed, lysis of adhesions and organ mobilization are performed to free the space between the stomach and the abdominal wall. Abdominal pressure is decreased down to 6–7 mmHg. PEG pull technique is now performed. Needle and tube insertion and stomach-to-wall approximation are controlled and confirmed under direct laparoscopic visualization. When needed, approximation can be facilitated by grasping the stomach to the abdominal wall. At the end, one or two fixation stitches can be laparoscopically positioned between the stomach and abdominal wall to decrease the risk of subsequent detachment. A limitation for this procedure is related to gastric inflation and subsequent downward carbon dioxide migration that can impair visualization of the whole abdominal cavity.

25.4.3 Laparoscopic Gastrostomy

Gastrostomy site is marked on the skin in the upper left quadrant. A 5 mm optical port is positioned through the umbilicus. After pneumoperitoneum's creation, the stomach is visualized. A 5 mm forceps is introduced trocarless through the gastrostomy site to grasp the anterior gastric wall. Before this manoeuvre, mild insufflation of the stomach by anaesthesiologist may help to avoid the accidental co-grasping of the posterior wall. Stomach is approximated to the abdominal wall corresponding to the gastrostomy site. Two fixation stitches are positioned in extracorporeal manner on both sides of this site. They are passed through the skin, abdominal wall and then internally through gastric wall under laparoscopic view. Stitches are then returned externally through abdominal wall. Once the stomach is secured to the abdominal wall, a Seldinger technique is used to introduce the gastrostomy tube. A needle is inserted in the stomach through the gastrostomy site, and a guidewire is passed. Gastrostomy site and gastric wall are progressively dilated with introducers up to the calibre of the tube which is at the end inserted. Correct positioning of the tube is assessed by injecting saline under direct laparoscopic view.

25.4.4 Laparoscopic Stamm Gastrostomy

A 5 mm optical port is positioned in the umbilicus. Two additional operative ports are positioned on the lower left and upper right quadrant. The stomach is visualized, and anterior antric/body wall of the stomach is approximated to the abdominal wall to identify the site of gastrostomy. Here a small incision is made on the skin and the wound undermined. Two fixation stitches are positioned between muscular wall and stomach above and on the left side of the insertion site. The strings are kept outside in a mosquito. A double purse string is fashioned laparoscopically around the insertion site on the gastric wall (Fig. 25.1). A gastrostomy tube is then passed through the site on the abdominal wall into the abdomen. An incision on the gastric wall is made in the middle of the purse string (Figs. 25.1 and 25.2), and the tube is then passed inside the stomach (Fig. 25.3). Purse strings are tightened laparoscopically around the tube (Fig. 25.3). Two additional fixation stitches are positioned between the abdominal wall and stomach below and on the right side of gastrostomy (Fig. 25.4). All fixation stitches are at the end tightened to securely approximate the stomach to the abdominal wall (Fig. 25.5). Threads are tied in the subcutaneous tissue. Figure 25.6 shows endoscopic view of the laparoscopic Stamm gastrostomy.

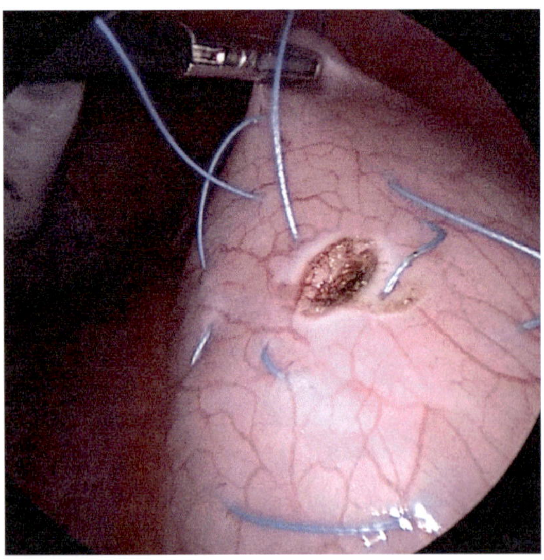

Fig. 25.1 The site for gastrostomy has been chosen; the purse string fashioned and a diathermy incision on the gastric wall are performed to lead the tube insertion

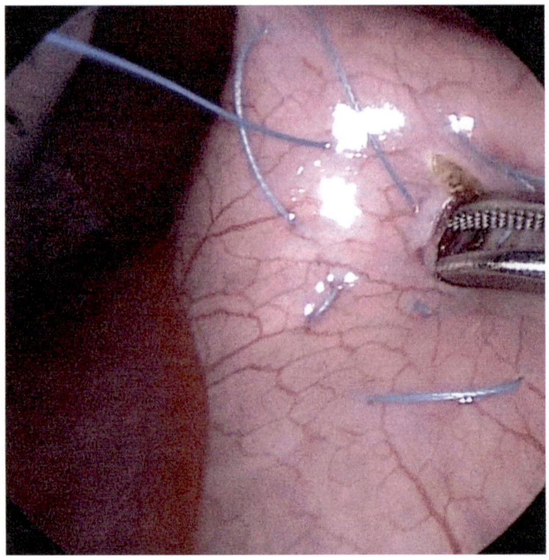

Fig. 25.2 Blunt dissection is required to reach the gastric cavity (the stomach is kept filled of air in order to early detect mucosal opening)

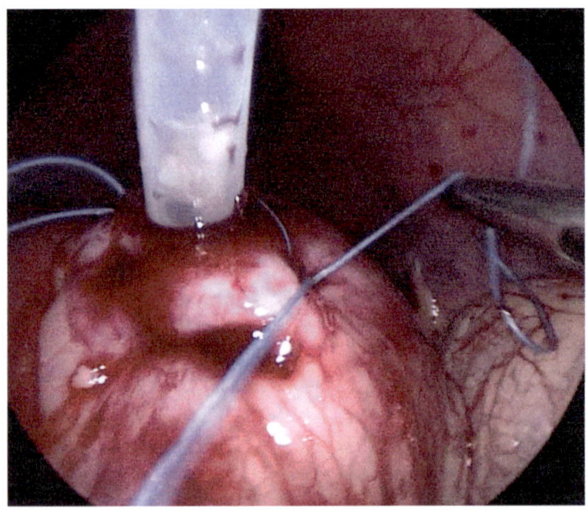

Fig. 25.3 Once the tube is inserted and the balloon inflated, the purse strings are sutured and tied to seal the gastrotomy

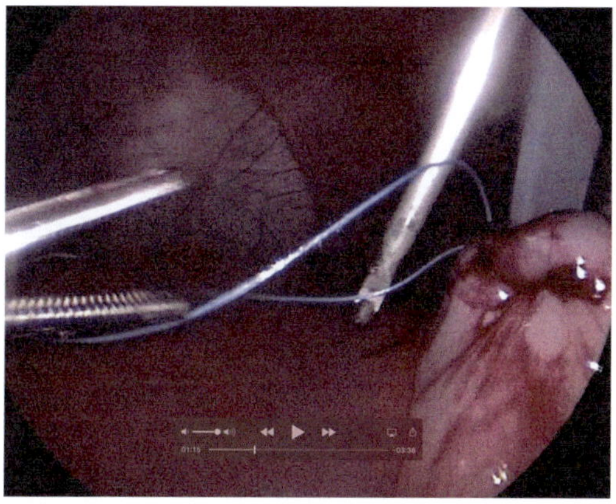

Fig. 25.4 An endoclose device is used to pull the sutures out of the abdominal wall

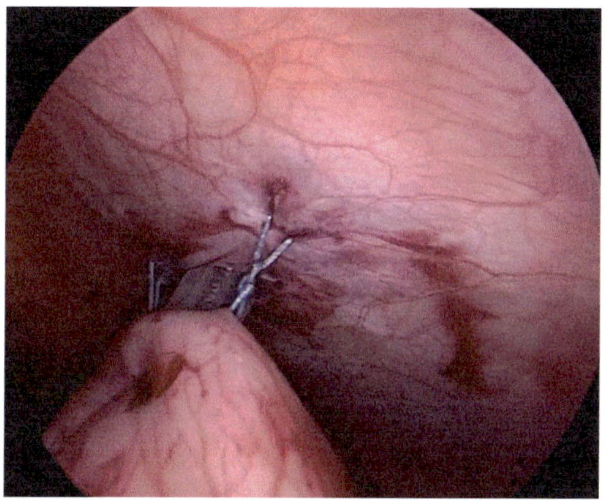

Fig. 25.5 The stomach is approximated to the anterior wall of the abdomen and tied strongly to allow fixation of the stomach

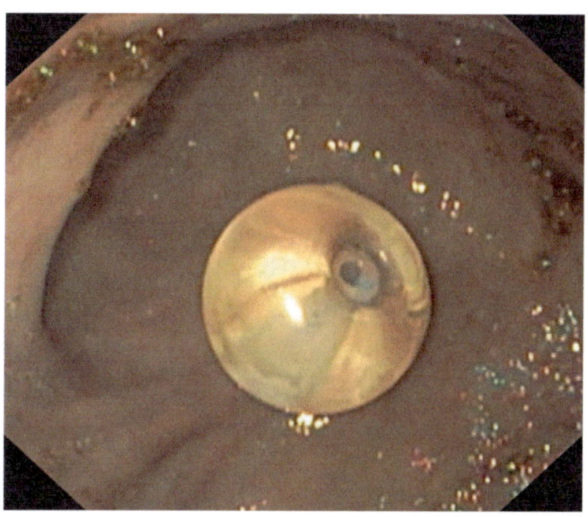

Fig. 25.6 Endoscopic view of the balloon inside the gastric cavity, well positioned and safe

25.5 Postoperative Care

For all gastrostomy techniques, feeding is allowed the day after surgery according to tolerance. It is preferable to start with small meals at low infusion rate to avoid stomach distension until a normal gastric motility is recovered. Meals' volume and infusion rate will be increased in 4–5 days to reach the full regimen according to tolerance. The presence of a gastrostomy doesn't exclude oral feeding when allowed. Patient can be discharged after 3–4 days or when full enteral tolerance is obtained. According to tolerance, a programme to increase infusion rate in order to reduce meals' duration and improve quality of life can be applied at home, after discharge.

The tension applied to the abdominal wall by gastric tube (or button) should be strictly assessed daily during first few days after surgery. Postoperatively tissues' oedema may lead to increased abdominal wall thickness. This issue can cause the balloon (or bumper) to sit on gastric mucosa. A well-balanced tension is needed to favour stomach-to-abdomen adhesion avoiding migration leading to "buried bumper syndrome". This is of utmost importance for dystrophic patient where tissues are weaker and thinner. Correct tube's placement can be assessed by its rotation and gentle movements through gastrostomy. Resistance to these movements and leakage from gastrostomy should rise the suspect of "buried bumper".

Gastrostomy can be kept cleaned using only saline. Few and small gauzes are sufficient to dress the gastrostomy during first weeks after surgery.

25.6 Brief Review of Literature and Discussion

Several diseases in children require a gastrostomy for enteral feeding. Among all, neurologic disabilities, intestinal failure, short gut syndrome and oesophageal obstruction are the most relevant. Advances led to development of minimally invasive techniques for gastrostomy formation. PEG described by Gauderer [1] was the first reported and gained popularity due to patient tolerance, minimally invasiveness and low cost. New laparoscopy-based techniques have been recently developed such as laparoscopic-assisted PEG (LAPEG), laparoscopic gastrostomy (LAP) and laparoscopic Stamm gastrostomy. PEG and its replacement, as well as all laparoscopic techniques are performed under general anaesthesia in most of cases. Completion rates are around 98–100%, and there are not significant differences between techniques [8, 9]. Of note, when addressing operative time under anaesthesia, one should consider that PEG requires two procedures. This will make PEG similar to others. Also, time to gain full enteral feed does not seem to be affected by the type of technique used for gastrostomy placement.

There is a debate on which of these techniques is the best option in children, and main discussions focus especially on differences between PEG and all laparoscopic approaches. Recently a meta-analysis has been published comparing laparoscopic versus endoscopic percutaneous gastrostomy in children [10]. Few studies in literature deeply investigated differences in outcome. PEG and laparoscopic techniques are extremely different due to the view under which the gastrostomy is created. PEG requires only one small skill incision, but the exclusive endoluminal view does not allow a totally safe control of bowel interposition with risk of perforation. Laparoscopic techniques require more incisions and pneumoperitoneum creation, but it is much safer towards risk of perforation due to the possibility to control stomach and bowel from outside the lumen.

A higher risk of major intra- and postoperative complications due to perforation of adjacent bowel has been demonstrated when using PEG technique [8, 9, 11]. This risk is irrelevant when laparoscopy is used. Moreover, using PEG, complications are usually detected postoperatively when faecal leakage, peritonitis or sepsis are present. This is very unlikely to happen with laparoscopic approaches as the eventual perforation would be identified and repaired intraoperatively avoiding worse morbidity.

Another comparative outcome related to complications is the rate of early tube dislodgments. Placement of PEG has been reported to have up to seven times higher risk of early dislodgments [10] which can result in main complications such as peritonitis due to intraperitoneal gastric leak [12]. Using laparoscopic techniques, gastropexy is always performed obtaining a firm attachment of the stomach to the abdominal wall. This technical aspect significantly reduces the risk of intraperitoneal leak in case of early tube dislodgment. Moreover, bedside tube replacement is likely to be successful without the need for a further anaesthesia which becomes necessary in those PEG cases where early dislodgment leads to stomach's detachment from abdominal wall [8, 11].

The risks of inadvertent bowel injury and early tube dislodgment are the reason why PEG is reported to carry a significantly higher reoperation rate when compared to laparoscopic techniques [10]. Similarly, major causes for reoperation for other techniques are mostly related to superficial stoma complications.

It has not been demonstrated which laparoscopic technique would be the preferable, yet. Indeed, as explained above, all of them carry common advantages towards risks of main intra- and postoperative complications thanks to the possibility of an extraluminal visualization and to gastropexy's feasibility. For this reason, the choice is mostly based on surgeon preferences and skills. As stated above, LAPEG may result in an inadequate visualization when the stomach is fully inflated. When performing LAP, visualization of the stomach and bowel is adequate, and gastropexy is easier. Anyway, LAP may not be indicated in older and heavier patients in whom it may be difficult to bring the stomach through a small incision. For this kind of patient, LAPEG may be considered the best option. The choice between LAP and laparoscopic Stamm gastrostomy resides mostly on surgeon's attitude and preference. Stamm procedure involves a higher number of intraperitoneal stitching manoeuvres and stomach opening inside the peritoneal cavity, making it more indicated for highly skilled surgeons [5].

Even if still under debate [13, 14], gastrostomy placement is often combined to gastric fundoplication in neurologic impaired patients with gastroesophageal reflux. In these cases, LAP or laparoscopic Stamm are the preferred technique due to the current ports' disposition. LAPEG or PEG should be avoided due to the need for transit of the endoscope and of the bumper through a just fashioned fundoplication.

PEG is still widely used in children due to its popularity, relative simplicity and (supposed) minor impact on patient due to minimal invasiveness. On the other hand, all the issues discussed above make laparoscopic procedures preferable in children when compared to PEG. Indeed, significantly, lower risks of complications are the main reasons to prefer a laparoscopic approach especially when advantages from the anaesthetic point of view are neither present. General anaesthesia may lead to complications, especially in patients with cardiac or respiratory disease [15]. If the choice of gastrostomy technique does not influence on general anaesthesia plan and procedure can be maintained relatively straightforward (based on surgeon's experience and skills), laparoscopic techniques should be preferred. All considerations reported above on several MIS techniques underline that all patients' characteristics are the most important indicator to choose the best gastrostomy technique.

References

1. Gauderer MW, Ponsky JL, Izant RJ. Gastrostomy without laparotomy: a percutaneous endoscopic technique. J Pediatr Surg. 1980;15:872–6.
2. Goretsky MF, Johnson N, Farrell M, et al. Alternative techniques of feeding gastrostomy in children: a critical analysis. J Am Coll Surg. 1996;182:233–40.
3. Rothenberg SS, Bealer JF, Chang JH. Primary laparoscopic placement of gastrostomy buttons for feeding tubes. A safer and simpler technique. Surg Endosc. 1999;13:995–7.
4. Jones VS, La Hei ER, Shun A. Laparoscopic gastrostomy: the preferred method of gastrostomy in children. Pediatr Surg Int. 2007;23:1085–9.
5. Vasseur Maurer S, Reinberg O. Laparoscopic technique to perform a true Stamm gastrostomy in children. J Pediatr Surg. 2015;50(10):1797–800.
6. Russell TR, Brotman M, Norris F. Percutaneous gastrostomy. A new simplified and cost-effective technique. Am J Surg. 1984;148:132–7.
7. Lopes G, Salcone M, Neff M. Laparoscopic-assisted percutaneous endoscopic gastrostomy tube placement. JSLS. 2010;14(1):66–9.
8. Akay B, Capizzani TR, Lee AM, Drongowski RA, Geiger JD, Hirschl RB, Mychaliska GB. Gastrostomy tube placement in infants and children: is there a preferred technique? J Pediatr Surg. 2010;45(6):1147–52.
9. Zamakhshary M, Jamal M, Blair GK, Murphy JJ, Webber EM, Skarsgard ED. Laparoscopic vs percutaneous endoscopic gastrostomy tube insertion: a new pediatric gold standard? J Pediatr Surg. 2005;40(5):859–62.
10. Suksamanapun N, Mauritz FA, Franken J, van der Zee DC, van Herwaarden-Lindeboom MY. Laparoscopic versus percutaneous endoscopic gastrostomy placement in children: results of a systematic review and meta-analysis. J Minim Access Surg. 2017;13(2):81–8.
11. Conlon SJ, Janik TA, Janik JS, Hendrickson RJ, Landholm AE. Gastrostomy revision: incidence and indications. J Pediatr Surg. 2004;39(9):1390–5.
12. Rosenberger LH, Newhook T, Schirmer B, Sawyer RG. Late accidental dislodgement of a percutaneous endoscopic gastrostomy tube: an underestimated burden on patients and the health care system. Surg Endosc. 2011;25(10):3307–11.
13. Viswanath N, Wong D, Channappa D, Kukkady A, Brown S, Samarakkody U. Is prophylactic fundoplication necessary in neurologically impaired children? Eur J Paediatr Surg. 2010;20:226–9.
14. Yap BK, Nah SA, Chen Y, Low Y. Fundoplication with gastrostomy vs gastrostomy alone: a systematic review and meta-analysis of outcomes and complications. Pediatr Surg Int. 2017;33(2):217–28.
15. LA G, Megison ML, Harmon CM, Chen MK, Anderson S, Chong AJ, Chaignaud BE, Beierle EA. Laparoscopic surgery in children with congenital heart disease. J Pediatr Surg. 2012;47(6):1084–8.

26 Laparoscopic Pyloromyotomy

Philippe Montupet, Ciro Esposito, and Mario Mendoza-Sagaon

26.1 Introduction

Little controversy still exists to establish the most appropriate treatment of hypertrophic pyloric stenosis (HPS) in neonates and infants. The nonoperative treatment with oral or intravenous atropine has low acceptance due to the overall success rate of 75–79%, the long-term therapy, and the collateral effects [1, 2]. Surgical treatment described in 1912 by Dr. Conrad Ramstedt remains the suitable standard management option due to the higher success rate (~100%), minimal complications, and shorter hospital stay [1, 3]. In recent years, pediatric laparoscopy and other minimal invasive techniques have found a place in the surgical therapy for HPS offering excellent results but creating some controversy about the benefits when comparing to the open approach [4–6].

HPS is the main cause of gastric outlet obstruction and one of the common pathologies requiring abdominal surgery within the first 2 months of life. It is characterized by hypertrophy of the circular muscle layer of the pylorus with a consequent narrowing and elongation of the pyloric channel. The exact etiology is unknown, but several studies have proposed a relation with genetic factors [8], maternal smoking during pregnancy, being first born, preterm delivery, small weight for gestational age, cesarean section [9], young maternal age [10], and exposure of erythromycin in the neonatal period [11, 12] . Positive family history has been reported in 17% with one family member and 3% in two or more family members [13]. The overall incidence in European countries is 2.0 per 1000 live births [10] and occurs with a fivefold male predominance [9]. The common onset of clinical features such as non-biliary progressive projectile vomiting, observing the gastric peristaltic waves, and palpation of the thickened (olive-shaped) pylorus occur between the third and the sixth week of age. Late-onset presentation has been described [14, 15]. Delay in the diagnosis and treatment causes dehydration, important electrolyte abnormalities such as hypokalemic/hypochloremic metabolic alkalosis, and in some cases jaundice and esophagitis [13].

P. Montupet
Department of Pediatric Surgery, University Hospital of Bicêtre, Paris, France

C. Esposito
Pediatric Surgery Unit, Department of Translational Medical Sciences (DISMET), University of Naples "Federico II", Naples, Italy
e-mail: ciroespo@unina.it

M. Mendoza-Sagaon (✉)
Department of Pediatric Surgery, Regional Hospital of Bellinzona-EOC, Bellinzona, Switzerland
e-mail: mario.mendozasagaon@eoc.ch

C. Esposito et al. (eds.), *ESPES Manual of Pediatric Minimally Invasive Surgery*,
https://doi.org/10.1007/978-3-030-00964-9_26

26.2 Diagnosis

A correct anamnesis and clinical examination allow to establish the diagnosis of HPS in the 75–80% of the cases, but in recent years, this is becoming a lost skill [13, 15].

Haller and Cohen in 1986 reported a pyloric diameter ≥15 mm, a pyloric wall muscle thickness ≥4 mm, and a pyloric channel length ≥18 mm as reliable ultrasound measurements to establish the diagnosis of HPS. Since then, ultrasound has gained popularity as a value tool in the diagnosis of HPS due to the excellent specificity and sensitivity and the ease of obtaining the noninvasive study. Forster et al. reported a sensitivity and specificity of pyloric muscle wall thickness of 91% and 85%, respectively, and sensitivity and specificity of pyloric muscle length of 76% and 85%, respectively [11]. Other authors have reported similar results modifying the US measurements of muscle wall thickness >3 mm, a pyloric diameter >10 mm, and a pyloric channel length >15 mm [12].

Upper GI series may be also helpful in the diagnosis of HPS and could exclude other pathologies. The characteristic features in HPS are delayed gastric emptying, the "string" sign (a single long central streak of contrast filling the pyloric channel), an up-turned pyloric curve, the "beak" sign (as contrast enters the proximal pyloric channel it forms a beak), and indentation of the base of the duodenal bulb by the pyloric muscle mass [14].

26.3 Preoperative Care

Before surgery, a complete stabilization and correction of the dehydration and electrolyte imbalance is mandatory to avoid complications with anesthesia and during the immediate postoperative period [2]. There is wide variance of protocols of fluid and electrolyte replacement in HPS, but typical regime includes correction with a solution containing 0.45% NaCl and 5 or 10% dextrose with KCl added at 10 mmol/500 ml. Controversy still exists regarding the benefits of nasogastric tubes for continuous decompression of the stomach preoperatively, the use of prophylactic antibiotics, and the use of antacids [9].

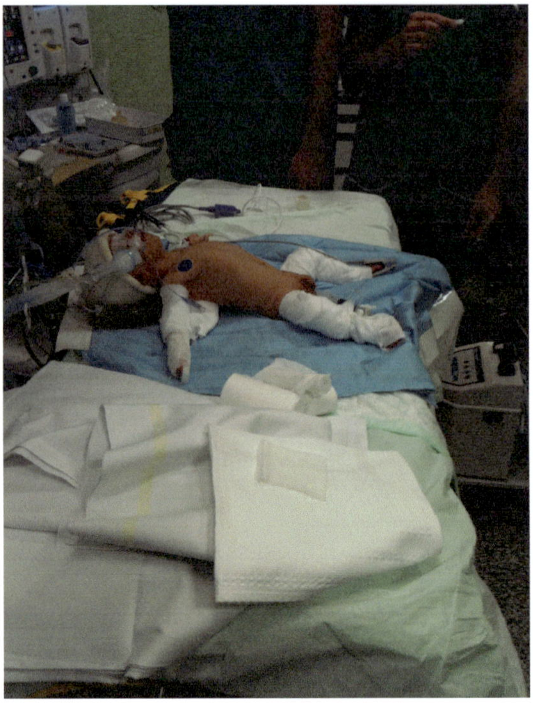

Fig. 26.1 Position

Small babies must be kept warm either with increase of the temperature in the operating room as well as with controlled temperature devices. For the laparoscopic approach, the small patient could be placed transversally in the operating table to facilitate the laparoscopic setting (Fig. 26.1). It is advised to place a nasogastric tube right before surgery to empty and to deflate the stomach and also could be used to exclude perforation of the mucosa during the pyloromyotomy [4].

26.4 Surgical Technique

Extramucosal pyloromyotomy described by Dr. Conrad Ramstedt in 1921 is the gold standard for the surgical treatment of HPS [4, 5]. Due to the higher success rate (~100%), shorter hospital stay, minimal complications, and nearly 100% survival, today, the surgical treatment for HPS is preferred in comparison with the conservative medical treatment. Moreover, in this new era with the concept of minimal invasive surgery, the classic open approach (right transverse supraumbilical minilaparotomy) to perform a Ramstedt's extramucosal pyloromyotomy (REP) has been losing popularity.

Patient positioning and laparoscopic setup are shown in Figs. 26.1 and 26.2. In our experience, the transverse position of the patient in the operating table allows better instrumentation settings and better ergonomic position to operate.

After disinfection and pose of sterile drapes, a small (~5 mm) curved upper or infraumbilical rim incision is performed. Incision of the aponeurosis and the peritoneum is performed. A U-shaped stitch of a 3-0 reabsorbed suture is placed in the aponeurosis. This suture will be use to fix the umbilical trocar to avoid displacement during surgery and to close the aponeurosis at the end of the procedure. A 5 mm trocar is placed in the umbilicus, and a 6–8 mmHg CO_2 pneumoperitoneum is applied. Special attention is recommended to purge very well the tube of the insufflator with CO_2 before to attach it to the trocar; this is performed to eliminate the room air in the system. Through this trocar, a 0° or 30° 5 mm telescope is inserted. The most common position of the other two trocars of 3 mm for instrumentation is one at the epigastrium and the other in the lateral part of the right hypochondrium (Fig. 26.3). With a 3-mm laparoscopic Babcock clamp, inserted in the right hypochondrium trocar, the hypertrophied pylorus is fixed and exposed. Through the epigastric trocar, a 3-mm laparoscopic retractable scalpel is inserted to perform the pyloromyotomy. The use of a laparoscopic electrocautery monopolar hook to perform the seromuscular pyloric incision has been also reported [6]. An incision is made over the anterosuperior part of the pylorus, beginning at the demarcated pyloroduodenal junction about 2 mm proximal to the pyloric vein and extending the incision onto the gastric antrum. Either with a special 3-mm laparoscopic pyloric spreader (Fig. 26.4) or with an atraumatic grasper, the pyloric muscle fibers are

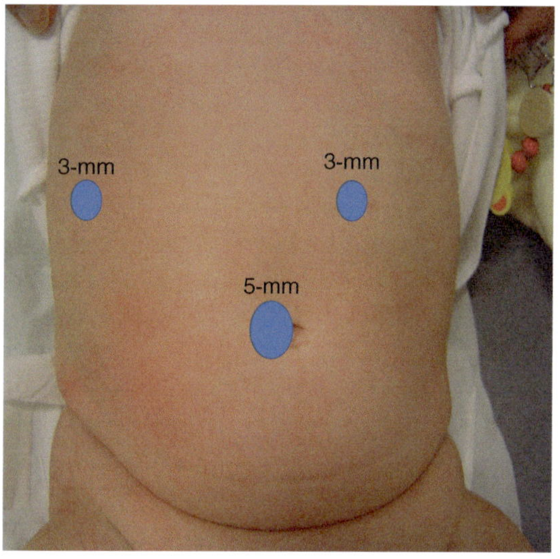

Fig. 26.3 Trocar position

Fig. 26.2 Setup

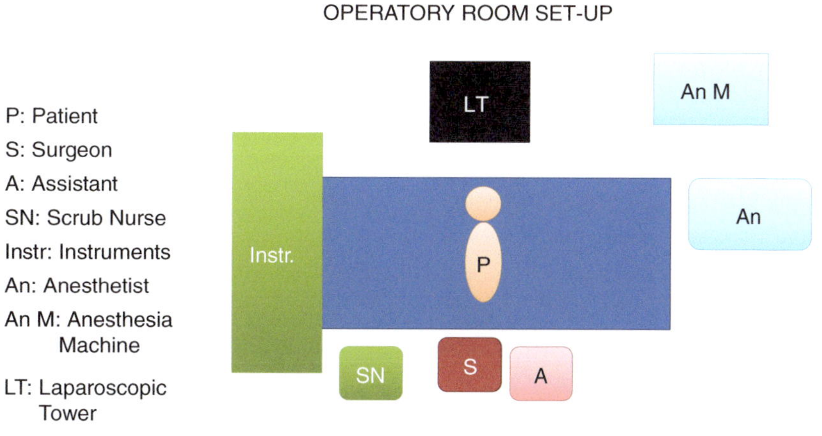

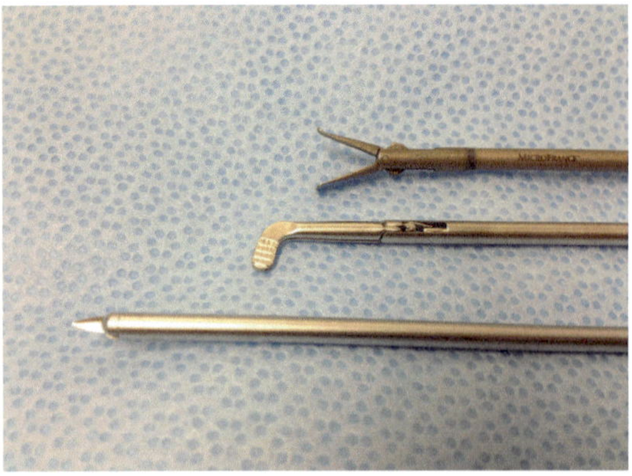

Fig. 26.4 Laparoscopic instruments for pyloromyotomy

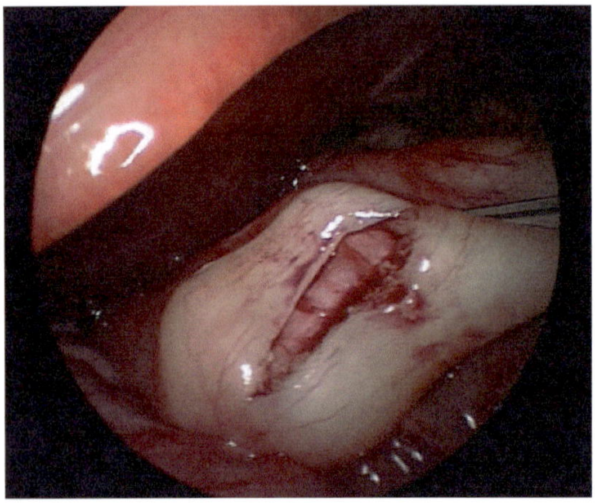

Fig. 26.5 Laparoscopic pyloromyotomy

then widely split until the mucosa is visible and bulging (Fig. 26.5). Hemostasis is assured. A perforation test could be performed dropping saline with a 3-mm laparoscopic irrigation system and insufflation of the stomach with air through a nasogastric tube, searching for bubbles. Although the absence of bubbles suggests a low suspicion of mucosal impairment, this technique does not exclude completely the possibility of perforation [2]. The pneumoperitoneum is evacuated, and the incisions of the trocars are closed with interrupted stitches of 4-0 absorbable sutures. The skin could be closed with rapid absorbable sutures or with glue.

26.5 Postoperative Care

Maintenance of intravenous fluids is continued until the patient is feeding satisfactorily. Most patients start oral feeds 4–6 h after surgery. Although several protocols to increase the volume and concentration of the meals for the reintroduction of oral feeds exist, some institutions advocate feeding *ad libitum* with excellent results [9]. Table 26.1 shows a common protocol of oral feeding. Most patients tolerate full feedings 24–48 h after surgery and could be discharged from the hospital [3]. Postoperative esthetics of the scars is very good (Fig. 26.6).

26.6 Complications

Randomized controlled trials comparing outcomes after open and laparoscopic pyloromyotomy have been published [6, 7]. These studies concluded that there were no statistically significant differences in complication rates.

Table 26.1 Feeding protocol 4–6 h after pyloromyotomy

Substance	Quantity	Time of interval	Times of administration
Pedialyte or water with 10% glucose	30 ml	Every 3 h	2
Half-strength formula or complete breast milk	30 ml	Every 3 h	1
Full-strength formula or breast milk	30 ml	Every 3 h	1
Full-strength formula or breast milk	60 ml	Every 3 h	2
Full-strength formula or breast milk	90 ml	Every 3 h	2
Full-strength formula or breast milk	*Ad libitum*	Every 3 h	

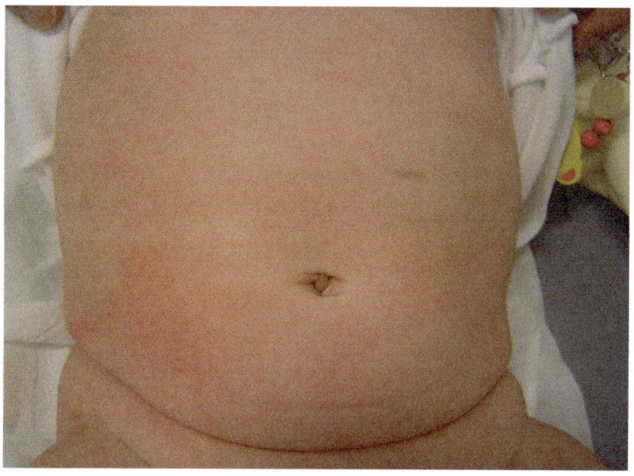

Fig. 26.6 Postoperative results of the scars

The rate of complications during or after pyloromyotomy is very low and generally related to the inexperience of the surgeon during the learning curve. Common major complications include mucosal perforation or incomplete pyloromyotomy. In both cases, the treatment of these complications should be performed with or by an experienced surgeon and could be performed by open or laparoscopic approach. Mucosal perforation occurs mainly secondary to excessive separation of the muscular fibers in the duodenal side of the pylorus; in this case, the perforation is closed with an absorbable suture, and a patch of omentum is applied over the suture. A new pyloromyotomy in the posterosuperior face of the pylorus may be performed. Incomplete pyloromyotomy is mainly secondary to a short incision or incomplete separation of the muscle fibers of the gastric side of the pylorus. In this case, a new intervention is necessary to complete the pyloromyotomy.

Other severe and very rare complications such as air or carbon dioxide embolism during laparoscopic pyloromyotomy have been reported [3].

26.7 Discussion

Diagnosis of HPS has made important changes since the introduction of ultrasound. Prompt diagnosis and stabilization of the dehydration and electrolyte imbalance allow a sooner surgical correction of the gastric outlet obstruction with a consequent better outcome. Regarding the surgical procedure, Ramstedt extramucosal pyloromyotomy is considered still the gold standard.

The randomized controlled trials existing in the literature, comparing the open and the laparoscopic pyloromyotomy, concluded that both approaches are equally safe and reproducible in experienced hands. From the cosmetic point of view, no real benefits exist between the transumbilical open approach and the laparoscopic approach. The surgeon must choose the best approach in base of his surgical experience and skills and in the resources of the institution where he works. Moreover, a close supervision by an experienced pediatric surgeon faculty is mandatory while training residents during an open or a laparoscopic pyloromyotomy to decrease the risk of major complications. Further randomized controlled trials regarding new techniques such as the needlescopic approach [6], single-incision approach [7], and the new endoscopic intraluminal pyloromyotomy [3] are necessary to evaluate their real benefits, complications, and contraindications in this domain.

Publications in the medical literature evaluating the long-term follow-up after pyloromyotomy are scanty. The outcome of the pyloric hypertrophy after a pyloromyotomy was studied in 103 infants by Muramori et al. [9]. They performed serial ultrasonographic measurements regarding channel length, muscle thickness, and diameter of the pylorus for a period of 1 year after surgery. In contrast to the prompt improvement of clinical symptoms, they found that the length of the pyloric channel reached a normal length (~12.7 ± 2.8 mm) around 4 months after surgery, the muscle thickness reached a normal range (~2 mm) until 8 months after surgery, and the pyloric diameter did not reach a normal diameter (~10–12 mm) even by the end of 1 year after surgery.

Walker et al. [3] analyzed the neurological development of infants operated for HPS and compare them with healthy control infants at 1 year of age. They found that the cognitive, receptive language and motor score were significantly lower in HPS infants than in controls. Other authors have reported chronic abdominal pain probably secondary to irritable bowel syndrome, functional dyspepsia, and functional abdominal pain in children operated of HPS in a mean follow-up period of 7 years when compared to healthy control children [4]. These findings raised concerns over the potential impact of HPS and its surgical treatment. Further studies are necessary to elucidate these results.

In conclusion, laparoscopic pyloromyotomy is safe and feasible and offers excellent postoperative results in neonates and infants with congenital pyloric stenosis. During the learning curve process of surgeons in training, a correct supervision by experienced laparoscopic surgeons is mandatory in order to decrease the risk of complications. Further studies regarding new techniques such as the needlescopic approach, the single-incision approach, and the endoscopic intraluminal pyloromyotomy are necessary to evaluate their real benefits, complications, and contraindications in this domain.

References

1. Aspelund G, Langer JC. Current management of hypertrophic pyloric stenosis. Semin Pediatr Surg. 2007;16(1):27–33.
2. Shaw A. Ramstedt and the centennial of pyloromyotomy. J Pediatr Surg. 2012;47(7):1433–5.
3. Sola JE, Neville HL. Laparoscopic vs. open pyloromyotomy: a systemic review and meta-analysis. J Pediatr Surg. 2009;44(8):1631–7.
4. Oomen MWN, Hoekstra LT, Ubbink DT, et al. Open versus laparoscopic pyloromyotomy for hypertrophic pyloric stenosis: a systematic review and meta-analysis focusing on major complications. Surg Endosc. 2012;26(8):2104–10.
5. Boybeyi O, Karnak I, Ekinci S, et al. Late-onset hypertrophic pyloric stenosis: definition of diagnostic criteria and algorithm for the management. J Pediatr Surg. 2010;45(9):1777–83.
6. Juang D, Adibe OO, Laituri CA, et al. Distribution of feeding styles after pyloromyotomy among pediatric surgical training programs in North America. Eu J Pediatr Surg. 2012;22(5):409–11.
7. Oomen MWN, Hoekstra LT, Baky R. Learning curves for pediatric laparoscopy: how many operations are enough? The Amsterdam experience with laparoscopic pyloromyotomy. Surg Endosc. 2010;24:1829–33.
8. Haricharan RN, Aprahamian CJ, Celik A, et al. Laparoscopic pyloromyotomy: effect of resident training on complications. J Pediatr Surg. 2008;43(1):97–101.
9. Taylor SP, Hoffman GM. Gas embolus and cardiac arrest during laparoscopic pyloromyotomy in an infant. Can J Anaesth. 2010;57(8):774–8.
10. Fischler M. Carbon dioxide embolism in a 3-week-old neonate during laparoscopic pyloromyotomy: a case report. J Pediatr Surg. 2009;44(9):1864.
11. Kudsi OY, Jones SA, Brenn BR. Carbon dioxide embolism in a 3-week-old neonate during laparoscopic pyloromyotomy: a case report. J Pediatr Surg. 2009;44(4):842–5.
12. Turial S, Enders J, Schier F, et al. Comparison of a novel technique of the microlaparoscopic pyloromyotomy to circumbilical and Weber-Ramstedt approaches. J Gastrointest Surg. 2011;15(7):1136–42.
13. Muensterer OJ, Adibe OO, Harmon CM, et al. Single-incision laparoscopic pyloromyotomy: initial experience. Surg Endosc. 2010;24(7):1589–93.
14. Zhang YX, Nie YQ, Xiao X, et al. Treatment of congenital hypertrophic pyloric stenosis with endoscopic pyloromyotomy. Zhonghua Er Ke Za Zhi. 2008;46(4):247–51.
15. Walker K, Halliday R, Holland AJ, et al. Early developmental outcome of infants with infantile hypertrophic pyloric stenosis. J Pediatr Surg. 2010;45(12):2369–72.

Laparoscopic Jejunostomy

27

Nikolaos Baltogiannis

27.1 Introduction

Enteral nutrition is defined as nutrition given through a feeding tube. This offers several advantages as compared to parenteral nutrition. Parenteral nutrition should only be used when nutritional requirements cannot be met via the gastrointestinal tract or when there is bowel dysfunction. Undoubtedly, enteral nutritional support is superior to total parenteral nutrition in terms of achieving nutritional goals, improving outcomes, maintaining gastrointestinal mucosal integrity, promoting immunosecretory function, and avoiding infectious complications.

Patients with a long-term need (>3 months) for enteric feeding are best managed with a gastrostomy or jejunostomy [1]. Jejunostomy is not commonly performed in children, but surgical feeding jejunostomy is an established feeding route in order to obviate gastric feeding intolerance [2, 3]. Jejunostomy feeding often starts with a transgastric jejunal tube placed distal to the ligament of Treitz; however, it is only a transitory choice due to its excessively high complication rate [2, 3]. Feeding via the jejunum was first described by Wilhelm Busch, who, in 1858, provided a diet of eggs, flour, meat, and broth to a woman through intermittent instillation with a jejunal fistula [4]. Since then, jejunostomy has been used for nutritional support in clinical situations wherein gastrostomy may be precluded or contraindicated. As a sole procedure, it is advised for congenital disorders and neurologic dysfunction presenting with persistent retching, sleep disturbance, and recurrent pneumonia in children with failure to thrive due to gastroparesis, uncorrected gastroesophageal reflux, postoperative feeding, anatomic or functional gastric outlet obstruction, or chronic pancreatitis [5, 6]. Most pediatric surgeons prefer the usage of more versatile gastrostomy for patients who require long-term enteric feeding; [5] moreover, we also primarily use gastrostomy over other methods for long-term enteral access.

The first jejunostomy, however, was not performed until 1878 by Surmay [7]. With the development of this technique and great demand for minimization of the surgical invasion and optimal cosmetic result, O'Regan and Scarrow pioneered laparoscopic jejunostomy in the 1990s [8]. After this initial effort, numerous surgical techniques for enteral feeding have evolved over the years: laparotomy including longitudinal and transverse Witzel [9], Roux-en-Y [10], "omega" jejunostomy tube [11], needle catheter technique [12], a percutaneous endoscopy [13], and laparoscopic-assisted jejunostomy [14] or totally laparoscopy [15]. The ideal jejunostomy technique depends on the material resources but more importantly on the experience of the pediatric surgeon. In

N. Baltogiannis (✉)
Surgical Department of Pediatric Center and Gaia Maternity Private Hospital of Athens Medical Group, Marousi, Greece

C. Esposito et al. (eds.), *ESPES Manual of Pediatric Minimally Invasive Surgery*,
https://doi.org/10.1007/978-3-030-00964-9_27

any case, endoscopic or laparoscopic surgery is a one-way road as all pediatric surgeons embrace minimally invasive surgery for various well-known reasons.

27.2 Operative Room Setup and Laparoscopic Instruments

The pediatric patient is placed in a supine position on the operating table. The surgeon and the camera operator are standing by the patient's right hip. The assistant may stand on the opposite side, whereas the scrub nurse is on the patient's right side near the foot of the table. The laparoscopy set is placed on the left side of the patient, near the child's left shoulder (Fig. 27.1a). The required laparoscopic instruments are the following:

- 0° or 30° laparoscope
- 5–10-mm trocar for laparoscope
- Two 3–5-mm trocars.
- Needle holder.
- Atraumatic or fenestrated bowel grasper.
- Scissors.
- Monopolar hook diathermy.
- Jejunostomy tube.

27.3 Trocar Placement

- 10-mm trocar for the camera in the umbilical region.
- First trocar in the right lower quadrant, near midline.
- Second trocar in the right upper quadrant (the position wherein the surgeon's left hand is located).
- Feeding jejunostomy is generally placed in the left upper quadrant, lateral to the rectus muscle sheath and slightly above the level of the umbilicus, and in a position not so cephalic as to interfere with a possible gastrostomy (Fig. 27.2).

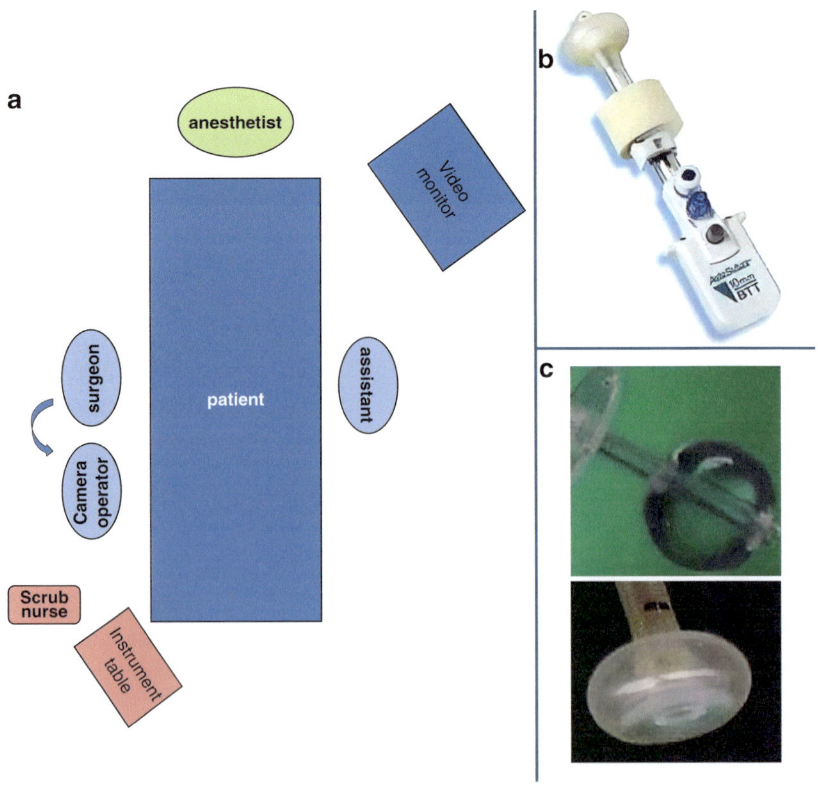

Fig. 27.1 (a–c) Operative room setup, laparoscopic optical trocar, and two types of low-profile balloon jejunostomy tubes

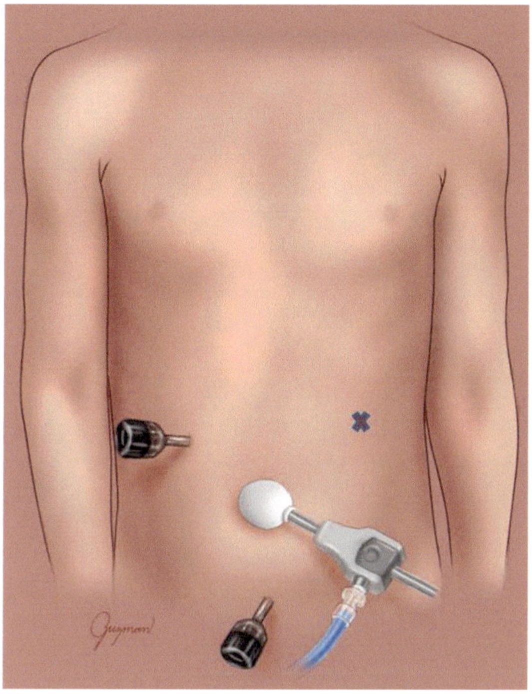

Fig. 27.2 Port placement for jejunostomy

27.4 Technique of Laparoscopic Jejunostomy

As with gastrostomy tube placement, no particular method of jejunostomy placement has been proven to be the best method.

- Under general anesthesia, the pediatric patient is placed in a supine position. All patients receive cefoxitin sodium intravenously prior to surgery as a prophylaxis. A nasogastric tube should be passed into the stomach before the procedure. The technique begins with a 10-mm semicircular or vertical incision in the umbilical fold that is wide enough to accommodate the diameter of the camera's trocar. We prefer the Hasson technique through open method to obtain intraperitoneal access at the umbilical port site. The trocar of the laparoscope needs not be fixed to the abdominal wall to prevent air leakages, as a balloon trocar is usually used (Fig. 27.1b). This device has a retention balloon that lies under the fascia and is filled with about 20 cm^3 of air. A moveable foam pad slides down the skin and is secured in place with an incorporated clasp to prevent air leakage. After carbon dioxide insufflation through the sleeve, the optical equipment is introduced in the usual manner, and the abdomen is surveyed in order to ensure no unexpected pathology or abnormalities. Subsequently, two ports must be placed under direct visualization for the working instruments. A 5-mm port is inserted into the right lower quadrant; another 5-mm port is inserted in the right upper quadrant where the surgeon's left hand is, lateral to the rectus abdominis muscle (Fig. 27.2). Proper trocar placement is essential for a successful laparoscopic surgery. The correct identification of the ligament of Treitz will aid in proper tube placement. Locating the ligament of Treitz is most easily accomplished by placing the patient in a slight reverse Trendelenburg position, reflecting the transverse colon and omentum superiorly and following the transverse colon mesentery to its posterior origin. The ligament of Treitz should be visualized just to the left of the midline in its posterior location. It is essential that the proximal jejunum is clearly identified. Once the loop is identified, a point that is approximately 30 cm from the duodenojejunal flexure is selected as the jejunostomy site. This is an appropriate distance for an ideal placement of jejunostomy, as malabsorption is possible if the tube is placed too distally. On the other hand, if the tube is too proximal, reflux may occur into the stomach via the duodenum and lead to aspiration.
- Once the appropriate point for the jejunostomy is identified, it has to be elevated to touch the left upper quadrant abdominal wall (Fig. 27.3). Moreover, it should be verified that there is no tension on the selected jejunal loop when brought up to the anterior abdominal wall.
- The jejunum is held at this point on its antimesenteric surface against the anterior abdominal wall. The first anchoring suture is placed just 1 cm cephalic to the point of the tube placement between the seromuscular layer of the antimesenteric border of the intestine and the abdominal wall adjacent to its entry site (Fig. 27.4). For this procedure, we use a 3–0 Vicryl suture.
- A small enterotomy is made with a monopolar hook diathermy, and if necessary, it is enlarged

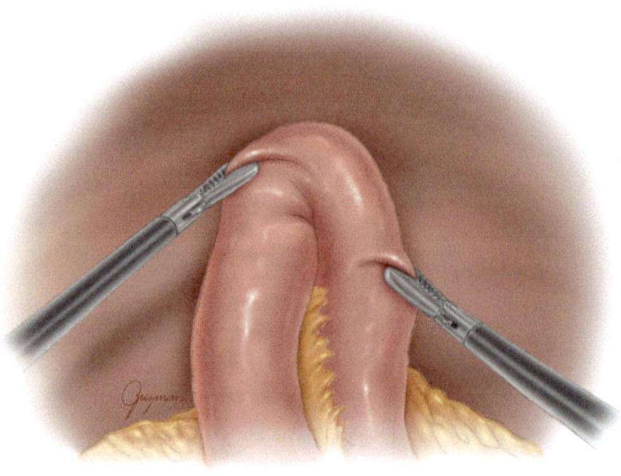

Fig. 27.3 The jejunum is elevated to touch the left upper quadrant abdominal wall

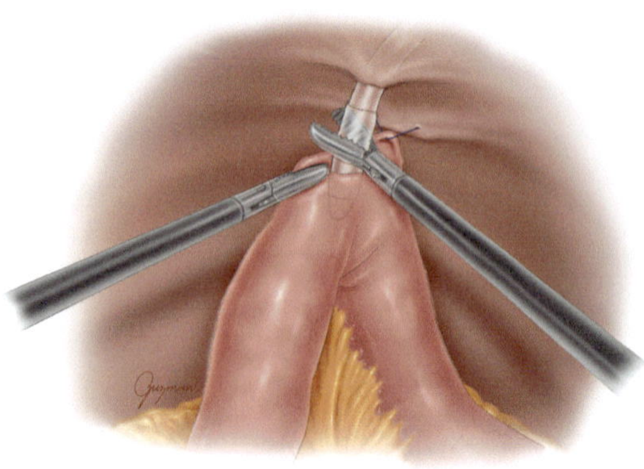

Fig. 27.5 The tube is passed into the jejunum

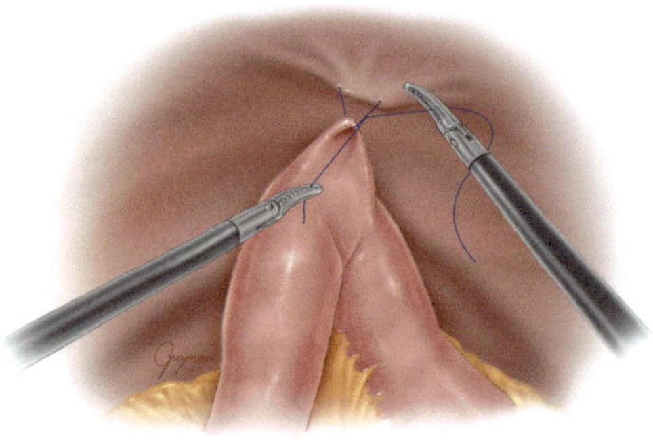

Fig. 27.4 The first suture is placed through the abdominal wall and jejunum

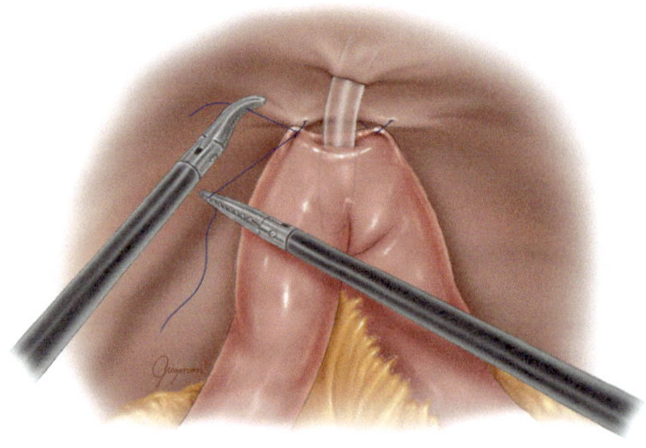

Fig. 27.6 The second suture is placed through the abdominal wall and the jejunum

with a laparoscopic dissector; however, this is not a common practice. The jejunostomy tube is inserted through the abdominal wall using an open technique and is passed into the jejunum under laparoscopic vision (Fig. 27.5).

- The second suture is placed symmetrically and similar to the first suture (Fig. 27.6).
- Inflate the balloon with 2–3 mL of saline, and ensure that the balloon will not cause intestinal obstruction. Note that the shape of the inflated balloon we use is not round as usual but is flat (Fig. 27.1c). Pull up the catheter so that the balloon will bring the jejunum firmly attached to the abdominal wall and push the outer flange against the anterior abdominal wall in order to anchor the tube to the skin. Through this, the absence of leakage can be ensured.
- If desired, additional 3–0 sutures may be placed to anchor the bowel wall to the underside of the abdominal wall at the left and right sides of the tube, as a safeguard against leakage. In cases of uncertainty, a seromuscular purse-string suture can be taken before creating the jejunal opening and be tied once the tube is in place.
- Test the catheter for ease flow of normal saline solution into the jejunum, and observe the resulting flow into the bowel with the laparoscope.
- Drip feeding is started 2–3 days after surgery at a slow rate and is gradually increased as tolerated by the patient.
- We prefer this technique over others because of its simplicity, versatility, and safety. However, since none has clearly shown supe-

riority, it remains a personal decision which one to use, and a pediatric surgeon should continue using the techniques which he is most comfortable with and according to the available resources.

27.5 Complications

The complications associated with jejunostomy include mechanical (tube occlusion, small bowel obstruction, volvulus, and leakage), infectious (perijejunostomy site infection, granulation tissue formation, and cutaneous or intra-abdominal abscesses), gastrointestinal (diarrhea, colic, nausea, vomiting, intestinal ischemia, and jejunal hematoma), and metabolic (hyperglycemia, hypokalemia, water and electrolyte imbalance, hypophosphatemia, and hypomagnesemia) complications.

27.6 Conclusion

Laparoscopic jejunostomy is a feasible and safe procedure that can be performed in patients who require alternative enteral feeding. It can be easily performed with basic laparoscopic skills regarding the surgeon's experience and with the use of standard laparoscopic equipment available in most hospitals. Like every other laparoscopic operation, it has its own benefits and limitations.

Acknowledgments I would like to offer my special thanks to William Guzman Jr., medical and biological illustrator, for his contribution to the fulfillment of this chapter with the designing of medical images.

References

1. Keith G. Laparoscopic versus open procedures for long-term enteral access. Supplement to NCP. 1997;12:S7–8.
2. Fascetti-Leon F, El Agami F, Gobbi D, et al. Feeding Jejunostomy: Is it a safe route in pediatric patients? Single institution experience. Eur J Pediatr Surg. 2018;28(03):293–6.
3. Egnell C, Eksborg S, Grahnquist L, et al. Jejunostomy enteral feeding in children: outcome and safety. JPEN J Parenter Enteral Nutr. 2014;38:631–6.
4. Busch W. Beitragzur physiology der verdauungsorgane. Virchow Arch Path Anat. 1858;14:140.
5. Georgeson KE. Laparoscopic Jejunostomy. In: Bax NMA, et al., editors. Endoscopic Surgery in Children. 1st ed. Berlin: Springer; 1999. p. 203–6.
6. Lightdale JR, Gremse DA. Gastroesophageal reflux: management guidance for the pediatrician. Pediatrics. 2013;131:e1684–95.
7. Surmay M. De l'enterostomie. Bull General Ther. 1878;94:445.
8. O'Regan PJ, Scarrow GD. Laparoscopic jejunostomy. Endoscopy. 1990;22(1):39–40.
9. Tapia J, Murguia R, Garcia G, et al. Jejunostomy: techniques, indications, and complications. World J Surg. 1999;23(6):596–602.
10. Neuman HB, Phillips JD. Laparoscopic Roux-en-Y feeding jejunostomy: a new minimally invasive surgical procedure for permanent feeding access in children with gastric dysfunction. J Laparoendosc Adv Surg Tech A. 2005;15(1):71–4.
11. Schlager A, Arps K, Siddharthan R, et al. The "omega" jejunostomy tube: a preferred alternative for postpyloric feeding access. J Pediatr Surg. 2016;51:260–3.
12. Ye P, Zeng L, Sun F, et al. A new modified technique of laparoscopic needle catheter jejunostomy: a 2-year follow-up study. Ther Clin Risk Manag. 2016;12:103–8.
13. Virnig DJ, Frech EJ, Delegge MH, et al. Direct percutaneous endoscopic jejunostomy: a case series in pediatric patients. Gastrointest Endosc. 2008;67:984–7.
14. Esposito C, Settimi A, Centonze A, et al. Laparoscopic assisted jejunostomy. Surg Endosc. 2005;19:501–5.
15. Georgeson KE. Laparoscopic jejunostomy. In: Holcomb GW, Georgeson K, Rothenberg S, editors. Atlas of pediatric laparoscopy and thoracoscopy. London: Saunders/Elsevier; 2008. p. 61–4.

Minimally Invasive Management of Duodenal and Jejunal Atresia

28

J. A. Sobrino and S. D. St. Peter

28.1 Introduction

Duodenal atresia occurs due to a failure of the lumen to recanalize during the 11th week of gestation. Over half of patients have an associated congenital anomaly with congenital heart disease, trisomy 21, malrotation, annular pancreas, and tracheoesophageal fistula among the most common. The classic presentation is a newborn with early bilious emesis. This finding is dependent on a post-ampullary obstruction, and a small percentage of cases may present with non-bilious emesis due to a pre-ampullary lesion [1]. Prenatal ultrasound often suggests obstruction due to dilated proximal small bowel and polyhydramnios. After birth, the classic imaging finding is the "double bubble" of stomach and duodenal bulb with an absence of distal gas; however, the presence of distal gas does not exclude atresia [2]. Gray and Skandalakis classified the types of duodenal atresia in 1972. Type I defects are the most common and contain a thin membranous separation between the two portions of bowel. In type II, an atretic, fibrous cord connects the two halves, and in type III the segments are entirely separated, and there is an adjacent mesenteric defect [3].

J. A. Sobrino · S. D. St. Peter (✉)
Department of Surgery, Children's Mercy Hospital, Kansas City, MO, USA
e-mail: sspeter@cmh.edu

Jejunal atresia is a separate entity and is thought to occur due to a late intrauterine vascular event that compromises the development of one or more sections of the midgut. Prenatal diagnosis is less common, though proximal lesions may present similar to duodenal atresia. Presentation may vary slightly based on location. Bilious emesis is a hallmark. Abdominal distension may not be present in proximal lesions due to the inability to sequester fluid throughout the intestines, but it is common in distal atresias. As such, distal atresias tend to present later as the child may tolerate the first few feedings. Associated congenital anomalies are far less common than in duodenal atresia, though defects related to the midgut are more common and severe. These include mesenteric defects with potential for internal hernias, volvulus, and multiple lesions accounting for significant bowel length. Supine and decubitus radiographs are generally adequate to confirm diagnosis and often display classic obstructive findings. The most commonly used classification system for distal intestinal atresias is the 1979 Grosfeld modification of the system originally described by Louw and Barnard (Fig.28.1) [4, 5]. Type I is a mucosal web or atresia with an intact bowel wall and mesentery. Type II is atretic bowel segments connected by a fibrous cord. Type IIIa is atretic bowel segments with a corresponding mesenteric defect, and IIIb is described as the apple peel atresia or Christmas tree defect. Type IV refers to multiple atretic defects.

C. Esposito et al. (eds.), *ESPES Manual of Pediatric Minimally Invasive Surgery*,
https://doi.org/10.1007/978-3-030-00964-9_28

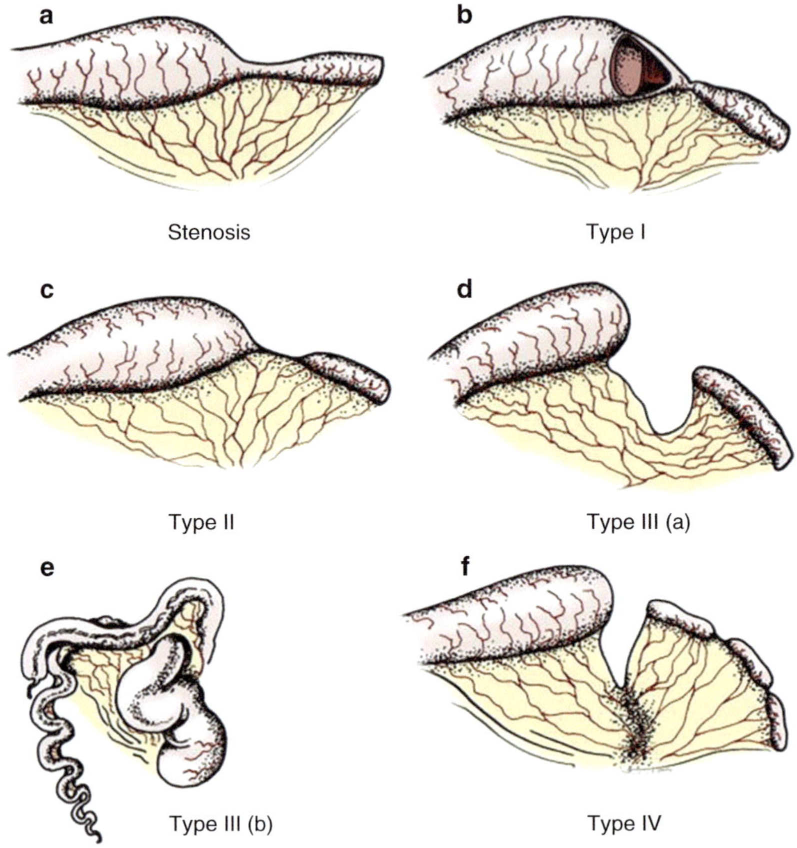

Fig. 28.1 Grosfeld classification system of jejunal atresias [14]

We describe in this chapter the minimally invasive approaches to duodenal and jejunal atresia.

Laparoscopic repairs have been shown to be at least as safe and efficacious as open repair [6, 7]. Some series demonstrate shorter hospital stays, time to initial feeding, and time to goal oral intake with the laparoscopic approach [8].

28.2 Preoperative Preparation

Neither of these conditions alone are surgical emergencies such that preoperative resuscitation and foregut decompression are the first objectives. Associated volvulus or internal hernias with strangulation are the only emergent indications for operation which can occur with more distal atresias.

With suspected duodenal atresia without clear radiographic evidence, we perform a limited upper gastrointestinal study by instilling just enough contrast volume to evaluate for malrotation and volvulus and evacuating any residual contrast. An echocardiogram should be obtained preoperatively in all cases, with additional workup electively and as clinically indicated.

Conversely, these measures may be selectively pursued as clinically indicated in jejunal atresia given the low incidence of associate anomalies. Unlike duodenal atresia, a water-soluble contrast enema is useful first to demonstrate microcolon from a small bowel obstruction, second to evaluate for concurrent distal atresia, and finally to evaluate associated Hirschsprung's disease or meconium ileus/plug. It is important to council families preoperatively that up to 15% of these cases may result in short bowel syndrome [9].

28.3 Positioning

The patient is positioned supine on the operating table with the arms tucked at their sides. Monitors for the surgeon and assistant are placed at the head of the bed. We usually accomplish this by turning the baby perpendicular to the table at the head of the bed and placing monitors opposite the surgeons. This requires passing the cords off the table over the opposite side of the baby from the head of the bed to avoid having the cords over the endotracheal tubing.

28.4 Instrumentation

A 5 mm trocar is used for the camera, and a 30°, 5 mm laparoscope is used for most cases with only 3 mm instruments. These can be place directly through the abdominal wall without ports using #11 blade to make the stab incisions.

28.5 Technique

The operation of choice for duodenal stenosis is a duodenoduodenostomy. Port placement may vary, and two options are shown in Fig. 28.2. In the upper abdomen, either a port or a transabdominal stitch through the falciform ligament can be used for liver retraction and exposure. The duodenum is mobilized sufficiently to identify the obstructing lesion and to create a tension-free anastomosis. A transverse enterotomy is made in the anterior wall of the dilated, proximal duodenum, and a longitudinal enterotomy is made on the antimesenteric border of the duodenum distal to the lesion (Fig. 28.3). Stay sutures placed at the corners can better align the bowel, and the back wall is sutured before the front in a single layer to create a diamond-shaped anastomosis, as seen in Fig. 28.4 [10]. Suture choice and interrupted vs.

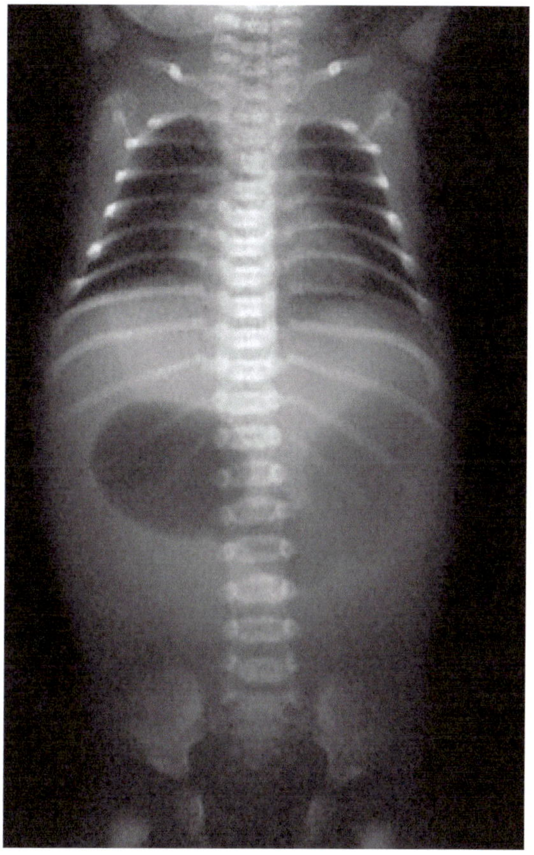

Fig. 28.2 Classic "double bubble" seen in duodenal atresia [14]

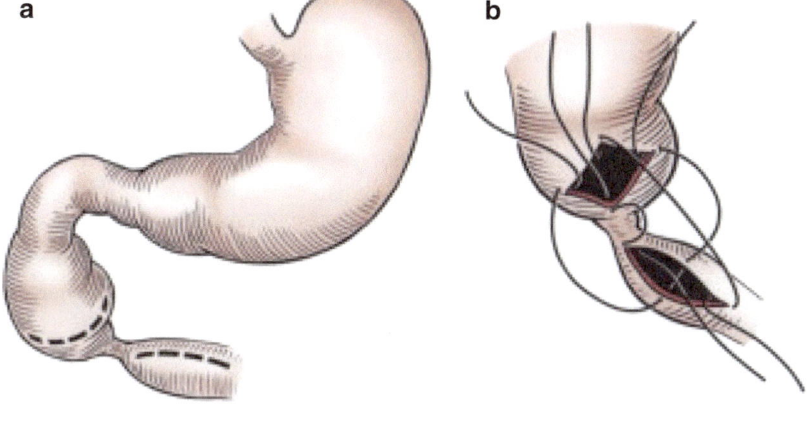

Fig. 28.3 Orientation for duodenoduodenostomy [14]

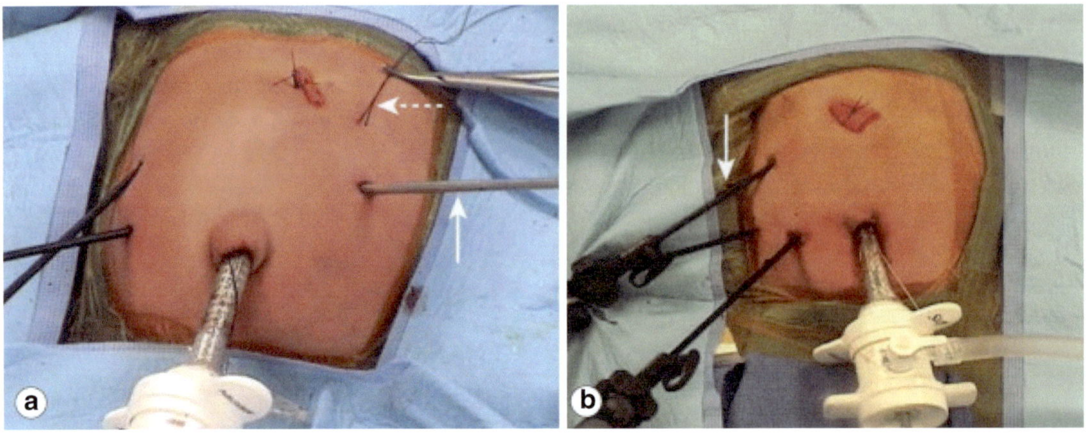

Fig. 28.4 Options for laparoscopic port placement [14]

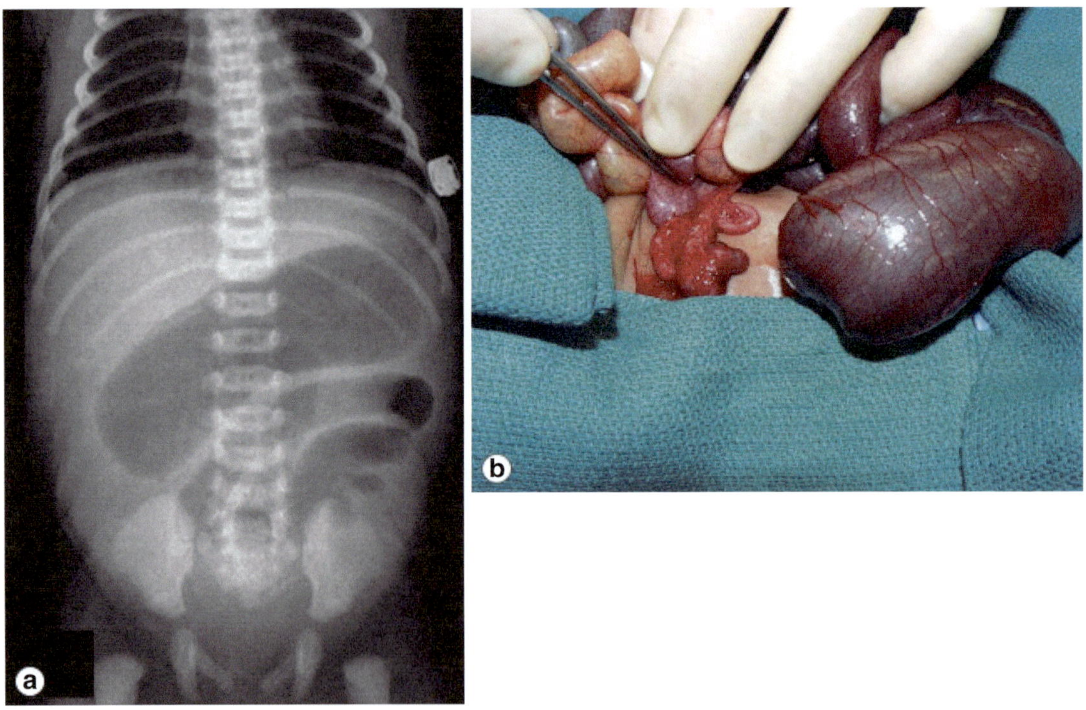

Fig. 28.5 Radiographic and intraoperative findings of jejunal atresia [14]

continuous technique do not seem to impact complication rates [7]. A tapering duodenoplasty is useful to accommodate a dramatic size mismatch.

Jejunal atresia is approached similarly, beginning with a broad survey of the abdomen contents. Any associated volvulus or internal hernia is reduced and bowel viability is assessed. The lesion is found by identifying the transition point between dilated proximal and normal or small-caliber distal bowels, and any adhesions are lysed to mobilize this segment (Fig. 28.5). Laparoscopy is often limited by intestinal distension in a small abdomen, and eviscerating via the umbilical incision, with or without an extension of the incision, is a useful adjunct. We frequently approach these by separating the cord vessels individually and eviscerating the bowel for an extracorporeal operation, which can be done without a cosmetic defect and avoiding the laparotomy. The overall goals are to maintain bowel length and establish continuity for enteral feeding. Size mismatch is routinely encountered and can be addressed by techniques such as tapering, elliptical anastomosis, or antimesenteric cutback anastomosis. Elliptical anastomoses are end-to-end reconstructions and are created by either cutting the distal bowel at an angle resecting more off the antimesenteric side or by cutting a slit in the antimesenteric border. Tapering is achieved by making an enterotomy in the distal end of the proximal dilated bowel and resecting antimesenteric bowel retrograde until more normal-caliber bowel. A 20–24 F rubber catheter can be placed in the lumen of the bowel to prevent narrowing. Grossly dilated small bowel is at high risk for dysfunctional motility and may need to be resected to prevent pseudo-obstruction and bacterial overgrowth. Type IIIb lesions place the patient at high risk for short bowel syndrome and have unique considerations. In these situations, absorptive surface area must be maximized, and therefore dilated, dysfunctional segments are tolerated. They may then be used in a taper or serial transverse enteroplasty.

28.6 Postoperative Care

In both conditions activity and bathing are not restricted after surgery. Acetaminophen is the primary analgesic with narcotics used for breakthrough pain.

In duodenal atresia, patients are kept NPO and on TPN, which is often initiated preoperatively, for 5 days. An orogastric tube is left in place to suction and may be transitioned to dependent drainage. On day 5, we perform an upper gastrointestinal contrast study. If no leak is identified and contrast empties beyond the anastomosis, the gastric tube is removed, and feeds are initiated. One series has suggested that a trans-anastomotic feeding tube can expedite time to initiation of feeds and time to goal feeds [11]. Traditional teaching suggested more proximal lesions resulted in longer time to return of bowel function. This was because it took weeks for the nasogastric tube to diminish the amount of bilious output. Early contrast may empty from the stomach, even with frank bilious output from teh gastric tube. This taught us that bilious output continues for so long with proximal lesions because of an incompetent pylorus allowing for suction of the duodenum, not because of inadequate bowel function.

Jejunal atresias follow standard postoperative advancement pathways based on return of bowel function, and these patients will likewise remain on TPN until then. High nasogastric output may require replacement.

28.7 Results

The average length of surgery is approximately 90–120 min. Complications include anastomotic leak, anastomotic stricture, missed obstruction, delayed gastric emptying, short bowel syndrome, dysfunctional bowel motility, and bacterial overgrowth. Operative mortality is low at ≤4% [1].

Surgical follow-up is not required in straightforward cases with patients on goal enteral feeds, particularly with duodenal atresia. Complicated cases and short bowel syndrome require specialized, multidisciplinary follow-up with the potential for surgical revision.

28.8 Tips and Tricks

- Be aware of the windsock deformity of a duodenal web or a diaphragm. If unrecognized an anastomosis may be created distal to the obstruction. Passage of a catheter proximally and distally can help exclude luminal obstruction.
- Identify the head of the pancreas and look for pancreatic tissue near the transition point, as a partial annulus can still the source of obstruction.
- In the case of premature infants, it is still worth mobilizing the duodenum completely and performing the anastomosis transumbili-

cally; this is also true when a tapering enteroplasty is used. We have done this for patients as small as 1 kg.
- Awaiting transition of orogastric tube output from bilious to clear and expecting traditionally normal volumes of output will delay progress after duodenoduodenoplasty. Patients will tolerate feeds well before this time.
- If a contrast enema is not obtained prior to operation for a distal small bowel atresia, ensure patency of the distal bowel by instilling saline antegrade through an enterotomy at the site of resection.
- Calcifications may be seen on radiographs and are concerning for in utero perforation, while displacement of the bowel loops by a gasless mass may indicate a meconium pseudocyst.

28.9 Discussion

Duodenal and jejunal atresias are intrinsic congenital intestinal obstructions and must be differentiated from both other intrinsic causes such as web or stenosis and extrinsic causes such as an annular pancreas. They are clinically distinct entities with different etiologies, associated congenital anomalies, and management strategies.

The presentation and management of duodenal atresia are generally more straightforward than jejunal atresias, and it is usually the associated disorders that require more involved evaluation. The operation is readily achieved laparoscopically, though a hybrid approach of laparoscopic mobilization with extracorporeal suture is a viable alternative. A criticism of the laparoscopic technique has been the inability to adequately evaluate for a concurrent distal atresia; however the rate of simultaneous lesions is less than 1% [12]. Thus, full inspection beyond what is capable laparoscopically is not necessary. Outcomes for duodenal atresia have been studied up to 30 years out, with a 9% revision rate. The late mortality rate was 6%, and the vast majority are due to comorbid conditions [13].

The complexity of jejunal atresias is in the operative decisionmaking, and the same principles may be applied to ileal atresia. The multitude of techniques can be used to achieve the primary goals of preserving bowel length and establishing enteral continuity for feeds. If both of these conditions are met, then minimizing the impact of dilated, dysfunctional bowel via tapering or resection can be entertained.

References

1. Dalla Vecchia LK, Grosfeld JL, West KW, Rescorla FJ, Scherer LR, Engum SA. Intestinal atresia and stenosis: a 25-year experience with 277 cases. Arch Surg 1998;133:490–6; discussion 496–497.
2. Grosfeld JL, Rescorla FJ. Duodenal atresia and stenosis: reassessment of treatment and outcome based on antenatal diagnosis, pathologic variance, and long-term follow-up. World J Surg. 1993;17:301–9.
3. Gray SW, Skandalakis JE. Embryology for surgeons: the embryological basis for the treatment of congenital defects. Philadelphia: Saunders; 1972.
4. Louw JH, Barnard CN. Congenital intestinal atresia; observations on its origin. Lancet Lond Engl. 1955;269:1065–7.
5. Louw JH. Congenital intestinal atresia and stenosis in the newborn. Observations on its pathogenesis and treatment. Ann R Coll Surg Engl. 1959;25:209–34.
6. Chung PHY, Wong CWY, Ip DKM, Tam PKH, Wong KKY. Is laparoscopic surgery better than open surgery for the repair of congenital duodenal obstruction? A review of the current evidences. J Pediatr Surg. 2017;52:498–503. https://doi.org/10.1016/j.jpedsurg.2016.08.010.
7. Mentessidou A, Saxena AK. Laparoscopic repair of duodenal atresia: systematic review and meta-analysis. World J Surg. 2017;41:2178–84. https://doi.org/10.1007/s00268-017-3937-3.
8. Spilde TL, St Peter SD, Keckler SJ, Holcomb GW, Snyder CL, Ostlie DJ. Open vs laparoscopic repair of congenital duodenal obstructions: a concurrent series. J Pediatr Surg. 2008;43:1002–5. https://doi.org/10.1016/j.jpedsurg.2008.02.021.
9. Stollman TH, de Blaauw I, Wijnen MHWA, van der Staak FHJM, Rieu PNMA, Draaisma JMT, et al. Decreased mortality but increased morbidity in neonates with jejunoileal atresia; a study of 114 cases over a 34-year period. J Pediatr Surg. 2009;44:217–21. https://doi.org/10.1016/j.jpedsurg.2008.10.043.
10. Rothenberg SS. Laparoscopic duodenoduodenostomy for duodenal obstruction in infants and children. J Pediatr Surg. 2002;37:1088–9.
11. Arnbjörnsson E, Larsson M, Finkel Y, Karpe B. Transanastomotic feeding tube after an operation

for duodenal atresia. Eur J Pediatr Surg. 2002;12:159–62. https://doi.org/10.1055/s-2002-32727.

12. St Peter SD, Little DC, Barsness KA, Copeland DR, Calkins CM, Yoder S, et al. Should we be concerned about jejunoileal atresia during repair of duodenal atresia? J Laparoendosc Adv Surg Tech A. 2010;20:773–5. https://doi.org/10.1089/lap.2010.0173.
13. Escobar MA, Ladd AP, Grosfeld JL, West KW, Rescorla FJ, Scherer LR, et al. Duodenal atresia and stenosis: long-term follow-up over 30 years. J Pediatr Surg. 2004;39:867–71; discussion 867-871.
14. Ashcraft KW, Holcomb GW, Murphy JP, Ostlie DJ, editors. Chapter 30: duodenal and intestinal atresia and stenosis. Ashcraft's pediatric surgery. 6th ed. New York: Saunders/Elsevier; 2014.

29 Minimally Invasive Surgery for Malrotation of the Intestine and Midgut Volvulus

Paul Philippe and Cindy Gomes Ferreira

29.1 Introduction

Malrotation is defined by an abnormal position and fixation of the bowel within the abdominal cavity.

In the early stage of embryologic development, the growing midgut (from the position of the hepatic bud to the area of the middle colic artery on the future transverse colon) elongates through the body stalk, outside of the abdominal cavity. Between week 7 and 10, the bowel reintegrates the abdominal cavity thanks to a precise folding: first to the right and then counterclockwise around the axis of the superior mesenteric artery. This results in the known retroperitoneal position of the second, third, and fourth portion of the duodenum and the fixation of the duodenojejunal junction at the Treitz angle, to the left of the vertebral colon. The future small bowel is the first to reintegrate the abdominal cavity. When the cecum and colon complete the reintegration at 10 weeks, it rotates to the right lower quadrant, where it contracts adhesions with the retroperitoneum. The ascending colon thus becomes "retroperitoneal," as its mesentery fuses with the posterior planes.

Whenever this process is incomplete or improper, various types or degrees of malrotation occur [1, 2].

They range from "incomplete" rotation to "non-rotation" with several variants. If the "non-rotation" state is usually asymptomatic, incomplete rotation with a narrow base of the mesentery to the midgut and tight attachment of the right colon to the right lateral retroperitoneum in front of the duodenum (Ladd's bands) can lead to severe and life-threatening complications.

Some abnormal rotation is present in abdominal wall congenital anomalies (congenital diaphragmatic hernia, omphalocele, gastroschisis) and can be associated with various other anomalies or syndromes. Congenital duodenal anomalies (atresia or intrinsic stenosis by a web) can coexist with malrotation and should not be overlooked.

The most dreaded complication of the abnormal fixation of the bowel is midgut volvulus, where the entire midgut loop, from the duodenum to the ascending colon, twists around the axis of the superior mesenteric artery, just below Ladd's bands. If not relieved urgently, this situation can lead to vascular compromise and necrosis of the entire small bowel with, if the patient survives, a major short bowel syndrome.

Intermittent or chronic (nonischemic) volvulus causes chronic or recurrent abdominal pain, with or without bilious emesis. Occasionally, duodenal compression by the bands can be symptomatic.

P. Philippe (✉) · C. Gomes Ferreira
Pediatric Surgery Service, KannerKlinik, Centre Hospitalier de Luxembourg, Luxembourg, Luxembourg
e-mail: philippe.paul@chl.lu

C. Esposito et al. (eds.), *ESPES Manual of Pediatric Minimally Invasive Surgery*,
https://doi.org/10.1007/978-3-030-00964-9_29

The work-up usually starts with a sonography, during which the respective position of the superior mesenteric artery and vein is evaluated: it is reversed in malrotation. The passage of the duodenum under the vascular axis and to the left of the vertebral column can sometimes be documented. A "corkscrew sign" can be seen in volvulus and is diagnostic.

Nonetheless, the echographic study can be impossible when air distention of the stomach or bowel is present and false-negative (as well as false-positive) results have been documented.

In adults, CT scan (or MRI) has been used to the same effect.

The gold standard remains the radiologic contrast upper GI study, which will demonstrate the duodenal shape and more precisely the position of Treitz angle.

Despite a high level of sensitivity, those tests are sometimes equivocal, and this could be an indication for diagnostic laparoscopy.

Ladd has outlined the principles of operative treatment of malrotation as early as 1938.

If present, a midgut volvulus should be untwisted counterclockwise. Then, all the preduodenal peritoneal attachments of the ascending colon (Ladd's bands) should be divided and the duodenum mobilized in order to bring the duodenojejunal junction to the right upper quadrant and to place the jejunum to the right side. The basis of the mesentery is widened by dividing all the peritoneal tissues between the duodenum and the colon until the superior mesenteric vein is exposed. This allows the placement of the "right" colon to the left and the ileocecal junction lying in the left lower quadrant. This maneuver creates a wider base of the mesentery, believed to be essential to minimize the risk of volvulus recurrence.

The intestines are thus placed in a non-rotated state, which carries no further risks of complications. An appendectomy can be added, as the appendix will lie in an unusual position.

This procedure is performed through a transverse or midline laparotomy and carries significant morbidity. Delayed return of bowel function and ability to feed are common. Late adhesive bowel obstruction is frequent (up to 15%). Thus, it was natural to seek an alternative, less invasive, and morbid approach. Laparoscopy aims at decreasing those sequelae but has to prove an equal efficiency on the correction of malrotation and recurrence of volvulus. Besides potential longer operating times and the potential metabolic implications of laparoscopy in infants, the expected advantage not to create adhesions and reduce the risk of late bowel obstruction could be a disadvantage, as those adhesion probably play a role in preventing recurrence of the volvulus.

29.2 Indication for Laparoscopy

With the progresses of neonatal minimally invasive surgery, age and weight are not limiting factors anymore.

Most infants come to surgery because of volvulus: a laparoscopy should be offered only to those that are fully resuscitated and stable. It is our belief that obvious signs of shock are associated with (impending) necrosis and an immediate laparotomy should be offered. Nonetheless, we had one such case where the bowel was healthy and in whom, on retrospect, a laparoscopy could have been performed.

Almost all infants are operated urgently, and a laparoscopy should be offered only if an entire team dedicated to neonatal minimally invasive surgery is available.

Uncomplicated malrotation is usually operated electively, based on symptoms. If a malrotation has been discovered incidentally, prevention of potential complications, including volvulus, is considered.

In other instances, the work-up is inconclusive, either to the presence of malrotation or to the risk of complications in an individual patient. In those cases, diagnostic laparoscopy is clearly indicated.

29.3 Preoperative Preparation

In elective cases, emptying the colon with an enema the night before could help provide more working space.

In emergency, such as volvulus, hemodynamic stabilization with intravenous fluids should be quickly performed before induction of anesthesia.

In infants, routine perioperative antibiotics are given, but not in elective, older patient cases.

29.4 Surgical Technique

29.4.1 Positioning

Under general endotracheal anesthesia with full relaxation and a nasogastric tube in place, the patient is positioned supine on the operating table. In infants, the patient is placed near the end of the table or obliquely, so the surgeon can stand at his feet. In older children, the frog or the "French" positions are used, so the surgeon can stand at the feet or between the legs of the patient.

We place a small roll under the back at the thoracolumbar junction to open up the epigastric space.

The monitor is placed above the head or right shoulder of the patient.

An anti-Trendelenburg (feet down) position is used, with tilting of the table to the side as necessary to help displace the bowel opposite to the working area.

Draping is wide as accessory trocars or suspension sutures, as well as conversion, could be necessary (Fig. 29.1).

29.4.2 Instrumentation

No specific instruments are required. A basic laparoscopy set with dissecting and grasping forceps, scissors, dissecting hook, and suction device is all that is mandatory. Three or 3.5 mm instruments are used in infants and 5 mm in the older child for ease of bowel grasping. Trocars are chosen according to the selected size of the instruments.

We usually use one or two fenestrated grasping forceps or Maryland dissectors, a hook with low-energy monopolar current, and curved scissors. Alternatively, one can use bipolar rotating instruments, such as RoBi® (Storz™), available in 3.5 mm.

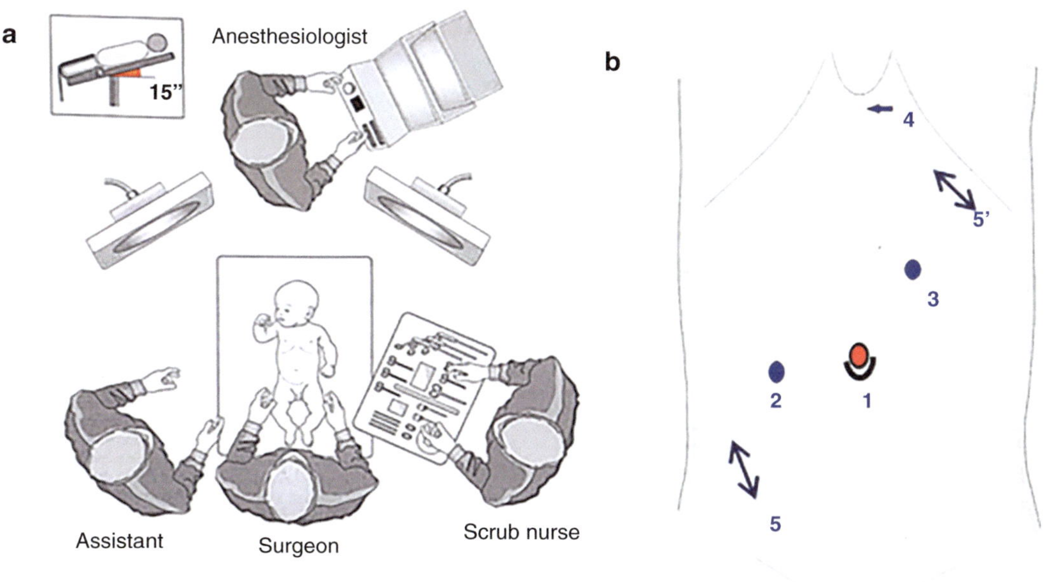

Fig. 29.1 Operating room setup: operating surgeon at the feet (or between the legs) of the patient, monitor above the head or right shoulder of the patient. Trocars position: (1) Umbilicus, 5 mm/30° telescope (option: 3.5 mm). (2 and 3) 3.5 mm instrumentation ports (option: 5 mm), adjusted to the length of the child. (4) Liver retraction: we currently use transparietal suspension of the falciform ligament. (5 and 5′) optional instrument ports for retraction, if necessary

We use a 5 mm, 30-degree telescope, placed through an umbilical port. A 3 mm can be used in small infants, with the advantage of being less space occupying, at the inconvenient of a lesser illumination and depth of visual field. Some of the perioperative illustrations in this chapter have been taken with such a telescope. Moreover, through the umbilical 5 or 7 mm port, one can introduce a small sponge (we use 1 × 1 cm neurosurgical patties or cottonoids, carefully counted not to leave any in the abdomen) that will be helpful during the dissection of the base of the mesentery.

29.5 Surgical Technique

Access to the peritoneal cavity is obtained through a small umbilical incision and an open technique in infants and small children. In older children, we use a Veress needle.

The carbopneumoperitoneum is established to a pressure as low as necessary to provide adequate visualization: 4–6 mmHg is often sufficient in infants, but a pressure of 12–14 can be necessary in the occasional teenager.

The main target organ will be the duodenum and the base of the mesentery, located in the medial right upper quadrant. Accordingly, two instrumentation ports are positioned, one at the lateral border of the right rectus muscle, below the umbilical line. In infants, we use 3.5 mm ports. These ports are sufficient for most older patients too but can be switched to 5 mm if necessary. Fixation of the trocars to the abdominal wall is very useful.

To retract the liver upward and provide easier access and better illumination, a third port for a retractor can be placed laterally in the right flank. Alternatively, we are currently using suspension sutures to fix the hepatic falciform ligament through or to the abdominal wall in the epigastrium, using either transparietal sutures or suturing it using self-locking sutures such as V-Lock® (Fig. 29.2).

An additional port can also be necessary, should an extra instrument become necessary to assist in bowel mobilization or exposure.

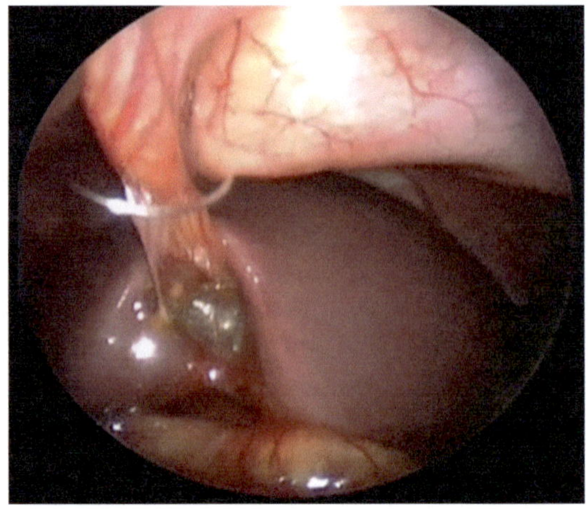

Fig. 29.2 Transparietal liver suspension is achieved with a 0 or 2.0 suture

No specific instruments are required. We usually use one or two fenestrated grasping forceps or Maryland dissectors, a hook with low-energy monopolar current, and curved scissors. Alternatively, one can use bipolar rotating instruments, such as RoBi® (Storz™), available in 3.5 mm.

29.5.1 Strategy

The operative steps vary according to the indication for surgery.

In suspected or uncomplicated malrotation, the first step is diagnostic.

It is important to remember that there is a spectrum of anatomy between the textbook anatomy and the non-rotated state. It is thus essential to recognize an anomaly and its pathological significance (Figs. 29.3 and 29.4).

In the unexpected presence of a volvulus, only small bowel will be visible at first, as the colon is twisted under the root of the mesentery and thus behind the ileum. In this circumstance, it is not always easy to identify the twist by following the anterior aspect of the pylorus and duodenum and gently retracting downward the whole bowel "en masse."

We start by identifying the location of the cecum and the ileocecal junction, as well as its mobility. We then control the attachments of

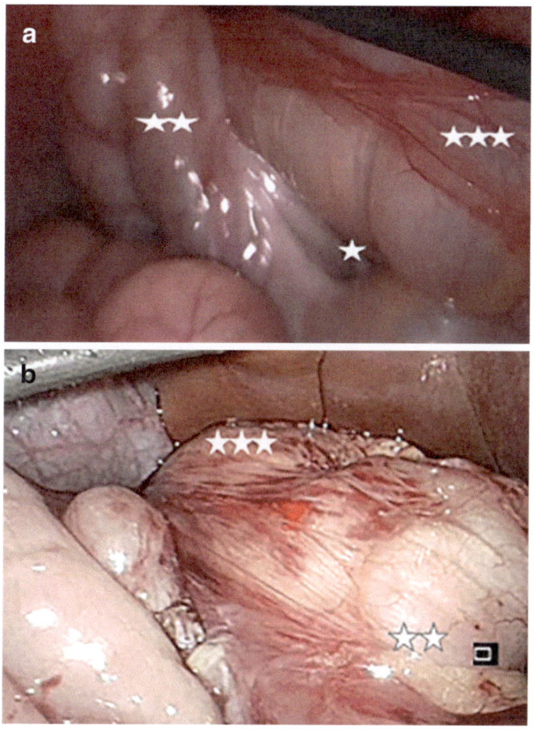

Fig. 29.3 Malrotation. (**a**) *Appendix and **Caecum below *Transverse colon. (**b**) *Ladd's bands from the **Ascending colon to the right, in front of ***Duodenum

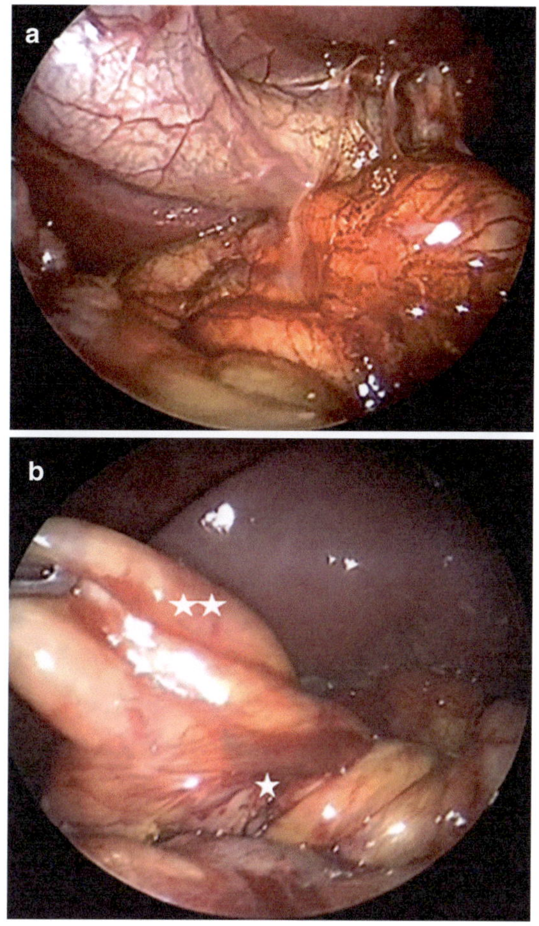

Fig. 29.4 Volvulus. (**a**) View of a Volvulus by pushing the small bowel mass downward. (**b**) *Ladd's bands, exposed before any attempt at undoing the Volvulus, by pulling the **Duodenum to the right

the ascending colon to the lateral abdominal wall (Toldt's fascia) and their relation to the duodenum.

We identify the Treitz ligament, by pulling up the transverse colon and inspecting its base: the duodenojejunal junction should be coming from under the mesocolon, to the left of the vertebral colon and to the left of the middle colic artery, confirming that the third duodenum does cross under the superior mesenteric artery.

When the diagnosis of malrotation is made, we proceed respecting the principles described by Ladd.

When a midgut volvulus has been confirmed preoperatively by sonography or radiologic studies, in a stable infant or child, the first step is to check for obvious necrosis, which we consider an indication for conversion to laparotomy. If the bowel is ischemic but not necrotic, and expertise with this approach is sufficient, an attempt at laparoscopic correction is safe but should be abandoned if no progresses are made in a reasonable time.

Undoing the volvulus in open surgery is straightforward, with two hands grasping the entire bowel mass and turning counterclockwise.

This is difficult if not impossible in laparoscopy.

As described by Bax and van der Zee [2], we have adopted a strategy that calls for the division of all Ladd's band first, followed by progressive detorsion of the bowel by simply pulling the jejunum to the right upper quadrant and progressively running it until the cecum is reached, which signs the completeness of the reduction of the volvulus (Fig. 29.5).

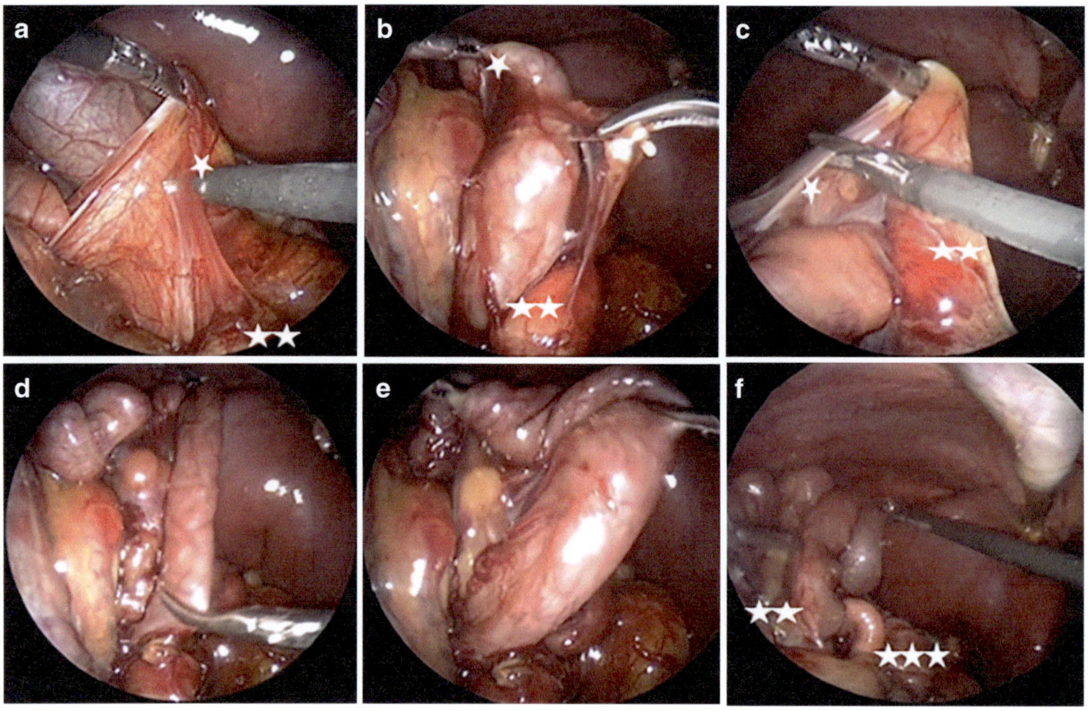

Fig. 29.5 Division of Ladd's bands and undoing of the Volvulus. (**a**, **b** and **c**) Division of Ladd's bands: * Duodenum; ** Colon. (**d**, **e** and **f**) Different stages of devolvulus; **Caecum and *** Terminal ileum freed

Thus, we start by identifying the pylorus under the liver. With tension on the duodenum or "hepatic flexure" of the colon, every peritoneal band in front of the anterior wall of the duodenum is divided using the hook as a dissector or curved scissors and only minimal amounts of monopolar energy always keeping the whole length of the metallic part of the instrument in view. Often, to achieve a complete dissection, tension will be placed alternatively to the left by pulling on the colon and to the right on the duodenum. The distal part of the duodenum has to be free in order for the jejunum to become loose and to be pulled up from left to right, undoing the volvulus in an anticlockwise fashion.

We recommend to slowly run the bowel with two graspers or gently handled forceps, paying attention that the instruments remain in the field of view and do not drop the bowel. If this happens, it is usually easier and safer to start all over again from the duodenum or the cecum, identifiable anatomical landmarks.

If this maneuver does not begin quite easily, residual bands are often found and have to be divided.

We usually run the bowel at least twice to confirm that no residual volvulus is present.

We then proceed with the widening of the base of the mesentery, freeing all the attachment between the mesentery (vascular plane) of the duodenum and the mesentery of the colon. Often, the superior mesenteric vein will be the posterior structure in this separation and should not be injured. At the end of this maneuver, the duodenum should run straight to the right subhepatic region with the jejunum, and the ascending colon should be placed on the left side, with the cecum in the left lower quadrant (Fig. 29.6).

An appendectomy is optional. We usually do it by dividing the mesoappendix with the hook and ligating the base of the appendix intracorporeally.

The pneumoperitoneum is carefully evacuated. The umbilical fascia is closed if a 5 mm or greater

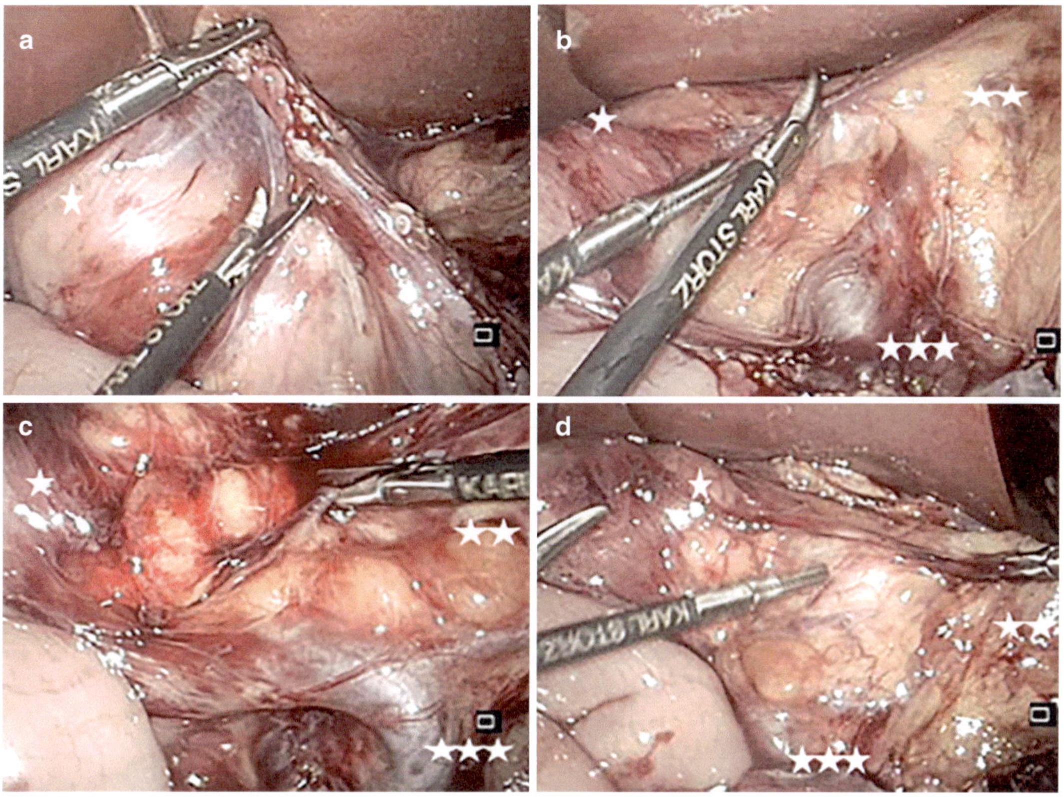

Fig. 29.6 (**a**, **b**, **c**) Steps of broadening of mesentery. ** Duodenum; ** Mesocolon;*** Superior mesenteric vein; (**d**) Final aspect; colon in the left flank

port has been used. On 3.5 mm trocar sites, we approximate the skin only with Steri-Strips.

The patient is discharged when tolerating full feeds.

29.6 Postoperative Care

Standard post-abdominal surgery care is initiated. When the procedure has been completed laparoscopically, we start enteral feedings as soon as the child asks for it. In newborns, trophic feeds are initiated on post-op day 1 and advanced as tolerated.

Pain control is obtained with a perioperative performed ultrasound-guided periumbilical or TAP block. WHO step 1 analgesics (paracetamol, non-steroidal anti-inflammatory drugs) are most often sufficient and can be discontinued after 1–3 days.

If no bowel injuries or compromise has been noticed, the antibiotics are discontinued at the end of surgery.

29.7 Results

Together with the groups of Strasbourg, Lausanne, and Montpellier, we published our results in neonates with acute midgut volvulus [3]. We compared 20 neonates (2–36 days) operated by laparoscopy to 20 matched historical controls. The average operative time was longer in the laparoscopy group (80 vs. 61 min.). Time to full-feed was shorter in the laparoscopy group: 4.7–6.7 days. Six (30%) laparoscopy patients vs. four (20%) needed reoperation for obstructive symptoms. In the laparoscopy group, it was always redone by the same technique. No case of recurrent volvulus was identified though two underwent further divisions of Ladd's band, and in at least two cases, the reoperation could have been avoided.

In addition to the cases included in this series, we have treated five further cases of infantile midgut volvulus, three late-presenting volvulus (6, 11, and 14 years old), among which the two older children had been under psychiatric care for 7 and 4 years, and nine radiologically suspected or incidentally discovered malrotation.

In our own case series in neonates, only the very first attempt at derotation of a volvulus needed conversion, before we adopted the described technique of "bands first." With this technique, nine consecutive infants with infantile volvulus have been successfully corrected. One (1/10) of them required redo laparoscopy for a suspected recurrence: we discovered an adhesive obstruction (entrapment of a loop under a band). One had been operated elsewhere by midline laparotomy at day of life 2 and found to have "segmental jejunal volvulus." At age 4 months, we confirmed a recurrent volvulus, and laparoscopy found a typical malrotation that was corrected as described.

We had no complications in older patients and elective cases. The two children under psychiatric care could discontinue this therapy after several months, to what could amount to a post-traumatic stress disorder caused by chronic and recurrent volvulus and chronic pain.

We have seen no recurrent symptoms in those children.

29.8 Discussion

The first attempt at laparoscopic correction of malrotation with volvulus was described in 1995 by Bax and van der Zee [4]. Thereafter, the diagnostic capability of laparoscopy was suggested by Gross et al. [5]. Since then, many case reports, series, and meta-analysis have been published.

The role of laparoscopy in the diagnosis and treatment of asymptomatic malrotation was assessed by the American Pediatric Surgical Association Outcomes and Evidence-Based Practice Committee [6]. It was found to be safe and accurate to determine if the patient has a high risk narrow mesenteric stalk, a non-rotation with a broad base at minimal risk for volvulus or an atypical anatomy with malposition of the duodenum. The Commitee found minimal evidence to support the use of laparoscopy in cases of midgut volvulus.

From a national database, Huntington et al. [7] identified 311 patients undergoing elective Ladd's operation. Fifty-eight had a laparoscopic procedure and 253 a laparotomy, including 22 converted from laparoscopy (27.5%). Urgent cases were excluded, as many surgeons would not consider laparoscopy in those circumstances. Though patient selection was probably biased, the more severely ill patients having more often open surgery, operative times were similar, and length of stay was shorter in the laparoscopy group. Nonsignificant advantages for laparoscopy were postoperative complications ($p = 0.08$) and blood transfusion ($p = 0.11$). The authors conclude that their study demonstrate the short-term safety and potential benefits of laparoscopy.

Though this study did not analyze the causes for conversions or recurrence after laparoscopic treatment, several others have.

Kinlin et al. [8] surveyed the attendees to the Canadian Association of Pediatric Surgeons. In the mind of the participants, incomplete procedure and lack of adhesions were the most likely causes of recurrences.

In 2010, Hagendoorn et al. [9] reported on 45 laparoscopy for suspected malrotation, in which the diagnosis was confirmed in 37. Only five presented with volvulus and four were corrected. Of the 37 malrotation cases, 9 required conversion, and 7 had to be operated for recurrent volvulus or malrotation. Most commonly, further Ladd's band had to be divided.

We found loss of orientation, mostly when trying to undo the volvulus by "en masse" mobilization of the bowel, to be the most common cause for conversion [3].

More recently, Reddy et al. [10] reviewed 41 cases: 6 were converted for loss of orientation or failure to progress. Nine required open reoperation, including five for incomplete correction, three for kinking of the duodenojejunal junction, and one for an unrecognized intrinsic duodenal stenosis.

Ooms et al. [11] reviewed all malrotations operated at their institution in a 7-year period and identified 50 laparotomy and 33 laparoscopy cases. Though one laparoscopy child was reoperated at 24 h for recurrent volvulus, nine laparotomy patients were reoperated for delayed adhesive bowel obstruction. In their hand, operative time was shorter in the laparoscopy group.

Thus, incomplete correction seems to be the leading cause for reoperation.

Reduction of the volvulus remains a technical challenge and the most common cause for conversion. Moving the entire mass of the bowel with two chopsticks is very difficult: orientation is lost; all the loops of bowel moving in front of the camera prevent correct viewing and orientation.

In 2017, Kisku [12] suggested an "orbit technique" in which he places a forceps on top of the bowel, introduced in the right lower quadrant and directed to the root of the mesentery. The bowel is then flipped from left to right over the axis represented by the forceps. He was successful in three older patients.

We believe that tight Ladd's bands are preventing the running of the bowel and that once completely divided, untwisting as described in the technique section is fairly straightforward.

Catania et al. [13] conducted a meta-analysis of studies comparing open versus laparoscopic Ladd's procedure in children. They identified only 9 studies matching their criteria and compared 744 patients with open surgery to 259 with laparoscopy. They found no prospective studies. They concluded that there is a lack of evidence to support either open or laparoscopic Ladd's procedure. In this study, most series approached volvulus openly. The conversion rate ranged from 25 to 50%, with a trend to be more frequent in the early experience. Laparoscopy was indeed associated with a shorter time to full-feed and a shorter hospital stay, though a bias in the selection of patients, the sicker getting open surgery, is acknowledged. The complication rate is higher in the open surgery patients (35%) than in laparoscopy (24%). Adhesive bowel obstruction was reported in 6 studies and was 22/207 in patient operated by laparotomy and 0/96 in those operated by laparoscopy, not a significant ($p = 0.07$) finding but in line with the expected benefits of laparoscopy.

They found that the rate of postoperative volvulus was 1.4% in the open group vs. 3.5% in the laparoscopy, reaching a significance ($p = 0.04$).

Thus the hypothesis to explain this risk is multiple: incomplete Ladd's band division or widening of the mesentery could be related to the difficult exposure, the limited experience of the surgeons at this stage (learning curve) and the development of less intraabdominal scaring and adhesions, beneficial in regard of adhesive obstruction, could here be detrimental.

Malrotation can be discovered in adults [14] incidentally or by its symptoms. A single-incision laparoscopy has been reported in an adult patient [15] but not yet in children.

29.9 Conclusion

A minimally invasive approach to the diagnosis of malrotation has become an accepted surgical strategy. Its exact role or limitations in the presence of established midgut volvulus remain to be established. Identifying the best way to reduce the volvulus and criteria to define the completeness of the release of Ladd's band and broadening of the mesentery is the next challenge. It is our belief that the surgical steps described in the chapter will help decrease the number of conversion and recurrences. Advanced skills in laparoscopy in infants and the ability to work in confined and limited space and to keep one's spatial orientation are mandatory to achieve success.

References

1. Dassinger M, Smith D. Disorders of intestinal rotation and fixation. In: Coran AJ, Adzick S, Krummel T, editors. Pediatric surgery. 7th ed: Mosby; 2012. p. 1111–25.
2. Bax KMA, van der Zee DC. Intestinal Malrotation. In: Bax KMA, Georgeson KE, Rothenberg SS, Valla JS, Yeung CK, editors. Endoscopic surgery in infants and children. Berlin: Springer; 2008.

3. Ferrero L, Ahmed YB, Philippe P, et al. Intestinal Malrotation and volvulus in neonates: laparoscopy versus open laparotomy. J Laparoendosc Adv Surg Tech A. 2017;27(3):318–21.
4. van der Zee DC, Bax NM. Laparoscopic repair of acute volvulus in a neonate with malrotation. Surg Endosc. 1995;9:1123–4.
5. Gross E, Chen MK, Lobe TE. Laparoscopic evaluation and treatment of intestinal malrotation in infants. Surg Endosc. 1996;10(9):936–7.
6. Graziano K, Islam S, Dasgupta R, et al. Asymptomatic malrotation: diagnosis and surgical management an American Pediatric Surgical Association outcomes and evidence based practice committee systematic review. J Pediatr Surg. 2015;50:1783–90.
7. Huntington JT, Lopez JJ, Mahida JB, et al. Comparing laparoscopic versus open Ladd's procedure in pediatric patients. J Pediatr Surg. 2017;52(7):1128–31. Epub 2016 Oct 30.
8. Kinlin C, Shawyer AC. The surgical management of malrotation: a Canadian Association of Pediatric Surgeons survey. J Pediatr Surg. 2017;52(5):853–8. Epub 2017 Jan 28.
9. Hagendoorn J, Vieira-Travasos D, van der Zee D. Laparoscopic treatment of intestinal malrotation in neonates and infants: a retrospective study. Surg Endosc. 2011;25:217–20.
10. Reddy AS, Shah RS, Kulkarni DR. Laparoscopic Ladd'S procedure in children: challenges, results, and problems. J Indian Assoc Pediatr Surg. 2018;23(2):61–5.
11. Ooms N, Matthyssens LE, Draaisma JM, et al. Laparoscopic treatment of intestinal malrotation in children. Eur J Pediatr Surg. 2016;26(4):376–81. Epub 2015 Jun18.
12. Kisku S. Orbit technique in malrotation with non-obstructive volvulus: a novel technique of devolvulation. Asian J Endosc Surg. 2017;10:213–5.
13. Catania VD, Lauriti G, Pierro A, et al. Open versus laparoscopic approach for intestinal malrotation in infants and children: a systematic review and meta-analysis. Pediatr Surg Int. 2016;32(12):1157–64. Epub 2016 Oct 5.
14. Frasier LL, Leverson G, Gosain A, et al. Laparoscopic versus open Ladd's procedure for intestinal malrotation in adults. Surg Endosc. 2015;29(6):1598–604.
15. Vassaur J, Vassaur H, Buckley P III. Single-incision laparoscopic Ladd's procedure for intestinal Malrotation. JSLS. 2014;18:132–5.

30 Laparoscopic Approach to Intestinal Duplication

Miguel Guelfand

30.1 Introduction

Congenital intestinal duplications (ID) are rare, having an incidence of 2/10,000 live newborns. It can occur from the base of the tongue to the rectum, but more than 50% of them are localized in the small bowel.

These malformations can be asymptomatic or present as non-specific symptoms such as recurrent abdominal pain, abdominal mass, vomiting, or sometimes as a life-threatening complication: intestinal hemorrhage, perforation, obstruction, and even malignant changes [1–9].

If not diagnosed antenatally, the majority present in the first 2 years of life. Up to one third of the patients with IDs can have associated anomalies such as spinal defects and lung and cardiac malformations [5–8].

The diagnosis can be made by antenatal or postnatal ultrasound, magnetic resonance imaging (MRI), computed tomography (CT), or technetium 99m pertechnetate scintigraphy (Tc99m scan). Occasionally it is made as an intraoperatively finding. In some cases, upper gastrointestinal contrast studies or endoscopy may be needed, mainly for gastric and duodenal duplications.

Any intestinal duplication should be resected after being diagnosed due to their potential for complications.

The laparoscopic approach to ID can be considered as the gold standard. Although there are no large series published, minimally invasive surgery provides the exact localization of the ID, which usually achieves complete resection, and provides a smaller incision than if a laparotomy was needed [5, 10].

30.2 Preoperative

Intestinal preparation is not needed. We suggest a clear liquid diet 24 h with 6 h of fasting prior to surgery. Patients receive preoperative intravenous antibiotic prophylaxis with metronidazole and amikacin.

30.3 Positioning

The patient is placed in the supine position near the bottom of the operating table. Proper fixation of the patient is recommended to allow mobilization of the operating table with no risk for the patient to slide. Ideally, two monitors will be needed for this operation, one on each side of the patient. This will allow a more ergonomic procedure, especially if the surgeon needs to run the intestine to localize the

M. Guelfand (✉)
Exequiel Gonzalez Cortes Childrens Hospital, Santiago, Chile

Las Condes Hospital, Santiago, Chile

University of Chile, Santiago, Chile
e-mail: mguelfand@clc.cl

C. Esposito et al. (eds.), *ESPES Manual of Pediatric Minimally Invasive Surgery*,
https://doi.org/10.1007/978-3-030-00964-9_30

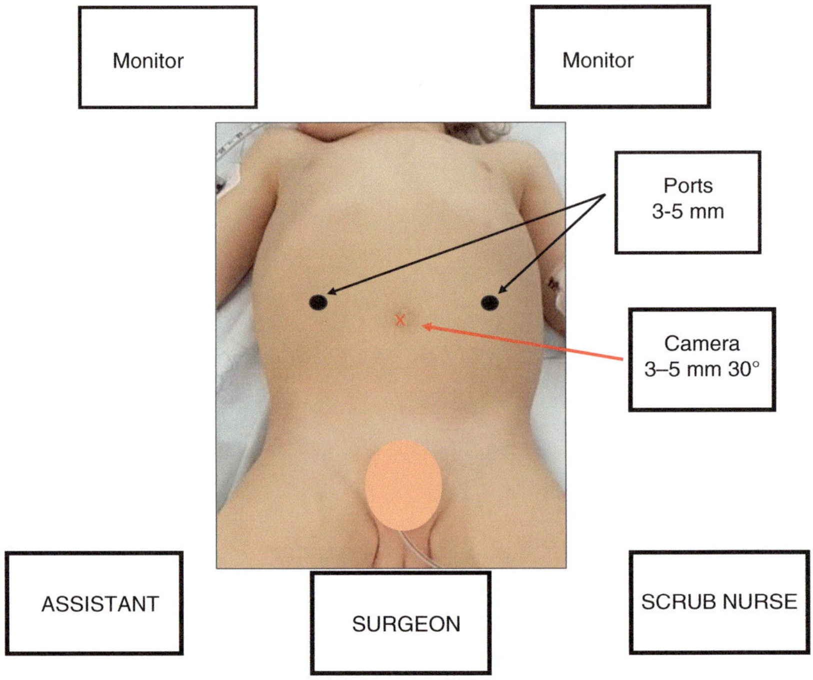

Fig. 30.1 Team position

duplication. The surgeon's position is at the foot of the patient, with the assistant to the left of the patient and the scrub nurse on its right (Fig. 30.1). This positioning and the two monitors will facilitate running the bowel if needed. The camera is placed through the umbilical cannula. Depending on the type of duplication and operation, the umbilicus could be the only trocar site (single incision laparoscopic surgery or trans-umbilical assisted resection) or one or two additional working ports can be placed on either or both sides of the umbilicus in the median axillary line, slightly cephalad to the umbilicus if needed.

30.4 Instrumentation

For the laparoscopic approach to an ID, including anything from a gastric duplication to a large bowel duplication, 3 millimeters(mm)–20 centimeters(cm) or 5 mm–30 cm (or similar) instruments will be needed depending on the size and weight of the patient. A curved and straight grasping forceps, bowel grasper, hook cautery, and curved scissors will be needed.

Also a 3–4 mm short or a 5 mm camera with a minimum of 30° will be necessary, again depending on the size of the patient.

It is important to have a CO_2 insufflator adjustable for neonates and small children as well.

The laparoscopic approach to IDs includes complete or partial resection of the duplication with or without intestinal resection and anastomosis. This will depend on the type, localization, and size. To accomplish this, the use of laparoscopic sealers or bipolar (3 or 5 mm), 5–12 mm staplers, and 5–10 mm clip appliers may be necessary at some point in the operation in some cases.

30.5 Technique

The technique used will depend on the position, size, and characteristics of the duplication. Most of the IDs are single, cystic, and with a widespread of sizes, although they can present as a tubular duplication, with or without communication with the adjacent bowel. They are typically located on the mesenteric side of the bowel, but not always.

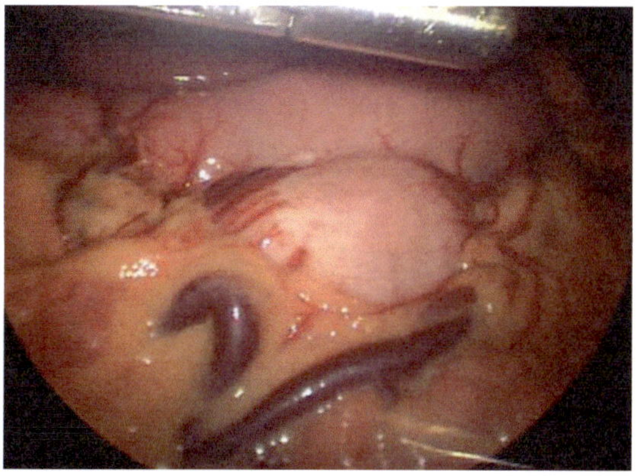

Fig. 30.2 Laparoscopic vision of a gastric duplication

Usually the gastric and duodenal duplications have a precise pre-surgical diagnosis (Fig. 30.2). The exact location of small and large bowel duplications can be difficult to pinpoint exactly prior to surgery.

First the umbilical port is introduced (Veress or Hasson technique). A laparoscopic evaluation is done to confirm the diagnosis or to assess the bowel to localize the duplication. Depending on the findings, the next steps are performed.

If a gastric or duodenal duplication is confirmed, usually two working ports will be necessary to complete the resection of the duplication. After that, it will be necessary to evaluate the anatomy of the duplication and its relation with the blood supply and the adjacent bowel. If no major vascular supply is involved (major mesenteric feeding vessel), a safe and complete resection/enucleation can usually be performed.

A complete resection is performed by first opening the serosa over the duplication to find the dissection plane. This is usually done with a hook cautery or monopolar scissors. Then the duplication is dissected within this plane from the adjacent bowel and mesentery with monopolar, bipolar, or sealing instruments. Major care has to be taken when the dissection takes place where a common wall may be identified. In these cases it is preferred to sacrifice part of the duplication wall, but not open the adjacent bowel.

In some cases, after the resection of the duplication, a seromuscular defect can be left, where the duplication shares a common wall with the native bowel. It will need to be repaired if possible with intra-corporeal suturing using an absorbable suture. If not possible, and the native mucosa is not harmed, the seromuscular defect can be left open. Cautery can be used for any bleeding.

If the duplication involves a large segment of bowel or is in a dangerous anatomic position such that its resection could compromise the adjacent bowel or blood supply, a partial resection should be considered, leaving part of the duplication attached to the segment with the common wall but with complete resection (if possible) or coagulation of the mucosa.

For resection of the gastric and duodenal duplications, usually two working ports are sufficient. Through one working port, a grasper will provide sufficient exposure, and, through the other port, a hook monopolar cautery, bipolar, or sealer will be helpful in the dissection of the duplication. In some cases, if better exposure is necessary, a percutaneous instrument or an extra port can be inserted.

During the resection, if possible, the duplication should not be opened. This will allow a better dissecting plane for a safer dissection and minimize the chance of entering the adjacent bowel.

For small and large bowel duplications, there are different approaches. These will depend on their location and size. After the umbilical laparoscope is introduced, and if the duplication is located in a mobile segment of the bowel, a complete laparoscopic or video-assisted resection can be performed (Figs. 30.3 and 30.4). If possible,

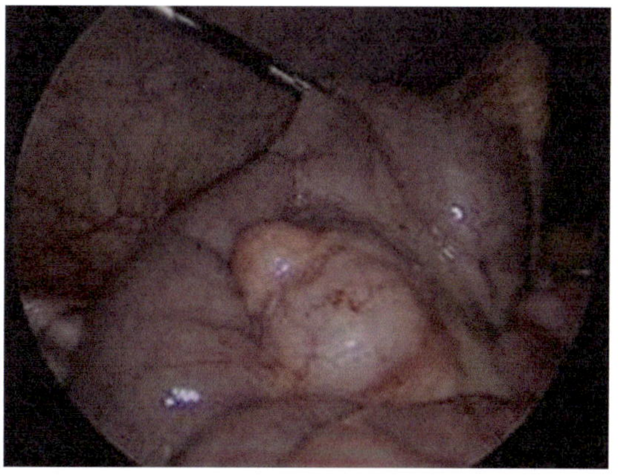

Fig. 30.3 Laparoscopic aspect of intestinal duplication

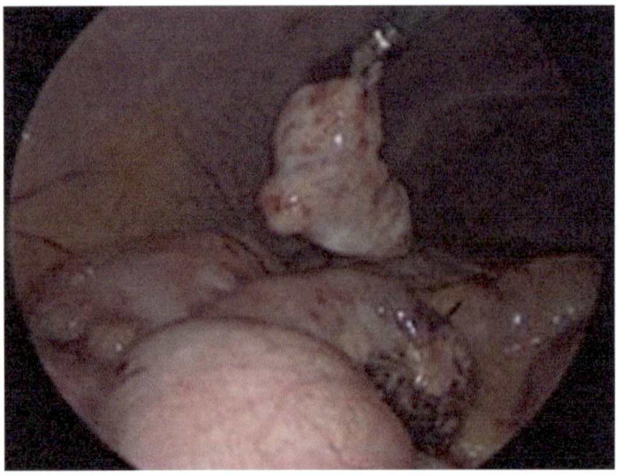

Fig. 30.4 Intestinal duplication specimen resected in laparoscopy

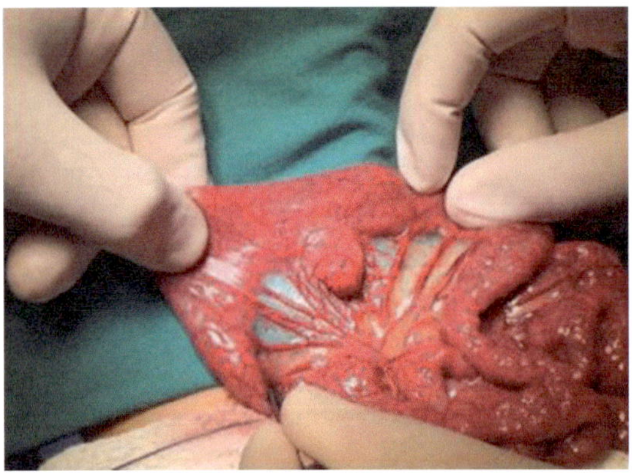

Fig. 30.5 Trans-umbilical extraction of the intestinal duplication

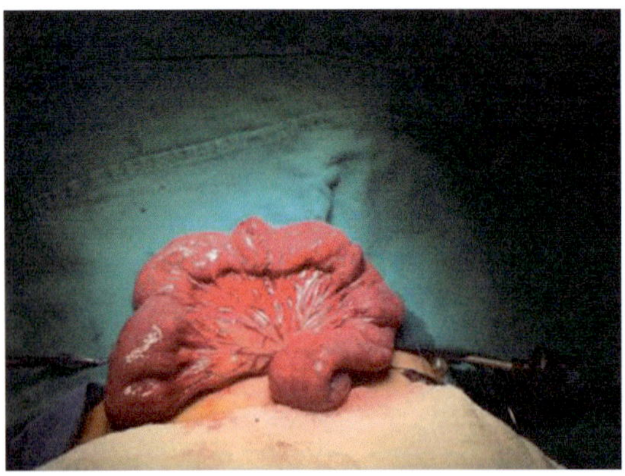

Fig. 30.6 Intestinal resection and end-to-end intestinal anastomosis outside the abdominal cavity

the duplication can be exteriorized by enlarging the umbilical incision (omega shape enlargement), and a complete resection, with or without bowel resection, can be performed (Figs. 30.5 and 30.6).

The large bowel duplications, depending on their location, can be resected with exteriorization or laparoscopically, depending on the size and mobility of the bowel segment.

If a bowel resection is needed in order to resect the duplication, a single-layer anastomosis is carried out or linear stapler can be used. Closing the mesenteric defect should be performed, too.

30.6 Postoperative Care

Patients without involvement of adjacent bowel can start feeding 4–6 h after the surgery and are discharged the next day.

Usually nonsteroidal analgesia is sufficient and is provided for the subsequent 24 h.

Those patients who had seromuscular compromise can be kept NPO (nothing by mouth) for 12–24 h depending on the extent of the resection. Patients with bowel resections will need to remain NPO for 1–3 days, depending on the level of resection. In selective cases, a nasogastric tube is indicated to avoid intestinal or gastric distension. Also they will require intra- and postoperative antibiotics.

30.7 Results

Patients with a duplication in a mobile segment of the bowel (jejunum, ileum, or ileocecal region) usually had a laparoscopic-assisted trans-umbilical resection. This operative approach usually takes between 45 and 90 min, including the time to identify the duplication laparoscopically, exteriorize the involved bowel, and perform the resection [11–13].

Depending on the nature of the duplication, and whether or not there is seromuscular involvement, and/or blood supply compromise, these lesions can often be resected completely with none or minimal seromuscular injury of the adjacent bowel. If a bowel resection is required, the anastomosis is usually performed hand sewn in a single layer with continuous or interrupted suture or with a bowel stapler.

Patients that had a complete resection of the intestinal duplication with no bowel compromise and/or minimum seromuscular involvement usually stay 1–3 days after the operation and start feeding 6–12 h postoperatively [12, 13].

After discharge they are followed up at week 1 and 4 weeks after surgery and then 2 and 4 months later. A follow-up ultrasound is performed only if symptoms develop.

30.8 Tips and Tricks

The first step in all cases should be the visualization of the abdominal cavity through the camera in the umbilical port. Once the duplication is seen, then it can be decided to carry out the operation only with the umbilical port or with one or more working ports. In all of our cases of gastric and duodenal duplications, we have used at least two working ports. Some of the duodenal cases have required an extra port or percutaneous instrument to have a better visualization of the dissection of the duplication.

Also, positioning of the table (Trendelenburg, Fowler, side inclination) can help to mobilize the bowel and assist in exposing the duplication. For some small bowel duplications, the localization can be sometimes difficult – requiring running the bowel from the ligament of Treitz to the cecum. This is done more ergonomically by using two working ports and two monitors as shown in Fig. 30.1. The first half of the running should be done looking to the monitor on the left at the top of the patient, and the second half the surgeon has to switch places to the left of the patient and look to the other monitor usually moving to the patient's lower body. It is important when running the bowel to visualize both sides of the bowel and the mesentery.

When an open resection through an enlarged umbilical incision is possible, it is important to allow enough space to return of the bowel after the resection without problems. This is more critical when the resection takes a longer time due to the natural edema of the bowel outside the peritoneal cavity.

Most of the cystic duplications are better resected using the tension of the duplication to allow a better plane of dissection. When the cyst is too big, interferes with a safe visualization of the dissection or difficult a trans-umbilical surgery, partial or complete aspiration of the cyst contents will be necessary. This is performed under laparoscopic view with a percutaneous needle or through the umbilical incision prior to externalizing the duplication.

30.9 Discussion

Intestinal duplications are a rare congenital anomaly that can be present at any level of the alimentary tract. In 1953, Ladd and Gross classified intestinal duplications requiring three essential characteristics that had to be present: (a) well-developed smooth muscle coat, (b) mucosal lining found within some portion of the alimentary tract, and (c) contiguity to any segment of the alimentary tract, although duplications can be located in the pancreas or biliary tract as well [11]. IDs usually have intestinal lining mucosa, but sometimes gastric or pancreatic mucosa can be present. Uncommonly, IDs communicate with the native intestinal lumen.

The main goal of the treatment is the resection of the duplication with as much conservation of the adjacent bowel as possible. Laparoscopy in intestinal duplications confirms the diagnosis in the cases in which imaging is unclear and also gives information as to the exact location of the malformation. With this information, different surgical approaches can be decided.

Although the complete removal of the duplication is the main objective, depending on the size, localization, and relation to the adjacent structures, this may not always be possible without compromising the adjacent bowel or surrounding structures.

There are different surgical strategies to deal with the widespread possibilities of intestinal duplications.

The standard approach is with a three-port technique: one 5 mm umbilical port for a 30-degree camera and two 3–5 mm working ports. If liver retraction is necessary, percutaneous liver retraction stiches can be placed or an extra port or a percutaneous laparoscopic instrument can be used. This approach is the most used in the non-mobile alimentary tract (esophagus, stomach, duodenum, colon, and rectum). In the mobile portions (jejunum, ileum, and ileocecal region), an assisted laparoscopic approach can be used – after identifying the duplication, it can be mobilized through an enlarged umbilical incision or a planned mini-laparotomy just over the duplication. A complete minimally invasive surgery (MIS) resection or MIS-assisted resection results in less pain, less bowel obstruction incidence, and better cosmetic results [11–13].

If it's not possible to do a complete and safe removal of the duplication, a partial resection can be performed – although this should be done with special consideration for the blood supply of the adjacent bowel. Minimal invasive surgery magnification helps in the identification of the blood supply during this approach with the advantage of less blood loss and reducing the chance of compromising the blood supply of the adjacent structures [4].

In a minority of cases, safe complete resection or enucleation is not possible. In these cases, the option is a partial resection or marsupialization, removing safely as much possible of the duplication, leaving the common wall with the adjacent bowel and main surrounding structures, and a complete stripping and/or coagulation of the mucosal layer. This approach is often used for duodenal duplications due to their relation with the pancreas and biliary tract [12, 13].

When a bowel resection is necessary for removal of the duplication, a complete resection and anastomosis can be performed laparoscopically. This can be performed with a hand-sewn or stapled (5–12 mm) anastomosis. However, if the duplication is in a mobile segment, a trans-umbilical MIS-assisted resection and anastomosis through the umbilicus is preferred.

30.10 Conclusion

IDs are uncommon. Nowadays, pre- and postnatal ultrasonographic investigation contributes to an earlier diagnosis of such pathology before the onset of the symptoms.

The laparoscopic approach to IDs allows confirmation of the diagnosis and defining precisely the anatomy, the nature, and the exact site and anatomical considerations of the duplication.

Laparoscopic surgery in ID can achieve the complete resection with the preservation of the adjacent bowel or allows a trans-umbilical video-assisted resection. If a laparotomy is needed, the MIS approach helps in achieving a smaller incision.

The laparoscopic approach has a diagnostic and therapeutic role in the management of IDs as well as effective and safe treatment.

References

1. Pintér AB, Schubert W, Szemlédy F, Göbel P, Schäfer J, Kustos G. Alimentary tract duplications in infants and children. Eur J Pediatr Surg. 1992;2(1):8–12.
2. Iyer CP, Mahour GH. Duplications of the alimentary tract in infants and children. J Pediatr Surg. 1995;30(9):1267–70.
3. Stern LE, Warner BW. Gastrointestinal duplications. Semin Pediatr Surg. 2000;9(3):135–40.
4. Royle SG, Doig CM. Perforation of the jejunum secondary to a duplication cyst lined with ectopic gastric mucosa. J Pediatr Surg. 1988;23:1025–6.
5. Lima M, Molinaro F, Ruggeri G, Gargano T, Randi B. Role of mini-invasive surgery in the treatment of enteric duplications in paediatric age: a survey of 15 years. Pediatr Med Chir. 2012;34:217–22.

6. Lister J. Lister J, Irwing M, editors. Duplications of the alimentary tract. Neonatal surgery, England, Butterworths. 1990; p. 474–84.
7. Catalano P, Di Pace MR, Caruso AM, De Grazia E, Cimador M. Ileal duplication cysts: is the loss of the valve always necessary? J Pediatr Surg. 2014;49:1049–51.
8. Laje P, Flake AW, Adzick NS. Prenatal diagnosis and postnatal resection of intraabdominal enteric duplications. J Pediatr Surg. 2010;45:1554–8.
9. Iyer CP, Mahour GH. Duplications of the alimentary tract in infants and children. J Pediatr Surg. 1995;30:1267–70.
10. Górecki W, Bogusz B, Zając A, Sołtysiak P. Laparoscopic and laparoscopy-assisted resection of enteric duplication cysts in children. J Laparoendosc Adv Surg Tech A. 2015;25(10):838–40.
11. Ladd WE, Gross RE. Surgical treatment of duplications of the alimentary tract: Enterogenous cyst, enteric cyst, or ileum duplex. Surg Gynaecol Obstet. 1940;70:295–307.
12. Guérin F, Podevin G, Petit T, Lopez M, de Lagausie P, Lardy H, Bonnard A, Becmeur F, Philippe P, Larroquet M, Sapin E, Kurzenne JY, le Mandat A, Francois-Fiquet C, Gaudin J, Valioulis I, Morisson-Lacombe G, Montupet P, Demarche M. Outcome of alimentary tract duplications operated on by minimally invasive surgery: a retrospective multicenter study by the GECI (Groupe d'Etude en Coeliochirurgie infantile). Surg Endosc. 2012;26:2848–55.
13. Ballehaninna UK, Nguyen T, Burjonrappa SC. Laparoscopic resection of Antenataly identified duodenal duplication cyst. JSLS. 2013;17:454–8.

31 Laparoscopy and Laparoscopic-Assisted Approach for Adhesive Small Bowel Obstruction

Illya Martynov and Martin Lacher

31.1 Introduction

The development of intestinal adhesions as result of transperitoneal surgery in neonates and children is common and may lead to adhesive small bowel obstruction (ASBO). In the first year after surgery, the incidence is estimated to be 2–5% with a lifetime risk of up to 30% [1–3]. Less commonly, ASBO is caused by congenital bands [4]. The clinical manifestation can vary depending on the type and extent of surgery. It ranges from mild symptoms including crampy abdominal pain, anorexia, emesis, and obstipation to lethargy and peritonitis [5]. The diagnosis of ASBO is usually based on physical examination combined with use of ultrasonography, plain radiographs, and in some cases cross-sectional imaging. The optimal management in children depends upon the extent of obstruction. Non-operative management is indicated in patients without signs of bowel ischemia and includes enteral decompression with a nasogastric tube, fluid resuscitation, and correction of electrolyte abnormalities [6]. However, patients who do not respond to conservative therapy require surgical intervention such as adhesiolysis and possible bowel resection [7, 8]. Both laparotomy and laparoscopic or laparoscopically assisted procedures can be used [9]. Laparoscopy was shown to be safe in management of acute and chronic ASOB and allows accurate diagnosis, quick recovery, and low morbidity [10]. However, due to extensive adhesions, the frequency of conversions to laparotomy ranges from 33 to 52% [9–11]. In this chapter, we aim to review the utilization of laparoscopic surgery for ASOB and to present our laparoscopic-assisted technique using single-incision laparoscopic surgery (SILS) with homemade glove port.

31.2 Preoperative Preparation

The extent of preoperative preparation depends on the presentation of the patient. The initial workup includes an ultrasound examination and plain abdominal radiographs. A nasogastric tube as well as a urinary catheter should be inserted and the output documented. Hypovolemia, electrolyte, and acid-base disturbances are to be corrected. Prophylactic antibiotics as a part of the perioperative management may be subject to local customs and personal preferences. General anesthesia with intubation and sufficient muscle relaxation for the establishment of optimal work place is essential, especially when bowel is dilated [12].

I. Martynov (✉) · M. Lacher
Department of Pediatric Surgery, University of Leipzig, Leipzig, Germany
e-mail: Illya.Martynov@medizin.uni-leipzig.de; martin.lacher@medizin.uni-leipzig.de

C. Esposito et al. (eds.), *ESPES Manual of Pediatric Minimally Invasive Surgery*,
https://doi.org/10.1007/978-3-030-00964-9_31

31.3 Positioning

In supine position the angle of the table is adjusted according to the localization of the adhesions. The surgeon stands on the left side of the patient, and an assistant on the same side to hold the camera. The monitor is placed opposite to the surgeon. The scrub nurse usually stands to the left of the surgeon.

Instrumentation

1. Wound retractor (Alexis, size XS, Applied Medical Resources Corp., Rancho Santa Margarita, CA), size 6.5 glove, 5-mm trocar (Karl Storz, Germany).
2. 5-mm 45-cm scope (Stryker Endoscopy, San Jose, CA)
3. 90° angulated light adapter (Karl Storz, Germany)
4. Straight laparoscopic instruments including atraumatic (bowel) graspers.
5. Bipolar electrocoagulation (optional).

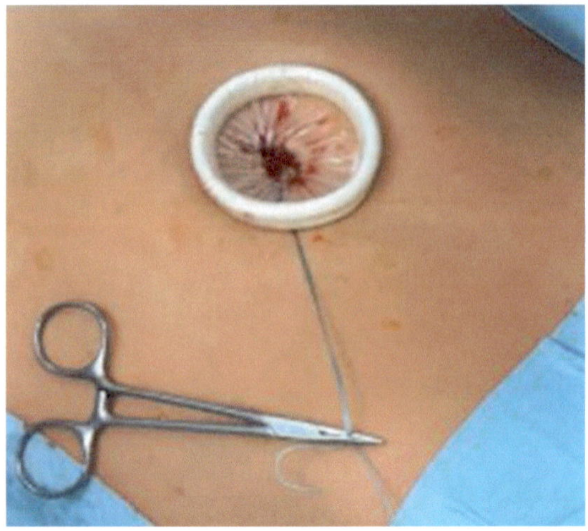

Fig. 31.1 Placement of an Alexis XS wound retractor through the umbilicus

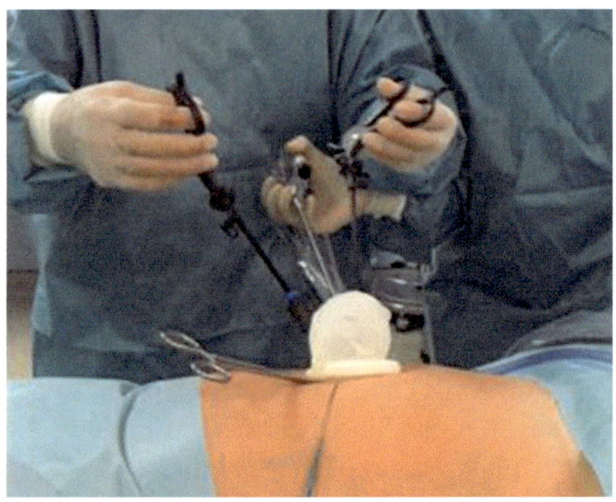

Fig. 31.2 5-mm straight laparoscopic instruments are introduced through tiny incisions in the fingertips of the glove port

31.4 Technique

Generally, the umbilicus is free of adhesions, and the wound retractor can be introduced transumbilically. A 2-cm vertical incision is made in the umbilicus, and the underlying midline fascia is opened over a variable length ranging from 1.5 to 2.5 cm to enter the peritoneal cavity. An Alexis XS wound retractor is placed directly through the fascia (Fig. 31.1), and a size 6.5 glove is connected to it. The thumb of the glove is cut off, and a 5-mm trocar is introduced and tied over this trocar enabling introduction of laparoscopic instruments (Fig. 31.2) [13, 14]. Additional ports can be placed depending on extension of adhesions under laparoscopic guidance. The laparoscopic exposition can be improved through changes in table position to allow distended bowel to fall away from the camera. First, the inspection of the abdominal cavity is performed. In early stages of ASBO, simple adhesions or isolated adhesive bands may be detected immediately making adhesiolysis a relatively straightforward procedure. However, in the case of extensive adhesions, the laparoscopic approach can be challenging due to dilated and inflamed bowel loops and therefore restricted vision. Short-term increase of CO_2 pressure and maneuvers to move bowel content from distal to proximal using atraumatic graspers may facilitate the procedure. Laparoscopic adhesiolysis can be performed using direct cutting with scissors or diathermy with bipolar forceps or sealing device. Impaired working space, multiple extensive adhesions, or iatrogenic collateral damage with traumatization of the obstructed bowel during laparoscopy may necessitate the conversion to open surgery. In our experience using a SILS technique, the initial dissection of adhesions and mobilization of bowel can be performed laparoscopically with or without the help of exteriorizing loops of bowel for dissection extracorporeally (Figs. 31.3 and 31.4).

Furthermore, bowel resection, if needed, can be performed using an open surgical approach through the Alexis port (Fig. 31.5). The fascial incision is approximated with a

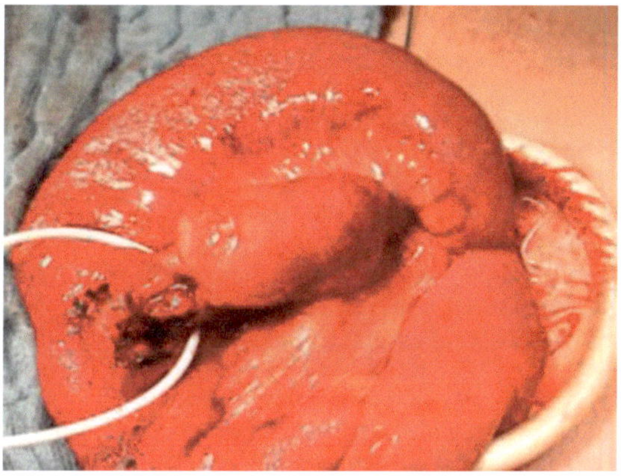

Fig. 31.3 External bowel preparation using a SILS approach in a 5-year-old boy with Meckel diverticulitis and adhesive small bowel obstruction. After laparoscopic adhesiolysis the perforated Meckel diverticulum is exteriorized through the umbilical incision

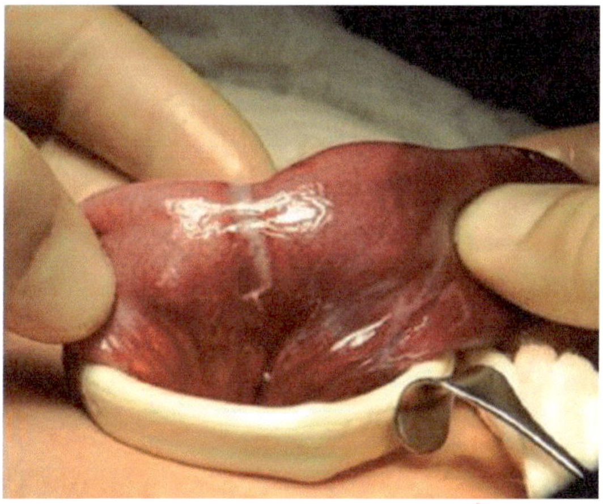

Fig. 31.4 Adhesive small bowel obstruction caused by an adhesive band leading to limited ischemia (perpendicular "whitish line" to the bowel loop). It may perforate within the following days and should therefore be resected at the time of adhesiolysis

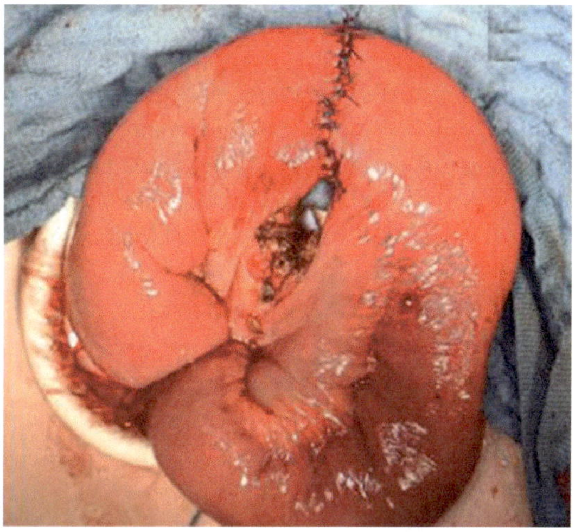

Fig. 31.5 After exteriorizing the Meckel diverticulum, a segmental small bowel resection is performed with end-to-end anastomosis

running 2-0 or 0 polyglactin suture. Finally, the skin incision is closed using interrupted subcuticular 4-0 poliglecaprone sutures.

31.5 Postoperative Care

Postoperative care varies depending on the preoperative condition of the patient and extent of the operation. In general, the nasogastric tube should stay and broad-spectrum antibiotics are administered. The Foley catheter is left in place for documentation of urinary output. A repeat abdominal examination is performed at regular intervals. Postoperative analgesia is adjusted based on clinical parameters. Oral feeding can be started after return of bowel function.

31.6 Results

Laparoscopy or laparoscopic-assisted approach to ASBO has been shown to be safe and feasible in patients with early stages of disease and low number of previous laparotomies [10]. The MIS approach allows a quick recovery with early discharge and low morbidity [9, 15]. However, the conversation rate to an open procedure remains as high as 33–52% [9, 10, 16, 17].

31.7 Tips and Tricks

1. Proper patient selection and good surgical judgment are the most important factors to successful outcome in laparoscopic treatment of ASBO [10]. Therefore surgeons starting MIS for ASBO should choose patients with an early diagnosis as laparoscopy is easier when the working space is not limited.
2. Patients with distal or complete small bowel obstruction have an exceeding bowel diameter and are therefore unlikely to be treated successfully by laparoscopy.
3. Use of ultrasonography may help to choose a safe site for the initial trocar insertion. We advocate the use of the open technique for trocar introduction.
4. Conversion to an open approach should not be considered as a surgeon's failure or complication but rather as the recognition of limitations of the technique and particular the disease process. Conversion should be done early and not late in the operative course.

31.8 Discussion

Postoperative small bowel obstruction due to development of adhesions is a frequent problem following abdominal surgery. The open surgical approach for ASBO has commonly been used during several years, whereas laparoscopy was considered contraindicated due to reduced working space and risk of bowel injury. However, the laparoscopic approach for ASBO has proven its benefits, safety, and feasibility [9]. Especially in early stages of ASBO, the laparoscopy is feasible as the working space is not limited by dilated bowel and the single band adhesions may be addressed relatively easy. Thus, initial attempt at laparoscopic approach in children is rewarding due to its association with quick postoperative recovery and early hospital discharge [9, 18, 19]. However, in cases of delayed diagnosis or extensive adhesions, the MIS approach can be challenging and require high expertise of the surgeon. At any time, the laparoscopic procedure can be augmented by a laparoscopic-assisted approach, minilaparotomy, or formal laparotomy.

References

1. Miller G, Boman J, Shrier I, Gordon PH. Natural history of patients with adhesive small bowel obstruction. Br J Surg. 2000;87(9):1240–7.
2. Ahlberg G, Bergdahl S, Rutqvist J, Soderquist C, Frenckner B. Mechanical small-bowel obstruction after conventional appendectomy in children. Eur J Pediatr Surg. 1997;7(1):13–5.
3. Dijkstra FR, Nieuwenhuijzen M, Reijnen MM, van Goor H. Recent clinical developments in pathophysiology, epidemiology, diagnosis and treatment of intra-abdominal adhesions. Scand J Gastroenterol Suppl. 2000;232:52–9.
4. Yang KH, Lee TB, Lee SH, Kim SH, Cho YH, Kim HY. Congenital adhesion band causing small bowel obstruction: What's the difference in various age groups, pediatric and adult patients? BMC Surg. 2016;16(1):79.
5. Choudhry MS, Grant HW. Small bowel obstruction due to adhesions following neonatal laparotomy. Pediatr Surg Int. 2006;22(9):729–32.
6. Lautz TB, Barsness KA. Adhesive small bowel obstruction--acute management and treatment in children. Semin Pediatr Surg. 2014;23(6):349–52.
7. Lautz TB, Raval MV, Reynolds M, Barsness KA. Adhesive small bowel obstruction in children and adolescents: operative utilization and factors associated with bowel loss. J Am Coll Surg. 2011;212(5):855–61.
8. Al-Salem AH, Oquaish M. Adhesive intestinal obstruction in infants and children: the place of conservative treatment. ISRN Surg. 2011;2011:1.
9. van der Zee DC, Bax NM. Management of adhesive bowel obstruction in children is changed by laparoscopy. Surg Endosc. 1999;13(9):925–7.
10. Farinella E, Cirocchi R, La Mura F, et al. Feasibility of laparoscopy for small bowel obstruction. World J Emerg Surg. 2009;4:3.
11. Aguayo P, Ho B, Fraser JD, Gamis A, St Peter SD, Snyder CL. Bowel obstruction after treatment of intra-abdominal tumors. Eur J Pediatr Surg. 2010;20(4):234–6.
12. Ledowski T. Muscle relaxation in laparoscopic surgery: what is the evidence for improved operating conditions and patient outcome? A brief review of the literature. Surg Laparosc Endosc Percutan Tech. 2015;25(4):281–5.
13. Martynov I. Homemade glove port for pediatric single-incision laparoscopic surgery (SILS)—how we do it. Eur J Pediatr Surg Rep. 2018; in press.
14. Lacher M, Muensterer OJ, Yannam GR, et al. Feasibility of single-incision pediatric endosurgery for treatment of appendicitis in 415 children. J Laparoendosc Adv Surg Tech A. 2012;22(6):604–8.
15. Miyake H, Seo S, Pierro A. Laparoscopy or laparotomy for adhesive bowel obstruction in children: a systematic review and meta-analysis. Pediatr Surg Int. 2018;34(2):177–82.

16. Chosidow D, Johanet H, Montariol T, et al. Laparoscopy for acute small-bowel obstruction secondary to adhesions. J Laparoendosc Adv Surg Tech A. 2000;10(3):155–9.
17. Young JY, Kim DS, Muratore CS, Kurkchubasche AG, Tracy TF Jr, Luks FI. High incidence of postoperative bowel obstruction in newborns and infants. J Pediatr Surg. 2007;42(6):962–5; discussion 5.
18. Franklin ME Jr, Gonzalez JJ Jr, Miter DB, Glass JL, Paulson D. Laparoscopic diagnosis and treatment of intestinal obstruction. Surg Endosc. 2004;18(1):26–30.
19. Sajid MS, Khawaja AH, Sains P, Singh KK, Baig MK. A systematic review comparing laparoscopic vs open adhesiolysis in patients with adhesional small bowel obstruction. Am J Surg. 2016;212(1):138–50.

MIS Management of Intussusception

32

Munther Haddad

32.1 Introduction

Intussusception is telescoping of a segment of the intestine into another adjacent distal segment. The word *intussusception is derived from the Latin **intus* (within) and **suscipere* (receive) (receive within).

It was first described by Hunter in 1793, and the first series of hydrostatic reductions of intussusception was reported by Hirschsprung in 1876, and Ladd reported the first radiograph of contrast enema in 1913.

Ravitch published a large series of successful barium enema reductions of intussusception with standard guidelines in 1948 [1–3].

Most cases occur in children between 5 and 10 months of age, common in males with 3:2 M:F ratio and two-thirds of children with intussusception being below the age of 1 year.

There are two types of intussusception:

Idiopathic with no distinct lead in most cases and usually starts at the ileocecal region.

Nonidiopathic secondary to a lead point which occurs in 2–12% of cases and seen in infants less than 3 months or older children above the age of 4 years, and the lead points may be:

- Meckel's diverticulum.
- Enlarged mesenteric lymph node.
- Benign or malignant tumours, i.e. lymphoma, polyp.
- Duplication cyst.
- Hamartomas associated with Peutz-Jeghers syndrome [3].

Most cases of intussusception occur at the ileocecal region. Small bowel intussusception is rare and usually secondary to a lead point and occasionally occurs in the postoperative period. Hydrostatic enema reduction is the preferred treatment unless there is evidence of perforation or dead bowel.

Minimally invasive approach is indicated when attempts at enema reduction have failed or where enema reduction is contraindicated; it can be also useful as a diagnostic tool when other modalities of investigations like ultrasound and contrast enema were inconclusive like intussusception of small bowel.

Minimally invasive approach is contraindicated in haemodynamically unstable child and where there is evidence of small bowel obstruction with marked abdominal distention and dilated bowel loops [4, 5].

32.2 Preoperative Preparation

Children often present acutely unwell over 24 h period or more. All children should be assessed

M. Haddad (✉)
Department of Paediatric Surgery, Chelsea and Westminster and St. Mary's Hospitals, London, UK

Faculty of Medicine, Imperial College London, London, UK
e-mail: m.haddad@imperial.ac.uk

C. Esposito et al. (eds.), *ESPES Manual of Pediatric Minimally Invasive Surgery*,
https://doi.org/10.1007/978-3-030-00964-9_32

regarding their haemodynamic status and sepsis. Appropriate resuscitation, i.e. intravenous fluids, is given as these children are often dehydrated (from vomiting and third space loss) and antibiotics given if the child looks septic. A plain abdominal X-ray is usually done before the enema reduction to check the degree of intestinal obstruction and to exclude free intraperitoneal gas. Ultrasound of the abdomen is usually a reliable diagnostic investigation. Once the diagnosis is confirmed, an enema reduction can be carried out according to enema reduction guidelines.

Surgery is indicated when enema reduction has failed.

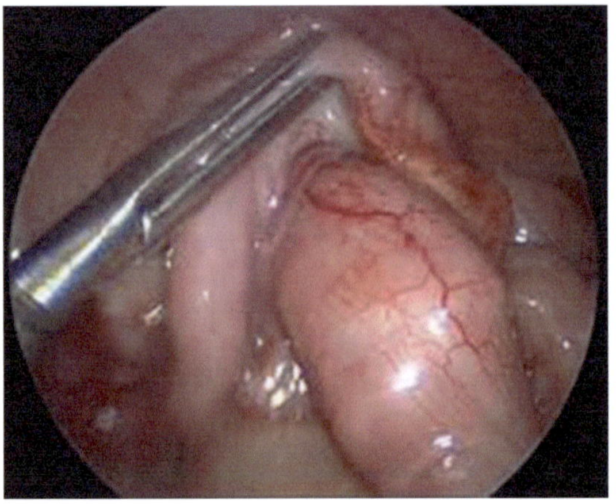

Fig. 32.1 The first step of the procedure is to identify the type and the extension of the intussusception

32.3 Positioning

The patient is positioned supine and towards the end of the operating table.

There are two monitors, the first one at the feet of patient to the left and the second one near the right patient's shoulder opposite the surgeon. The surgeon's position is on the left side of the patient with a nurse on his side, and the cameraman is in front of the surgeon.

Instrumentation

- 5 mm 30 degree scope
- 3–5 mm (Hasson) trocars
- Two atraumatic bowel graspers.
- 3–5 mm Maryland dissector
- 3–5 diathermy device
- 3–5 mm suction irrigation device.

32.4 Technique

The procedure is carried out under general anaesthesia with endotracheal intubation and muscle relaxant. A nasogastric tube should be inserted to decompress the upper gastrointestinal tract if there is intestinal distention.

The primary port is inserted through the umbilicus under direct vision (Hasson technique); CO_2 is used to insufflate the abdominal cavity up to 10 mmHg. The technique is divided in two phases, the diagnostic phase and the therapeutic phase. In the diagnostic phase, initial intra-abdominal inspection and assessment are carried out to determine:

- The feasibility of proceeding according to the degree of bowel distention.
- Identification of the intussusception and its extent (Fig. 32.1).
- Assessment of the degree of bowel ischemia and the likelihood of success with MIS.
- Assessment of the degree of peritoneal contamination.

This may need the help of other ports, usually two, which are inserted under direct vision, and their placement usually depends on the examination under anaesthesia carried out earlier and helped by the preoperative enema localizing the intussusception, as in most cases the incomplete reduction of the intussusception is localized as far as the ileocecal region or the ascending colon. Two ports should be inserted on the left side of the abdomen, one above and one below the level of the umbilicus or both below it. A third port might need to be inserted in the right side of the abdomen to help with the reduction of an intussusception in the left upper quadrant and to avoid overlap clashing of the instruments and the scope.

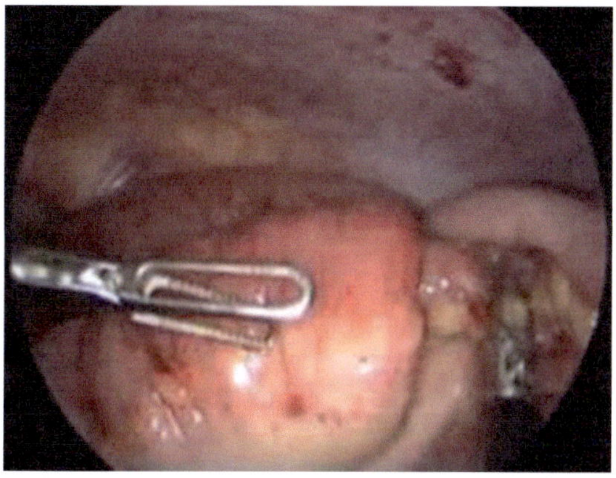

Fig. 32.2 The reduction can be achieved by application of balanced combination of traction and steady eversion pressure

Similar to open surgery, milking the intussusception proximally is the ideal and safest way, but this may be difficult with the laparoscopic approach due to bowel distention, poorer control (compared with the hand) and limited space. Milking alone may not be effective so proximal traction to the bowel is used to help with the reduction.

Reduction at the ileocecal valve is usually the most difficult part, and care should be taken not to cause any injury of the bowel wall, and reduction can be achieved by application of balanced combination of traction and steady eversion pressure, and it may be necessary to introduce a non-crushing grasper via a third working port to assist with the reduction (Fig. 32.2).

Following reduction the bowel is assessed for viability, the presence of any injury to the bowel wall or perforation and to exclude any lead point.

The abdominal cavity is then cleaned by irrigation of normal saline and suctioning.

The ports are removed, the abdomen is deflated, and the port site wounds are closed with absorbable sutures.

32.5 Postoperative Care

In the postoperative period, non-opiate analgesia is all what is needed, and opiate analgesia is only required occasionally. The analgesic requirement (paracetamol every 6 h) is generally limited to the first 24 postoperative hours.

In the majority of cases, oral intake is started soon after recovering from anaesthesia, and when they are no longer nauseated and able to tolerate fluids, they can restart full oral feeding few hours after surgery; this may be delayed if there has been significant bowel manipulation or bowel obstruction with dilated proximal bowel loops.

Most children are usually discharged home within 24 h, or maximum on the second postoperative day, unless there has been a need for resection and reanastomosis.

32.6 Tips and Tricks

- Examination of the abdomen under anaesthesia will help in placing the ports according to the location of intussusception to give maximum ergonomic advantage [6, 7].
- The use of 30 degree scope will provide better vision and access.
- Consider introduction of an additional port when needed.
- Be patient, and do not rush the reduction; apply a balanced traction and controlled steady pressure [8].
- Conversion to open technique should be considered early if reduction has failed.

32.7 Complications

Failure of laparoscopic reduction is not a complication.

*Bowel perforation due to the procedure or due to ischaemia preceding the procedure.

*Postoperative recurrence usually occurs within 24–48 h. Ultrasound may confirm that air enema can be reattempted unless there are signs of peritonitis.

*Pathological lead point may be difficult to recognize or missed [9].

References

1. Apelt N, Featherstone N, Giuliani S. Laparoscopic treatment of intussusception in children: a systematic review. J Pediatr Surg. 2013 Aug;48(8):1789–93. https://doi.org/10.1016/j.jpedsurg.2013.05.024.
2. Sklar CM, Chan E, Nasr A. Laparoscopic versus open reduction of intussusception in children: a retrospective review and meta-analysis. J Laparoendosc Adv Surg Tech A. 2014 Jul;24(7):518–22.
3. Charles T, Penninga L, Reurings JC, Berry MC. Intussusception in children: a clinical review. Acta Chir Belg. 2015 Sep-Oct;115(5):327–33.
4. Wei CH, Fu YW, Wang NL, Du YC, Sheu JC. Laparoscopy versus open surgery for idiopathic intussusception in children. Surg Endosc. 2015 Mar;29(3):668–72.
5. Hill SJ, Koontz CS, Langness SM, Wulkan ML. Laparoscopic versus open reduction of intussusception in children: experience over a decade. J Laparoendosc Adv Surg Tech A. 2013 Feb;23(2):166–9.
6. Alemayehu H, Stringel G, Lo IJ, Golden J, Pandya S, McBride W, Muensterer O. Laparoscopy and complicated meckel diverticulum in children. JSLS. 2014 Jul-Sep;18(3):e2014.00015.
7. Honjo H, Mike M, Kusanagi H, Kano N. Adult intussusception: a retrospective review. World J Surg. 2015 Jan;39(1):134–8.
8. Kao C, Tseng SH, Chen Y. Laparoscopic reduction of intussusception in children by a single surgeon in comparison with open surgery. Minim Invasive Ther Allied Technol. 2011 May;20(3):141–5.
9. Esposito C, Giurin I, Farina A, Ascione G, Miele E, Staiano A, Di Benedetto V, Settimi A. Blue rubber bleb nevus: an uncommon cause of intestinal intussusception. Eur J Pediatr 2012;171(7):1139–1140 2012.

Current Operative Management of Meckel Diverticulum

33

J. A. Sobrino and G. W. Holcomb III

33.1 Introduction

Meckel diverticulum is a true diverticulum, containing all layers of the bowel wall. It results from failure of the omphalomesenteric duct to regress. The incidence is estimated to be 1–2%, though the true rate is unknown as only approximately 4% are symptomatic and the risk of developing symptoms decreases with age. While the actual values vary, the often taught "rule of 2s" remains useful: the incidence is 2%, the male to female ratio is 2:1, the presentation is mostly before 2 years of age, the location is within 2 ft. (60 cm) from the ileocecal valve, and they are approximately 2 cm in diameter and 2 in (5 cm) long and can contain two types of heterotopic mucosa [1].

Although open excision is still used, most pediatric surgeons now utilize the laparoscopic approach which carries the advantage of being diagnostic and potentially therapeutic for other etiologies of abdominal symptoms [2, 3]. In this chapter, we describe our laparoscopic approach for resection of a Meckel diverticulum (Fig. 33.1).

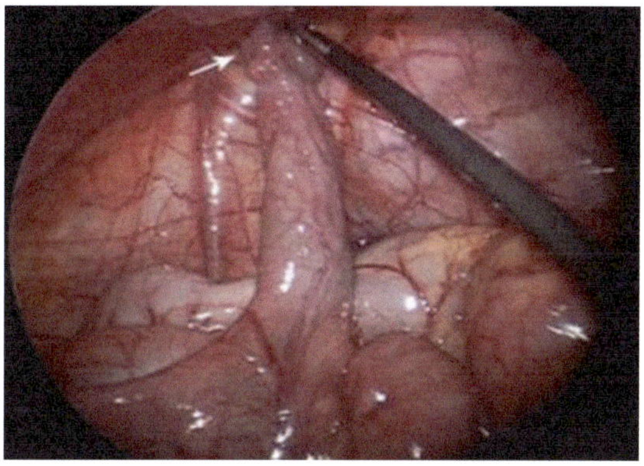

Fig. 33.1 Laparoscopic view of a Meckel diverticulum (From Holcomb GW, Murphy JP, Ostlie DJ, eds. Ashcraft's Pediatric Surgery. Sixth Edition. London; New York: Saunders/Elsevier; 2014. Reprinted with permission)

33.2 Preoperative Preparation

Different presentations will have unique preoperative requirements. The bleeding diverticulum may require transfusion, while the obstructed or perforated patient is likely to require intravenous rehydration, electrolyte correction, antibiotics, and gastric decompression. Informed consent is obtained and should include both diverticulectomy and small bowel resection. General endotracheal anesthesia with muscular relaxation is utilized.

J. A. Sobrino · G. W. Holcomb III (✉)
Department of Surgery, Children's Mercy Hospital, Kansas City, MO, USA
e-mail: gholcomb@cmh.edu

C. Esposito et al. (eds.), *ESPES Manual of Pediatric Minimally Invasive Surgery*,
https://doi.org/10.1007/978-3-030-00964-9_33

33.3 Positioning

The patient is positioned supine with the arms tucked. Two monitors are positioned at the front of the bed on either side of the patient for the surgeon and assistant. A urinary catheter may be needed, depending on the patient's condition or at the discretion of the surgeon or anesthetist. Ports are placed beginning with a 12 mm cannula at the umbilicus with the remaining port positioning dictated by the pathology. In the setting of an isolated Meckel diverticulum, two 5 mm cannulas or two 3–5 mm stab incisions are placed in the left lower quadrant (Fig. 33.2f). An intussusception due to a Meckel diverticulum may require alternative placement based on the extent of involved bowel. Intracorporeal and laparoscopic-assisted extracorporeal variations of the procedure exist.

33.4 Instrumentation

A 30°, 10 mm laparoscope and 3–5 mm bowel graspers are useful for initial inspection. Additional equipment, such as gastrointestinal staplers and sutures, will vary based on the operative findings and the decision for diverticulectomy or small bowel resection.

33.5 Technique

The surgeon should begin by surveying the abdomen for abnormalities. Next, the cecum should be identified followed by the small bowel, working distal to proximal. For intussusception, laparoscopic reduction can be attempted by applying gentle traction to the proximal segment to reduce it from the distal bowel. After identifying the diver-

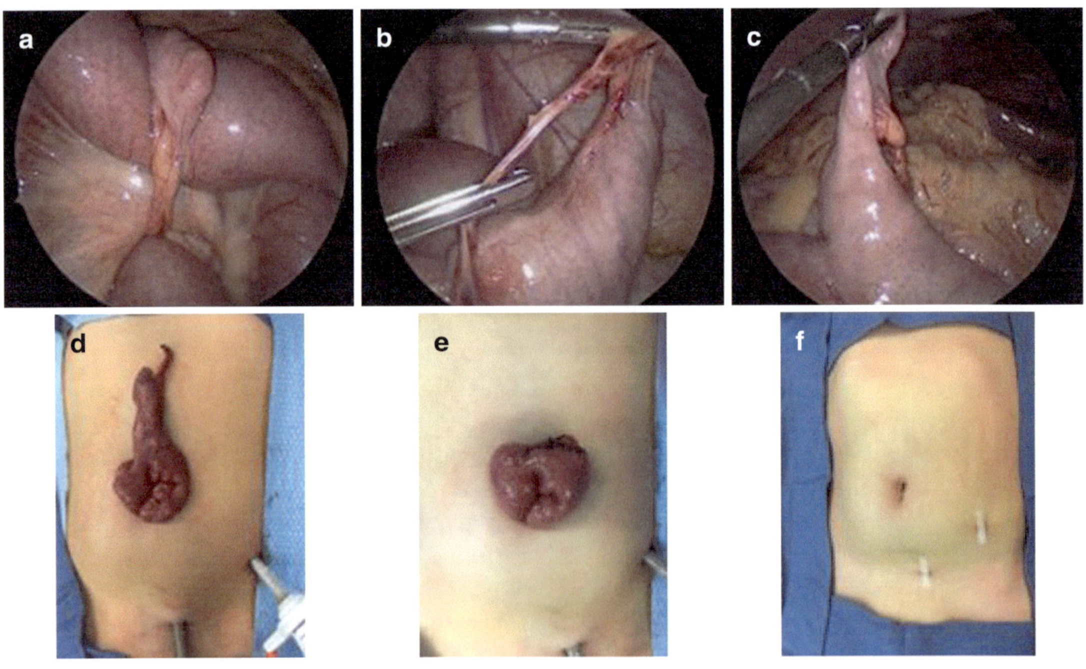

Fig. 33.2 Three-incision approach in a child presenting with a small bowel obstruction. A loop of small bowel is seen incarcerated in an adhesive band running from the tip of the Meckel diverticulum to the base of the mesentery (**a**). The bowel is reduced and the band divided (**b**, **c**). The diverticulum is then exteriorized via the umbilical incision (**d**), resected (**e**), and the bowel is then returned to the abdominal cavity. The incisions are then closed (**f**) (From Holcomb GW, Murphy JP, Ostlie DJ, eds. Ashcraft's Pediatric Surgery. Sixth Edition. London; New York: Saunders/Elsevier; 2014. Reprinted with permission)

ticulum as the lead point, the decision is made to continue laparoscopically or to externalize the bowel through an enlarged umbilical incision.

If no intussusception is seen, the next decision is whether to perform an intracorporeal or a laparoscopic-assisted extracorporeal diverticulectomy. We prefer to perform an extracorporeal diverticulectomy (Fig. 33.2). We enlarge the umbilical incision enough to exteriorize the diverticulum. The diverticulum is grasped using a grasper inserted through one of the accessory ports, and the diverticulum is maneuvered toward the umbilicus. The umbilical port and telescope are removed, and the diverticulum is seen and grasped and exteriorized through the umbilicus. The plane of resection for diverticulectomy is parallel to the bowel along the base of the diverticulum. If performing a stapled diverticulectomy, it may be helpful to orient the staple line obliquely to the bowel to avoid narrowing the lumen (Fig. 33.3), although data are lacking about whether this oblique orientation of the stapler is necessary. Excision and hand-sewn closure is achieved by resecting the diverticulum in a wedge shape directed from the anti-mesenteric border toward the mesentery. This partial enterectomy is then be closed similar to a small bowel anastomosis. If desired, a small bowel resection for Meckel diverticulum can be performed in the standard fashion. The bowel is then returned to the abdomen and the umbilical fascia and skin are closed.

33.6 Postoperative Care

Postoperative pain control is similar to other laparoscopic operations. There are no activity or bathing limitations. A nasogastric tube is not needed, and a diet may begin once there are signs of returning bowel function.

33.7 Results

The average length of operation is about 1 h. Complications are rare but include staple or suture line leak, anastomotic obstruction, and

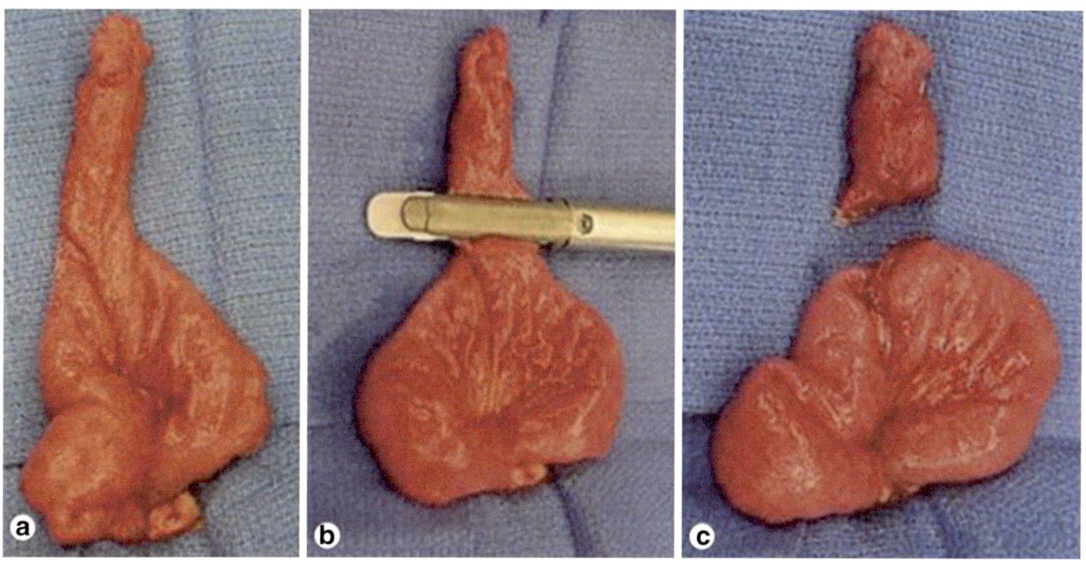

Fig. 33.3 Extracorporeal stapled resection of a Meckel diverticulum. Although difficult to see, the stapler was placed slightly obliquely across the base of the diverticulum in order not to obstruct the bowel at the site of the diverticulectomy (From Holcomb GW, Murphy JP, Ostlie DJ, eds. Ashcraft's Pediatric Surgery. Sixth Edition. London; New York: Saunders/Elsevier; 2014. Reprinted with permission)

ongoing bleeding due to incomplete resection. A single follow-up visit is usually adequate.

33.8 Tips and Tricks

- The laparoscopic-assisted extracorporeal technique is helpful in all patients, but especially in smaller patients due to limited operational domain, particularly if a stapler is used.
- Vertically oriented umbilical incisions are easily extended to facilitate evisceration of the small bowel with minimal postoperative scarring.
- For bleeding, it is useful to open the diverticulectomy specimen to confirm resection of the bleeding ulcer.

33.9 Discussion

Bleeding, obstruction, and inflammation of the diverticulum are the most common presentations of Meckel diverticulum. Less common presentations include perforation (more commonly seen in neonates) or incarceration in an abdominal wall hernia (Littré hernia). Laparoscopy has been effective in the management of these unusual or difficult presentations as well [4]. Bleeding classically presents as episodic, painless hematochezia, though slower bleeding may not be clinically apparent apart from anemia. Ectopic gastric mucosa producing mucosal ulceration is commonly found in a bleeding Meckel diverticulum. Obstruction most commonly arises via intussusception or volvulus. The diverticulum may act as a lead point for the intussusceptum of an obstructing ileoileal or ileocolic intussusception. Volvulus, on the other hand, may occur around the axis of a fibrous vitelline remnant and can lead to bowel ischemia. Meckel diverticulitis is often mistaken for appendicitis given the proximity of the diverticulum to the ileocecal valve.

The preoperative diagnosis of a Meckel diverticulum is relatively uncommon. For example, an intussuscepted diverticulum is most likely to be diagnosed intraoperatively after reduction or in the pathological specimen after resection. Patients who undergo successful enema reduction in the setting of a Meckel diverticulum may not fully reduce or, if they do, may recur. Subacute gastrointestinal bleeding is more likely to yield a preoperative diagnosis as the work-up to localize the bleeding may lead to a Meckel scan (technetium-99m pertechnetate radionuclide study). This isotope is selectively taken up by gastric mucosa and visualized on scintigraphy. While the Meckel scan is highly specific with a high positive predictive value, the sensitivity has been reported to be between 60 and 100% in various series. Given these values and that non-gastric mucosa does not take up the isotope, a negative scan cannot exclude a Meckel diverticulum.

Laparoscopic management of Meckel diverticulum is now the preferred approach, particularly given the ease of hybrid techniques that eviscerate the diverticulum through an extension of the umbilical extension. These patients have similar outcomes with shorter lengths of stay [2, 5].

References

1. Holcomb GW, Murphy JP, Ostlie DJ. Ashcraft's pediatric surgery. 6th ed. London: Saunders/Elsevier; 2014.
2. Ezekian B, Leraas HJ, Englum BR, Gilmore BF, Reed C, Fitzgerald TN, et al. Outcomes of laparoscopic resection of Meckel's diverticulum are equivalent to open laparotomy. J Pediatr Surg. 2019;54(3):507–10.
3. Shalaby RY, Soliman SM, Fawy M, et al. Laparoscopic management of Meckel's diverticulum in children. J Pediatr Surg. 2005;40:562–7.
4. Chan KW, Lee KH, Mou JWC, et al. Laparoscopic management of complicated Meckel's diverticulum in children: a 10-year review. Surg Endosc. 2008;22:1509–12.
5. Ruscher KA, Fisher JN, Hughes CD, et al. National trends in the surgical management of Meckel's diverticulum. J Pediatr Surg. 2011;46:893–6.

Bariatric Surgery for Paediatric Patients

34

Jennifer Billington and Ashish Desai

34.1 Introduction

Morbid obesity amongst paediatric patients is a growing problem that represents a formidable global health challenge. In the past three decades, prevalence of childhood obesity has tripled [1]. The WHO estimates that worldwide, there are currently 41 million children ≤5 years old who are overweight or obese.

Though initially managed with lifestyle changes, surgical options in morbidly obese children are shown to have most sustained weight loss [2]. However, it should always be performed in multidisciplinary team (MDT) in centres that routinely perform the same. There are three main surgical options: Roux-en-Y bypass surgery (RYGB), sleeve gastrectomy (SG) and Laparoscopic Gastric Band (LGB). Sleeve gastrectomy is now one of the most commonly performed surgeries in children. Hence we shall describe surgical technique for the same.

J. Billington · A. Desai (✉)
Department of Paediatric Surgery, King's College Hospital, London, UK
e-mail: ashishdesai@nhs.net

34.2 Eligibility for Surgery

Patient selection is very important and should be a joint decision from a MDT consisting of paediatrician, surgeon, dietician and psychologist.

Before decision-making, patients are thoroughly investigated to identify any underlying condition causing obesity, e.g. hypothyroidism or Prader-Willi syndrome (PWS). Investigations also look for any obesity-related co-morbidities. Blood investigations include full blood count, urea and electrolytes, liver function and metabolic profile to look for non-alcoholic hepatic steatosis or type 2 diabetes. A sleep study should also be performed to diagnose obstructive sleep apnoea. Apart from this, baseline anthropometric measurements, an ECG, echocardiogram, and ambulatory blood pressure monitoring are also performed.

Input from paediatric gastroenterology, respiratory and endocrinology physicians are essential in the amelioration of such conditions prior to surgery.

As per recently published guidelines from the American Society of Metabolic and Bariatric Surgery (ASMBS) 2018, criteria are as per Table 34.1.

C. Esposito et al. (eds.), *ESPES Manual of Pediatric Minimally Invasive Surgery*,
https://doi.org/10.1007/978-3-030-00964-9_34

Table 34.1 Indications and contraindications for adolescent metabolic and bariatric surgery (MBS) [3]

Indications for adolescent MBS include
• BMI ≥35 kg/m² or 120% of the 95th percentile with clinically significant co-morbid conditions such as obstructive sleep apnoea (AHI 45), T2D, IIH, NASH, Blount's disease, SCFE, GERD or hypertension or BMI ≥40 kg/m² or 140% of the 95th percentile (whichever is lower) • A multidisciplinary team must also consider whether the patient and family have the ability and motivation to adhere to recommended treatments pre- and postoperatively, including consistent use of micronutrient supplements
Contraindications for adolescent MBS include
• A medically correctable cause of obesity • An ongoing substance abuse problem (within the preceding year) • A medical, psychiatric, psychosocial or cognitive condition that prevents adherence to postoperative dietary and medication regimens • Current or planned pregnancy within 12–18 months of the procedure

BMI Body Mass Index; *T2D* Type 2 Diabetes; *NASH* Nonalcoholic Steato-Hepatitis; *SCFE* Sliiped Capital Femoral Epiphysis; *GERD* Gastro-Esophageal Reflux Disease

34.3 Surgical Approach

34.3.1 Preoperative Preparation

When a patient has been deemed suitable for surgical intervention, a liver shrinking diet is recommended. It comprises of a 14-day period of high-protein, low-carbohydrate milkshake replacement for meals, which aims to reduce weight and size of the liver, making the laparoscopic access to the stomach easier.

34.3.2 Patient Positioning

The most important consideration for patients undergoing LSG is the proper positioning on the operating table. Ideally patients can walk into theatre and be anaesthetised on the table, eliminating the need to move from trolley to table. If this is not possible, an inflatable hover mattress can be utilised.

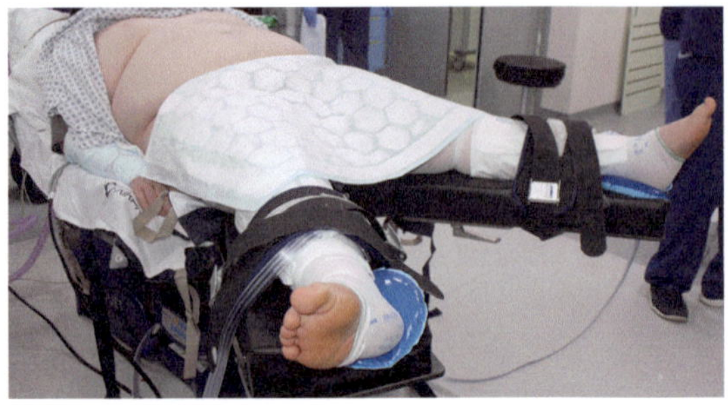

Fig. 34.1 Position of the patient with appropriate padding to protect pressure points

A number of anaesthetic considerations must be noted for the obese patient. IV access may prove difficult due to excessive subcutaneous fat. Obese patients have decreased functional reserve, and a period of prolonged preoxygenation may prevent rapid desaturation following administration of induction agents. A short thick neck often makes visualisation of the larynx difficult, a problem which can be remedied by a glidoscope.

Patient positioning is imperative to ensure good body mechanics of the operating surgeon and ensuring the patient is secure on the operating table. A sufficient number of staff should be present to assist in securing the patient. In our institution, patients are placed in a supine position, with their legs apart. The legs are secured with straps, and where necessary, breast tissue is taped away from the operative field (Fig. 34.1). Finally, a head up, hips up position ensures the abdominal field is best exposed with minimal skin fold creases. Arms should be tucked in.

Thorough attention to detail for skin assessment and padding ensures no pressure sores are encountered. All patients, unless contraindicated, should have TED stockings and inflatable boot devices applied. Patients receive intraoperative broad spectrum antibiotics and further two doses in the post-operative period.

34.3.3 Instrumentation

– 5 ports—12, 12, 5, 5, +/5 fifth 5—Visiport technique

- 10 mm camera
- Harmonic scalpel
- GIA linear stapler device

34.3.4 Surgical Technique

- An OGD is performed and gastric/oesophageal biopsies taken to look for evidence of any pathology, gastro-oesophageal reflux and *H. pylori* infection.
- Following safe and appropriate set-up of the patient, a pneumoperitoneum is created using a Visiport in supraumbilical region (Fig. 34.2). The remaining ports are inserted under direct visual guidance.
- The position of ports is illustrated in Figs. 34.2 and 34.3.
- A liver lift is inserted to elevate the liver and allow stomach to be seen. A laparoscopic grasper can also be used; however, we feel liver lift offers better visualisation.
- The greater and lesser curves are visualised, as is the pylorus.
- Using a harmonic device, the greater curvature is devascularised from 5 cm proximal to the pylorus up to gastro-oesophageal junction (GOJ) until the diaphragmatic crus is visualised. Care should be taken to ensure the GOJ is well vascularised.
- An appropriately sized bougie is placed endoscopically to ensure an adequately sized stomach remains. In our centre we use a size 36–38 bougie.

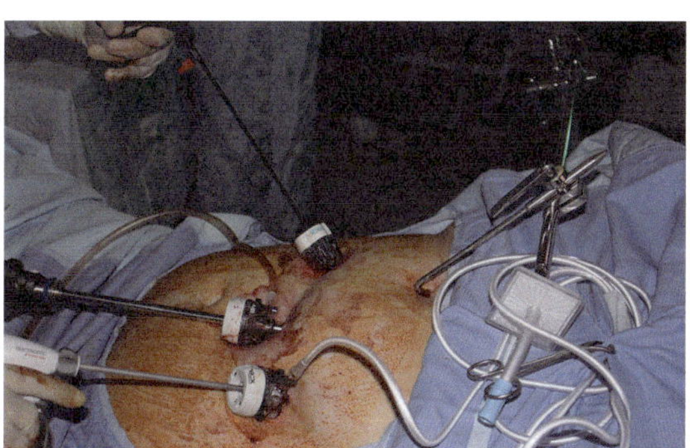

Fig. 34.2 Port placement

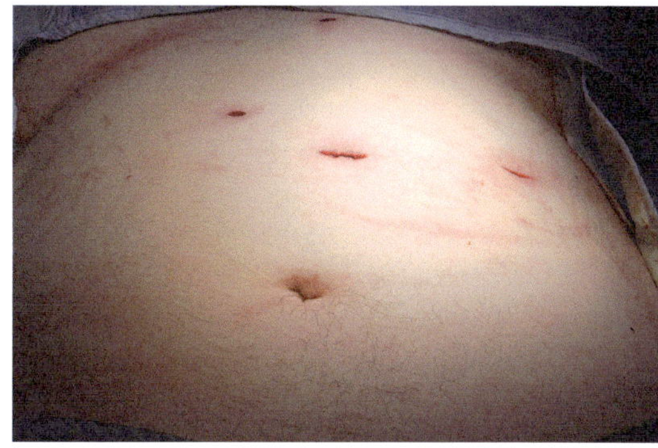

Fig. 34.3 Position of ports after port removal

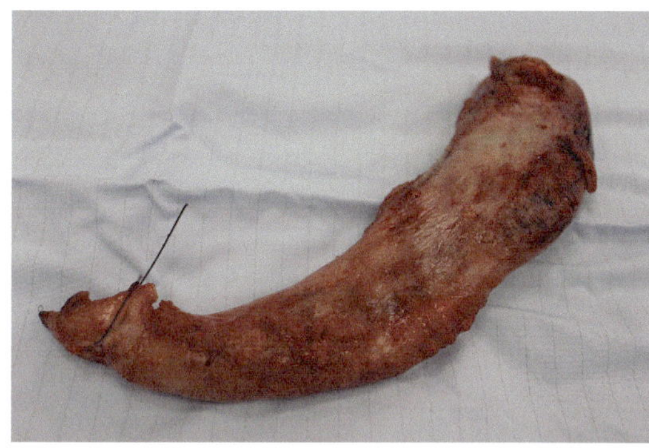

Fig. 34.4 Resected specimen

- Using the bougie as a guide, a linear stapler allows excision of the greater curvature and tubularisation of the stomach.
- Commencing at the proximal staple line at the gastric antrum, a running stitch of 4/0 PDS may be used to re-enforce the staple line.
- The suture line is tested laparoscopically, and a check for haemostasis is performed.
- The stomach is removed from the supraumbilical port (Figs. 34.3 and 34.4).
- We routinely perform trucut biopsy from liver under direct visualisation to grade hepatic steatosis.
- Closure of wounds using 1/0 Vicryl J needle and glue for skin.

34.3.5 Procedure-Specific Complications

- Bleeding from suture line or liver
- Inability to complete due to large liver

- Damage to spleen
- Pneumothorax
- Deep vein thrombosis and pulmonary embolism
- Leakage from the staple line
- Failure to lose weight or weight regain
- Gastro-oesophageal reflux

34.4 Post-operative Care

Below is a sample protocol, similar to what we use for the post-operative management of patients at our institution (Table 34.2).

34.5 Results

A recent retrospective review of our 7-year institutional experience of performing LSG in morbidly obese teenagers has demonstrated good medium-term weight loss. Within our institution, the average age for patients undergoing LSG is 16 years of age (16.8, 13–19). Mean preoperative weight was 140.25 kg, with a mean BMI of 51.26 kg/m^2.

Table 34.2 Post-operative bariatric surgical protocol

Post-operative bariatric surgical protocol
Diet – Free fluids (Week 1 and 2) – Pureed food (Week 3 and 4) – Normal diet (Week 4 onward)
Medications on discharge – 1 g paracetamol PO QDS – 50 mg diclofenac PO TDS – 30 mg lansoprazole OD x 3/12 – Ursodeoxycholic acid 650 mg nocte × 6/12
Vitamin and mineral supplementation
Anti-thrombotic treatment – TEDS (4 weeks) – Enoxaparin <100 kg 40 mg OD for 4 weeks 100–150 kg 40 mg BD for 4 weeks >150 kg 60 mg BD for 4 weeks
Laboratory investigations – 3, 6, 12 months then annually → U&E, LFT, bone profile, Vit D, PTH, FBC, ferritin, folate, Vit B12, INR, HBA1c, FBG, FPI, lipid
Additional – CLO test – If positive, HeliClear when on pureed diet

The procedure takes approximately 90 min, which has reduced slightly with the learning curve within our institution. Patients with an uncomplicated post-operative course usually are discharged home on day 1 or 2 post-operatively.

Within our cohort, complications have included staple line haemorrhage, inadvertent stapling of a nasogastric tube and post-operative collection with pleural effusion. In the longer term, a proportion of our patients have developed GI symptoms such as nausea and vomiting which have responded to medical management. We have had no readmissions and no mortality within our cohort of patients

At 1-year follow-up, our patients achieve on average loss of >50% of excessive body weight. Our patients are being followed up in the longer term and data is being collected on reduction in BMI, management of obesity-related co-morbidities and general wellbeing of the patient post-operatively.

34.6 Tips and Tricks

- Ensuring proper time and manpower for patient position is fundamental in performing this procedure with ease. We recommend a 'heads up, hips up' position, which prevents a flexed upper torso. Without this position, we have found the folds of abdominal skin often impede the visual field.
- Port position, as demonstrated in Fig. 34.2, ensures no camera clash and adequate triangulation of instruments.
- Removal of nasogastric tube and bougie before commencing stapling of the stomach is essential to prevent inadvertent stapling.

34.7 Discussion

Surgical treatment of paediatric obesity is not routinely accepted as it is considered as lifestyle condition. Being a relatively new procedure in paediatric population, doubts are also raised about its possible safety profile. However, recently there has been surge in publications reporting safety and efficacy.

Adolescents Morbid Obesity Study (AMOS) is a randomised control trial between RYGB and lifestyle intervention in 13–18 years old. Out of 81 patients operated, there was no mortality either intraoperatively or within 30 days of surgery [3]. Similar results were also demonstrated by Inge et al. while reporting multisite, observational study Teen-Longitudinal Assessment Study (Teen-LABS) with 242 patients having had surgery [4].

Surgery provides the most clinically significant short-term weight loss, with 50–60% excess weight lost in the first year in most case series. In the adult cohorts, long-term studies suggest the excess weight loss persists beyond 10 years.

Alqhatani et al. demonstrated a loss of 64.9% of excess body weight over 3 years in 108 paediatric patients. He also demonstrated 90% resolution of various co-morbidities like OSA, hypertension, type 2 diabetes and dyslipidaemia [5, 6].

In the Teen-LABS study, mean weight reduced by 28% in RYGB and 26% in SG which was sustained for 3 years. This study also demonstrated remission of diabetes in 95% and improved kidney function in 86%. In this series, 8% patients suffered a major complication. Major complications in this cohort included reoperation for bowel obstruction/intra-abdominal sepsis/bleeding and thromboembolic disease.

The AMOS study also demonstrated weight loss of 32% with 100% resolution of type 2 diabetes and hypertension. There was 92% improvement in abnormal liver function [4].

However, there is concern about vitamin and micronutrient deficiency post-operatively in these patients. Hence it is imperative that these children are treated with lifelong vitamin and micronutrient supplements.

The need for a further surgery is mainly seen after RYGB; however it is also seen to be the case for all procedures. These procedures are mainly endoscopy, cholecystectomy and diagnostic laparoscopy.

34.8 Conclusion

Bariatric surgery is slowly getting acceptance in paediatric population. Sleeve gastrectomy is most commonly performed procedure. It is a relatively safe procedure. Selection is a key factor and should be made in MDT setting. In view of risk of trace elements and vitamin deficiency in long term, these patients need long-term follow-up.

References

1. Paulus GF, et al. Bariatric surgery in morbidly obese adolescents: a systematic review and meta-analysis. Obes Surg. 2015;25(5):860–78.
2. Black JA, et al. Bariatric surgery for obese children and adolescents: a systematic review and meta-analysis. Obes Rev. 2013;14(8):634–44.
3. Janey, et al. ASMBS pediatric metabolic and bariatric surgery guidelines, 2018. Surg Obes Relat Dis. 2018;14(7):882–901.
4. Olbers, et al. The Adolescent Morbid Obesity Surgery (AMOS) study: five year outcomes following laparoscopic Roux-en-Y gastric bypass in a Swedish nationwide study. Obes Facts. 2016;9:158.
5. Inge, et al. Perioperative outcomes of adolescents undergoing bariatric surgery: the Teen-Longitudinal Assessment of Bariatric Surgery (Teen-LABS) study. JAMA Pediatr. 2014;168(1):47–53.
6. Durkin N, Desai AP. What is the evidence for paediatric/adolescent bariatric surgery? Curr Obes Rep. 2017;6(3):278–85.

35 Laparoscopic Liver Surgery

Orkan Ergün

35.1 Introduction

Minimally invasive surgery (MIS) has shown a dazzling evolution in the recent two decades. Although most of the developments initially targeted general surgery and adult patient population, the rapid introduction of smaller instruments for pediatric age group, despite some limitations, has provided pediatric surgeons to adapt and improve their skills in neonatal and pediatric MIS. Currently, pediatric surgeons worldwide perform laparoscopic procedures in almost every field of pediatric surgery. However, the same progress has not been achieved in pediatric laparoscopic liver surgery (LLS), and the trend for performing LLS in liver diseases of childhood has been relatively slow and hesitant [1, 2].

This chapter aims to present the considerations, technical aspects, implementation, and the limitations of LLS in pediatric surgery.

35.2 Indications and Considerations

Indications for LLS are similar and not quite diverse from those for open surgery [2–9]. Cystic and solid benign lesions as well as malignancies and lesions with diagnostic uncertainty may be managed successfully by laparoscopic approaches. One should bear in mind that liver surgery is a complex procedure, and attempting LLS requires expertise in both open liver surgery and advanced laparoscopic techniques [1, 3, 10]. Formal training in hepatobiliary surgery, being familiar with parenchymal transection techniques as well as sectional relationship of anatomical structures such as vascular and biliary tree, and hemostasis principles are of utmost importance before considering performing LLS [10].

35.2.1 Tumor Size and Location

Preoperative evaluation is similar to open surgery; however, technical feasibility should be assessed thoroughly, and tumor size, location, and pathology must be taken into consideration [3–9].

Tumor size less than 5 cm in diameter and those that are located in the anterolateral segments (segments II and VI; called laparoscopic segments) are the best indications for laparoscopic approach [3, 5, 6, 10–12]. Similarly, segments III and V and inferior part of segment IV are easily accessible locations. Exophytic lesions (even those exceeding 5 cm in size) which seem to be easily resectable in preoperative imaging may also be considered for laparoscopic resection provided that the surgeon feels

O. Ergün (✉)
Department of Pediatric Surgery, School of Medicine, Ege University, İzmir, Turkey
e-mail: orkan.ergun@ege.edu.tr

C. Esposito et al. (eds.), *ESPES Manual of Pediatric Minimally Invasive Surgery*,
https://doi.org/10.1007/978-3-030-00964-9_35

confident in adequate handling of the mass and bleeding control [5, 9, 13, 14]. Right hepatectomy could be procedure of choice for those lesions located in the right lobe and allowing for safe tumor margins [3]. Following the mobilization of the liver, ligation of right hepatic artery and right portal vein at the level of hepatic hilum and ligation and division of right hepatic vein prior to starting parenchymal dissection for right hepatectomy may facilitate obtaining a bloodless dissection plane during transection. The exceptions to patient assignment for right hepatectomy are the lesions in the hepatic hilum and hepatocaval junction due to risk of injury to major vascular and biliary structures [7, 15].

Patients with lesions occupying segments I, VII, and VIII (non-laparoscopic segments, poorly accessible locations), or close to hepatic hilum and vena cava, confluence of major hepatic veins and major biliary structures, and tumor size exceeding 10 cm are not considered good candidates for LLS [1, 7, 15]. Tumors larger than 5 cm have the possibility of tumor rupture and spillage during mobilization, retraction, or resection [11].

35.2.2 Technical Considerations

Laparoscopic parenchymal dissection can be performed by pure laparoscopy, hand-assisted laparoscopic approach, or a hybrid technique which is laparoscopy-assisted open procedure [1, 7, 16, 17].

"Pure laparoscopic technique" incorporates parenchymal dissection, vascular control, and resection solely performed by laparoscopy. This technique requires placement of an umbilical trocar and pneumoperitoneum by CO_2 insufflation. Depending on the tumor location, and the type of resection planned, three or four additional working ports are required. The number and site of the trocars are determined according to the patient size and the location of the lesion. The insufflation pressures are maintained between 8 and 10 mmHg in children and 4 and 6 mmHg in infants [11] to prevent or minimize the risk of gas embolism [1, 3, 11, 18]. Nevertheless, gas (CO_2) embolism in clinical setting is very rare and usually without significance in majority of cases [19].

Bleeding during parenchymal transection may challenge the surgeon since it is not easy to control it during laparoscopy. A dry, bloodless operative field may be obtained by controlling the inflow by Pringle maneuver at the level of porta hepatis, outflow by decreasing the central venous pressure (by the anesthesiologist), and utilization of useful devices and appropriate techniques [10, 11].

The superficial parenchyma of the liver is best managed by "harmonic dissector." The availability of "laparoscopic cavitron ultrasonic surgical aspirator (CUSA)" at the operative field facilitates clean and clear parenchymal dissection and transection [10]. Division of minor vasculature may be done by harmonic dissector or vascular sealing devices; however, special care must be given to identifying biliary structures and clipping them before dividing since division of bile ducts by sealing devices may not be safe and end up in bile leaks. Division of major vascular structures is best achieved and facilitated by linear vascular staplers.

For deep lesions invisible through the outer margins of the liver parenchyma, incorporation of laparoscopic ultrasonography to delineate the margins of the tumor and to identify the relationship of the mass with the vascular and biliary structures may guide and facilitate safe dissection and vascular control [18]. Recently, radiofrequency (RF) precoagulation utilizing 50 W electrical power for approximately 40 min has been proposed to create a zone of coagulation necrosis around the tumor margins before the liver transection. Utilization of RF precoagulation in LLS for malignant tumors resulted in favorable blood loss and no tumor recurrence [13].

"Hand-assisted laparoscopic procedure" is performed through a small incision below the xiphoid process to allow insertion of the surgeon's hand inside the abdomen. A hand port is then introduced through this incision. Following the creation of pneumoperitoneum, the inserted fingers or hand through the hand port offers the advantage of tactile feedback, while it facilitates laparoscopic dissection by retraction, mobilization, and control of bleeding if necessary. After the completion of dissection, the hand port is removed, and the specimen is extracted through the incision [3, 8].

"The hybrid procedure," which incorporates the advantages of minimally invasive techniques and smaller incisions for better cosmesis and faster recovery, involves mobilization of the liver by pure laparoscopy or hand-assisted technique after which either a small 8–12 cm midline incision is made or hand port removed if the latter technique is utilized. Then, the traditional open techniques are used for parenchymal transection, hilar dissection, and extraction of the specimen [6].

35.2.3 Conversion to Open Surgery

The need for conversion to open surgery basically is quite similar to conventional MIS; poor quality of view, inadequacy of exposure, inefficient dissection, fragile mass, prolonged operative time with the inability of making progress of the surgery, massive bleeding, and inability of control of bleeding or oozing are the main reasons for conversion to laparotomy [3]. The conversion rates are around 5–15% in the literature [3, 5, 6].

35.3 LLS for Cystic Lesions of the Liver

Cystic lesions of the liver may be congenital (nonparasitic) or acquired (parasitic, malignant, or traumatic).

Congenital hepatic cysts (CHCs) are very rare and tend to remain asymptomatic until adulthood. Therefore, the exact frequency of these lesions in pediatric age group is difficult to calculate [11, 16]. They are either discovered incidentally or if they cause symptoms, and it is estimated that only 10–40% of congenital cysts become symptomatic. Typical CHC is a solitary unilocular cyst located at segment V of the right lobe [16], but they can be multiple and/or multilocular as well. CHCs occur as a result of the abnormal development of the biliary tree; however, only 25% of them communicate with the bile system [10]. Unlike polycystic liver disease, CHCs do not have a genetic basis. Pathogenesis involves fluid accumulation and inflammation due to secretory epithelium [16]. Symptoms may vary depending on the location and the size of CHCs and include pain, nausea, as well as space-occupying symptoms such as gastroesophageal reflux, abdominal distention, obstructive jaundice, cholangitis, and even portal hypertension [18, 19].

Although CHCs are being increasingly recognized owing to widespread use of imaging modalities such as ultrasonography, asymptomatic and small lesions do not require treatment [11]. Despite they are benign in nature, CHCs need to be followed closely for their growth and risk of malignant transformation [18]. Needle puncture and aspiration in an attempt for nonoperative treatment of CHCs are ineffective and associated with a 100% recurrence rate [1, 3] and should only be considered as a temporizing measure in the presence of acute and severe symptoms such as respiratory distress and infection [16].

Surgical options include fenestration, enucleation, resection, and internal drainage. The principle is to eliminate fluid-secreting epithelium that can be achieved by either complete removal of the cyst walls or by internal drainage (i.e., cystogastrostomy or cystojejunostomy) if the cyst communicates with the biliary tree. Fenestration is a reasonable option provided that the cyst is close to the surface of the liver and has no connection with the biliary system. In this case, the fluid is absorbed by the peritoneum. This is a simple procedure that does not require parenchymal dissection and is associated with low morbidity and recurrence rate which is reported to be around 0–38%. Adding omentoplasty for the residual cavity reduces the recurrence rate [13].

Enucleation of liver cyst involves removing all the cyst epithelium. Puncture and aspiration of the cyst content under laparoscopic vision before starting enucleation reduces the pressure inside the cyst and may help identify the plane between the cyst and the parenchyma and ease the dissection (Fig. 35.1 and 35.2). Usually, there is a clear plane between the cyst and liver parenchyma (Fig. 35.3), and dissection is relatively simple once in the correct plane, and complete removal of the cyst is curative. Keeping close to the margins of the cyst wall during dissection and adhering to basic principles for hemostasis using adequate instruments allow for safe and bloodless surgery (Fig. 35.4).

Relative contraindications for LLS for CHCs include deeply located lesions within parenchyma not visible from the surface and association with hilar structure due to increased risk of bleeding or injury to biliary system [17, 18].

Parasitic cysts of the liver mainly include *Echinococcus granulosus* infection, namely, hydatid cysts, and the manifestation is endemic in some countries in the Middle East and Asia. The hydatid liver cysts have a combined

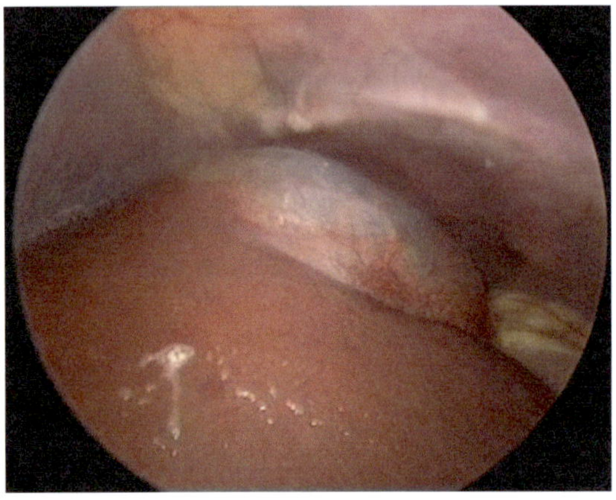

Fig. 35.1 An exophytic large, unilocular congenital liver cyst at the lateral sector of the liver

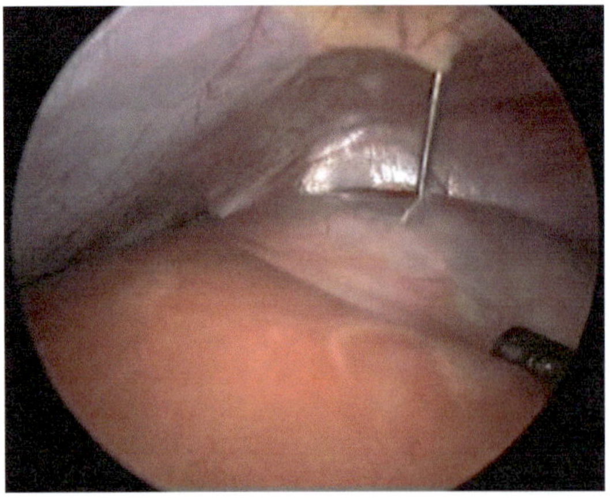

Fig. 35.2 Puncture of the cyst through the abdominal wall to aspirate and reduce the pressure inside the cyst to ease the dissection

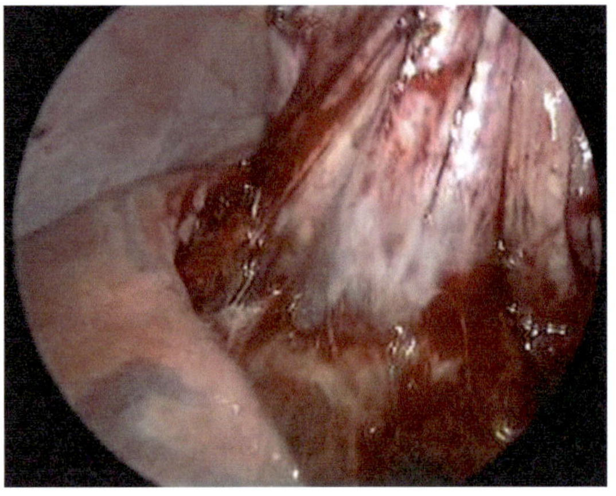

Fig. 35.3 The clear plane between the cyst wall and the liver parenchyma can be easily seen and dissected once in the correct plane

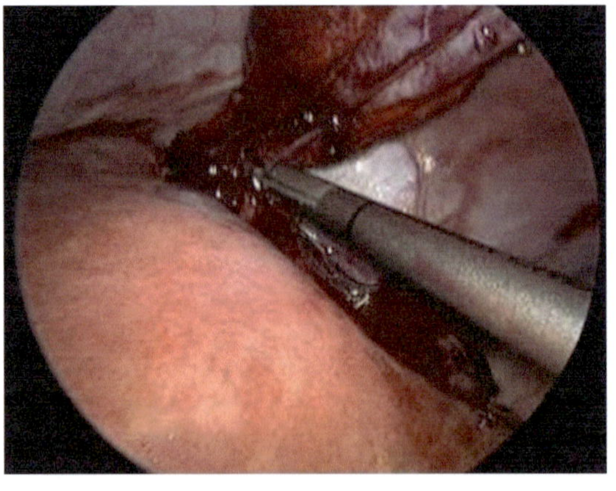

Fig. 35.4 Complete removal of the cyst

management with albendazole and ultrasonography-guided PAIR (**P**uncture-**A**spiration-**I**njection of a scolicidal agent-**R**easpiration) techniques. However, indications for PAIR are limited, and not all hydatid cysts are suitable for this technique. Laparoscopic surgical treatment is applicable in selected cases and involves injection of scolicidal agent under laparoscopic vision followed by opening of the cyst cavity, aspiration of its content, removal of the germinative membrane, and inspection of the residual cavity for biliary leaks. The procedure may be performed using multi-port or single-incision laparoscopic surgical techniques [14] depending on the site and the size of the cyst and the preference and the experience of the surgeon.

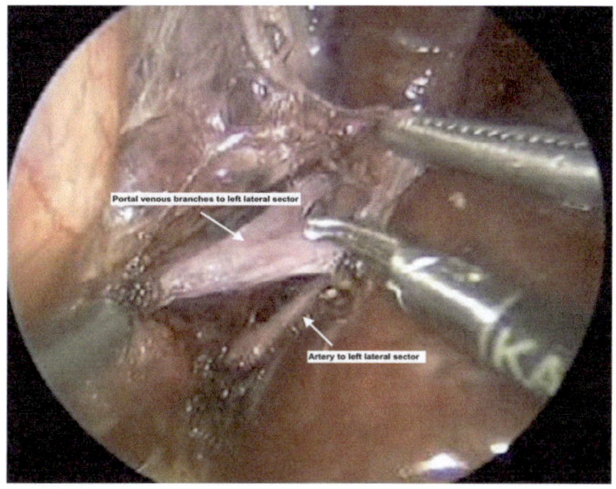

Fig. 35.5 Exposing the vascular supply to the left lateral sector of the liver

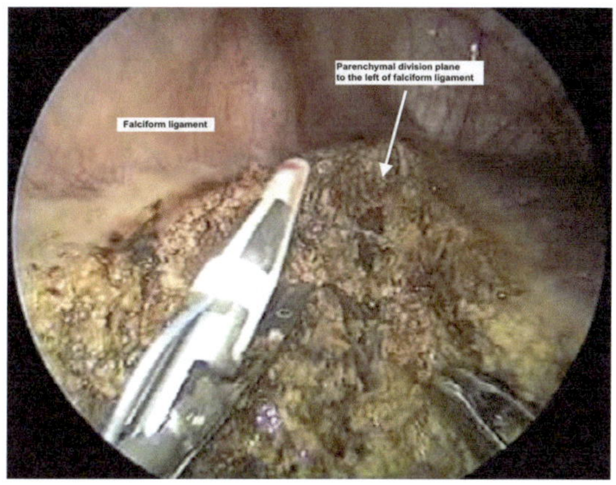

Fig. 35.6 Division of the liver parenchyma staying to the left of the falciform ligament

35.4 Left Lateral Sectionectomy

Lateral section (segments II and III) of the left lobe has a relatively smaller volume, unique and independent vascular anatomy, and more easily accessible position in the abdominal cavity. Therefore, left lateral sectionectomy represents one of the most common laparoscopically performed liver resection procedures especially in adult series including for living related donor hepatectomies [5, 7]. Moreover, some go even one step further to propose laparoscopic approach as a gold standard for left lateral sectionectomy [3].

For the left lateral sectionectomy procedure, the patient is given a 30° reverse Trendelenburg position. Left triangular and coronary ligaments are mobilized, and the round ligament is divided. Dissection of the left portal vein along the incisure of the round ligament exposes portal venous branches and artery to segments II and III (Fig. 35.5) that are clipped and divided. Parenchymal dissection keeping to the left of the falciform ligament is carried out by harmonic scalpel, vascular sealing devices, and/or CUSA, and bipolar cautery facilitates the hemostasis (Fig. 35.6). Left hepatic vein is divided by using endovascular GIA stapler (Fig. 35.7a, b).

A recent meta-analysis looking into the place of left lateral sectionectomy in the treatment of lesions occupying the left lateral sector has found that there were no significant differences in the operative time between open and laparoscopic procedures. On the other hand, blood loss and the need for blood transfusion were significantly lower, and hospital stays were significantly shorter in laparoscopic lateral sectionectomies. This also reflected to postoperative morbidity and mortality [15].

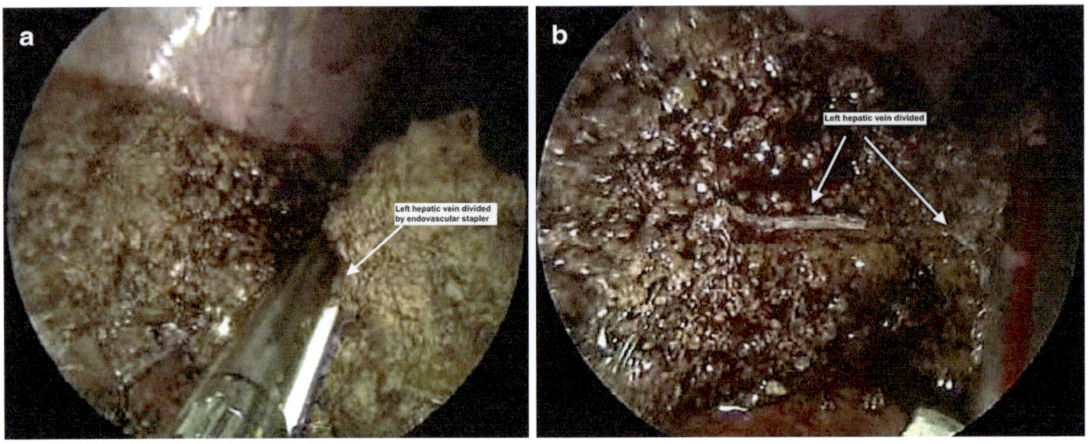

Fig. 35.7 (**a**) Division of the left hepatic vein by endovascular stapler. (**b**) The left hepatic vein divided

35.5 Conclusion

The adoption of laparoscopic liver resections in pediatric surgery has been much slower than all other laparoscopic procedures given the fact that LLS requires expertise in both advanced minimally invasive techniques and liver surgery, the risk and difficulty of controlling the bleeding as well as oncological drawbacks. However, with the introduction of adequate instruments and growing evidence concerning the benefits of LLS, the number of patients offered laparoscopic liver resections for benign and malignant conditions is increasing. Similarly, left lateral sectionectomy has become the procedure of choice for various conditions owing to its unique anatomical features. Within the last two decades when first laparoscopic liver resection was attempted in 1992, pediatric surgeons have become more and more interested in LLS, and the number of large pediatric series of laparoscopic liver resections is progressively increasing.

References

1. Veenstra MA, Koffron AJ. Minimally-invasive liver resection in pediatric patients: initial experience and outcomes. HPB. 2016;18:518–22.
2. Vibert E, Perniceni T, Levard H, et al. Laparoscopic liver resection. Br J Surg. 2006;93(1):67–72.
3. Buell JF, Thomas MT, Rudich S, et al. Experience with more than 500 minimally invasive hepatic procedures. Ann Surg. 2008;248(3):475–86.
4. Wei J, Feng J. Laparoscopic treatment of liver diseases in children. Front Med. 2011;5(4):388–94.
5. Cherqui D. Laparoscopic liver resection. Br J Surg. 2003;90(6):644–6.
6. Belli G, Fantini C, D'Agostino A, et al. Laparoscopic versus open liver resection for hepatocellular carcinoma in patients with histologically proven cirrhosis: short- and middle-term results. Surg Endosc. 2007;21(11):2004–11.
7. Huang MT, Lee WJ, Wang W, Wei PL, Chen RJ. Hand-assisted laparoscopic hepatectomy for solid tumor in the posterior portion of the right lobe: initial experience. Ann Surg. 2003;238(5):674–9.
8. Koffron AJ, Kung RD, Auffenberg GB, et al. Laparoscopic liver surgery for everyone: the hybrid method. Surgery. 2007;142:463–8.
9. Han H-S, Cho JY, Yoon Y-S. Techniques for performing laparoscopic liver resection in various hepatic locations. J Hepato-Biliary-Pancreat Surg. 2009;16:427–32.
10. Farges O, Jagot P, Kirstetter P, et al. Prospective assessment of the safety and benefit of laparoscopic liver resections. J Hepato-Biliary-Pancreat Surg. 2002;9(2):242–8.
11. Rahusen FD, Cuesta MA, Borgstein PJ, et al. Selection of patients for resection of colorectal metastases to the liver using diagnostic laparoscopy and laparoscopic ultrasonography. Ann Surg. 1999;230:31–7.
12. Min SK, Han HS, Kim SW, et al. Initial experiences with laparoscopy-assisted and total laparoscopy for anatomical liver resection: a preliminary study. J Korean Med Sci. 2006;21:69–74.
13. Linden AF, Pulcrano ME, Duffy BJ, et al. Laparoscopic excision of congenital hepatic cysts in the pediatric population: a case series and literature review. J Laparoendosc Adv Surg Tech A. 2016;26(6): 493–7.

14. Charles AR, Gupta AK, Bhatnagar V. Giant congenital solitary cyst of the liver: report of a case. Surg Today. 2001;31:732–4.
15. Morino M, DeGiuli M, Festa V, Garrone C. Laparoscopic management of symptomatic non-parasitic cysts of the liver: indications and results. Ann Surg. 1994;219:157–64.
16. Shankar SR, Parelkar SV, Das SA, Mathure AB. An antenatally-diagnosed solitary, non-parasitic hepatic cyst with duodenal obstruction. Pediatr Surg Int. 2000;6:214–5.
17. Acharya H, Agrawal V, Tiwari A, Sharma D. Single-incision trocar-less endoscopic management of giant liver hydatid cyst in children. J Minim Access Surg. 2018;14(2):130–3.
18. Buell JF, Cherqui D, Geller DA, et al. The international position on laparoscopic liver surgery: the Louisville Statement, 2008. Ann Surg. 2009;250:825–30.
19. Wakabayashi G, Cherqui D, Geller DA, et al. Recommendations for laparoscopic liver resection: a report from the second international consensus conference held in Morioka. Ann Surg. 2015;261:619–29.

Laparoscopic Management of Choledochal Cyst

36

Omid Madadi-Sanjani, Claus Petersen, Christoph Zoeller, Benno M. Ure, and Joachim F. Kuebler

36.1 Introduction

Choledochal cysts are rare congenital malformations with an incidence of approximately 1:100.000–1:150.000 in Western countries and high geographical variations with a reported incidence of 1:1.000 in Asian populations [1]. Diagnosis can be made during episodes with abdominal symptoms or as an incidental finding during abdominal ultrasound, and few reports on antenatal detections are available [2]. Diagnostics include laboratory controls of inflammatory and cholestasis parameters as well as sonography, CT scan, hepatobiliary scintigraphy with Technetium 99 (HIDA), MRCP, or ERCP [1]. In our institution abdominal ultrasound is the only essential imaging. MRCPs are included in our diagnostic protocols in unclear cases, and ERCP and potential stenting are mainly restricted to patients with acute obstruction [3].

Acute symptoms of choledochal cysts include biliary obstruction and jaundice, cholangitis, and pancreatitis [4]. Besides the acute symptoms, there is an increased risk of malignant transformations with an elevated incidence of cholangiocarcinoma and gallbladder carcinoma in patients with choledochal cysts [5]. Untreated patients have a lifetime risk of up to 30% [6], but this risk is significantly reduced by complete resection of the cyst. Nonetheless, the risk of malignant transformation is not restricted to the cystic area of the pancreatobiliary duct system and remains elevated especially in patients with resection of the cyst in adolescence or adulthood.

In 1995 the first case report of laparoscopic choledochal cyst excision with reconstruction via hepatico-jejunostomy was published [7]. Since then, multiple reports have demonstrated that laparoscopic approaches are feasible and safe [8, 9]. Biliodigestive anastomosis can be done with hepatico-jejunostomy or hepatico-duodenostomy, with no evidence of the superiority of any technique. Hepatico-duodenostomy is technically easier and faster but might be associated with a slightly higher risk of postoperative inflammation, i.e., due to biliary reflux [10]. As we consider chronic inflammation as the main culprit of the increased malignant transformation, hepatico-jejunostomy is the preferred method in our institution.

Cyst excision should be performed shortly after diagnosis and in young children from 3 months of age.

We recommend cyst excision in an interval without inflammation when no complications (e.g., cyst perforation, peritonitis) are present.

O. Madadi-Sanjani (✉) · C. Petersen · C. Zoeller
B. M. Ure · J. F. Kuebler
Center of Pediatric Surgery Hannover, Hannover Medical School, Hannover, Germany
e-mail: madadi-sanjani.omid@mh-hannover.de; petersen.claus@mh-hannover.de; zoeller.christoph@mh-hannover.de; ure.benno@mh-hannover.de; kuebler.joachim@mh-hannover.de

C. Esposito et al. (eds.), *ESPES Manual of Pediatric Minimally Invasive Surgery*,
https://doi.org/10.1007/978-3-030-00964-9_36

Patients with cholangitis or pancreatitis should undergo broad-spectrum antibiotics, and in cases of obstruction, ERCP and stenting has been helpful. Between inflammation and operative approach, a minimum interval of 6–8 weeks should be waited.

36.2 Preoperative Preparation

Informed consent includes counseling the parents of the increased lifetime risk of malignant transformation. Few hours prior to premedication, patients receive bowel preparation with enemas to reduce the colonic content. During anesthetic induction antibiotic prophylaxis with ampicillin and sulbactam is given. Operation is performed under general anesthesia and endotracheal intubation. A NG tube is placed for stomach decompression. A transurethral catheter is optional.

36.3 Positioning

The infant patient is placed in supine position at the end of the operating table in a frog-leg position, with minimal reclination at position of the xiphoid sternum (Fig. 36.1). Patients older than 2 years are placed in supine position with lower limbs apart. The surgeon is positioned at the end of the operating table and in older patients stands between the legs. The cameraman is sitting on the left side of the surgeon, and the second assistant and the nurse are on the right side of the surgeon.

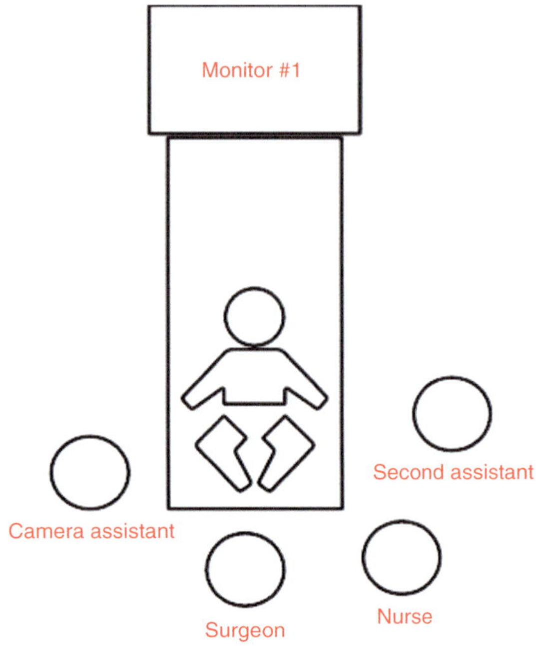

Fig. 36.1 Child is placed at the lower end of the operating table in a frog-leg position, with the surgeon positioned at the end of the operating table and in older patients stood between the legs. The second assistant is optional

36.4 Instrumentation

A 30° endoscope is preferred for camera visualization, which is inserted through an umbilical 5 or 10 mm port, depending on patient's age. Three additional ports (3.5 mm) are placed in the right abdomen, the left upper abdomen, and subxiphoid. Instruments for conventional, open surgery should always be present in the OR, for the case of a necessary quick conversion.

36.5 Technique

Open insertion of a 5–10 mm umbilical trocar: we usually use a disposable balloon trocar. Insufflation with CO_2 to establish a capnoperitoneum of 8 mmHg throughout the operation. Insertion of the right abdominal trocar and the trocar in the left upper abdomen. The ligamentum teres is then fixed to the ventral abdominal wall with a transcutaneous stay suture to elevate the liver, and a subxiphoid trocar is inserted (Fig. 36.2). During the first steps, the cranial adhesions of the ligamentum hepatoduodenale are released, and, thus, in a slight reverse Trendelenburg position of the patient, the space for the further preparation is created. When we have exposed the cyst, careful preparation usually with monopolar hook cautery along the cystic wall from ventral to dorsal takes place until the cyst is released at its back side (Fig. 36.3). During this step one has to be aware that the common hepatic artery usually runs medially adjacent

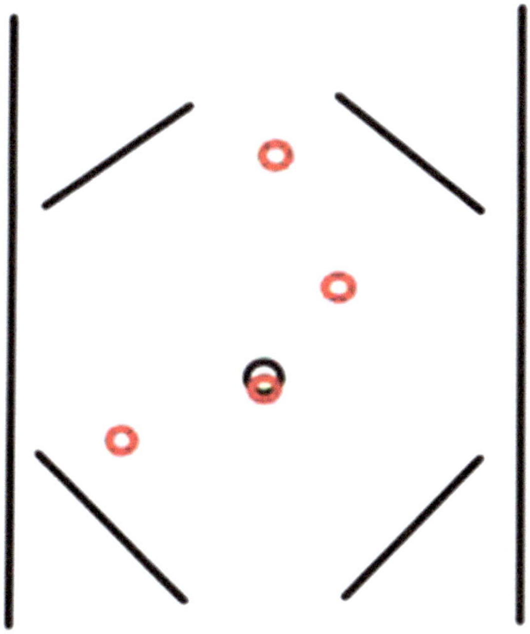

Fig. 36.2 Trocar positions as preferred at our institution

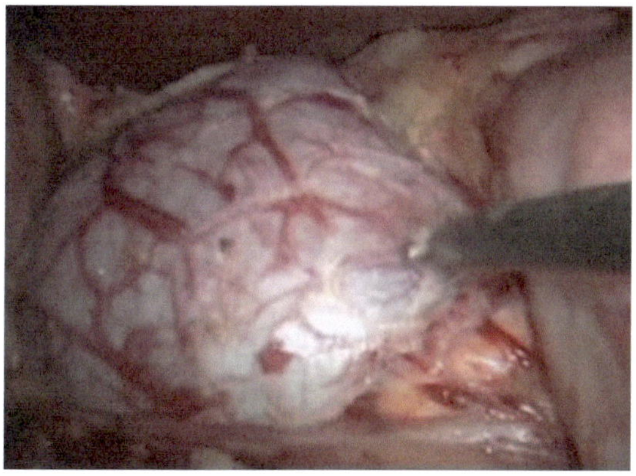

Fig. 36.3 Mobilization of the choledochal cyst with monopolar hook cautery

to the cyst, but variants, i.e., with a proximal separation and the left hepatic artery on the medial side and the right hepatic artery on the ventrolateral side, frequently exist. On the dorsal side of the cyst, the preparation and separation from the portal vein can be difficult, especially in large cysts. In some cases it can be helpful to elevate the medial and lateral corner of the cyst with traction sutures. During this step cyst content is released and the cyst shrinks. With the traction sutures or after the complete circumference of

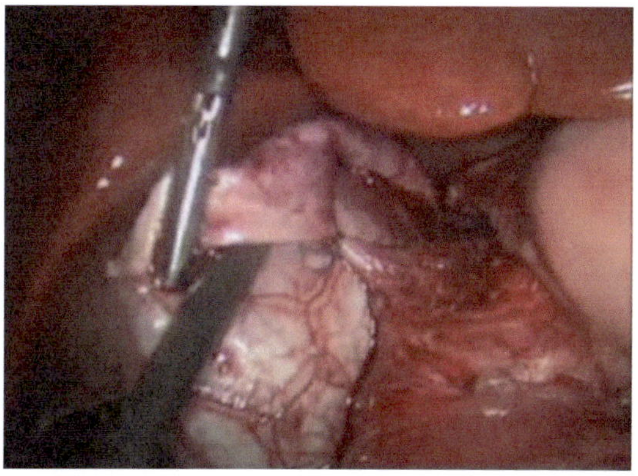

Fig. 36.4 Distal part of the cyst with narrowing to the pancreas before dissection

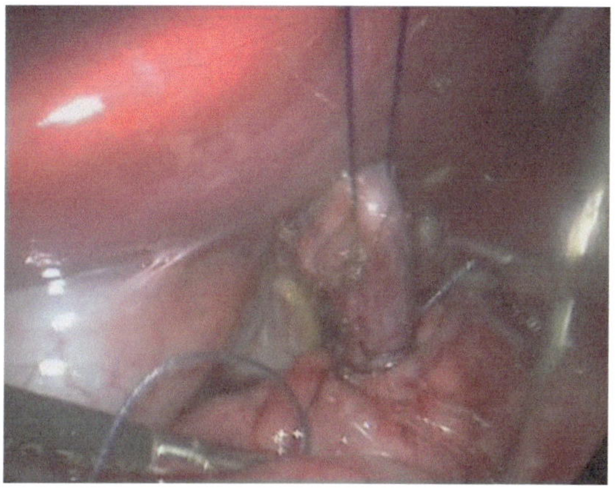

Fig. 36.5 Complete (long-distance) mobilization of the hepatic duct

the cyst has been freed, the cyst can be lifted up to completely mobilize it out of the pancreas (Fig. 36.4). This frequently involves mobilization of the cyst from the surrounding pancreatic tissue. The thin distal choledochus is then closed with a ligature and cut. The cystic artery is ligated, and the gallbladder and cystic duct are completely mobilized. Then, the proximal part of the cyst is mobilized, and the hepatic duct is cut proximal to the cyst but with a little distance to the liver parenchyma. While cutting the duct tissue, we usually pull it away from the liver, and one has to be aware that the tissue afterward retracts (Fig. 36.5). If the cyst reaches into the liver parenchyma, we resect as much as possible and perform the anastomosis on the hepatic surface, similar to a Kasai portoenterostomy. If we are suspicious on stones or sludge, a small endoscope can be inserted into the bile duct, and an inspection and lavage are performed. However, in our patient collective stones are rare. The completely mobilized cyst is dissected from the hepatic duct and is then placed on the liver, for later removal.

For the creation of the Roux-en-Y loop, we identify a suitable part of the jejunum, approximately 10 cm distal to the ligament of Treitz. A polyglactin suture is placed to facilitate exteriorization of the loop and to mark the oral direction. The suture is grasped with an instrument introduced via the umbilical trocar, and on the trocar, the umbilical incision is enlarged to easily exteriorize the intestinal loops. This has to be generous, as during the following steps, the temporarily impaired venous reflux results in an edematous swelling of the bowel. The jejunum is exteriorized. The Roux limb is ligated and the suture is left long. The jejuno-jejunostomy is performed extracorporeally approximately 20–30 cm distally. Care has to be taken to prevent misalignment, as orientation can be difficult. The antimesenteric opening of the loop is closed, and the intestine is repositioned in the abdominal cavity. Then, the fascia around the umbilicus is partially closed and the trocar is reinserted. After re-insufflation, the Roux limb is identified by the long suture. To facilitate the retrocolic pull through of the Roux limb, the mesenterium of the transverse colon is incised with the monopolar hook, and through this opening, a grasper holding the long suture is introduced and pushed through the mesenterium. Another instrument takes the suture cranial of the transversum, and the opened grasper is retracted to create a sufficient opening for the Roux limb. The limb is then approximated to the porta hepatis. In cases with anastomosis of the right and left hepatic ducts with the loop, both ducts are first attached to each other and then are anastomosed to the loop. The end-to-site hepatico-jejunostomy is started at the lateral position and is the performed with interrupted, counterclockwise polyglactin 5/0 sutures (Fig. 36.6). At this stage it is important to be aware of the hepatic bifurcation, as sometimes the distance is quite close and a suture could potentially obstruct one of the ducts.

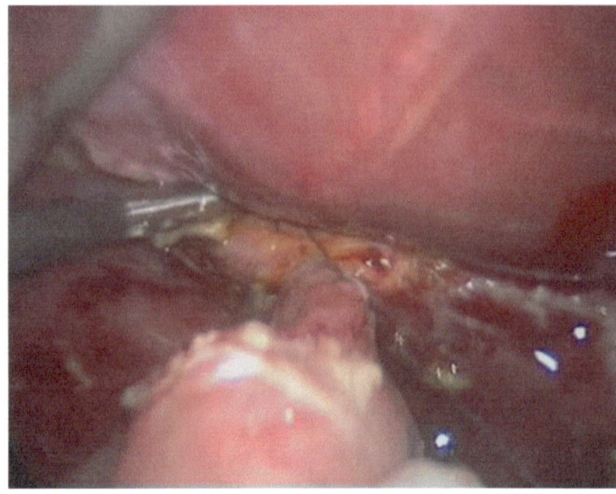

Fig. 36.6 Performing the end-to-site hepatico-jejunostomy

Sometimes, a lateral incision of the hepatic duct allows for an adequate width of the anastomosis, preventing an anastomosis stenosis. Finally, removal of the excised cyst and gallbladder through the umbilicus.

36.6 Postoperative Care

Following operation patients are referred to intermediate care unit in our institution. After an uneventful period of 24 h, patients are transferred to the pediatric surgical ward. Enteral nutrition is started on the first postoperative day. Intravenous antibiotic therapy is continued until the third postoperative day, and an oral antibiotic (penicillins with beta-lactamase inhibitors) is continued for another week. Analgetics are carefully reduced, and patients regularly show fast reconvalescence. Patients are regularly discharged on the thirdtofourth postoperative day. The first follow-up with the local pediatrician during the first week after hospital discharge includes abdominal ultrasound and laboratory controls of cholestasis parameters.

36.7 Results

Laparoscopic choledochal cyst resection with Roux-en-Y limb is the standard technique in our institution. The average length of surgery is about 240 min. Numerous reports have shown equivalent results in postoperative bile leak and anastomotic strictures comparing hepatico-jejunostomy and hepatico-duodenostomy following choledochal cyst excision. However, a recent meta-analysis by Narayanan et al. presented higher rates of cholangitis and bile reflux following hepatico-duodenostomy [10]. Conversion rates in large cohorts were lower than 1% [12]. In conclusion, laparoscopic cyst excision has proven to be a safe and feasible technique with a high learning curve.

36.8 Follow-Up

The Hannover follow-up protocol includes yearly follow-ups during childhood with clinical check-ups and laboratory controls such as cholestasis parameters and abdominal ultrasound in a specialized pediatric gastroenterology center. Entering adulthood, laboratory parameters should include yearly CA 19-9 controls for early diagnostics of malignant transformation [11].

36.9 Tips and Tricks

The trocars should not be positioned caudal of the umbilicus to facilitate exposition of the distal part of the cyst.

An adequate expansion of the umbilical incision is recommended. We perform an S-shaped transumbilical incision with which the fascial opening can be further stretched. Alternatively, an infraumbilical approach can be used.

Traction sutures on the edges of the cyst may facilitate the preparation on the dorsal side of the cyst and help to mobilize the cyst out of the pancreas.

Marking the Roux limb with a long suture simplifies finding the window through the transverse mesocolon.

36.10 Discussion

Since the first description of laparoscopic choledochal cyst excision, multiple advances in technique and equipment have made it the standard technique in centers of excellence. Various retrospective analyses since then have reported on the advantages of laparoscopic cyst excision such as a shorter hospital stay, faster recovery of bowel functions, and a lower rate of intraoperative (e.g., bleeding and blood transfusion) and postoperative complications (e.g., pancreatitis) compared to open, conventional surgery. However, the operation time was longer in laparoscopy [8, 9].

Today, both hepatico-jejunostomy and hepatico-duodenostomy are regularly performed in different centers, and high-level evidence recommending one or the other is lacking. Although hepatico-duodenostomy is faster compared to the hepatico-jejunostomy, in a recent review, data showed equivalent outcomes for postoperative bile leak and anastomotic strictures, while rates of cholangitis and bile reflux were higher following hepatico-duodenostomy [10, 12, 13]. An important aspect of the outcome after resection of a choledochal cyst is the increased rate of malignant transformations [14]. While it was hypothesized that complete cyst excision eliminates cancer risk, reports on malignancies decades after (complete) cyst excision cumulate [15]. As we consider chronic local inflammation of the main culprit of the increased risk of delayed malignancies, we prefer in our institution the reconstruction via hepatico-jejunostomy.

As a caveat, the interval between resection and malignancy is quite long, and therefore follow-up reports on malignancies following cyst excision during infancy are missing. No malignant transformation after laparoscopic approach is known; nonetheless regular and lifelong follow-ups are necessary for early identification of potential cancer manifestations [11].

Several modifications of the laparoscopic techniques have been reported to be feasible, such as single-incision laparoscopic cyst excision and robotic-assisted cyst excision, but are not yet widely applied [16, 17].

In conclusion, laparoscopic resection of a choledochal cyst is a safe and feasible technique showing excellent results in the hand of laparoscopic experienced surgeons.

References

1. Soares KC, Goldstein SD, Ghaseb MA, Kamel I, Hackam DJ, Pawlik TM. Pediatric choledochal cysts: diagnosis and current management. Pediatr Surg Int. 2017;33(6):637–50.
2. Weng R, Hu W, Cai S, Guo X, Luo Q. Prenatal diagnosis and prognosis assessment of congenital choledochal cyst in 21 cases. J Obstet Gynaecol. 2016;36(3):324–7.
3. Tsuchiya H, Kaneko K, Itoh A, Kawashima H, Ono Y, Tainaka T, et al. Endoscopic biliary drainage for children with persistent or exacerbated symptoms of choledochal cysts. J Hepatobiliary Pancreat Sci. 2013;20(3):303–6.
4. Muthucumaru M, Ljuhar D, Panabokke G, Paul E, Nataraja R, Ferguson P, et al. Acute pancreatitis complicating choledochal cysts in children. J Paediatr Child Health. 2017;53(3):291–4.
5. Sastry AV, Abbadessa B, Wayne MG, Steele JG, Cooperman AM. What is the incidence of biliary carcinoma in choledochal cysts, when do they develop, and how should it affect management? World J Surg. 2015;39(2):487–92.
6. Jabłońska B. Biliary cysts: etiology, diagnosis and management. World J Gastroenterol. 2012;18(35):4801–10.
7. Farello GA, Cerofolini A, Rebonato M, Bergamaschi G, Ferrari C, Chiappetta A. Congenital choledochal cyst: video-guided laparoscopic treatment. Surg Laparosc Endosc. 1995;5(5):354–8.
8. Shen H-J, Xu M, Zhu H-Y, Yang C, Li F, Li K, et al. Laparoscopic versus open surgery in children with choledochal cysts: a meta-analysis. Pediatr Surg Int. 2015;31(6):529–34.
9. Zhen C, Xia Z, Long L, Lishuang M, Pu Y, Wenjuan Z, et al. Laparoscopic excision versus open excision for the treatment of choledochal cysts: a systematic review and meta-analysis. Int Surg. 2015;100(1):115–22.
10. Narayanan SK, Chen Y, Narasimhan KL, Cohen RC. Hepaticoduodenostomy versus hepaticojejunostomy after resection of choledochal cyst: a systematic review and meta-analysis. J Pediatr Surg. 2013;48(11):2336–42.
11. Madadi-Sanjani O, Wirth TC, Kuebler JF, Petersen C, Ure BM. Choledochal cyst and malignancy: a plea for lifelong follow-up. Eur J Pediatr Surg. 2019;29(2):143–9.
12. Liem NT, Dung LA, Son TN. Laparoscopic complete cyst excision and hepaticoduodenostomy for choledochal cyst: early results in 74 cases. J Laparoendosc Adv Surg Tech A. 2009;19(Suppl 1):S87–90.
13. Yeung F, Chung PHY, Wong KKY, Tam PKH. Biliary-enteric reconstruction with hepaticoduodenostomy following laparoscopic excision of choledochal cyst is associated with better postoperative outcomes: a single-centre experience. Pediatr Surg Int. 2015;31(2):149–53.
14. Ten Hove A, de Meijer VE, Hulscher JBF, de Kleine RHJ. Meta-analysis of risk of developing malignancy in congenital choledochal malformation. Br J Surg. 2018;105(5):482–90.
15. Ohashi T, Wakai T, Kubota M, Matsuda Y, Arai Y, Ohyama T, et al. Risk of subsequent biliary malignancy in patients undergoing cyst excision for congenital choledochal cysts. J Gastroenterol Hepatol. 2013;28(2):243–7.
16. Tang Y, Li F, He G. Comparison of single-incision and conventional laparoscopic cyst excision and Roux-en-Y hepaticojejunostomy for children with choledochal cysts. Indian J Surg. 2016;78(4):259–64.
17. Dawrant MJ, Najmaldin AS, Alizai NK. Robot-assisted resection of choledochal cysts and hepaticojejunostomy in children less than 10 kg. J Pediatr Surg. 2010;45(12):2364–8.

37 Laparoscopic Cholecystectomy

Naved Kamal Alizai

37.1 Introduction

The first ever cholecystectomy on record was performed on July 15, 1882, by Carl Johann August Langenbuch (1846–1901) at Lazarus Krankenhaus in Berlin [1]. Few years earlier, on July 15, 1867, John Stough Bobbs of Indianapolis had performed a cholecystostomy on a 30-year-old woman with ovarian cancer [2]. It was over 100 years later, in Germany again, that Erich Mühe of Boblingen performed the first laparoscopic (Fig. 37.1) cholecystectomy [3]. This was a turning point for minimal access approach in general surgery. Another major advance, which helped the surgeons, was the development of a laparoscopic clip applicator with multiple clips. Dr. Mühe had to overcome a lot of hurdles before his technique was being recognised and adopted by other surgeons. He submitted his article to *The American Journal of Surgery* in 1990 but was rejected. His article never got published in English literature. The procedure was performed on September 12, 1985, with the help of a side-viewing endoscope and an instrumentation channel through the umbilicus. Eventually, his work was rewarded by him receiving the German Surgical Society Anniversary Award with praises

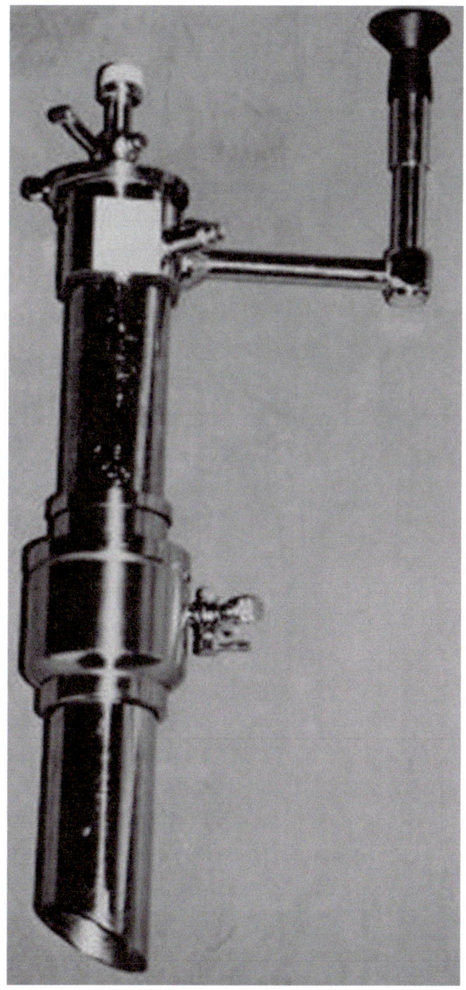

Fig. 37.1 Galloscope-Laparoscope invented by Erich Muhe and used in the first Laparoscopic Cholecystectomy

N. K. Alizai (✉)
Leeds General Infirmary, Leeds Teaching Hospitals NHS Trust, Leeds, United Kingdom
e-mail: Naved.Alizai@nhs.net

C. Esposito et al. (eds.), *ESPES Manual of Pediatric Minimally Invasive Surgery*,
https://doi.org/10.1007/978-3-030-00964-9_37

like "One of the greatest achievements of German medicine in recent history."

Over the years laparoscopic cholecystectomy has become the rule rather than the exception. Since the advent of laparoscopic cholecystectomy, where the first procedure took many hours and an inpatient hospital stay, it has become a day-case procedure with an operating time of literally a few minutes in experienced hands. The complication rates reported for laparoscopic cholecystectomy are reassuringly low. In adult practice, this procedure is the cardinal procedure used for teaching and training, and most laparoscopic cholecystectomies are performed by trainees as an emergency procedure, just the way an appendicectomy is performed in paediatric practice.

In paediatric practice gall bladder disease is not common, and a laparoscopic cholecystectomy procedure is considered to be a moderately complicated procedure. Paediatric cholecystectomies are generally performed by the consultants or trainees, supervised by a consultant.

37.2 Indications of Cholecystectomy

The remit of this chapter does not include a detailed discussion of the pathology and indications for a cholecystectomy. Gall bladder disease in children may be picked up incidentally or may present with symptoms of gall bladder disease or as with a complication. The commonest indication for cholecystectomy in the paediatric group is symptomatic gall stones. However, cholecystectomy may be required for gall bladder polyps (larger than 1 cm) and biliary dyskinesia (very rare). The patient may present with acute or chronic symptoms. Cholecystectomy may also be required for acalculous cholecystitis, Mirizzi's syndrome and suspected gall stone pancreatitis, even if there are no more stones left in the gall bladder following the episode of pancreatitis.

Absolute contraindications (gall bladder carcinoma, uncorrected coagulopathy) are very rare in paediatric practice, while relative contraindications (previous abdominal surgery, Mirizzi's syndrome type 2, porcelain gall bladder, cholecystoenteric fistula) depend on the experience of the operator.

In author's department, cholecystectomy is not offered for incidentally picked up asymptomatic cholelithiasis. In his experience (unpublished data), between 7 and 10% of asymptomatic gall stone patients will present with symptoms at some stage, requiring cholecystectomy.

37.3 Preoperative Considerations

Most paediatric laparoscopic cholecystectomy procedures are elective procedures. It is less common to perform emergency cholecystectomy in paediatric practice.

Once the patients are placed on the waiting list, they are assessed for any possible comorbidities and anaesthetic risks. Most patients will have investigations looking for the cause of underlying pathology requiring necessitating cholecystectomy. In general we perform a full blood count, coagulation screen and liver function test prior to the surgery. A group and save is usually not required. However, in units where cholecystectomy is not performed routinely or there is a risk of delay in arranging blood for transfusion, a group and save or cross-match may be required.

Most children would have had at least an ultrasound of their biliary system at some stage. In author's unit, it is a routine practice to perform a preoperative biliary ultrasound in symptomatic patients to confirm or exclude biliary duct stones. This scan is performed the day before or in the morning of the surgery. In asymptomatic patients an ultrasound is not required in the immediate preoperative period.

Antibiotics are not generally used. However, if there is a need for exploration of the ducts or operative cholangiogram, then either cephalosporin or co-amoxiclav is the antibiotic of choice.

It is crucial for the anaesthetist to pass a reasonable size nasogastric tube. As for any other laparoscopic procedures, we request our anaesthetist to relax the patients and avoid bagging on induction. The nasogastric tube is aspirated regularly and put on free drainage. The nasogastric tube should not be left spigotted. It is also important to make sure that the nasogastric tube is not passed too far into the stomach or the duodenum as the curve of the nasogastric tube can make the duodenum bulge towards the porta hepatis, which affects the field of view during surgery. During the procedure, if the stomach is seen to be distended, the anaesthetist is asked to aspirate the nasogastric tube. These measures keep the stomach empty and stop the gas passing into the small and large bowel, which can make the procedure difficult.

37.4 Instrumentation

A combination of reusable or disposable instruments can be used. The author prefers to use a size 10 telescope as it provides a far superior image as compared to size 5. Depending upon the size of the patient, 5- or 3-mm instruments are used. The main instruments generally used for a laparoscopic cholecystectomy include the following:

- Maryland forceps
- Johann's graspers
- Hook dissector
- Scissors
- Clip applicator
- Snake retractor and/or fixed retraction (Nathanson liver retractor—Cook Medical)
- 5 or preferable 10 mm 30° telescope
- Cannulae and obturators

37.5 Procedure

The patient is placed supine on the table. Some surgeons prefer to break the table at the xiphisternum level or place a bag under the lower thoracic region. However, in author's opinion, such measures can make the procedure difficult. However, raising the head-end of the table does help to encourage the bowel to migrate towards the pelvis. If a fixed retraction is used, it is important to tilt the table first before fixing the arm to the table because some tables may not move in harmony

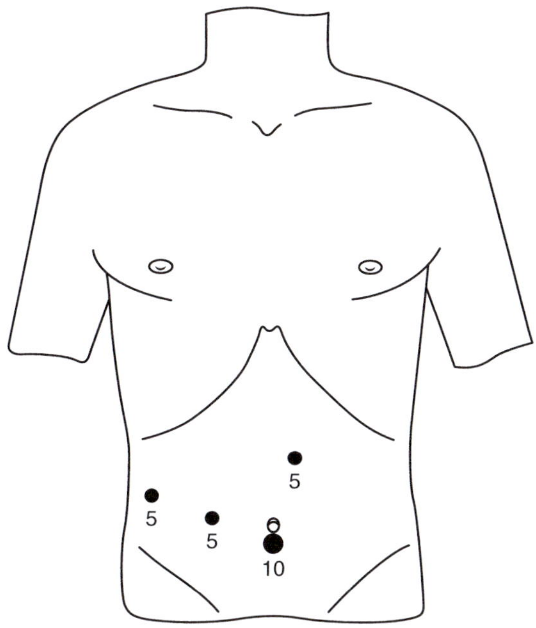

Fig. 37.2 Trocar position to perform a laparoscopic cholecystectomy

with the arm of a fixed retractor, which can cause damage to the tissues being retracted. It is wise to place the patient on the table in a way which will allow imaging, in case an on-table cholangiography is performed, even if one was not deemed necessary.

The conventional approach involves four ports (Fig. 37.2). The primary port insertion is through an infra-umbilical curved incision using Hasson's (open) technique. The abdominal pressure is kept between 8 and 12 mmHg. The insufflation rate depends on the size of the patient. It is a safe practice to keep the insufflation rate low, between 0.5 and 1.5 L/min. If the equipment is used jointly by adult surgeons or the gynaecologist, it is not unusual for the insufflation pressures to be set at high, and it is crucial for the paediatric surgeons to check the insufflation rate and pressures before each use. The other three ports are inserted under direct vision. Two of the ports are for the operator and the third port is for retraction. The position of the working ports depend on the size of the patient. In an adult size patient, the port used for operator's right hand is below the costo-chondral junction to the left side of the midline, and the left-hand port is in the mid-clavicle line at a level midway between the costal margin and the level of the umbilicus. In a small child, the right-hand port is moved further laterally and inferiorly, and the left-hand port can also be moved further down to give more operating space.

The retraction can be performed using a snake retractor, which is held by an assistant, or attached to a fixed arm. If using an assistant to hold the snake retractor, the port is inserted near the right iliac fossa with the port insertion facing towards the gall bladder so that there is no traction and displacement of the tissues when the port is being held with the retractor. If the port insertion direction is not in the direction where the port will be facing during surgery, it can cause undue traction on the wound and increased pain and worse scarring.

The surgeon stands on the left side of the patient. The assistant stands on the right side and can hold the camera in the right hand and the retractor in the left hand. If the assistant is not experienced, then two separate assistants may be required: one to hold the camera, who can stand on the left side of the patient behind the surgeon, and the other assistant, holding the retractor, will stand on the right side of the patient. The nurse can stand on the right side of the patient as there will be more space for the nurse and the trolley on the right side.

If using a fixed retraction, a Nathanson retractor can be used. The Nathanson comes with different size blades and is inserted through the right subcostal stab incision. The angled part of the retractor lifts the right lobe and porta and should be positioned so that it does not impinge on the gall bladder. In our experience dynamic snake retractor is more versatile since it can be moved to where more retraction is required; however, it does need an assistant.

In adult practice surgeons prefer retraction using Johann's grasping forceps. The grasping forceps holds the fundus of the gall bladder and pulls it above the liver, thus retracting the gall bladder and the liver and opening the triangle of dissection. In author's opinion, this technique, known as the Reddick-Olsen [4], is a potentially unsafe technique in the paediatric group. In adult patients most of the cholecystectomies are performed for cholecystitis, in which the gall bladder wall is fairly thick. In the paediatric group, most of the cholecystectomies are performed for gall stones or possibly gall bladder polyps in which the gall bladder wall is not thick. If the gall bladder fundus is held by Johann and pushed above the liver to retract the liver, the gall bladder can rupture. In most cases this retraction is performed by a junior doctor, and the camera and operator are not looking at this site as they will be concentrating on the dissection which starts in the porta hepatis. The retraction of the fundus is out of the field of view of the camera, and any undue push by Johann's grasper will damage the gall bladder. Having said that, in some situations Hartmann's pouch may not be obvious or can be quite oedematous and thick because of infection or it could be compacted with stones, which will make it impossible to hold. In this scenario the body or fundus retraction may be necessary.

The surgery proceeds with initial evaluation of the abdomen and pelvis, and the dissection starts by retraction of Hartmann's pouch performed by operator's left hand using Johann's grasper. The lateral GB traction with a grasper and countertraction of the liver with the liver retractor opens Calot's triangle and the triangle of the dissection. The triangle of the dissection is the area between the liver and the gall bladder and the upper margins of the cystic artery and sometimes cystic duct. The operator starts by removing any congenital or inflammatory adhesions between the omentum and the gall bladder by using with monopolar hook dissector. Scissors may be used, on a monopolar with spreading and cutting. The visceral peritoneal layer is incised close to Hartmann's pouch and the underlying fat dissected to expose the cystic duct and the cystic artery. In most cases the cystic duct is inferior to the cystic artery and can be exposed before the cystic artery. It is quite common for the cystic duct to take a tortuous course, where it arises towards the porta hepatis, before turning inferiorly to join the common hepatic duct. It can travel adjacent to the right hepatic duct. The pulsations of the cystic artery may be visible and guide the operator. The cystic artery usually arises from the right hepatic artery and divides into the anterior and posterior cystic arteries. It is not unusual for it to arise from the left or even the main hepatic artery. On occasions the anterior and posterior cystic arteries arise separately from different sources. It is important for the operator to be aware of the possible variations anomalies. It is useful to expose the cystic artery and the cystic duct before ligating/stapling or cutting.

It is crucial to confirm that the cystic duct is connected to Hartmann's pouch. The dissection should stay close to Hartmann's pouch where it joins the cystic duct. It is not uncommon for the cystic duct to be very short and stubby, and performing dissection away from Hartmann's pouch carries a danger of incorrectly assuming that the duct entering that area is the cystic duct as in cases of a short cystic duct the common hepatic duct may give the impression that it is a cystic duct and can be ligated or damaged inadvertently. Depending upon the availability of the instrumentation and experience of the surgeon, the cystic duct and cystic artery can either be clipped using commercially available clip applicators, they can also be ligated or transfixed. If using clip applicators, most applicators are inserted through a 5-mm port. Some of the clip applicators can fire clips which although can be inserted through a 5-mm port but fire 8-mm clips, which is useful for a dilated cystic duct. If the cystic duct is large, it can be ligated first and then clipped. Ligation helps to reduce the size of the duct. There are single mounted clips which can go around bigger ducts.

Once the cystic duct and cystic artery is clipped and cut, the rest of the dissection involves lifting the gall bladder from the gall bladder fossa. The safest and easiest way is to use a monopolar hook. The dissection is facilitated by retraction of the gall bladder. If the gall bladder is not retracted appropriately to make the tissues tense, the monopolar dissector will cause charring and will not cut properly. Charring of the tissues will make the anatomy obscure. It is important to stay close to the wall of the gall bladder if possible. This is to avoid damage to the duct of Luschka, which if present travels in the gall bladder fossa and can enter the right hepatic duct, the left hepatic duct and sometimes the cystic duct. If the duct of Luschka gets damaged, it may not be apparent straight away, and it can cause bile leak in the post-operative period. The left-hand grasper holding the gall bladder can be rolled, known as the spaghetti manoeuvre [5] which reduces the need to pull the hand too far away from the gall bladder fossa to apply appropriate traction.

Once the gall bladder is detached from the gall bladder fossa, examination of the gall bladder fossa and porta hepatis is performed. Any small bleeding areas on the liver surface can be touched with diathermy. It is important to examine the cystic duct and cystic artery to make sure that the clips have not been dislodged during the dissection.

The gall bladder can be removed using a commercially available retrieval bag. In author's department, we tend not to use a bag unless necessary. The author removes the gall bladder through the umbilical port site, which is the biggest of all. The neck of the gall bladder is held by Johann's forceps and directed towards the camera port while looking at it with the telescope. Once the neck or the instrument is in the port, the port is gradually pulled out, and the gall bladder neck held with a clip externally and gradually pulled out on the surface. If the gall bladder is large, it can be aspirated by opening or with a syringe, making sure not to drip any bile into the wound or in the abdomen. The wound can be packed with a gauze swab. Sometimes, the gall bladder is full of stones which can be removed under vision using a small forceps before gradually pulling the gall bladder out completely. The umbilical port is closed using a box stitch for the fascia with 2/0 (or smaller) absorbable multifilament suture. The 5-mm ports are removed, and deep muscle stitches placed using absorbable multifilament sutures. If there has been any bleeding during surgery that can be sucked out or washed with a warm saline. A nasogastric tube is left in for the post-operative period, which can be removed on the ward once the child is able to drink and eat. Most children are able to drink, eat and mobilise the same day.

37.6 Single-Port Cholecystectomy [6]

Over the years there has been an increased interest and experience in single-port cholecystectomy. Single-port technique employs the use of commercially available gel ports which are inserted through a 2.5 cm incision. One of the limitations of single-port technique is the fact that the instruments which are curved have to be inserted to a certain length for them to be effective. If the abdominal cavity is small, it makes the use of crossed/curved instruments difficult. Stab wounds to the umbilical fascia for curved or straight instruments is an option. The use of straight instruments requires quite intricate movements which are difficult to learn, however feasible in experienced hands. The fact that most of the dissection is performed in a very small area makes this procedure suitable for a single-port technique using straight instruments.

37.6.1 Notes

Natural Orifice Transluminal Endoscopic Surgery was actively taken up by some progressive people. However, it is too early to say whether this approach will be used in paediatric practice. Although gastrointestinal system has been used for a NOTES cholecystectomy, most NOTES cholecystectomies are performed through a transvaginal approach. The first transvaginal cholecystectomy was performed by Zorrón et al. in 2007, from Rio de Janeiro [7]. A recent article published in Gastrointestinal Endoscopy compared transvaginal NOTES cholecystectomy with laparoscopic cholecystectomy and found that patients experienced less pain with NOTES [8]. However, there was an increased risk of adverse events following NOTES (bleeding in two patients, gall bladder rupture in one). Although transvaginal NOTES cholecystectomy is gaining increasing acceptance in adult practice and is an attractive alternative to cholecystectomy in female patients, it is unlikely that it will be adopted in the paediatric population.

37.7 Small Calibre Instrument Cholecystectomy [9]

The advantages of minimal access surgery are in part due to its minimal invasiveness. If procedures could be performed using finer-caliber instruments, these advantages could be amplified. In 1998 Kimura developed 3-mm caliber instruments and performed laparoscopic cholecystectomy in 20 patients using one 5-mm and two 3-mm instrument ports. The results were retrospectively compared with those of standard laparoscopic cholecystectomies. The operating time was 107.2 ± 50.0 min, there were no complications, the number of doses of analgesia required was 0.80 ± 0.83, and post-operative hospital stay was 4.9 ± 1.2 days, which was not significantly different from the standard laparoscopic cholecystectomy. At 6 months post-operatively, the scars were smaller. They did not find that the surgery using fine-caliber instruments was more difficult than standard laparoscopic procedure.

37.8 Difficult Situations

It is imperative that the surgeon performing laparoscopic cholecystectomy is familiar with biliary anatomy and its variations and anomalies. The reader is referred to the Atlas of Biliary Anatomy. Difficult or challenging situations may arise during cholecystectomy due to a variety of reasons. The difficulties can be due to patient factors like obesity, aberrant biliary or vascular anatomy, heterotaxia and situs inversus, preduodenal portal vein, difficult acute pathology and on occasions non-availability or inappropriate size of the instruments, especially for small children.

Bleeding: One of the drawbacks of minimal access approach is the fact that any bleeding visualised by the camera is exacerbated because of the enlarged picture. Although injury to major vasculature is possible, most bleeding happens from small vessels which can be stopped with diathermy or pressure. It is always useful to clip and cut the cystic artery before dissecting the gall bladder. In the event of bleeding from a branch of a cystic artery on the gall bladder wall, away from the porta hepatis, which can be encountered in a difficult case and retrograde dissection, the bleeding area can be held with an instrument and diathermy applied blindly. In situations where a bleeding point is close to the porta hepatis or not visualised and/or obscured by a pool of blood pressure can be applied with a swab inserted through one of the ports. It is possible to insert a 5 × 5 swab or a dental pack through the port. The pressure can be applied for few minutes after which the area is washed and sucked to visualise. Another option is to use a haemostatic agent which works on intrinsic and extrinsic mechanisms for haemostasis. This approach will also require pressure on the area for a few minutes. After waiting for few minutes, the excess material can be washed away and dissection completed. On very few occasions where the surgeon finds it difficult to stop the bleeding, pressure should be applied using a small swab, while help should be asked for, and conversion to open technique is recommended.

Infection: In a very small percentage of children, a cholecystectomy is performed for acute or chronic cholecystitis. The role of antibiotics in acute cholecystitis is not clearly established; however, our practice is to give antibiotics at the time of diagnosis of the acute condition. The antibiotics are continued for a period of 48–72 h after surgery. In adult practice there is evidence from meta-analysis that the complication rates in patients undergoing early operation for acute cholecystitis are not significantly different to the ones undergoing late procedures [10].

In acute or chronic cholecystitis, it may be difficult to dissect cystic duct and cystic artery. In such conditions retrograde cholecystectomy approach can be employed. If performing a retrograde (fundus-down/fundus-first) cholecystectomy, it is crucial to continually evaluate and examine the relationship of the porta hepatis and dissection, as it is not difficult to dissect too far towards the porta hepatis without realising. In extreme conditions, where neither retrograde nor antegrade dissection is possible, the technique of sub-total cholecystectomy, used in open surgery, can be adopted for laparoscopic cholecystectomy. In this technique the gall bladder is aspirated and opened. If there are any stones in the gall bladder, it is advisable to insert a small bag or finger of a glove to catch all the stones in the bag. The gall bladder is cut in the middle using a diathermy. The wall of the gall bladder attached to the liver can be left in place. The gall bladder is visualised from inside and dissection of the wall extended slowly towards the cystic duct entry site. Once the cystic duct entry site is reached, a non-absorbable purse string suture can be applied from within the gall bladder to occlude the lumen of the cystic duct. In this approach it is not necessary to dissect the cystic artery, since the small branches of the cystic artery would have been occluded and dissected while cutting the gall bladder wall with the diathermy.

Biliary Problems: Bile ducts can be injured during cholecystectomy. In paediatric practice the ducts are fairly small in size. Although repair of a duct is possible, especially if only one side of the wall is breached, there is a high risk of biliary leak and stricture. T-tube repairs are not frequently employed in paediatric practice; however, it is a time-proven technique, which can be used in such situations. In paediatric practice the size limitations of T-tube is a drawback. If the injury happens due to diathermy, it can be quite extensive. The safest approach to repair a damage to the common bile duct, hepatic ducts or the common hepatic duct is to create a Roux-en-Y hepatico-jejunostomy. In experienced hands this can be performed by laparoscopic techniques; however, if the surgeon has not performed laparoscopic choledochal cyst procedures, the safest approach would be to convert and perform hepatico-jejunostomy as an open procedure.

Access: Paediatric patients come in all sizes and shapes, ranging from very emaciated children who have thin abdominal wall and limited fat in their omentum to obese teenagers who have the physical attributes of large adults. All techniques need to be adjusted according to their size and habitus of the patient. In difficult cases it is recommended to insert further ports to retract and help the dissection.

Biliary Stones: In author's department, all symptomatic children undergoing

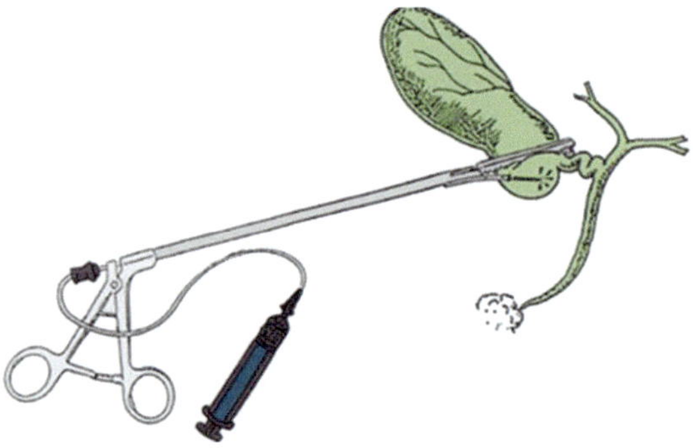

Fig. 37.3 An operative cholangiogram can be performed by using a Kumar clamp®(KC-002 Fig. 1) (Nashville Surgical Instruments) which consists of a Johann-shaped grasper with a lumen for a cholangiogram catheter. The lumen is directed such that once the grasper is applied at Hartmann's pouch the catheter inserted through the channel will enter Hartmann's pouch for the injection of the contrast

cholecystectomy undergo a preoperative ultrasound following admission for cholecystectomy. If stones are noted in the bile ducts, the simplest approach to deal is to perform cholecystectomy and ERCP at two separate settings. It is not necessary to be regimental about the sequence of the ERCP and cholecystectomy procedures. The sequence may depend upon the local condition in the department. The author prefers to perform cholecystectomy first, simply because it may be possible to flush the biliary duct stones at the time of cholecystectomy. The instruments available for bile duct exploration are large in size and not suitable in paediatric practice. There is a high risk of damage to the biliary duct by the blind use of forceps. Flushing the duct using saline may flush the sludge and dislodge the stones. A gentle suction using a nasogastric tube inserted through the cystic duct can also suck sludge and the stone and/or may push the stone through the sphincter into the duodenum. Any attempts at laparoscopic bile duct exploration should be taken with extreme precaution and only by highly experienced surgeons [11].

An operative cholangiogram can be performed by using a Kumar clamp® (KC-002 Fig. 37.3) (Nashville Surgical Instruments) which consists of a Johann-shaped grasper with a lumen for a cholangiogram catheter (Fig. 37.3). The lumen is directed such that once the grasper is applied at Hartmann's pouch the catheter inserted through the channel will enter Hartmann's pouch for the injection of the contrast. The grasper stops the contrast from entering the gall bladder. If a Kumar clamp is not available, Johann's grasper could be inserted through a 5-mm port. The Johann should be applied at the junction of Hartmann's pouch and the gall bladder and can be left to stand on its own on a ratchet. Following this, a catheter or a long (spinal) needle can be inserted directly through the abdominal wall and with the help of another instrument can be guided into Hartmann's pouch for the injection of the contrast. It is important to make sure there are no air bubbles in the catheter or the syringe, and the catheter and the syringe and the needle are pre-flushed with the contrast material.

Carcinoma: Carcinoma of the biliary system and gall bladder is extremely rare in paediatric practice. The author has the experience of one patient who presented with a carcinoma of the cystic duct, blocking the gall bladder. In a situation like this, there may be unusual findings in the ultrasound, which may include space-occupying lesion or a mass filling the lumen of the gall bladder or the biliary ducts. The gall bladder wall or the biliary duct wall may be thickened. Calcifications may be noted in the wall of the biliary system. In most cases the gall bladder cancers are discovered in the operating theatre [12].

37.9 Outcomes

A large review based on 80,000 cases worldwide between 1990 and 1998 has suggested an overall mortality rate of 1.2% following laparoscopic cholecystectomy. The morbidity rate was around 7%, while 5% of the cases were converted to open based on the 14 studies reviewed. The mean length of stay was 1.8 days with a mean return-to-work time of 6 days [12].

In another review in 2005 of 1674 consecutive laparoscopic cholecystectomies, Misra [13] and colleagues reported the following complications:

- Cystic duct leaks 0.63%
- Duct of Luschka leaks 0.52%

- Post-operative haemorrhage 0.42%
- Wound infection 0.94%
- Wound herniation 1.4%
- Deep vein thrombosis 0.31%

The serious complications of laparoscopic cholecystectomy include bile duct injury, bile duct leaks, bleeding and bowel injury. Most of these complications happen because of poor patient selection, surgical inexperience or technical constraints. One should know their limits, and if a safe dissection cannot be ensured laparoscopically, early conversion to an open approach should be accepted as the proper course.

A national survey of 2292 hospitals, performed in the USA, analysing over 77,000 cases, suggested that laparotomy was required for the treatment of complication in 1.2% of cases [14]. The mean rate of bile duct injury was 0.6% and was significantly lower at institutions that had performed more than 100 cases. In half of the cases, bile duct injuries were recognised in the post-operative period and frequently required anastomotic repair. Intraoperative cholangiography was practised selectively by 52% of the respondents and routinely by 31%. Bowel and vascular injuries occurred in 0.14% and 0.25% of cases, respectively, and were the most lethal complications. Post-operative bile leak was recognised in 0.3% of patients, most commonly originating from the cystic duct. Eighteen of 33 post-operative deaths resulted from operative injury. Data suggested that cholecystectomy performed laparoscopically was associated with a low risk of morbidity and mortality but a significant rate of milder injury. It also suggested that there is limited scope for an occasional surgeon to perform biliary procedures.

37.10 In Summary

Laparoscopy has revolutionised cholecystectomy. The technique has a low risk of complications, which is further lowered if the surgeons performing the technique have high throughput of cases.

The spectrum of cholelithiasis and cholecystitis is changing in children, and cholecystectomy is becoming an increasingly common procedure in children [15]. In paediatric practice we cannot apply the same techniques of dissection used for adult patients. In centres with access to robotic programme, cholecystectomy is being performed robotically with superior outcomes (personal experience).

References

1. Morgenstern L. Carl Langenbuch and the first cholecystectomy. Surg Endosc. 1992;6(3):113–4.
2. Bobbs JS. Case of lithotomy of the gallbladder. Trans Indiana Mod Soc. 1868;18:68.
3. Reynolds W Jr. The first laparoscopic cholecystectomy. JSLS. 2001;5:89–94.
4. Reddick EJ, Olsen DO, Span A, et al. Safe performance of difficult laparoscopic cholecystectomies. Am J Surg. 1991;161:377–81.
5. Durai R, Ng PC. "Spaghetti technique"-novel technique to facilitate laparoscopic appendicectomy and cholecystectomy. J Laparoendosc Adv Surg Tech A. 2009;19(5):667–8. https://doi.org/10.1089/lap.2009.0024.
6. Piskun G, Rajpal S. Transumbilical laparoscopic cholecystectomy utilizes no incisions outside the umbilicus. J Laparoendosc Adv Surg Tech A. 1999;9(4):361–4.
7. Zorrón R, Filgueiras M, Maggioni LC, Pombo L, Lopes Carvalho G, Lacerda Oliveira A. NOTES. Transvaginal cholecystectomy: report of the first case. Surg Innov. 2007;14(4):279–83.
8. Benhidjeb T, et al. Laparoscopic cholecystectomy versus transvaginal natural orifice transluminal endoscopic surgery cholecystectomy: results of a prospective-comparative single-center study. Gastrointest Endosc. 2018;87(2):509–16.
9. Kimura T, Sakuramachi S, Yoshida M, Kobayashi T, Takeuchi Y. Laparoscopic cholecystectomy using fine-caliber instruments. Surg Endosc. 1998;12(3):283–6. (ISSN: 0930-2794).
10. Gurusamy KS, Samraj K. Early versus delayed laparoscopic cholecystectomy for acute cholecystectomy. Cochrane Database Syst Rev. 2006;(4):CD005440.
11. Shah RS, Blakley ML, Lobe TE. The role of laparoscopy in the management of common bile duct obstruction in children. Surg Endosc. 2001;15:1353–5.
12. Harris HW. Chapter 47: biliary system. In: Norton JA, Barie PS, et al., editors. Surgery: basic science and clinical evidence. 2nd ed. New York: Springer; 2008. p. 911–42.
13. Misra M, Schiff J, Rendon G, Rothschild J, Schwaitzberg S. Laparoscopic cholecystectomy after

the learning curve: what should we expect? Surg Endosc. 2005;19:1266–71.
14. Deziel DJ, Millikan KW, Economou SG, Doolas A, Ko S-T, Airan MC. Complications of laparoscopic cholecystectomy: a national survey of 4,292 hospitals and an analysis of 77,604 cases. Am J Surg. 1993;165(1):9–14.
15. Waldhausen JH, Benjamin DR. Cholecystectomy is becoming an increasingly common operation in children. Am J Surg. 1999;177(5):364–7.

Laparoscopic Pancreatic Surgery 38

David C. van der Zee

38.1 Introduction

Pancreatic tumors in children are rare [1]. A 38-year retrospective single-institute study revealed only 14 patients with pseudopapillary neoplasms being the most frequent with 6 cases, followed by insulinoma ($N = 3$). There were two neoplastic tumors. Furthermore focal or diffuse hyperinsulinism in infancy may be encountered [2, 3].

Depending on the underlying tumor, symptomatology may vary from pain to symptoms related to hypoglycemia, such as lethargy, seizures, and drowsiness [4].

Diagnostic assessment comprises ultrasound and CT scan preferably combined with 18FDOPA-positron emission tomography (PETscan) [5].

In children with congenital hyperinsulinism initially, medical treatment may be undertaken with diazoxide and/or octreotide, but in case of failure of medical treatment, surgical approach is warranted [1, 2, 4].

38.2 Preoperative Preparation

All patients receive a rectal washout or clysma the evening before surgery to empty the fore lying colon. The procedure is performed under general anesthesia with muscle relaxants to ensure proper insufflation without too high pressures. If necessary for frequent glucose determination, an arterial line is added. A urine catheter is inserted when a prolonged procedure is to be expected. No antibiotics are indicated.

38.3 Positioning

The patient is placed in a supine position, in smaller children at the lower end of the table with the legs bent in a frog position. The surgeon stands at the feet of the operating table with the assistant at his right side and the scrub nurse on his left. The monitor is above the head of the patient.

38.4 Instrumentation

A 5 mm trocar is placed in the umbilicus for the camera. Two to three 3½ mm reusable trocars and instruments are used: two Maryland graspers, monopolar hook, scissors, flexible retractor if necessary, and suction device. In more extensive dissections/resections, a 3 or 5 mm sealing device

D. C. van der Zee (✉)
Department of Pediatric Surgery, Wilhelmina Children's Hospital, University Medical Center Utrecht, Utrecht, The Netherlands
e-mail: d.c.vanderzee@umcutrecht.nl

C. Esposito et al. (eds.), *ESPES Manual of Pediatric Minimally Invasive Surgery*,
https://doi.org/10.1007/978-3-030-00964-9_38

can be used and a retrieval bag for taking out the specimen. Nowadays also a 5 mm stapler is available.

38.5 Technique

The first 5 mm trocar is placed in the lower crease of the umbilicus through an open technique to allow later retrieval of the specimen. The trocar is fixed to the fascia with a suture Vicryl 2×0. A silastic tubing can be placed over the trocar to prevent sliding of the trocar.

Under direct vision two additional 3 mm trocars are placed in the left and right mid abdomen. After making a small stab incision, the defect can be enlarged with small mosquitos to facilitate the trocar placement (Fig. 38.1).

After identifying the stomach, two stay sutures can be placed in the larger curvature to lift up the stomach and allow entry of the bursa omentalis through the gastrocolic ligament (Fig. 38.2). After creating a large enough window, the pancreas can be seen. The large magnification of the endoscope sometimes allows for the (endocrine) tumor to be identified immediately. In case of a solitary tumor, the tissue can be dissected with the 3 mm diathermia hook, which allows very selective dissection (Fig. 38.3). The tissue can be placed in a glove finger and sent for frozen section determination. If the DOPA-PET scan has detected only a solitary hot spot, the procedure can be terminated with removal of trocars under direct vision and closure of all defects.

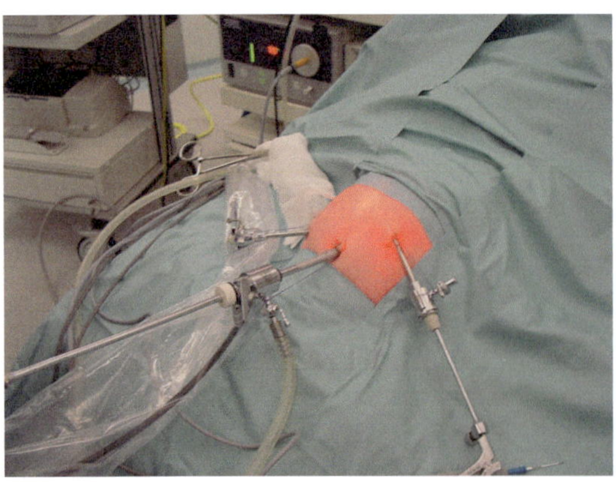

Fig. 38.1 Position of trocars in laparoscopic approach of pancreatic lesion in infant

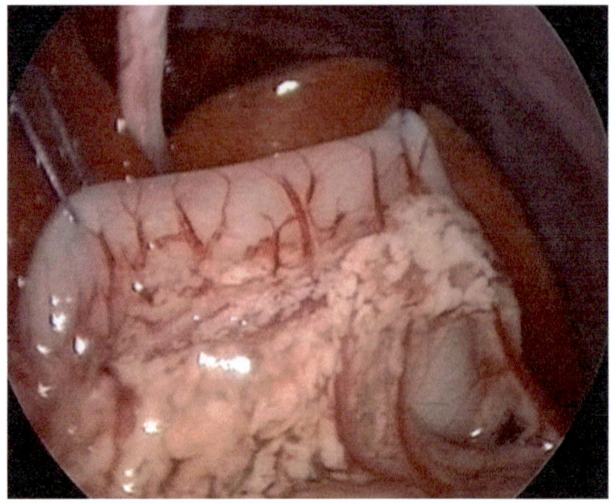

Fig. 38.2 Stay sutures in greater curvature of the stomach to lift the stomach up in order to get entry into the bursa omentalis

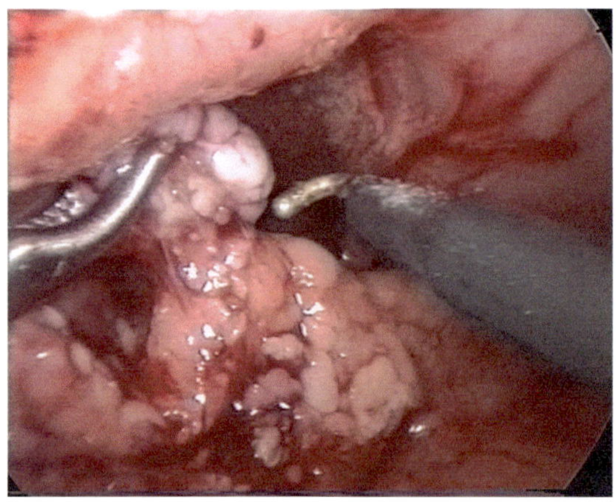

Fig. 38.3 Resection of focal lesion in infant with hyperinsulinism

In case of a more diffuse lesion, the dissection is started at the tail of the pancreas with meticulously taking down all small vessels arising from the splenic vein with the 3 mm diathermia hook, making sure the splenic vein is spared. Working from the tail toward the head of the pancreas until the choledochal duct is reached. The pancreatic duct is closed with a transfixing suture or a clip and transected (Fig. 38.4). In case of a subtotal resection, the dissection is continued until only a rim along the descending

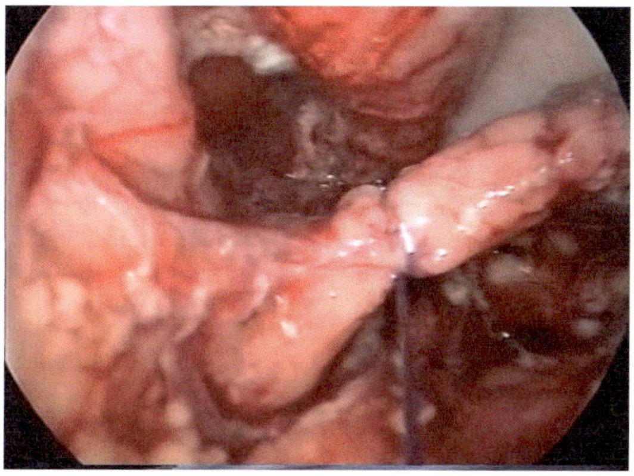

Fig. 38.4 Resection of pancreas tail in more diffuse lesion of hyperinsulinism

duodenum is left. The specimen can be taken out with a retrieval bag by slightly enlarging the subumbilical incision. As usually little cicatrization is formed during laparoscopic dissection, it can be decided to initially leave a little more tissue in place and see if insulin levels normalize postoperatively. If further excision is necessary, this can easily be carried out laparoscopically at a later stage.

38.6 Postoperative Care

Monitoring of glucose levels continue until they have stabilized. Oral feeds can be resumed a few hours after surgery. Most patients will have caudal analgesia for the first 24 h and continue on paracetamol on indication. Discharge is dependent on the stability of glucose levels. The first 5 days, the child can be washed and rinsed of. Thereafter they may bath again.

38.7 Results

All focal lesions in neonates were cured in one session.

A few of the cases with multiple focal lesions needed two procedures to remove all lesions.

The cases with diffuse lesions underwent a subtotal pancreatectomy. In one patient thrombosis of the splenic vein occurred.

38.8 Discussion

In children pancreatic tumors are usually of benign origin, although some malignant tumors have been described [6, 7]. Congenital hyperinsulinism in infancy is more common in children and is characterized by inappropriate oversecretion of insulin, resulting in hypoglycemia [8]. If medical care is not sufficient, surgical management is warranted. It is sometimes difficult to determine the appropriate level of resection to cure the disease and not induce diabetes [9].

To determine the extent of the lesion, the additional use of 18FDOPA-PET scan has proven to be useful [5]. With the use of this technique, we were able to find and treat the focal lesions.

The use of laparoscopy in children was first described by Bax et al. [2]. The advantage of laparoscopy is the huge magnification of 18×, which is much more than can be achieved with binoculars. Also the minimal incisions and no-touch technique causes much less cicatrication and therefore leaves room for a more conservative initial resection in order to avoid diabetes. Later re-resection does not cause much problems.

Although the procedure is straight forward, it is advisable to concentrate the surgical management for these lesions in high-volume centers of expertise [4].

References

1. Nasher O, Hall NJ, Sebire NJ, De Coppi P, Pierro A. Pancreatic tumours in children: diagnosis, treatment and outcome. Pediatr Surg Int. 2015;31:831–5.
2. Bax NM, van der Zee DC, de Vroede M, Jansen M, Nikkels J. Laparoscopic identification and removal of focal lesions in persistent hyperinsulinemic hypoglycemia of infancy. Surg Endosc. 2003;17(5):833.
3. Bax KN, van der Zee DC. The laparoscopic approach toward hyperinsulinism in children. Semin Pediatr Surg. 2007;16(4):245–51.
4. Esposito C, De Lagausie P, Escolino M, Saxena A, Holcomb GW 3rd, Settimi A, Becmeur F, van der Zee D. Laparoscopic resection of pancreatic tumors in children: results of a multicentric survey. J Laparoendosc Adv Surg Tech A. 2017;27(5):533–8.
5. Laje P, States LJ, Zhuang H, Becker SA, Palladino AA, Stanley CA, Adzick NS. Accuracy of PET/CT

scan in the diagnosis of the focal form of congenital hyperinsulinism. J Pediatr Surg. 2013;48:388–93.

6. Namgoong JM, Kim DY, Kim SC, Kim SC, Hwang JH, Song KB. Laparoscopic distal pancreatectomy to treat solid pseudopapillary tumors in children: transition from open to laparoscopic approaches in suitable cases. Pediatr Surg Int. 2014;30:259–66.
7. Verhoef S, van Diemen-Steenvoorde R, Akkersdijk WL, Bax NM, Ariyurek Y, Hermans CJ, van Nieuwenhuizen O, Nikkels PG, Lindhout D, Halley DJ, Lips K, van den Ouweland AM. Malignant pancreatic tumour within the spectrum of tuberous sclerosis complex in childhood. Eur J Pediatr. 1999;158(4):284–7.
8. Pierro A, Nah SA. Surgical management of congenital hyperinsulinism of infancy. Semin Pediatr Surg. 2011;20:50–3.
9. Menni F, de Lonlay P, Sevin C, Touati G, Peigne´ C, Barbier V, Nihoul-Fékété C, Saudubray JM, Robert JJ. Neurologic outcomes of 90 neonates and infants with persistent hyperinsulinemic hypoglycemia. Pediatrics. 2001;107:476–9.

Laparoscopic Splenectomy

39

Catarina Barroso and Jorge Correia-Pinto

39.1 Introduction

In the pediatric age group, splenectomy has been performed mostly for hematologic disorders, such as hereditary spherocytosis, idiopathic thrombocytopenic purpura, and sickle cell anemia. Throughout the history of splenectomy, two major events influenced clinical practice to what it is today. Those were (1) the realization of children's susceptibility to infection after splenectomy, by King and Shumaker in 1952, leading pediatric physicians to embrace conservative approaches for splenic diseases and injuries [1], and (2) the advent of laparoscopic splenectomy first described for adults, by Delaitre in 1991 [2], and then for children, by Tulman in 1993 [3]. Reduced postoperative pain, shorter length of stay, and improved cosmesis made laparoscopic splenectomy the standard of care when spleen removal is indicated [1, 2]. Over the years, there were reports of increased costs (for longer operative time) and inadequate detection of accessory spleens and splenosis [2, 3]. These were overcome by more recent studies, including a meta-analysis from 2016, revealing lower overall costs (considering shorter hospitalization), less blood loss, similar rate of removal of accessory spleens, and postoperative complications. Conversion rates in pediatric series range from 0 to 6% and have been mainly for bleeding and splenomegaly [1, 2]. Nevertheless, similar postoperative outcomes have been reported for enlarged spleens, except for operative time.

39.2 Anatomical Considerations

Anatomic relations and attachments of the spleen must be understood to perform a safe splenectomy. Lying in the upper quadrant of the abdomen, between the diaphragm and the stomach, the spleen is in close contact to the colon, pancreas, and left kidney whose impressions are marked in its visceral surface (inferiorly and medially). Three attachments hold the spleen in its position: splenorenal, splenocolic, and gastrosplenic ligaments. Between the two layers of the splenorenal ligament, there are the hilum splenic vessels and also the tail of the pancreas. The gastrosplenic ligament is likewise composed of two layers, between which the short gastric arteries and left gastroepiploic artery course.

C. Barroso · J. Correia-Pinto (✉)
Pediatric Surgery Department, Hospital de Braga, Braga, Portugal

Life and Health Sciences Research Institute (ICVS), School of Medicine, University of Minho, Braga, Portugal

ICVS/3B's—PT Government Associate Laboratory, Braga/Guimarães, Portugal
e-mail: catarina.barroso@hospitaldebraga.pt; jcp@med.uminho.pt

C. Esposito et al. (eds.), *ESPES Manual of Pediatric Minimally Invasive Surgery*,
https://doi.org/10.1007/978-3-030-00964-9_39

39.3 Indications for Splenectomy

Over the years, there has been a change in the paradigm of the treatment of splenic conditions. Considering the risk of postoperative overwhelming sepsis, especially among children under 1-year-old, the indications for splenectomy have become more and more restricted. With the tremendous improvement in pediatric trauma care, we now know that an emergent splenectomy is hardly required, as nonoperative treatment is successful in 95–100% of blunt splenic lesions [1]. Even in hematologic conditions, the development of new medical therapies led to the replacement of an early surgical approach to a "wait and see" attitude, by postponing or avoiding splenectomy. Listed below are the most common conditions requiring splenectomy nowadays.

39.3.1 Hereditary Spherocytosis (HS)

HS is a genetic condition, with autosomal dominant transmission. A deficiency of spectrin, a cytoskeletal protein of the red blood cell, leads to a membrane abnormality resulting in spherical, small erythrocytes, susceptible of entrapment and destruction in the spleen. Hemolytic anemia with jaundice and splenomegaly should spur the diagnosis, which ought to be confirmed by a peripheral blood smear with spherocytes, increased reticulocyte count, and negative Coombs test. Splenectomy reduces the rate of hemolysis leading to anemia resolution [1].

39.3.2 Idiopathic Thrombocytopenic Purpura (ITP)

ITP is an autoimmune disorder defined by a transient or persistent reduced platelet count (<100,000/μL) and increased risk of spontaneous bleeding. While the physiopathology is not well understood, it includes impaired platelet production and T-cell-mediated actions [1]. Children with ITP mostly experience spontaneous resolution, whereas 20% develops chronic disease. Despite the paucity of guidelines for the treatment of this condition, it is consensual that splenectomy should be performed (1) in life-threatening hemorrhage complicating acute ITP and (2) in chronic ITP with significant bleeding, who do not respond or cannot tolerate other therapies (corticosteroids, immunoglobulin, anti-D) [1]. Following splenectomy, approximately two thirds of the patients achieve complete response with normalization of platelet count and require no additional therapy [2].

39.3.3 Sickle Cell Anemia (SCA)

SCA is an autosomal recessive disease involving a mutated form of hemoglobin, the hemoglobin S (HbS). Under low oxygen arterial pressure, the abnormal hemoglobin polymerizes and distorts the red blood cell into a sickle shape. The sickled erythrocytes will block small blood vessels resulting in tissue damaging. Also, there is erythrocyte entrapment in the spleen (splenic sequestration) causing enlargement, pooling, and destruction of the sickle red blood cells leading to anemia. SCA usually manifests early in childhood. Presentation may occur with vaso-occlusive crisis causing episodes of pain, chronic hemolytic anemia, splenic sequestration, increased risk of infection particularly by encapsulated bacteria, and acute chest syndrome (chest pain, fever, cough, tachypnea, leukocytosis, and pulmonary infiltrates in the upper lobes). Diagnosis is confirmed by an electrophoresis identifying a homozygous HbS. Splenectomy is indicated in the presence of one major or two minor crisis of acute splenic sequestration, once it is associated with a high mortality rate. In children with hypersplenism, splenectomy decreased transfusion requirements and eliminated discomfort caused by the enlarged spleen. Moreover, autosplenectomy can occur in SCA patients due to splenic infarctions secondary to vaso-occlusion which is not uncommon. Children with SCA are likely to develop cholelithiasis; thus they should undergo routine abdominal ultrasound preoperatively, and if gallstones are identified, a concomitant cholecystectomy is advocated [1].

39.3.4 Other Indications

Other indications for splenectomy in children are β-thalassemia, Hodgkin's disease, Gaucher's disease, splenic abscess, leukemia, or lymphoma [1, 2].

39.4 Preoperative Management

All children undergoing a splenectomy should receive vaccinations for *Streptococcus pneumoniae* and *Neisseria meningitidis*, at least 2 weeks before surgery. *Haemophilus influenzae* type B is now part of routine childhood immunizations, and an additional immunization is not usually required. A preoperative abdominal ultrasonography should be done in children with hemolytic anemia to evaluate the presence of gallstones and need for concomitant cholecystectomy. There is some debate on whether imaging for accessory spleens is necessary. It does not seem to be useful as sensitivity and specificity of computed tomography for detecting accessory spleens are 60% and 95.6%, respectively, whereas of laparoscopy are 93.3% and 100%, respectively [2]. Children with SCA should be prepared for surgery with adequate hydration with intravenous fluids since the night before surgery and red blood cell transfusions to increase the hemoglobin level to 10–12 g/dL. In splenomegaly, if conditions are available, perioperative spleen embolization might decrease splenic volume and facilitate dissection. Despite minor postoperative complications, possibly due to the microparticle injection, it is believed to reduce intraoperative blood loss, conversion to open surgery, and the need for transfusion [1, 2].

39.5 Surgical Technique

39.5.1 Laparoscopic Splenectomy

The procedure is performed under general anesthesia, with the patient positioned in right lateral decubitus, at approximately 45°. The surgeon stands in front of the patient, with the assistant at his right side. The monitor is placed at the patient's back. A 5 mm trocar (30° optics) is placed at the umbilicus, followed by a 12 mm port in the left lower quadrant and one or two 3 mm ports throughout the epigastric midline. Insufflation pressure should be between 8 and 12 mmHg depending on the patient's age. The gastrosplenic ligament is divided at first. By grasping the stomach with an atraumatic grasper, the gastrosplenic ligament is retracted enabling the division of the short gastric vessels. This should be performed using a *LigaSure*, an *Ultracision* or by isolating each vessel and applying clips. After dividing the short gastric vessels, retraction of the spleen to the right will expose splenocolic attachments that should be divided, allowing inferior mobilization of the colon. Posterolateral fascial attachments are then divided. By then, the remaining vascular supply of the spleen is the splenic hilar vessel, within the splenorenal ligament. Gentle dissection is used to identify and isolate the splenic artery and vein (Fig. 39.1). Extreme caution should be taken not to harm the tail of the pancreas just behind the hilum. Each vessel should be applied a double clip or ligature before division (Fig. 39.2). Alternatively, an endoscopic stapler (12 mm trocar) can be used or a bipolar device in small children (Fig. 39.3). Dividing the attachments at the upper pole of the spleen will free the spleen. An endoscopic bag is introduced through the 12 mm trocar and the spleen is placed into the sac (Fig. 39.4). The neck of the sac is exteriorized and opened to access the spleen. Using finger or

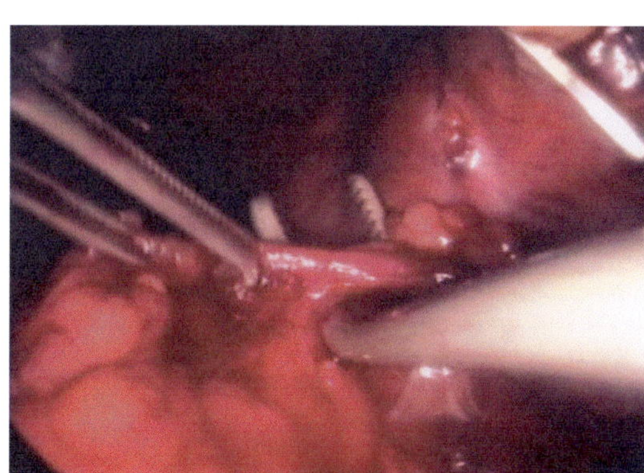

Fig. 39.1 A gentle dissection is used to identify and isolate the splenic artery and vein

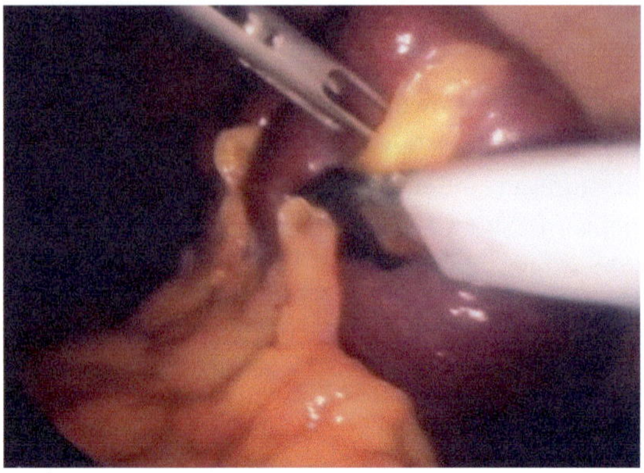

Fig. 39.2 Splenic hilar vessel should be treated using clips, ligature, or sealing devices

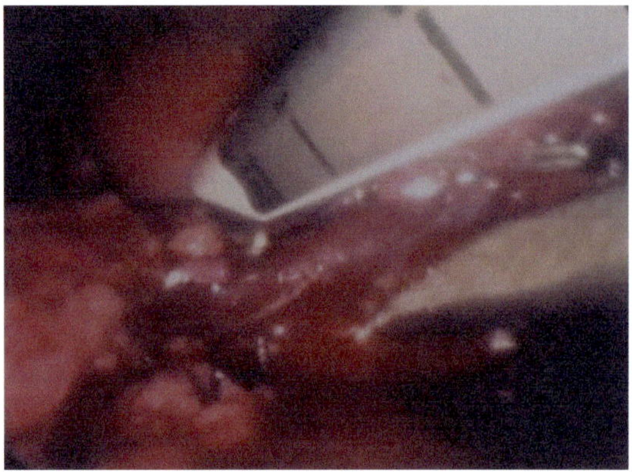

Fig. 39.3 Alternatively, in case of large vessels, an endoscopic stapler can be used

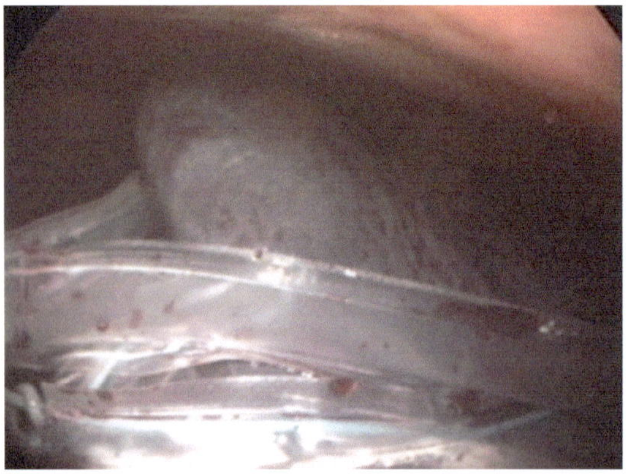

Fig. 39.4 An endoscopic bag is introduced through the 12 mm trocar, and the spleen is placed into the sac and then exteriorized through the umbilicus

ring forceps, the spleen should be morcellated in order to be withdrawn through the trocar site, taking care not to tear the bag as this could seed the abdomen with splenic tissue. The 12 mm trocar is replaced and pneumoperitoneum induced again. Hemostasis should be confirmed, and the peritoneal cavity is inspected for accessory spleens, namely, the area of the pancreatic tail, kidney, bowel mesentery, omentum, gastrosplenic ligament, and pelvis. The ports are closed with absorbable suture and covered with a waterproof dressing.

The authors have performed 20 laparoscopic splenectomies using this technique, with no intraoperative complications. In 11 patients, the spleen was removed in an *endobag* after morcellation, while in 9 children a mini-pfannenstiel incision was required to exteriorize the spleen. One patient, with the diagnosis of PTI, required a second laparoscopy for accessory spleen removal that was found in the greater omentum.

39.5.2 Perioperative Complications

It is consensual nowadays that laparoscopic splenectomy is a safe procedure; nevertheless it does not lack intraoperative complications. Intraoperative hemorrhage is the main reported complication and the most frequent reason for conversion to open surgery. It usually results of a lesion of the hilar or short gastric vessels, splenic capsule or splenic parenchyma and commonly occurs during the dissection and ligation of the hilum vessels. Lesion of adjacent organs and structures can also occur. The tail of the pancreas is especially susceptible during dissection and ligation of the hilum vessels considering its proximity. Pancreatic fistula would be the resulting complication [1].

39.5.3 Variations of the Technique

An attempt to reach the least invasive surgery encouraged surgeons to reduce and even abolish abdominal trocar incisions for splenectomy. The single-incision laparoscopic surgery (SILS) for splenectomy, first described in 2009 [3–5], offered potential for improved cosmesis without increased risk of complications. The SILS uses a convenient umbilical incision where multiple laparoscopic instruments are introduced, enabling complex surgical procedures to be performed by a single abdominal port [4, 5]. There are some major challenges associated with SILS: the absence of triangulation, lack of space, and clashing of the instruments. Still, early literature has suggested shorter hospital stay, fewer postoperative complications, better pain control, and improved cosmesis. Standardization of SILS splenectomy technique and better patient selection criteria are still required [5–7]. The natural orifice transluminal endoscopic surgery (NOTES) accesses body cavities through natural openings, like the mouth or vagina, meaning that a splenectomy may performed without external incisions. Even though NOTES was extensively studied, there are not enough evidence of its safety as it involves viscerotomy, requires appropriate advanced instruments, and provides reduced operative exposure, which hampered this technique to be widely embraced [7, 8].

39.6 Postoperative Care

Some hours after surgery, the patient is offered liquids and, when tolerated, solid food. Pain control should be assured according to each institution postoperative protocol. Antibiotic prophylaxis with penicillin should be employed for at least 1 year after surgery and until the age of 5 years. Some authors recommend lifelong prophylactic penicillin [8–10].

39.7 Postoperative Complications

Early postoperative complications include postoperative bleeding, intra-abdominal abscess, pancreatic fistula, ileus, and wound infection which are widely accepted to have reduced with laparoscopic splenectomy [6, 7]. Special considerations should be made for the risk of postoperative portal vein thrombosis, overwhelming sepsis, and recurrence of the hematologic disease.

39.7.1 Portal Vein Thrombosis (PVT)

PVT is a rare but potentially lethal complication after splenectomy. The incidence of PVT varies between 0 and 6%. It mainly occurs during the first postoperative week and presents with abdominal pain and fever, although it can be asymptomatic. Abdominal ultrasonography confirms the diagnosis. Complicated portal hypertension is a known consequence of PVT. The identified risk factors are female gender, decreased levels of coagulation inhibitors, splenomegaly, thrombocytosis, and concomitant cholecystectomy [11]. No difference was noticed between open and laparoscopic splenectomy [12]. In the presence of risk factors, prophylactic antiplatelet and antithrombotic therapy should be considered after splenectomy [13, 14].

39.7.2 Overwhelming Postsplenectomy Infection (OPSI)

The incidence of OPSI ranges from 2 to 12% depending on the preventive strategy used and primary disease. The risk is greater if the splenectomy is performed in the first few years of life and within the 2 years following operation, although it remains increased for more than 10 years and probably for life. The microorganism most commonly implicated is *Streptococcus pneumoniae*, followed by *Haemophilus influenzae* and *Neisseria meningitidis*. Increased susceptibility to *Salmonella* infections has also been noticed [14].

39.7.3 Recurrence of the Hematologic Disease

An unseen accessory spleen may lead to failed hematologic response, namely, in patients with PTI. The incidence of accessory spleens varies between 4 and 16% in the general population, and 10 and 30% in splenectomized patients, according to autopsy series [13–15]. The identification rate is similar in both open and laparoscopy splenectomies. Whenever a retained accessory spleen is suspected, it can be removed laparoscopically [15].

Conflicts of Interest Jorge Correia-Pinto is an international Karl Storz Gmbh & Co. KG consultant for training and education in minimally invasive pediatric surgery.

References

1. King H, Shumacker HB. Splenic studies. I. Susceptibility to infection after splenectomy performed in infancy. Ann Surg. 1952;136(2):239–42.
2. Delaitre B, Maignien B. Splenectomy by the coelioscopic approach: report of a case. Presse Med. 1991;20:2263.
3. Tulman S, Holcomb GW III, Karamanoukian HL, Reynhout J. Pediatric laparoscopic splenectomy. J Pediatr Surg. 1993;28(5):689–92.
4. Rescorla FJ, Engum SA, West K, Tres Scherer LR III, Rouse TM, Grosfeld JL. Laparoscopic splenectomy has become the gold standard in children. Ann Surg. 2002;68(3):297–301.
5. Janu PG, Rogers DA, Lobe TE. A comparison of laparoscopic and traditional open splenectomy in childhood. J Pediatr Surg. 1986;31(1):109–14.
6. Feng S, Qiu Y, Li X, et al. Laparoscopic versus open splenectomy in children: a systematic review and meta-analysis. Pediatr Surg Int. 2016;32(3):253–9.
7. Rescorla FJ, Breitfeld PP, West KW, Williams D, Engum SA, Grosfeld JL. A case controlled comparison of open and laparoscopic splenectomy in children. Surgery. 1998;124(4):670–6.
8. Coccolini F, Montori G, Catena F, et al. Splenic trauma: WSES classification and guidelines for adult and pediatric patients. World J Emerg Surg. 2017;12(1):1–26.
9. Bruzoni M, Dutta S. Single-site umbilical laparoscopic splenectomy. Semin Pediatr Surg. 2011;20(4):212–8.
10. Al-Salem AH. Indications and complications of splenectomy for children with sickle cell disease. J Pediatr Surg. 2006;41(11):1909–15.
11. Wu Z, Zhou J, Pankaj P, Peng B. Comparative treatment and literature review for laparoscopic splenectomy alone versus preoperative splenic artery embolization splenectomy. Surg Endosc. 2012;26(10):2758–66.
12. Garey CL, Laituri CA, Ostlie DJ, et al. Single-incision laparoscopic surgery in children: initial single-center experience. J Pediatr Surg. 2011;46(5):904–7.
13. Owusu-Ofori S, Riddington C. Splenectomy versus conservative management for acute sequestration crises in people with sickle cell disease. [Review]. Cochrane Database Syst Rev. 2017;(11):CD003425.
14. Soyer T, Ciftci AO, Tanyel FC, Şenocak ME, Büyükpamukçu N. Portal vein thrombosis after splenectomy in pediatric hematologic disease: risk factors, clinical features, and outcome. J Pediatr Surg. 2006;41(11):1899–902.
15. Luoto TT, Pakarinen MP, Koivusalo A. Long-term outcomes after pediatric splenectomy. Surgery. 2016;159(6):1583–90.

Laparoscopic Partial Splenectomy 40

François Becmeur and C. Klipfel

40.1 Introduction

Primarily, partial splenectomy was introduced as an alternative to total splenectomy to avoid post-splenectomy sepsis in children <5 years of age [1, 2].

But the hematologists are mostly able to manage patients with congenital hemolytic anemias until they are older. Most of our patients now are well >10 years old and have done reasonably well with a few blood transfusions.

Potential benefits of partial splenectomy also included avoidance of thromboembolic events, incomplete immunization, and non-compliance with antibiotic prophylaxis.

Risk of splenic regrowth and the possibility of a required completion splenectomy have to be evaluated with a long-term follow-up [3]. Among patients operated on by laparotomy [4], rate of accidental total splenectomy during an attempt to perform partial splenectomy was 4%, and risk for total secondary completion splenectomy was 10% with a 12-year follow-up. Such a long follow-up in laparoscopic partial splenectomy series has not yet been reported.

Several questions remain about the amount of splenic parenchyma that has to be left. What is a good definition for a partial splenectomy for congenital hemolytic anemias?

Is it a 1/3 partial splenectomy? Probably not: the risk of completion splenectomy seems to be high with a short follow-up (around 2 years). This partial splenectomy is insufficient to reduce the hemolytic rate. And the risk of cholelithiasis remains.

Is it a subtotal splenectomy or more, a near total splenectomy [5]? Is the amount of splenic parenchyma enough to work as a normal spleen to maintain a good immune function?

Several studies concluded that 75–90% [4, 6] of the enlarged splenic tissue had to be removed for hematological cases to ensure a satisfying result. It means that less than 25% of the normal spleen volume is retained [4].

The circumstances are totally different in case of a splenic cyst or a tumor. In these cases, partial splenectomy is a focal splenectomy, removing the cyst or the tumor. We have clinical experiences like a hemangioma of the spleen (Fig. 40.1a, b) and a littoral cell angioma (Fig. 40.2a, b).

F. Becmeur (✉) · C. Klipfel
Pediatric Surgery Unit, University of Strasbourg, Hôpital de Hautepierre, Strasbourg Cedex, France
e-mail: francois.becmeur@chru-strasbourg.fr

C. Esposito et al. (eds.), *ESPES Manual of Pediatric Minimally Invasive Surgery*,
https://doi.org/10.1007/978-3-030-00964-9_40

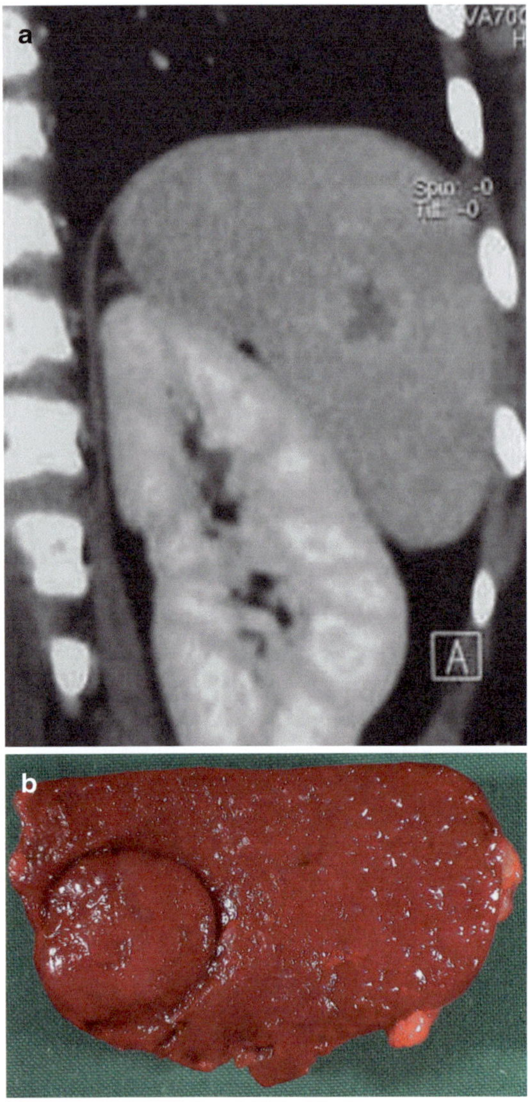

Fig. 40.1 Hemangioma allowing removing the lower third of the spleen (**a**). Hemangioma, the sample (**b**)

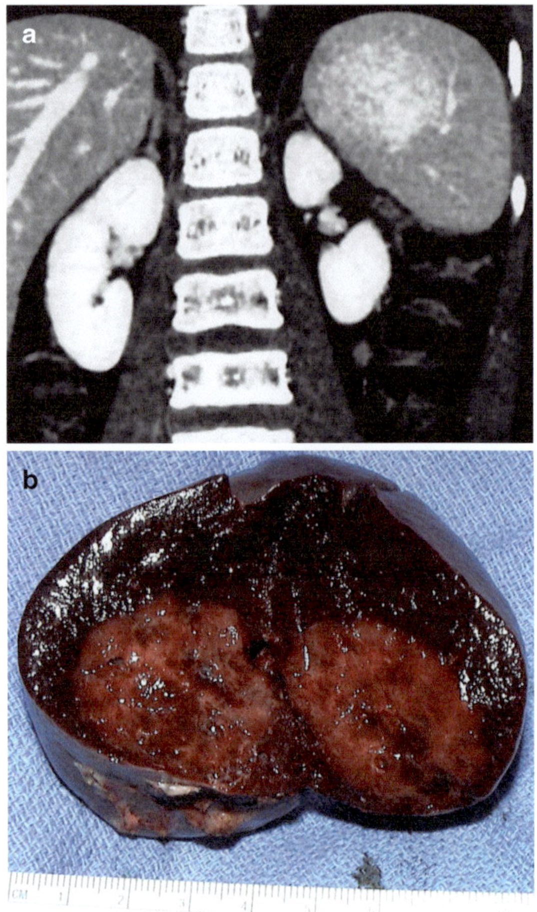

Fig. 40.2 Littoral cell angioma requiring removing the superior part of the spleen (**a**). Littoral cell angioma, the sample (**b**)

40.2 Preoperative Preparation

Patients should be immunized preoperatively with pneumococcal and meningococcal vaccines. Vaccination for *Haemophilus influenzae* is required as well. Even in case of a successful partial splenectomy, patients will receive prophylactic penicillin during 2–3 years after surgery [7].

40.3 Positioning

The patient is lying in a right semi-lateral decubitus (45°). Monitor is placed on the left side of the patient at the level of the thorax. The surgeon is standing on the patient's right side in front of the lower right iliac fossa, facing the monitor [8]. The assistant is on the left side of the surgeon and the scrub nurse on his right side.

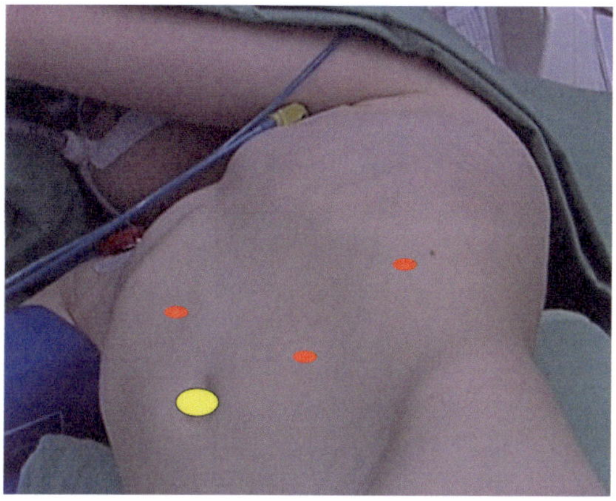

Fig. 40.3 One 10 mm 30° telescope through the umbilicus and three additional trocars

40.4 Instrumentation

One optical trocar and a 30° telescope are needed; it will be a 5 or 10 mm trocar depending on the size of the child. We know that the color of the splenic tissue reduces the light inside the peritoneal cavity. That is why a 10 mm telescope is mostly preferred to have a perfect lighting. Three additional 5 mm trocars are needed (Fig. 40.3). Two atraumatic forceps, one dissector, and scissors are required; 3-0 or 2-0 Vicryl thread is needed when the option is to ligate the vessels. A vessel loop will allow doing Blalock loop on the main artery to secure splenic vessels division. Sealing devices are used for dissection, cutting short gastric vessels, and dividing splenic parenchyma. Argon beam laser may be useful to cauterize the raw edge of the spleen, but it is not essential. We do not use endostaplers and fibrin glue. But they may be an option to treat, respectively, the main vessels and the raw edge of the spleen [9].

40.5 Technique

An open laparoscopy is performed with a 10 mm 30° telescope through the umbilicus. Three additional 5 mm ports are placed: one between the xiphoid cartilage and the umbilicus; one lower or at the level of the umbilicus, on the left mid-clavicular line; and the third one in the left flank for the spleen retractor or suction device.

40.5.1 Subtotal Splenectomy in Congenital Hemolytic Anemias

40.5.1.1 First Step

The short gastric vessels are divided leaving the last upper vessels to preserve a remaining blood supply on the upper part of the spleen. This first step will allow a good exposure of the main splenic vessels.

40.5.1.2 Second Step

Main artery is then dissected and isolated to place a Blalock loop using a vessel loop. This precaution was adopted to secure the following dissection of the hilum.

40.5.1.3 Third Step

Secondary arteries going into the splenic parenchyma are progressively divided along the spleen, nearby the parenchyma, beginning by the lower vessels and going up to the top of the spleen. Veins are then divided. Intracorporeal knots or Hem-o-lok clips are used depending on the size of the vessels. It is necessary to free the pancreatic tail with caution avoiding damaging it in order to prevent postoperative pancreatic leakage. At least it is important to ligate arteries first to obtain a satisfying washout of the blood retained in the parenchyma. Thereby we insure less bleeding and reduce blood loss.

40.5.1.4 Fourth Step

A delimitation line will appear on the splenic surface. Then, it becomes possible to tattoo and draw the future section line on the splenic capsule with a monopolar hook, 1 cm afar from the delimitation line in the ischemic part of the spleen (Fig. 40.4). The section of the parenchyma is then performed using a sealing device such as LigaSure or a Harmonic scalpel. A suction device

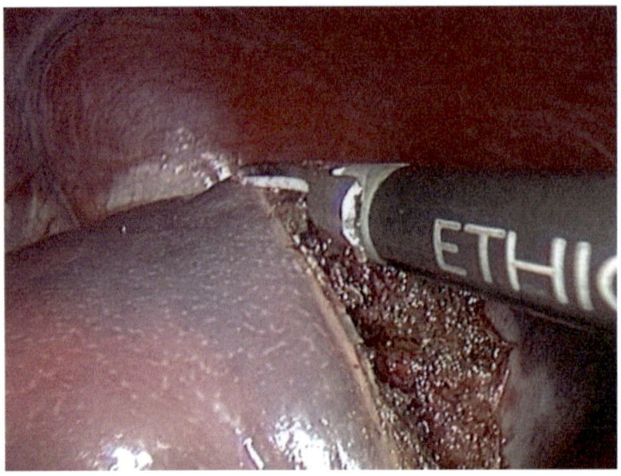

Fig. 40.4 Section of the spleen 1 cm far from the delimitation line in the dark zone

is introduced through the external left operative trocar to wash the surface of the severed spleen and to suck up blood and smoke.

40.5.1.5 Fifth Step

Hemostasis is controlled. Bipolar coagulation or argon beam laser is used. Then, great omentum may be used to cover the raw edge. The aim of this maneuver is to avoid bowel adhesion. Fibrin glue is rarely required, as it is expensive and not easy to put on the irregular section surface of the spleen.

Removal of the main part of the spleen from the abdomen needs an endobag. To be able to open the endobag, it is pushed inside through the umbilicus or a short left inguinal approach depending of the size of the abdominal cavity. The subtotal spleen is morcellated using a finger and a good suction device, avoiding any traumatic instruments that may rip the endobag and induce a spillage of splenic tissue in the peritoneal cavity. Drainage is unnecessary at the end of the procedure.

40.5.2 Partial Splenectomy to Remove a Cyst or a Tumor

40.5.2.1 First Step

The short gastric vessels are divided (Fig. 40.5a) leaving vessels to preserve a remaining blood supply on the part of the spleen that will be left in

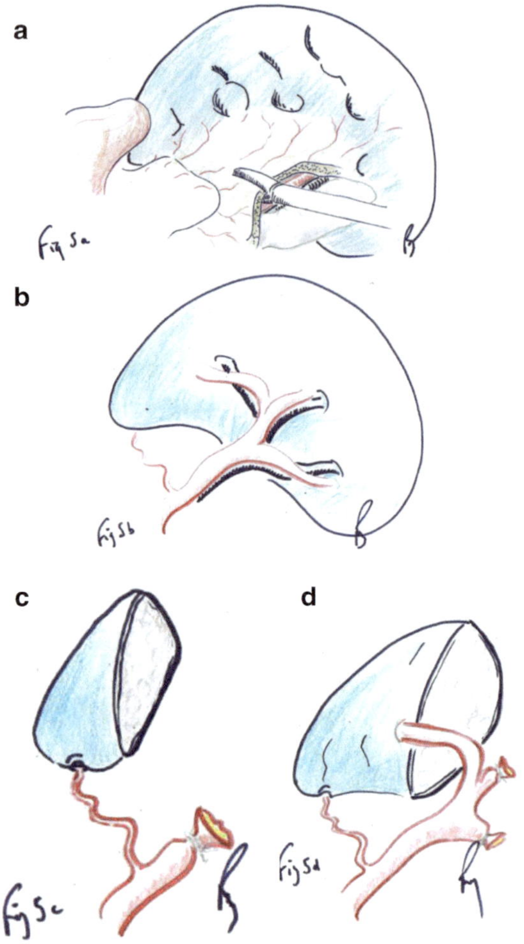

Fig. 40.5 Section of the short gastric vessels (**a**); exposure of the main splenic vessels (**b**); subtotal splenectomy removing 80% of the spleen (**c**); partial splenectomy removing 2/3 of the spleen (**d**)

place. This first step will allow a good exposure of the main splenic vessels.

40.5.2.2 Second Step

Main artery is then dissected and isolated to place a Blalock loop using a vessel loop. This precaution was adopted to secure the following dissection of the hilum.

40.5.2.3 Third Step

Secondary vessels going toward the lesion are progressively divided along the spleen, nearby the parenchyma. Intracorporeal knots or Hem-o-lok clips are used depending on the size of the vessels.

Cyst dissection should remove a thin splenic parenchymal part surrounding the lesion.

40.5.2.4 Fourth Step

The cyst is then released from any adhesion along the surface of the diaphragm, the liver, or the omentum. The cyst is then emptied from its content and is widely opened to check the section of the parenchyma easily. The parenchymal section is done, close to the parietal wall of the cyst to ensure a complete ground resection: the cyst and surrounding parenchyma. This resection is performed using a sealing device such as LigaSure or a Harmonic scalpel. A suction device is introduced through the external left operative trocar to wash out the surface of the severed spleen and to suck up blood and smoke.

40.5.2.5 Fifth Step

Hemostasis is controlled. Bipolar coagulation or argon beam laser is used. Then, great omentum may be used to cover the raw edge. The aim of this maneuver is to avoid bowel adhesion. Fibrin glue is rarely required, expensive, and not easy to put on the irregular section surface of the spleen.

Removal of the cyst from the abdomen requires an endobag. To be able to open the endobag, it is pushed inside through the umbilicus or a short left inguinal approach depending on the size of the abdominal cavity. Drainage is unnecessary at the end of the procedure.

40.6 Postoperative Care

Antibiotic prophylaxis began at the beginning of the procedure. Oral antibiotic prophylaxis will be carried out for 2 or 3 years.

No transfusion is required during surgery or after.

The mean hospital stay has to be sufficient to be sure no postoperative bleeding occurs. We consider these patients as those who are managed in the ICU for a non-operative treatment after a spleen trauma. Nevertheless, it depends on the surgical team, and length hospital stay differs from one study to another [3, 6–8].

Abdominal ultrasonography allows excluding any blood collection in the peritoneal cavity. Doppler analysis of the splenic tissue allows checking spleen blood supply and to be sure that spleen vascularization is well preserved in the first postoperative days. Main veins (splenic vein, superior mesenteric vein, portal vein) are controlled as well, to prevent any thromboembolic event.

In case of congenital hemolytic anemias, hematological outcome requires to control values for hemoglobin, platelet count, and reticulocyte count. Spleen size and the occurrence of hemolytic anemia crisis are regularly controlled.

In case of a splenic cyst, late ultrasonography, 1 year after surgery, allows to be sure there is no recurrence.

Radionuclide spleen scan may be done in case of any doubt about the remnant spleen vitality.

40.7 Results

The effectiveness of partial splenectomy is evaluated on the hematological outcomes. Most studies reported an increase in hemoglobin level with a decrease in reticulocytes, transfusions, and anemic crisis [2, 3, 9, 10]. A law rate of total splenectomy, after earlier partial splenectomy, is considered by many clinicians, as the best measure of long-term success for partial splenectomy. However this outcome is not frequently reported and has a wide variation depending on length of follow-up. For example, six studies reported a conversion rate of 0–15% at 1–6 years of follow-up, and one study reported a rate of 40% at 2 years of follow-up [2]. Obviously, the actual reported follow-up is too short.

The risk of conversion of laparoscopy to laparotomy in different types of splenectomy was reported in several studies and ranged from 1.8 to 11% [2].

The risk of intraoperative conversion from partial to total splenectomy ranged from 4 to 6.9% [2]. That gives reason for invariable vaccination before surgery.

In our own experience, the risk of intraoperative conversion from partial to total splenectomy is minimal. If anatomical local conditions are not favorable for a subtotal splenectomy, one must not hesitate to perform a total splenectomy. We report ten subtotal splenectomies for spherocytosis with a mean follow-up of 6.5 years (from 2 to 12). Only one totalization required, 6 years after the first procedure.

40.8 Discussion

40.8.1 Congenital Hemolytic Anemias

The aim of partial splenectomy is to decrease the risk for anemic crisis. That is why 80–90% of splenic parenchyma should be removed to be effective (Fig. 40.5c). But, at the opposite, the aim of partial splenectomy is to preserve enough splenic tissue, in order to prevent post-splenectomy infections.

Preservation of immune function is assessed using the sepsis rate after total splenectomy [3]. The long-term risk of lethal infection after total splenectomy could be around 0.73/1000 patient-years [11]. There is no study about the estimated risk of sepsis after partial splenectomy. The only issue we have is about the size of the remnant spleen and its blood supply.

Further studies are required to assess long-term splenic function in terms of immunization, after partial splenectomy. We have no idea at all about the remaining splenic immune function. Generally, the upper pole of the spleen is left. The native adhesion to the diaphragm can lower the risk of wandering remnant spleen.

40.8.2 Nonparasitic Splenic Cysts

Only symptomatic and >5–10 cm diameter non-parasitic splenic cysts have to be operated on.

To facilitate partial splenectomy in case of cysts or tumors (benign tumors like rare hemangioma), 3D virtual rendering can be useful to guide the surgical procedure, allowing to foresee which vessels supply the lesion [12].

Unroofing results in a high rate of recurrence: 11/15 patients in [12]. Recurrences occurred after a mean postoperative follow-up of 8.7 months (range 1–42.7).

Unroofing plus ground resection seems to have good results. But Shier [13] wrote "also argon laser treatment of the ground surface of the cyst resulted in recurrence."

When feasible, laparoscopic partial splenectomy (Fig. 40.5d) is the technique of choice [14]. If not, total splenectomy is required.

References

1. Tchernia G, Gauthier F, Mielot F, Dommergues JP, Yvart J, Chasis JA, Mohandas N. Initial assessment of the beneficial effect of partial splenectomy in hereditary spherocytosis. Blood. 1993;81:2014–20.
2. Rice HE, Crary SE, Langer JC, Kemper AR. Comparative effectiveness of different types of splenectomy for children with congenital hemolytic anemias. J Pediatr. 2012;160:684–9.
3. Seims AD, Breckler FD, Hardacker KD, Rescorla FJ. Partial versus total splenectomy in children with hereditary spherocytosis. Surgery. 2013;154:849–53.
4. Tchernia G, Bader-Meunier B, Berterottiere P, Eber S, Dommergues JP, Gauthier F. Effectiveness of partial splenectomy in hereditary spherocytosis. Curr Opin Hematol. 1997;41:36–41.
5. Stoehr GA, Stauffer UG, Eber SW. Near-total splenectomy. A new technique for the management of hereditary spherocytosis. Ann Surg. 2005;241:40–7.
6. Hery G, Becmeur F, Mefat L, Kalfa D, Lutz P, Lutz L, Guys JM, de Lagausie P. Laparoscopic partial splenectomy: indications and results of a multicenter retrospective study. Surg Endosc. 2008;22:45–9.
7. Al Salem AH. Splenectomy for children with thalassemia: total or partial splenectomy, open or laparoscopic splenectomy. J Pediatr Hematol Oncol. 2016;38:1–4.
8. Cai H, An Y, Wu D, Chen X, Zhang Y, Zhu F, Jiang Y, Sun D. Laparoscopic partial splenectomy: a preferred method for select patients. J Laparoendosc Adv Surg Tech A. 2016;26:1010–4.
9. Pugi J, Caracao M, Drury LJ, Langer JC. Results after laparoscopic partial splenectomy for children with hereditary spherocytosis: are outcomes influenced by genetic mutation? J Pediatr Surg. 2018;53(5):973–5. pii: S0022-3468(18)30081-2.
10. Englun BR, Rothman J, Leonard S, Reiter A, Thornburg C, Brindle M, Wright N, Heeney MM, Jason Smithers C, Brown RL, et al. Hematologic outcomes after total splenectomy and partial splenectomy for congenital hemolytic anemia. J Pediatr Surg. 2016;51:122–7.

11. Schilling RF. Estimating the risk for sepsis after splenectomy in hereditary spherocytosis. Ann Intern Med. 1995;122:187–8.
12. Delforge X, Chaussy Y, Borrego P, Abbo O, Sauvat F, Ballouhey Q, Irtan S, Arnaud A, Ibtissan K, Panait N, et al. Management of nonparasitic splenic cysts in children: a French multicenter review of 100 cases. J Pediatr Surg. 2017;52:1465–70.
13. Schier F, Waag KL, Ure B. Laparoscopic unroofing of splenic cysts results in a high rate of recurrences. J Pediatr Surg. 2007;42:1860–3.
14. Lima M, Reinberg O, De Buys Roessingh AS, Gargano T, Soler L, Mogiatti M, Cantone N. 3D virtual rendering before laparoscopic partial splenectomy in children. J Pediatr Surg. 2013;48:1784–8.

41 Minimal Invasive Management of Lymphatic Malformations

Gabriela Guillén, Sergio López-Fernández, José Andrés Molino, and Manuel López

41.1 Introduction

"Vascular anomalies" is a term used to denominate a wide group of conditions that include vascular malformations and proliferating tumors. Currently, the classification system from the International Society for the Study of Vascular Anomalies (ISSVA), first developed in 1996 and updated in 2014, is the gold standard for most authors [1]. The classification is based on physical examination, disease course, vascular flow characteristics, and histopathology. The establishment of a correct diagnosis, based on multidisciplinary evaluation of each particular case, is the key to provide an adequate treatment [2].

According to this classification, lymphangiomas or, more accurately, lymphatic malformations (LMs) are considered "low-flow vascular malformations". However, they can show mixed features, being classified as "complex combined vascular malformations" which include capillary-lymphatic malformations, lymphatic-venous malformations, and capillary-lymphatic-arteriovenous malformations, and this can have therapeutic implications. Their incidence is low, and it is estimated between 1:2000 and 100,000 newborns [3]. As a rule, it is imperative to identify precisely the nature of the lesion before proposing any treatment. Even more, differential diagnosis must be established with other soft-tissue conditions that can mimic lymphatic malformations, as can be other congenital malformations (bronchogenic cysts, branchial cysts, intestinal duplications, etc.) and some malignant tumors (infantile fibrosarcomas and other soft-tissue sarcomas). Sometimes, only a biopsy or a complete resection provides a definitive diagnosis.

Although LMs are benign, they can produce severe complications, cosmetic sequelae, and functional compromise, mostly due to compression of nearby structures, infection, and bleeding, which can even be life-threatening. Diagnosis can happen prenatally on ultrasound or after birth. Their finding can be incidental or after having developed any symptoms (most commonly bulging, infection, compression, pain, or bleeding). LMs can invade nearby structures and organs. Ascites and chylothorax are infrequent findings, but typically associated with abdominal or thoracic lesions, respectively. It is well known that some cases can even disappear after spontaneous episodes of bleeding or infection.

Most of them occur in the head and neck or axillary region. However, they can affect almost any soft tissue, including thoracic and abdominal locations, that together make 20% of cases [3]. Less than 1% of LMs occur at the mesentery or the retroperitoneum [4]. Mediastinal lymphatic

G. Guillén (✉) · S. López-Fernández · J. A. Molino
M. López
Pediatric Surgery Department, Hospital Universitari Vall d'Hebron—Universitat Autònoma de Barcelona (UAB), Barcelona, Spain
e-mail: gguillen@vhebron.net

C. Esposito et al. (eds.), *ESPES Manual of Pediatric Minimally Invasive Surgery*,
https://doi.org/10.1007/978-3-030-00964-9_41

malformations are uncommon and can be related to cervical or axillary lesions.

Traditionally, open surgical excision was the mainstream for treatment, although it can be associated with severe complications and sequelae. During the last two decades, image-guided percutaneous sclerotherapy with different agents has gained popularity, with excellent results for pure lymphatic macrocystic lesions in most anatomic locations, but disappointing in the microcystic ones. On the other hand, minimal invasive surgery, through its different modalities, offers an interesting approach for some selected cases.

41.2 Preoperative Preparation

Diagnosis of low-flow vascular malformations, including lymphatic malformations (LMs), is based on clinical history, physical examination, Doppler ultrasound, and magnetic resonance imaging [5]. Magnetic resonance imaging (MRI) is the preferred diagnostic tool because it provides information that allows diagnosis and treatment planning. Macrocystic and microcystic LMs show different features on MRI, and some lesions can present mixed findings. Sometimes, if there is concern or doubt about possible involvement of hollow viscera (such as the esophagus or the stomach), endoscopic ultrasound can provide very valuable information for treatment. In the setting of an emergency (bleeding, infection), CT scan is the most efficient and available image modality. When image tests show atypical findings, the study work-up must be extended and might include biopsies.

Each case should be discussed by a multidisciplinary team constituted, at least, by pediatric surgeons, plastic surgeons, interventional radiologists, dermatologists, pediatricians, pediatric oncologists, pediatric radiologists, and pathologists; in order to reach a diagnostic consensus, consider the actual need of treatment and select the most appropriate modality. In 2005, Lee proposed some absolute and relative indications for treatment of vascular malformations [6]. Some of them can be applied to LMs: hemorrhage and lesions in a life-, vital function-, or limb-threatening location are considered absolute indications, and disabling or discomfort, functional impairment or disability, severe cosmetic deformity and/or psychological impact, location at site of high risk of complications, and recurrent infection or sepsis are considered relative indications.

Depending on the anatomic origin of the lesion, if intestinal or pulmonary resections are foreseen, antibiotic prophylaxis according to each center protocols is recommended. Otherwise, antibiotics are not required. If there is any possibility of performing a splenectomy, adequate preoperative immunization should be completed. Red blood concentrates should be available at the OR. If any sclerosing agent is going to be used, alone or in combination of minimal invasive surgery, allergies must be ruled out.

41.3 Positioning

Positioning varies depending on anatomic location of the LM. However, adequate triangulation, optimum cosmetic positioning of the port through which the surgical specimen will be retrieved and planned incision in case of conversion to an open surgery, must be the standard for every procedure.

41.4 Instrumentation

Number and size of trocars will depend on the localization of the lesion. Generally, at least two 5 mm trocars will be needed, one for the optics and the other for an energy sealing device. The LigaSure™ 23 cm Maryland jaw sealer (Covidien, Medtronic) offers an excellent control of bleeding and allows dissection thanks to the shape of the tip. The Harmonic ACE™ +7 23 cm scissors (Ethicon, Johnson & Johnson) shows similar advantages and is our preferred instrument for small working spaces, as it does not produce smoke. However, care must be taken with the active blade that can inadvertently burn the surrounding structures. For grasping and bipolar coagulation, 3 mm instruments are optimal.

41.5 Technique

Some of the most frequent locations that are amenable to an endoscopic or combined approach are summarized below:

41.5.1 Thoracoscopy for Mediastinal LMs

Many macrocystic thoracic LMs are easily amenable to percutaneous sclerotherapy, although care should be taken as chylothorax is a possible complication and compression of thoracic structures can occur. For microcystic lesions and macrocystic lesions not amenable to puncture, thoracoscopy is an excellent approach. Most lesions develop in the mediastinum, and special attention has to be taken in order to avoid damage to the main vessels, nerves, esophagus, and thoracic duct. The pericardium is usually respected by the lesion and provides a good plane for dissection (Fig. 41.1). If total resection carries a high risk of damaging any of these structures, then a subtotal resection must be favored, combined, or not with sclerotherapy performed under direct vision. Blood concentrates and open thoracotomy instruments must be immediately available in case any surgical complication happens.

41.5.2 Laparoscopy for Abdominal and Retroperitoneal LMs

It is estimated that around 20% of all LMs happen in the abdomen [3]. Omentum, mesentery, and retroperitoneum are the most common locations, but abdominal viscera can also be affected. Abdominal LMs can develop complications (most frequently bleeding or infection, but also intestinal occlusion and even volvulus), and it's our common practice to treat them when diagnosed. However, if the lesion is in the mesenteric root or the retroperitoneum and is asymptomatic, we favor a conservative management as other authors suggest [7].

An initial laparoscopic approach should be the preferred elective surgical procedure for almost every abdominal LM, in our opinion. Depending on the affected organs and localization, trocar number and positioning will vary. There are even some reports of single-port procedures, when the lesion is mobile and well defined. The exact origin of the LM can be difficult to determine, making an initial thorough inspection of the peritoneal cavity a key point of the surgery. Bowel resection and, in some cases, splenectomy must be anticipated in terms of preoperative immunization and prophylactic antibiotic administration. If great vessels or solid viscera are involved, blood concentrates must be available at the OR. When the LM shows an intimate relation with vital structures, a laparoscopic subtotal resection can be safely performed and total resection completed through a minilaparotomy, avoiding larger incisions. The largest cysts can be emptied before starting the excision, but it's our practice to delay it as possible to appreciate more clearly the limits of the lesion. Laparoscopically assisted bowel resection—if needed—is another interesting option in mesenteric LMs, enlarging one of the incisions (usually, the umbilical port) and performing an extracorporeal resection and anastomosis, as reported by Tran [8].

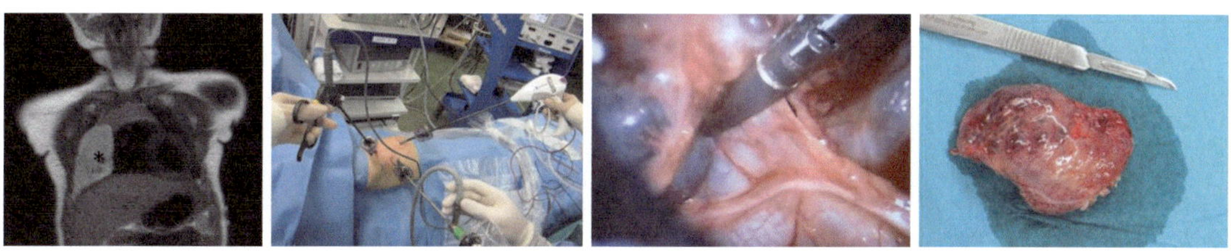

Fig. 41.1 Prenatally diagnosed mediastinal mass that happened to be a microcystic lymphangioma, in a 1-year-old child. (**a**) Thoracic MRI, Haste coronal. Large thoracic-mediastinal mass in the right hemithorax (asterisk). (**b**) Port placement. (**c**) Excision of the lesion from the pericardium (respecting the phrenic nerve). (**d**) Final surgical specimen

There are few reports on minimal invasive treatment of retroperitoneal LMs in children [9, 10], but, when feasible, it provides some important benefits (less recurrence if total resection is achieved, less pain, direct control of vital structures). Most authors choose a laparoscopic transperitoneal approach. Some maneuvers can facilitate the procedure, like placing the patient on a lateral position and catheterizing the ureters through cystoscopy. A particular care with major vascular structures must be considered in this anatomic location.

41.5.3 Subcutaneoscopy for LMs

During the last year, we have started to use a new approach for subcutaneous thoracic and abdominal microcystic lymphatic malformations that do not infiltrate the skin (unpublished results). It is inspired in the endoscopic subcutaneous mastectomy, a technique recently described for male gynecomastia [11]. The patient is placed in an adequate position, depending on the anatomical site. The limits of the lesion are drawn with a marker pen, and a tight adhesive tape is placed around, in order to limit the CO_2 emphysema. The port incisions must be placed far enough to allow the movement of the instruments, but as near as possible from the cavity that the surgeon will create. To do so, at least 50 cc of physiologic serum are injected around the lesion, to separate it from the surrounding tissues, creating a virtual working space (Fig. 41.2).

Gas is insufflated with moderate pressure (10–15 mmHg), to avoid skin necrosis, and flow is set at 5–10 lpm. We use two 5 mm ports for camera and for the Harmonic ACE™ +7 23 cm scissors (Ethicon, Johnson & Johnson). A third 3 mm trocar is placed for grasping and/or bipolar coagulation. Trocars are secured to the skin with flanges and silk sutures (Fig. 41.3).

The lesion is first separated from the underlying muscular plane and the surrounding fat tissue, using the ultrasonic device (Fig. 41.4). We have chosen to use this energy instrument because it doesn't generate smoke, which is important in this small working field. Then, the lesion is separated from the skin, with care not to damage it. One helpful maneuver at this point is to push the lesion from the outside with one hand.

41.5.4 Combined Endoscopic Management

Different endoscopic techniques (like esophagogastroscopy, fiber optics, or rigid bronchoscopy/laryngoscopy) can provide very valuable information regarding compression or transmural involvement, for diagnostic and therapeutic purposes (Fig. 41.5). The combination with endoscopic ultrasound can help in decision-making in some difficult cases. These techniques allow a successful direct sclerotherapy under visual control for some difficult locations or can be combined with other approaches (like percutaneous sclerotherapy).

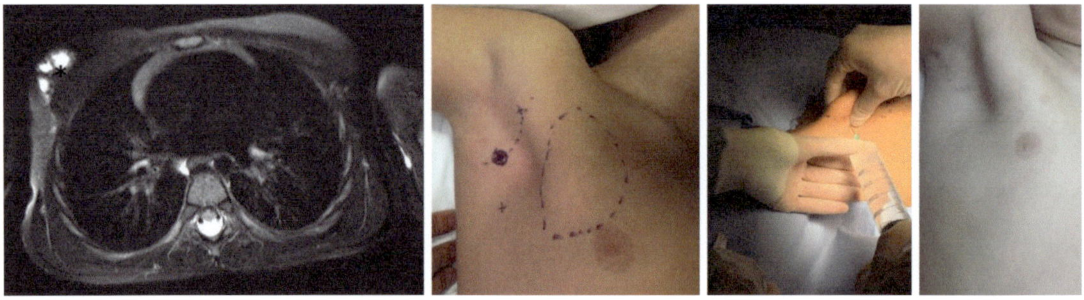

Fig. 41.2 Subcutaneoscopy for resection of a right-sided thoracic wall macro-/microcystic LM (asterisk) that persisted after two sclerotherapy sessions with OK432. (**a**) MRI, T2 axial view. (**b**) The lymphangioma is located above the nipple. Port placement is set on demand. An axillary incision is planned in case conversion is needed. (**c**) Physiologic serum is injected to create a virtual cavity around the lesion. (**d**) Final result

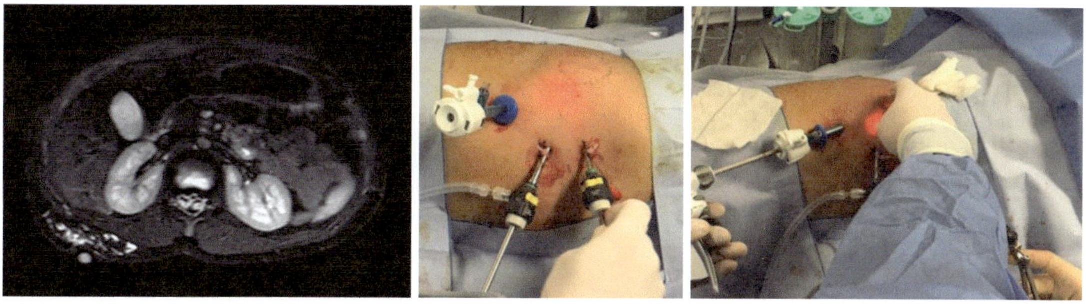

Fig. 41.3 Subcutaneoscopy for resection of a lumbar wall microcystic lymphangioma. (**a**) MRI, STIR axial view. (**b**) Port placement is set on demand. Steel trocars are secured with flanges and silk stitches to the skin. (**c**) While holding the ultrasonic device with the left hand, the lesion is mobilized from the outside with the right hand

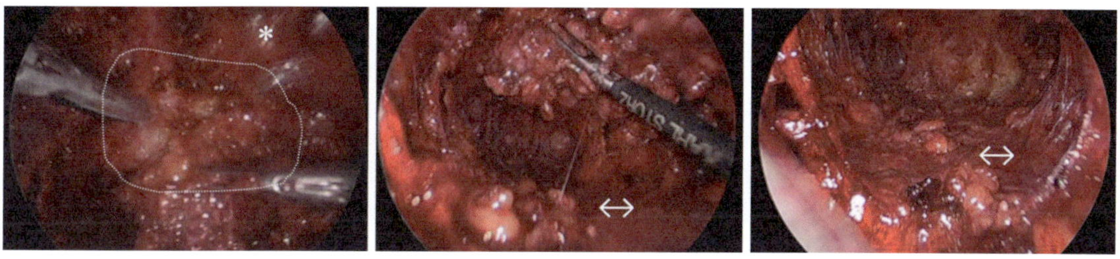

Fig. 41.4 Endoscopic view of the case in Fig. 41.3. (**a**) Resection of a LM (dotted line), which has been separated from the muscle (↔) and now is being dissected from the skin (asterisk). (**b**) View with the lesion completely enucleated, taken with a grasper. (**c**) Final result

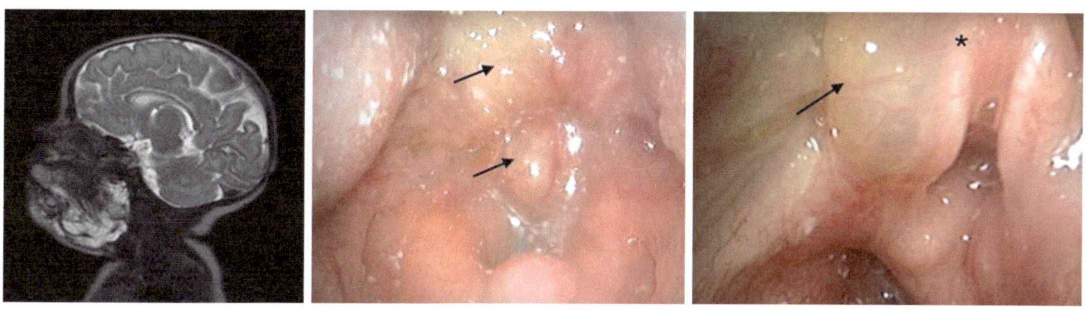

Fig. 41.5 (**a**) Cervical LM diagnosed after birth. Despite the child initially showed no respiratory distress, MRI proved a diffuse infiltration of the tongue and airway compromise. Laryngoscopy demonstrated extensive pharyngeal and laryngeal involvement. (**b**) Pharynx with multiple cysts (arrows). (**c**) Larynx with cysts that even affect the epiglottis (asterisk). A prophylactic tracheostomy was performed before starting treatment (OK432 sclerotherapy of the largest cysts and, later on, sirolimus). Tracheostomy was successfully removed after 1 year and a half

41.5.5 Fetal Treatment and Perinatal Management

Despite not being the focus of this chapter and that fetal surgery will be further discussed in this book, prenatally diagnosed LMs deserve a special mention. LMs can be diagnosed during gestation, generally around the second or third trimester [4, 12]. In most cases these lesions do not require any intervention before birth, but when located in the head and neck region or the mediastinum, the risk of upper airway obstruction at birth must be considered. The EXIT (*Ex Utero Intrapartum Treatment*) procedure provides an excellent opportunity of securing the neonatal airway by means of tracheal intubation or tracheostomy in hands of highly trained teams, as we reported in 2010 [13]. However, it can be associated with severe complications.

Two minimally invasive interventions can be especially helpful when managing these cases, in order to avoid more aggressive approaches:

- Prenatal ultrasound-guided percutaneous puncture, shunting, or even sclerosis with OK432 of macrocystic lesions. This management can be useful also in large LMs in other anatomical locations that can pose a risk of dystocia. However, this management can be impossible in certain situations.
- Fetal endoscopic tracheal intubation (FETI) has been recently described [14]. It consists of an orotracheal intubation performed though fetoscopy to prenatally secure the airway and could successfully avoid some EXIT procedures.

41.6 Postoperative Care

Pain control with conventional analgesia is usually enough. Antibiotic prophylaxis or treatment should be followed according to each center protocol. Drainages and/or compressive dressings are highly recommended in subcutaneous lesions and should be kept in place for at least 24–48 h. Patients can be discharged on the same operative day, if there is no risk of bleeding. Otherwise, 24 h of hospital stay are recommended. A chest X-ray before discharge is advisable after excision of intrathoracic lesions, as chylothorax is a possible complication. Chylous ascites can happen in mesenteric LMs, but usually it's better tolerated than in the thorax. Our common practice in mesenteric LMs is to recommend a low-fat diet during the first week and to perform an outpatient abdominal ultrasound 7–10 days after the surgery. It is our common practice to perform an MRI 1 year after surgery, to confirm that there is not relapse.

41.7 Results

A formal Vascular Anomalies Committee was constituted in our center in 2009; since then, most cases of vascular anomalies are discussed in a multidisciplinary basis. During the period January 2009–May 2018, 388 patients with vascular anomalies were treated by the committee. From these, 23% of cases had some lymphatic malformation (72 patients with pure LMs and 18 patients with lymphatic-venous malformations), excluding other complex cases. A total of 26 patients underwent surgical resection, only 7 patients through a minimal invasive approach. Other five cases required some endoscopic procedure to help in diagnosis and/or treatment.

A laparoscopic approach was performed in three patients, with conversion to minilaparotomy in two: in one, due to risk of damaging main vascular structures (the inferior vena cava and the root of the mesentery), and in the other, due to the large size of the lesion. LMs were omental (two cases) and mesenteric (one case). There were no complications or relapses in this group, with a mean follow-up of 18 months. During the same period, three patients underwent resection through laparotomy due to preoperative clinical findings. Two of them debuted as massive intralesional bleeding with anemia and hemodynamic instability, and the last one had a large microcystic LM that surrounded the superior mesenteric artery and was causing crisis of pain. We must remark that none of the abdominal LMs treated in this period required any intestinal resection, even when the mesentery was involved in 3/6 cases (2 small bowel, 1 colon), thanks to a very careful dissection and maintenance of at least one peritoneal sheet. This is not a common finding compared to other authors [7, 8], in whose larger experience bowel resection is not an uncommon procedure.

Regarding thoracoscopy, two procedures were performed. Both were mediastinal LMs, not amenable to percutaneous treatment. One of them presented with intracystic bleeding and was adherent to the superior vena cava (SVC), making difficult to identify the cyst walls; during the resection, a lesion of the SVC happened. The patient underwent an emergency thoracotomy and the bleeding

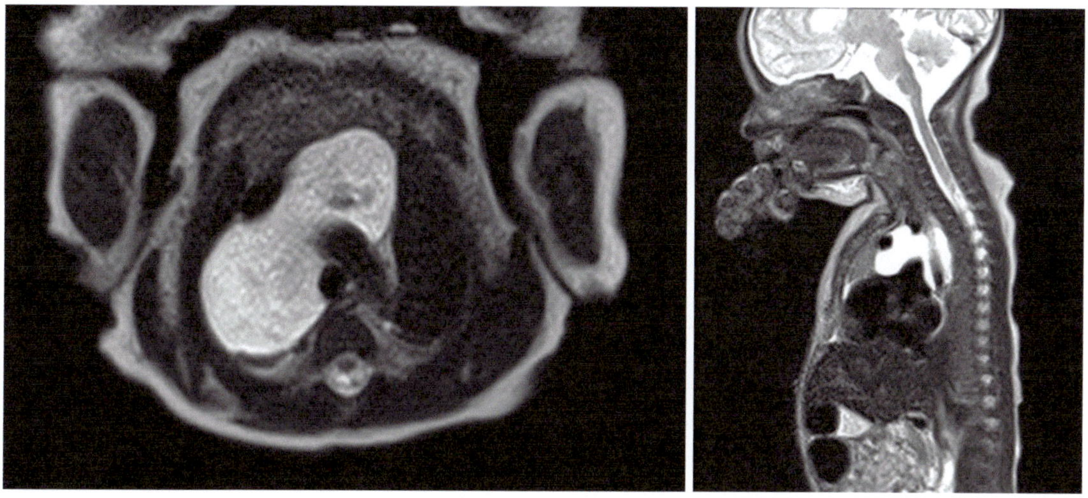

Fig. 41.6 Prenatally diagnosed mediastinal LM that produced tracheal collapse and deviation in prenatal US and MRI. An EXIT procedure was performed, to allow a secure airway. The pictures show the postnatal MRI, before surgical resection via sternotomy. Sclerotherapy was not considered in this case due to risk of compression of main vascular and airway structures

was controlled. This highlights the importance of foreseeing possible complications in certain locations and disposing adequate measures to treat them. The other patient was prenatally diagnosed as a CPAM, but thoracoscopy showed a large mediastinal microcystic LM, occupying the right hemithorax that was resected uneventfully.

Two subcutaneoscopies were performed; as there was no preliminary experience of this approach in LMs, parents received informed consent that this was an experimental procedure. Both cases corresponded to lesions with macro- and microcystic features. Sclerotherapy had failed twice in the first case, so we looked for a more definitive treatment modality with minimal scarring. After a short follow-up (7 and 3 months, respectively), there is no sign of local relapse, and excellent cosmetic results have been achieved in both patients. Although it seems a promising technique, more cases and a longer follow-up are needed to confirm its results and determine adequate patient selection criteria.

During the same period, only one patient required an EXIT procedure due to a prenatal diagnosis of a large mediastinal LM that compressed the trachea. Due to the location of the cysts (surrounding the main thoracic vessels and airway), in utero puncture was discarded (Fig. 41.6). After cesarean section, placental support time was maintained for 10 min, during which nasotracheal intubation and a minimally invasive percutaneous ultrasound-guided puncture and voiding of the cysts were performed. The patient underwent elective complete resection via sternotomy 3 days later. There were no maternal or child complications.

Five cases underwent some endoscopic procedure, with diagnostic or therapeutic intention. One patient with a cervical LM underwent a tracheostomy after laryngoscopy confirmed a massive involvement of the upper airway, and another patient with an oral, lingual, and pharyngeal lymphatic-venous malformation underwent sclerotherapy though a combined endoscopic and percutaneous approach. One patient was diagnosed of a bleeding gastric lymphatic-venous malformation thanks to an esophagogastroscopy. Two other patients were diagnosed of lymphatic enteropathy, in the context of massive mesenteric LMs.

41.8 Tips and Tricks

- When bleeding occurs inside a macrocystic LM, the cyst walls can be difficult to distinguish from the vessels (particularly, from the veins). Extreme care should be taken in order to avoid any serious vascular lesion.

- If major vascular structures are involved, an open surgery table with adequate instruments should be prepared in case an emergent conversion is needed.
- When there is a serious possibility of damaging any major structure (vascular, nervous, or any high-risk anatomic structure—i.e., esophagus, pancreas), then a subtotal resection should be favored, combined if necessary with sclerotherapy in the remaining cysts.
- Some difficult cases might benefit from a combined approach, using different techniques and even systemic treatments (i.e., sirolimus). This can avoid performing unnecessary mutilating resections, like in extensive mesenteric lesions.

41.9 Discussion

Current studies prove that LMs show excellent results, in terms of cure and symptoms relief, when managed by means of multiple sessions of sclerotherapy with different agents (OK432, bleomycin, doxycycline) [5]. However, this might not be a realistic approach for certain anatomic locations and for microcystic lesions that respond to sclerotherapy in a much lesser percentage. In these cases, a minimal invasive surgical approach might be a more definitive treatment as a single procedure; it can also be combined with sclerotherapy in certain situations. However, most evidence is reduced to small case series and case reports, without large prospective studies, but the usual benefits of MIS (reduced pain and scars, reduced bowel adhesions, less bleeding) can be found.

Thoracic LMs are very uncommon, and, therefore, there are few case reports of thoracoscopically resected lesions, most of them in adult population. Enomoto et al. [15] reported one mediastinal lesion in a child treated through thoracoscopy. We have treated two of such cases, and one of them suffered a massive bleeding due to an unnoticed lesion of the superior vena cava. This highlights the importance of an adequate preoperative work-up and intraoperative anticipation of possible severe complications. Conversion to open surgery and blood concentrates must be available in the shortest possible time.

Abdominal lymphatic malformations can develop intraperitoneally or extraperitoneally, including the retroperitoneum and the root of the mesentery. Their typical debut forms are signs and symptoms of acute abdomen due to infection or bleeding and bulging; however, US incidental finding is becoming more and more common.

Laparoscopic resection of abdominal LM has proved to be safe and effective. In a series of patients from two pediatric hospitals over a 5-year period, published by Lagausie et al. [3] in 2005, only 9 out of 15 abdominal lymphatic malformations treated surgically were considered amenable to a laparoscopic approach; from these, three patients were converted to an open approach due to different technical difficulties. With a mean follow-up of 35 months, no recurrences were reported.

In 2012, Tran and Nguyen [8] reviewed the largest series of patients published to date, 47 cases treated during a 4-year period, either laparoscopically or laparoscopically assisted (which included bowel resections). Seventy-five percent of patients presented mesenteric lesions; the remaining 25% were omental. Conversion to open approach was required in only 6.4% of cases, without any reported complications. With a variable follow-up, only one recurrence happened in a complex mesenteric lesion.

Retroperitoneal LMs are uncommon. When symptomatic, surgical treatment with complete resection, if possible, is the preferred treatment. However, often this is not feasible as they commonly infiltrate multiple vital structures. In that case, sclerotherapy through a drainage catheter might be a better treatment option. Nevertheless, severe complications have been reported with sclerotherapy too, particularly in adult population. A limited number of published reports on laparoscopic resection of retroperitoneal LMs in children offer good results in terms of few local relapses and complications.

Lymphatic malformations can be diagnosed prenatally, usually during second trimester. Perinatal complications must be anticipated, depending on the location and size of the malformation, like polyhydramnios, hydrops, and mechanical dystocia [12]. In these cases, different minimal invasive alternatives of prenatal or intrapartum interventions can be considered in order to prevent life-threatening events for both mother and child.

Advances in technology and instruments are making minimal invasive surgery a very attractive and more definitive approach than sclerotherapy for certain LMs. Minimal invasive techniques, including endoscopic techniques, provide a wide range of benefits that come from diagnostic to therapeutic. The pediatric surgeon must be familiar with the diagnostic and therapeutic criteria of LMs and must consider all the currently available therapeutic armament.

References

1. ISSVA classification for vascular anomalies. 20th ISSVA workshop, Melbourne; 2014.
2. Wassef M, Blei F, Adams D, Alomari A, Baselga E, Berenstein A, et al. Vascular anomalies classification: recommendations from the International Society for the Study of Vascular Anomalies. Pediatrics. 2015;136(1):e203–14.
3. de Lagausie P, Bonnard A, Berrebi D, Lepretre O, Statopoulos L, Delarue A, et al. Abdominal lymphangiomas in children: interest of the laparoscopic approach. Surg Endosc. 2007;21(7):1153–7.
4. Surico D, Amadori R, D'Ajello P, Vercellotti E, Surico N. Antenatal diagnosis of fetal lymphangioma by ultrasonography. Eur J Obstet Gynecol Reprod Biol. 2013;168(2):236.
5. Legiehn GM, Heran MKS. A step-by-step practical approach to imaging diagnosis and interventional radiologic therapy in vascular malformations. Semin Interv Radiol. 2010;27(2):209–31.
6. Lee B. New approaches to the treatment of congenital vascular malformations (CVMs)—a single centre experience. Eur J Vasc Endovasc Surg. 2005;30(2):184–97.
7. Chiappinelli A, Forgues D, Galifer RB. Congenital abdominal cystic lymphangiomas: what is the correct management? J Matern Fetal Neonatal Med. 2012;25(7):915–9.
8. Tran NS, Nguyen TL. Laparoscopic management of abdominal lymphatic cyst in children. J Laparoendosc Adv Surg Tech A. 2012;22(5):505–7.
9. Wildhaber BE, Chardot C, Le Coultre C, Genin B. Total laparoscopic excision of retroperitoneal cystic lymphangioma. J Laparoendosc Adv Surg Tech A. 2006;16(5):530–3.
10. Singh RR, Govindarajan KK, Bowen C, Chandran H. Retroperitoneal cystic lymphangioma: a rare presentation in childhood, treated laparoscopically. J Laparoendosc Adv Surg Tech A. 2009;19(2):249–50.
11. Cao H, Yang Z-X, Sun Y-H, Wu H-R, Jiang G-Q. Endoscopic subcutaneous mastectomy: a novel and effective treatment for gynecomastia. Exp Ther Med. 2013;5(6):1683–6.
12. Arisoy R, Erdogdu E, Kumru P, Demirci O, Yuksel MA, Pekin O, et al. Prenatal diagnosis and outcome of lymphangiomas and its relationship with fetal chromosomal abnormalities. J Matern Fetal Neonatal Med. 2016;29(3):466–72.
13. Molino JA, Guillén G, Peiró JL, García-Vaquero JA, Marhuenda C, Carreras E, et al. Cervical cystic lymphangioma: still a challenge. Cir Pediatr. 2010;23(3):147–52.
14. Cruz-Martinez R, Moreno-Alvarez O, Garcia M, Méndez A, Pineda H, Cruz-Martinez MA, et al. Fetal endoscopic tracheal intubation: a new fetoscopic procedure to ensure extrauterine tracheal permeability in a case with congenital cervical teratoma. Fetal Diagn Ther. 2015;38(2):154–8.
15. Enomoto T, Hashimoto T, Tsuchida M, Yamato Y, Hayashi J. Mediastinal lymphangioma treated under video-assisted thoracic surgery. Kyobu Geka. 2003;56(3):255–7.

42 Laparoscopic-Assisted Endorectal Pull-Through in Hirschsprung's Disease and Familial Adenomatous Polyposis

G. Mattioli, M. G. Faticato, and M. C. Y. Wong

42.1 Introduction

Hirschsprung's disease (HD) is a congenital rare condition characterized by the absence of ganglion cells in the myenteric and submucosal plexuses, and it is one of the most common causes of intestinal obstruction in the newborn. The disease occurs as a consequence of abnormal migration/differentiation of neural crest-derived neuroblasts into the developing gut that determines absence of intestinal intramural ganglia. In most of the cases, the aganglionosis involves the rectum or rectosigmoid tract, but it may extend proximally involving the whole colon or even a tract of the small bowel. The incidence of HD is approximately 1:5000 live births with male preponderance [1]. The usual presentation of a neonate affected by HD is intestinal obstruction during the first few days of life. The most feared complication is enterocolitis. The gold standard for the diagnosis of HD is rectal suction biopsy [2].

Familial adenomatous polyposis (FAP) is an autosomal dominant inherited syndrome characterized by multiple adenomatous polyps, predisposing to colorectal cancer development.

Surgical treatment is mandatory in HD and FAP. In HD the main goal is to remove the aganglionic segment and pull down the normoganglionic bowel. Many techniques have been described, both with open and laparoscopic approaches. In the last 20 years, minimally invasive approach has gained popularity, and HD treatment changed accordingly. Also Robot-Assisted Soave Procedure was described [3].

In this chapter, we describe the main laparoscopic approach performed in our institution: the Soave-Georgeson endorectal pull-through (ERPT) [4].

G. Mattioli (✉) · M. G. Faticato · M. C. Y. Wong
Pediatric Surgery Unit, IRCCS Giannina Gaslini Institute, DINOGMI, University of Genoa, Genoa, Italy
e-mail: girolamomattioli@gaslini.org

42.2 Preoperative Preparation

All patients and their parents have to sign a specifically formulated informed consent before the procedure. Bowel nursing with enema is usually recommended for at least 2 days before the operation. A diet with clear liquids is generally indicated for 24–48 h before the operation. Preoperative intravenous antibiotics are administered at least 30 min before the incision. The surgical procedure is performed under general anesthesia. A nasogastric tube is positioned to decompress the stomach.

42.3 Positioning

The patient is placed in lithotomy position along the long axis of the table, with a slight Trendelenburg and left side up, in order to allow the access to both the abdomen and the perineum.

C. Esposito et al. (eds.), *ESPES Manual of Pediatric Minimally Invasive Surgery*,
https://doi.org/10.1007/978-3-030-00964-9_42

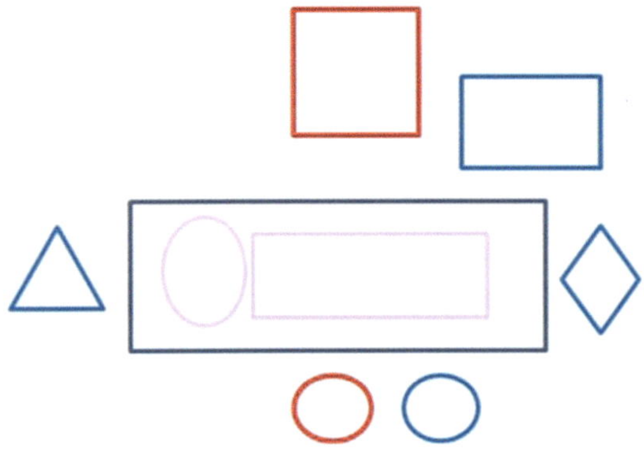

Fig. 42.1 Team position. Red ring is the first surgeon, blue ring is the assistant surgeon, rumble is the scrub nurse, triangle is the anesthetist, red square is the video monitor, and blue rectangle is the scrub table

Skin preparation is performed, and the operative field is prepared from nipples to toes, in order to include the whole abdomen and perineum, allowing to switch position in a sterile way. Buttocks and legs are cleaned circumferentially to the toes and sterile stockings are placed on both legs. Also the lower part of the back is sterilely prepared. A urinary catheter is inserted by the surgeon.

The video monitor is positioned on the left side of the patient toward the feet. For the laparoscopic step, the surgeon and cameraman stand on the right side of the bed with the scrub nurse on the same side (Fig. 42.1). A quality controlled timeout checklist is always performed before incision to avoid the risk of incomplete compliance.

42.4 Instrumentation

The first port is placed on the right hypochondrium in the anterior axillary line. This port is usually 5 mm for the infants and 12 mm for older children. A 5 mm 30° scope is placed in infants, and a 12 mm 30° scope is preferred in older children. Intra-abdominal pressure of 6–12 mmHg is used to create the pneumoperitoneum. Other two ports are inserted: one 5 mm in the right iliac region and one 3 mm trocarless in the left lumbar region. When the aganglionic segment is long, a fourth 5 mm trocar can be added in the left iliac region (Fig. 42.2).

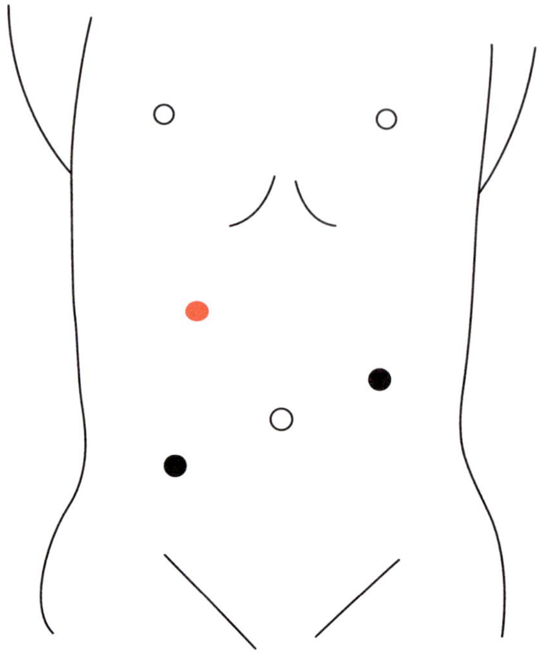

Fig. 42.2 Position of port sites. Red point: scope port (12 mm or 5 mm); black points: 5 mm port in the right iliac region and 3 mm port in the left lumbar region

The laparoscopic instrumentation consists of one 5 mm grasper and one 3 mm grasper, one 5 mm scissor, one 5 mm sealing/dividing forceps, one 5 mm hook, and one 5 mm needle holder.

In addition you need a standard set of instruments for traditional open surgery and electric cautery.

42.5 Technique

The technique is divided into two phases, the diagnostic and the therapeutic one.

In the diagnostic phase, the aim is to identify the colonic transition zone in order to pull through the normoganglionic colon. Seromuscular biopsy is performed with scissor proximal to the dilated colon and sent immediately for the extemporaneous histological examination. The specimen is obtained grasping the colon and cutting along the length of the colon (Fig. 42.3). Biopsy site is closed with a nonabsorbable suture. If the biopsy results show an aganglionic bowel, it is mandatory to repeat a biopsy in the upstream colon. It is important to wait for the biopsies results before proceeding with the dissection and mobilization of the rectum and the colon, if a transition zone is not clear.

Once the ganglionic bowel is determined, the therapeutic phase can start. A window through the rectosigmoid mesocolon is performed with sealing/dividing forceps or with hook monopolar (Fig. 42.4), paying attention to stay close to the colon wall in order to preserve the vascularization. In fact, the marginal artery provides the vascular supply to the segment which will be pulled down. Inferior mesenteric pedicle has to be preserved to keep a good vascularization to the rectal cuff.

The window is widened distally until the peritoneal reflection in the pelvis. During the dissection, it is important to detect ureters and vas deferens (in males). When the transition zone is found in the superior part of the sigmoid colon, or descending colon or in the transverse colon, a colon pedicle is required. The rectal dissection is performed circumferentially with the monopolar hook (Fig. 42.5).

The last abdominal step is the evaluation of sufficient colon mobilization by trying to reach the pelvis; if it is insufficient, laparoscopic mobilization should continue.

When the colon mobilization and rectal dissection end, the pneumoperitoneum is evacuated, laparoscopic instruments are removed, and trocars are left in place for a second look after the pull-through in order to check possible colon torsion.

Once the laparoscopic phase has been completed, the perineal step starts by switching the position in a gynecological one. Skin stiches are placed in order to expose the anal canal up to the pectinate line (Fig. 42.6). Traction sutures are placed in the four cardinal points in the proximal rectal mucosa, and mucosal dissection starts 5 mm above the dentate line with blunt and sharp

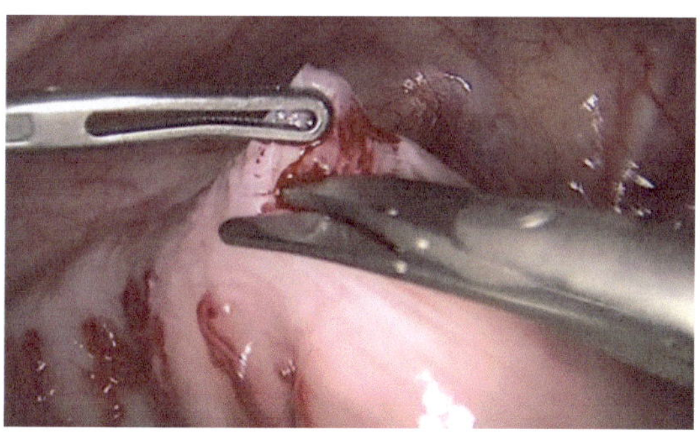

Fig. 42.3 Seromuscular biopsy is performed with scissor, grasping the colon by its taenia coli, and it is obtained by cutting along the length of the colon. The biopsy site is closed with a nonabsorbable suture

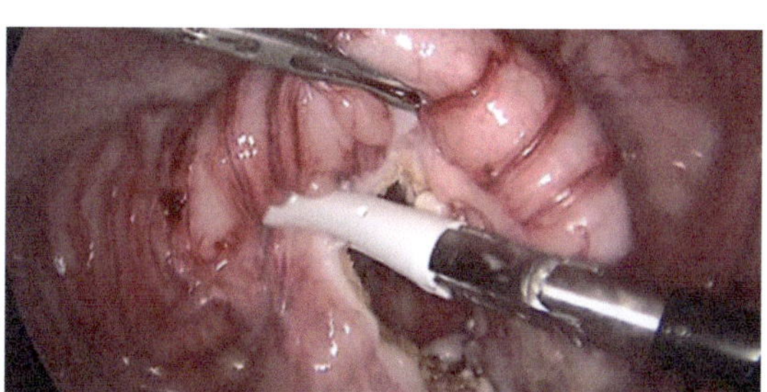

Fig. 42.4 The rectosigmoid mesocolic window is created using sealing/dividing forceps

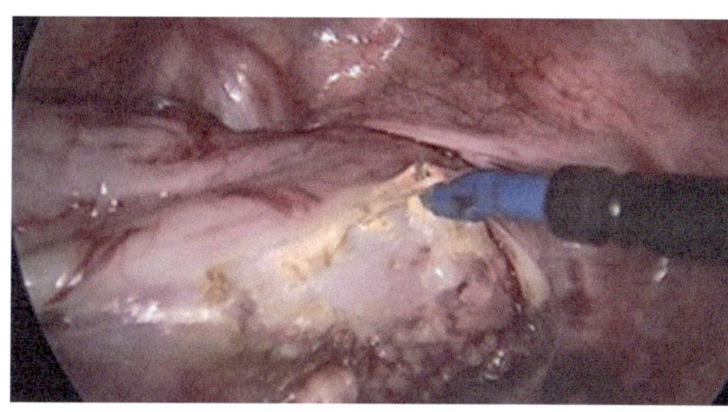

Fig. 42.5 Rectal circumferential dissection with monopolar hook is performed paying attention to ureters and vas deferens. Rectal dissection continues distally in order to obtain a complete mobilization

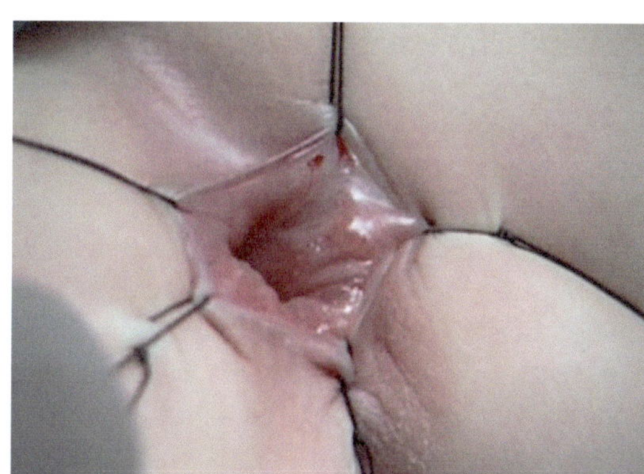

Fig. 42.6 Skin stitches are put in order to expose the anal canal up to the pectinate line

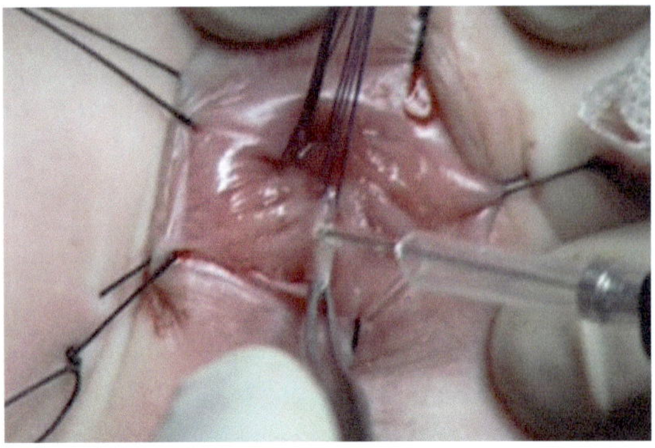

Fig. 42.7 Traction sutures are put in the proximal rectal mucosa to help the surgeon during the dissection and mucosal dissection starts with blunt and sharp electrocautery

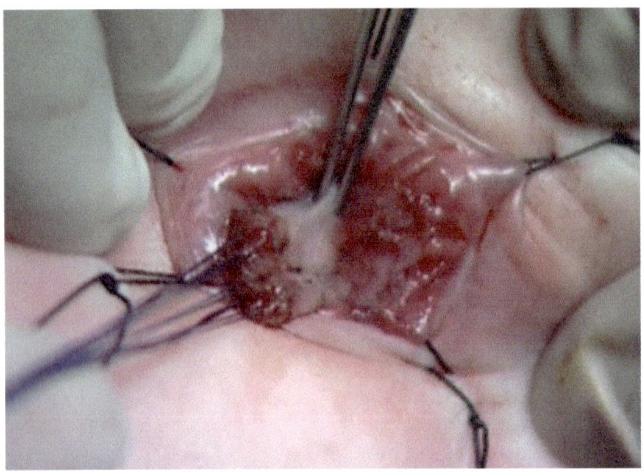

Fig. 42.8 The plane between submucosal and circular smooth muscle is started laterally and then continued circumferentially

electrocautery (Fig. 42.7). Traction sutures help the surgeon to retract the mucosa during the circumferential dissection.

The plane between submucosal and circular smooth muscle should be started laterally and then continued circumferentially (Fig. 42.8). The submucosal dissection continues proximally until the smooth muscle cuff is achieved and the colorectum prolapses, indicating that the internal perirectal dissection has been reached. When the perineal dissection plane joins the laparoscopic one, the short muscular rectal cuff is split with cautery posteriorly in the midline 1–2 cm above the dentate line, in order to provide space for neorectal reservoir. The cuff is pushed back into the pelvis, and the aganglionic bowel is pulled through the anal

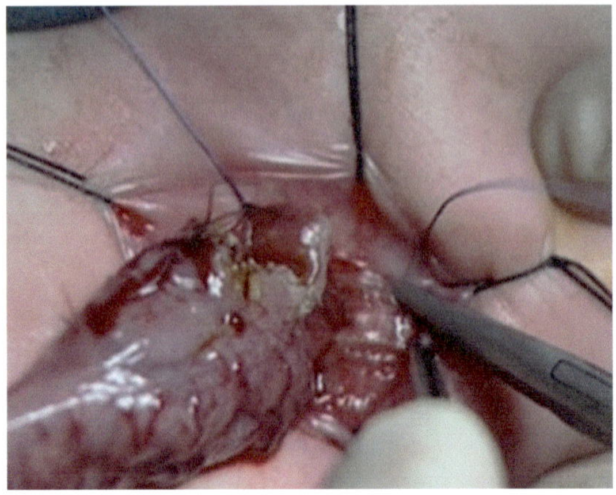

Fig. 42.9 The anterior half of the pull-through bowel is incised, and absorbable stitches are placed at 12 o'clock, 9 o'clock, and 3 o'clock positions

canal until the most proximal biopsy site, previously marked with recognizable suture.

Before performing the anastomosis, it is important to inspect the internal cuff and straighten it if necessary.

The anastomosis between anal canal and normoganglionic bowel can now be performed. The anastomosis must always be done proximally to the biopsy site. The anterior half of the pull-through bowel is incised, and separate absorbable 5-0 or 6-0 stitches are placed at 12 o'clock, 9 o'clock, and 3 0'clock positions (Fig. 42.9). The pull-through bowel is then completely transected, and a single stitch at 6 o'clock site is put. The anastomosis is ended with other separate stitches in each quadrant (Fig. 42.10). A total of eight stitches are usually added (two for each quadrant).

The pneumoperitoneum is reintroduced in order to check the correct orientation of the vascular pedicle and to exclude internal herniation, then the pneumoperitoneum is evacuated, the ports are removed, and the port sites are closed with fascial and skin stitches.

42.6 Postoperative Care

In the postoperative period, the patients can keep a normal decubitus. Nasogastric tube is removed at the end of the operation. The urinary catheter

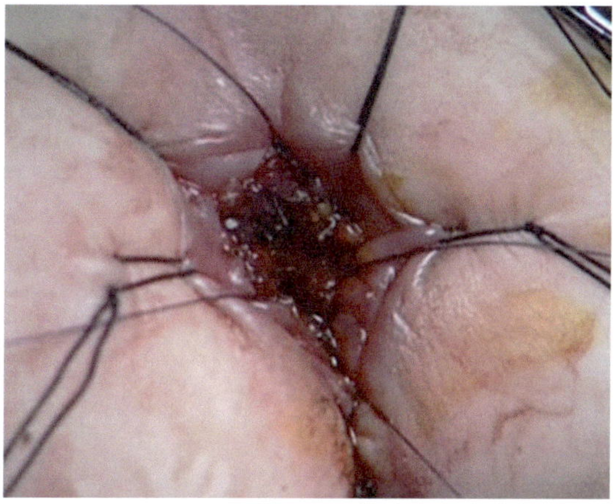

Fig. 42.10 End of the anastomosis

is left in place until opioid analgesics are used. Otherwise, the urinary catheter can be removed after 24 h.

Oral feeding can restart when there is evidence of bowel function. Antibiotic prophylaxis is continued for 24 h after surgery. The analgesic therapy is managed by a specialized team which follows the patient daily.

All patients are discharged on the third–fourth postoperative day, if the course is uneventful.

No shower is admitted for 1 week after surgery.

Narcosis visit in the operation theater is planned after 3–4 weeks from the pull-through for the rectal examination to check the anastomosis, in particular the presence of stenosis. If the anastomosis is felt tight, weekly dilatation is supported.

42.7 Results

In the last 10 years (2007–2017), we performed the Soave-Georgeson technique in 91 patients. The average age at surgery was 21.5 months (range 1.58–223.34 months).

The median length of surgery was about 190 min (range 80–525 min). In three patients, the operation was performed with robotic da Vinci assistance, with longer operative time. No intraoperative complications occurred, but in three cases the conversion to open surgery was necessary for long aganglionic bowel (beyond the transverse colon).

The median time to return to full daily activities was 6 days (range 4–18).

Follow-up is usually carried out by clinical examinations at 1 month, 6 months, and then annually. In our series, within 91 patients, no recurrence was recorded. Anastomosis stricture occurred in two patients, who underwent two dilatations with success result. Cuff stricture occurred in two patients, who underwent two dilatations with failure, and, later, a laparoscopy was indicated for cuff dissection.

42.8 Tips and Tricks

When placing the first trocar with Veress needle technique, it is important to pay attention to liver injuries, especially in neonates. In fact, in newborns the inferior liver margin extends far from the costal margin.

During the laparoscopic perirectal dissection, the surgeon must take care during the lateral and anterior dissection, in order to avoid damage to the nervi erigentes, deferens, and vagina which can result in impotence or bladder dysfunction.

When a vascular pedicle is performed, the surgeon should always assess the length of the pedicle, ensuring that the segment of bowel is sufficiently mobile to reach the deep pelvis without tension.

The posterior split of the rectal cuff has to be always performed, for the high risk of cuff retraction and stricture.

In case of very dilated colon up to the transition zone, it is recommended to remove normoganglionic bowel, so that the coloanal anastomosis involves normal, non-dilated colon wall.

Ischemia, torsion, tension, and cuff stricture must be avoided as they lead to complications, with necessity of re-intervention.

42.9 Discussion

For many decades surgical treatment of HD was characterized by staged procedures, while in recent years many surgeons have preferred one-stage pull-through operations with minimal morbidity rates and encouraging results [5–8]. A lot of studies demonstrate the importance of minimal access approach to treat HD [9–11]. The first description of laparoscopic-assisted endorectal pull-through was reported by Georgeson in 1995 [4].

The Soave-Georgeson endorectal pull-through provides important advantages compared to other procedures. First of all, the mobilization of the colon pedicle with a laparoscopic approach allows to reduce peritoneal trauma and subsequent adherence formation. Second, the laparoscopic approach permits a less bloody perirectal dissection compared to open procedure [12]. Third, with laparoscopic assistance, clear delineation of pelvic structures, faster postoperative recovery, and better cosmetic results have been described [13–15]. Moreover, compared to totally transanal endorectal pull-through, the Soave-Georgeson technique allows to better assess the colon pedicle tension, to avoid colon twisting, and to perform intraoperative colon biopsies before starting endorectal dissection and mesocolic vessel division.

Finally, current literature shows that mini-invasive procedures provide advantages over open surgery in terms of operative time, intraoperative blood loss, postoperative hospital stay, soiling/incontinence, and constipation. In contrast, no differences are present for enterocolitis occurrence and anastomotic stricture [16, 17]. We cannot compare the laparoscopic ERPT with the total transanal ERPT and Duhamel operation as in our institute we do not perform these techniques.

References

1. Suita S, Taguchi T, Ieiri S, Nakatsuji T. Hirschsprung's disease in Japan: analysis of 3852 patients based on a nationwide survey in 30 years. J Pediatr Surg. 2005;40(1):197–201; discussion 201–2.
2. Friedmacher F, Puri P. Rectal suction biopsy for the diagnosis of Hirschsprung's disease: a systematic review of diagnostic accuracy and complications. Pediatr Surg Int. 2015;31(9):821–30.
3. Mattioli G, Pio L, Leonelli L, Razore B, Disma N, Montobbio G, Jasonni V, Petralia P, Pini Prato A. A provisional experience with robot-assisted soave procedure for older children with Hirschsprung disease: back to the future? J Laparoendosc Adv Surg Tech A. 2017;27(5):546–9.
4. Georgeson KE, Fuenfer MM, Hardin WD. Primary laparoscopic pull-through for Hirschsprung's disease in infants and children. J Pediatr Surg. 1995;30(7):1017–21; discussion 1021–2.
5. So HB, Schwartz DL, Becker JM, Daum F, Schneider KM. Endorectal "pull-through" without preliminary colostomy in neonates with Hirschsprung's disease. J Pediatr Surg. 1980;15(4):470–1.
6. Cilley RE, Statter MB, Hirschl RB, Coran AG. Definitive treatment of Hirschsprung's disease in the newborn with a one-stage procedure. Surgery. 1994;115(5):551–6.
7. Wilcox DT, Bruce J, Bowen J, Bianchi A. One-stage neonatal pull-through to treat Hirschsprung's disease. J Pediatr Surg. 1997;32(2):243–5; discussion 245–7.
8. Coran AG, Teitelbaum DH. Recent advances in the management of Hirschsprung's disease. Am J Surg. 2000;180(5):382–7.
9. Georgeson KE, Cohen RD, Hebra A, Jona JZ, Powell DM, Rothenberg SS, Tagge EP. Primary laparoscopic-assisted endorectal colon pull-through for Hirschsprung's disease: a new gold standard. Ann Surg. 1999;229(5):678–82; discussion 682–3.
10. Thomson D, Allin B, Long AM, Bradnock T, Walker G, Knight M. Laparoscopic assistance for primary transanal pull-through in Hirschsprung's disease: a systematic review and meta-analysis. BMJ Open. 2015;5(3):e006063.
11. Tomuschat C, Zimmer J, Puri P. Laparoscopic-assisted pull-through operation for Hirschsprung's disease: a systematic review and meta-analysis. Pediatr Surg Int. 2016;32(8):751–7.
12. Mattioli G, Pini Prato A, Giunta C, Avanzini S, Della Rocca M, Montobbio G, Parodi S, Rapuzzi G, Georgeson K, Jasonni V. Outcome of primary endorectal pull-through for the treatment of classic Hirschsprung disease. J Laparoendosc Adv Surg Tech A. 2008;18(6):869–74.
13. Georgeson KE, Robertson DJ. Laparoscopic-assisted approaches for the definitive surgery for Hirschsprung's disease. Semin Pediatr Surg. 2004;13(4):256–62.
14. Murphy F, Menezes M, Puri P. Enterocolitis complicating Hirschsprung's disease. In: Puri P, editor. Hirschsprung's disease and allied disorders. 3rd ed. Berlin: Springer; 2008. p. 138–9.
15. Craigie RJ, Conway SJ, Cooper L, Turnock RR, Lamont GL, Baillie CT, Kenny SE. Primary pull-through for Hirschsprung's disease: comparison of open and laparoscopic-assisted procedures. J Laparoendosc Adv Surg Tech A. 2007;17(6):809–12.
16. Gosemann JH, Friedmacher F, Ure B, Lacher M. Open versus transanal pull-through for Hirschsprung disease: a systematic review of long-term outcome. Eur J Pediatr Surg. 2013;23(2):94–102.
17. Zhao B, Liu T, Li Q. Comparison of the efficacy and safety of laparoscopic-assisted operations and open operations for Hirschsprung's disease: evidence from a meta-analysis. Int J Clin Exp Med. 2015;8(8):12963–9, eCollection 2015.

Laparoscopic Approach to Anorectal Malformations

43

Alejandra Vilanova-Sánchez, Richard J. Wood, Rebecca M. Rentea, and Marc A. Levitt

43.1 Introduction

Anorectal malformations (ARM) are relatively common in children, affecting 1/5000 live births. Since the description of the posterior sagittal anorectoplasty (PSARP), the rectum is most often easily reachable from a posterior sagittal approach [1]. However, there are some malformations in which the rectum is located high in the pelvis and can benefit from a combined abdominal and perineal approach [2]. It is important to understand that if the fistula is low in the pelvis, below the peritoneal reflection (low rectoprostatic or rectobulbar or low rectum without a fistula), it may be more difficult to mobilize the very distal rectum away from the urinary/gynecologic tract utilizing an abdominal approach. Inadequate ligation of the fistula results in a retained remnant of the original fistula (ROOF) [3].

In this chapter we describe the indications, preoperative and postoperative considerations, surgical steps, and useful tips and tricks for utilizing laparoscopy for the primary repair of ARM.

A. Vilanova-Sánchez (✉)
Pediatric Surgery, Colorectal Unit, University Hospital La Paz, Madrid, Spain
e-mail: alejandra.vilanova@salud.madrid.org

R. J. Wood · R. M. Rentea · M. A. Levitt
Center for Colorectal and Pelvic Reconstruction, Nationwide Children's Hospital, Columbus, OH, USA

43.2 Preoperative Preparation

All patients must have a complete VACTERL (vertebral, anal, cardiac, tracheoesophageal, renal, and limb) screening work-up. This includes chest X-ray and abdominal X-ray, AP and lateral sacrum X-ray, spinal U/S or MRI, echocardiogram, and renal U/S. Urological assesment by a pediatric urologist should be also performed in all patients with anorectal malformations.

Before the procedure a high-pressure distal colostogram should also be completed in order to identify position and length of the distal rectum. This study will help the surgeon decide whether the patient requires a posterior sagittal approach only or one combined with a laparoscopic/abdominal assisted pull-through.

A useful rule to assist the surgeon on whether or not a laparoscopic approach can be taken is to draw a line from the tip of the coccyx to the very next structure one would find via a posterior sagittal approach. If the structure which the line touches on the contrast enema is the rectum, then the rectum is reachable from below. If that structure which the line touches is the bladder, urethra, or vagina, then laparoscopy will be needed in order to dissect the rectum intra-abdominally (Fig. 43.1a, b). Patients do not need any bowel preparation before surgery as all of them have a colostomy. Broad-spectrum antibiotics are given immediately prior to incision.

C. Esposito et al. (eds.), *ESPES Manual of Pediatric Minimally Invasive Surgery*,
https://doi.org/10.1007/978-3-030-00964-9_43

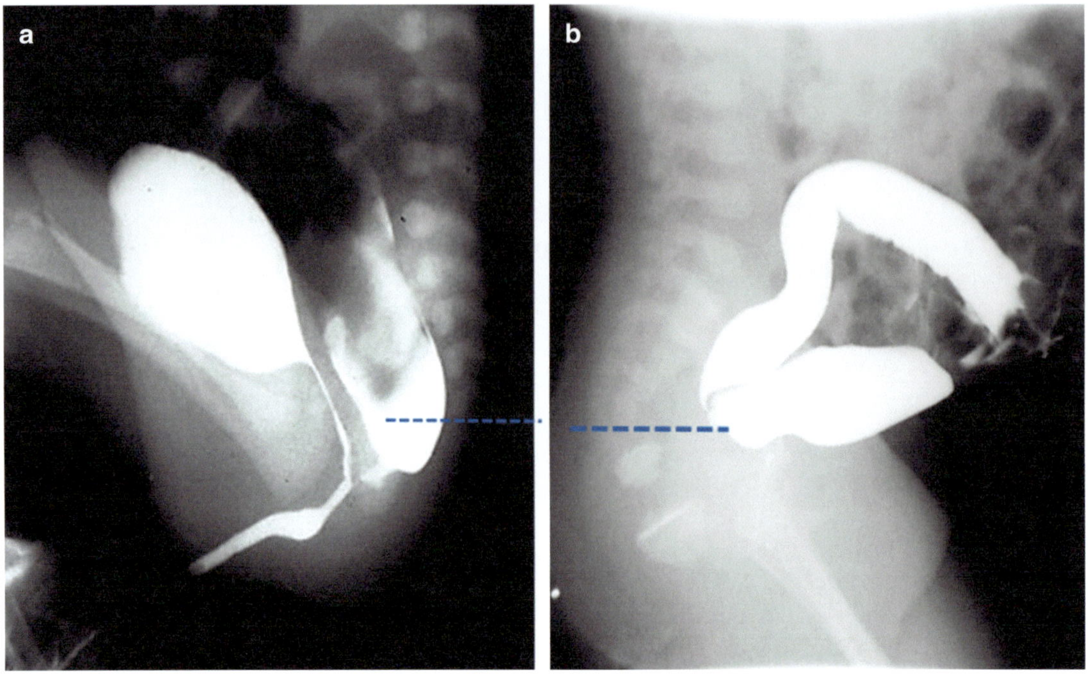

Fig. 43.1 (**a**) Line from coccyx touches the rectum first—case can be done posterior sagittally. (**b**) Line from coccyx touches urinary tract first—case needs laparoscopy

43.3 Positioning

The patient is placed in supine position.

43.3.1 Total Body Preparation

We firstly perform a total body preparation; two people are needed to complete the prep; one person preps the patient, while the other (wearing sterile gloves on) lifts the patient. Once the entire patient is prepped from the toes to the nipples, the prep person pulls the 3/4 sheet out from under the patient, and the scrub nurse places sterile 3/4 sheet under the patient, and then legs are laid down. The patient is the placed through the circular hole of a large sterile drap. The legs are wrapped in sterile dressing (sterile cotton and Coban) up to the buttock crease. The Coban should have a "toe flap" (so that it can later have a clamp on it without crushing the toes or falling off).

The stoma should be covered by a sponge and sterile tape. A coude tip urethral catheter must be placed to drain the bladder on sterile field. A wide tip 60-mL syringe should be connected to the coude (coude tip catheter is easier to insert in patients with anorectal malformation and recto-urinary fistula) catheter for urine collection during the procedure.

43.3.2 Trocar Positioning

A 5-mm umbilical access is used to start the pneumoperitoneum with 8–10 mmHg of pressure. 4-mm trocars in the right upper quadrant and right mid abdomen are placed. The right upper quadrant port is for the camera access. The right lower quadrant port is for the surgeon's right hand and the umbilicus is for the left hand. If needed a left upper quadrant port can be placed to help retract the sigmoid and used to place the endoloop to ligate the fistula (Fig. 43.2a, b). Once the abdominal portion is completed, the patient's legs are elevated in order to have access to the perineum. We are able to elevate the legs by clamping with a mosquito clamp the toe flap of the Coban dressing and then utilizing an S-shape

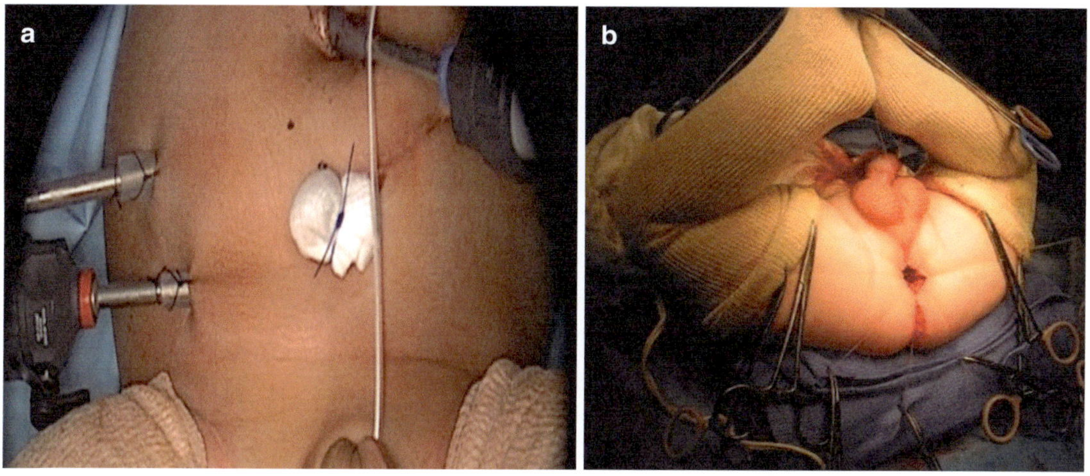

Fig. 43.2 (**a**) Trocar positioning in a laparoscopic assisted anorectoplasty for ARM. (**b**) Positioning for the posterior sagittal approach portion of the procedure

retractor to hang the mosquito onto the anesthesia screen bar. A small roll in the distal lumbar area is placed to elevate the buttocks.

43.4 Instrumentation

A 5-mm 30° camera and 4-mm trocars (2 or 3) are utilized as the instruments (5-mm trocars are also accepted). Hook electrocautery and a 3-mm endosealer are utilized to avoid thermal spread when approaching the bladder/vagina. A 3-mm grasper in the upper left quadrant can be utilized in the left upper quadrant to provide additional traction.

In recto-bladder fistula if the bladder anatomy of the patient blocks the view of the distal dissection of the rectum going into the bladder, a transcutaneous stitch to elevate the bladder could be also performed to improve posterior bladder visualization. To ligate the fistula, a preloaded endoloop with 2/0 absorbable monofilament works well. Staplers should be avoided on bladder and vaginal sutures. For the posterior anal portion of the case, a nerve stimulator is utilized to identify the anterior and posterior limits of the sphincter mechanism. For the rectal dissection, fine electrocautery tip (Colorado tip or Olsen tip) results in the most precise dissection. In addition, a standard set of open instruments is needed, and also a traditional monopolar cautery.

43.5 Technique

Once the trocars are placed and pneumoperitoneum achieved, we identify the rectum in the pelvis going down to the pelvis inlet. The first step (if necessary) is to fix the bladder to the anterior abdominal wall with a transcutaneous stay suture to have better exposure of the pelvis.

The distal rectum is then mobilized using an energy device in a circumferential fashion, starting with the anterior attachments and working laterally until the posterior attachments are able to be visualized and released. While doing this dissection, both ureters and vas deferens were identified and avoided. The 3-mm endosealer is very helpful for attachments near the bladder as it avoids thermal spread. Great care needs to be taken to preserve the IMA and its branches which provide intramural blood supply to the distal rectum. Once the fistula is dissected circumferentially, a fourth 3-mm instrument assists with division of the fistula. Once the fistula is dissected circumferentially, at the point of maximal tapering near the bladder, the fistula is divided. The distal fistula should be dissected to the size whereby a 3-mm grasper can completely traverse it. The bladder side is secured with a grasper and a preloaded endoloop used to close the fistula site (Fig. 43.3).

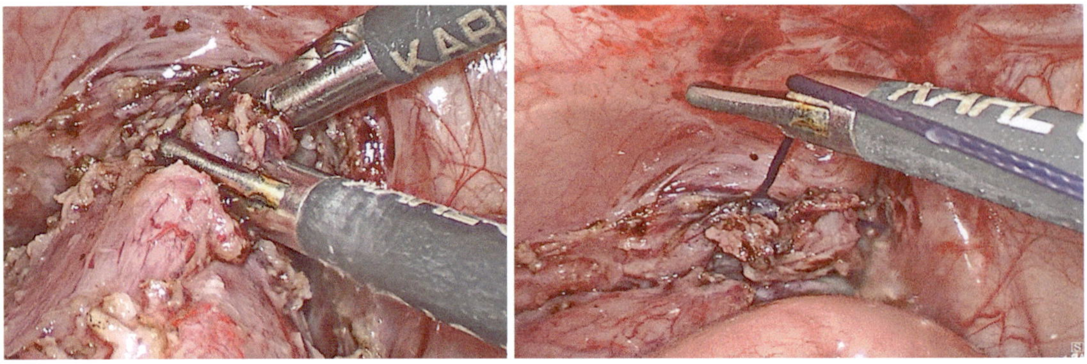

Fig. 43.3 Ligation of the rectourethral fistula

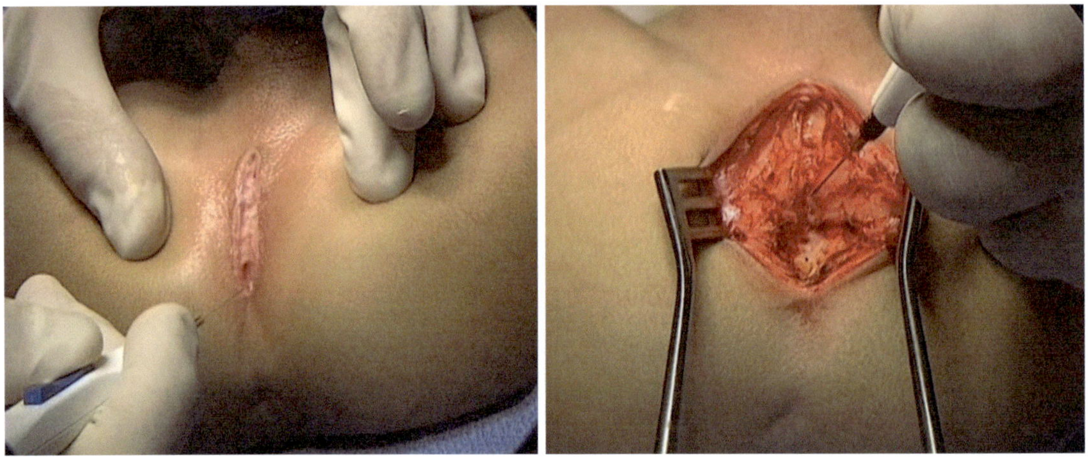

Fig. 43.4 Limited perineal incision, patient is in supine position

Once there is sufficient rectal length, the patient's legs are elevated. There is no need for prone positioning. The muscle complex is defined (anterior and posterior limits are noted and marked) with the nerve stimulator, and a limited posterior sagittal incision is made (Fig. 43.4). The incision is opened with electrocautery and with blunt dissection in order to reach the peritoneal reflection (Fig. 43.5). We then tack the muscles to the pulled through rectum to avoid prolapse and perform an anoplasty with 16 interrupted sutures. The perineal incision is closed with interrupted sutures as well (Fig. 43.6).

43.6 Postoperative Care

In the postoperative period, the patient can be maintained in a supine position. We recommend avoiding any buttock spreading the first 2 weeks following surgery. Nasogastric tube is not required in the postoperative period. Full oral feeds can be initiated immediately following surgery as the child has a colostomy. Postoperative antibiotics can be limited to two postoperative doses. The analgesic requirement is generally limited to the first 48 postoperative hours.

The coude catheter is kept in place for 1 week in patients with recto-bladder or rectourethral fis-

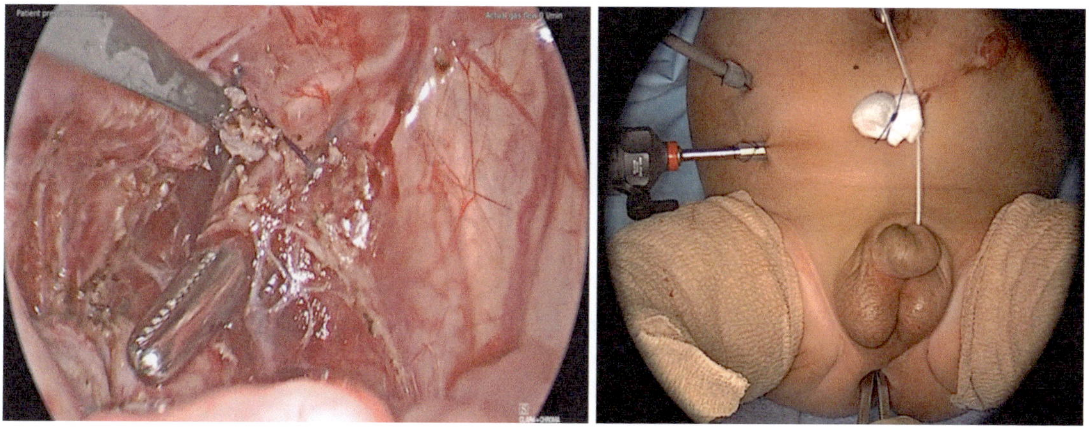

Fig. 43.5 Obtaining access to pelvis via the perineal incision

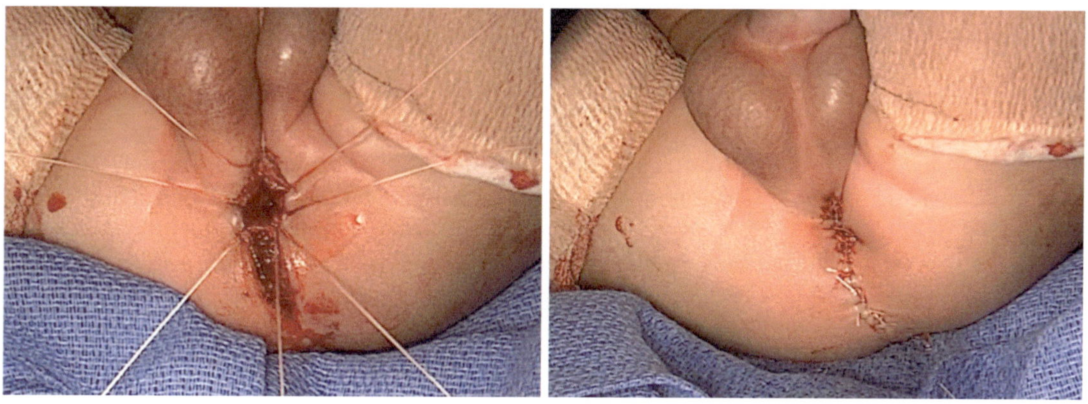

Fig. 43.6 Tacking of the rectum, anoplasty, and perineal closure

tula. In females with rectovaginal fistula, it is kept 1–2 days. In cloacas it will determined by the urethral work done during the procedure after the laparoscopic dissection. The catheter can be placed between two diapers to allow the infant more comfort and mobility. Patients are usually discharged on the second to third postoperative day. Before discharge the posterior sagittal wound as well as the anoplasty should be carefully inspected at the bedside in order to rule out dehiscence or mucosal traction at the anoplasty site. In the postoperative period and upon discharge, the wound should be washed with soap and water, wiping should be avoided and the area should be patted dry. No creams or ointments should be applied on sutures or incision. Tub bath should be avoided for a week after surgery. The patient will need to be examined in clinic 2 weeks after surgery to assess the need for anal dilations. Once the ideal Hegar size for age is reached, the colostomy can be closed, usually 2–3 months after the procedure.

43.7 Results

The average length of surgery is about 3–4 h for bladder neck fistulas and high rectovaginal fistulas. For cloacas it will depend on the anatomy of the cloaca (length of the common channel, length of the urethra, and need for vaginal replacement). Follow-up is carried out by clinical examinations at 2 weeks to assess anal dilations, 2–3 months after for colostomy closure, and every 6 months–1 year for general follow-up and assessment of constipation or incontinence.

In our series from June 2014 to May 2018, we have performed 20 laparoscopic assisted PSARP for ARM: 16 recto-bladder neck, 2 rectovaginal, and 2 high rectums in cloaca. No complications occurred relating to the laparoscopic approach or mini-posterior sagittal approach. Sixteen of the patients required anal dilations and four did not. There was one postoperative stricture that required revision. There was no rectal prolapse.

43.8 Tips and Tricks

1. Review the high-pressure distal colostogram prior to deciding posterior vs. abdominal (laparoscopic) approach.
2. Draw a line from the tip of the coccyx to the very next structure one would find via a posterior sagittal approach. If the structure on the contrast enema is the rectum, then the rectum is reachable from below.
3. Identify the vas deferens and ureters during pelvic dissection.
4. Rectal dissection should be kept immediately outside the muscle wall of the rectum.
5. Mark the sphincter complex with its anterior and posterior limits both before administering paralytics and prior to making a limited posterior incision.
6. Utilize a limited posterior incision instead of serial trocar dilations as the rectum can then be pexied to the muscle complex, preventing future prolapse, and it is a safer way to find the path into the pelvis.

43.9 Discussion

Malformations such as perineal, vestibular, rectobulbar, and low rectoprostatic are easy to repair with a posterior sagittal approach. The ARMs, which benefit from laparoscopy, include high prostatic or bladder neck fistula in males and congenital high rectovaginal fistula or cloacas with high rectum in girls [3]. It is important to understand that if the fistula is low in the pelvis (low rectoprostatic or rectobulbar, below the peritoneal reflection), it is much more difficult to ligate the fistula close to the urinary/gynecologic tract from an abdominal approach. Inability to perform close ligation to the urinary/gynecologic structures results in a remnant of the original fistula (ROOF) being left behind causing future problems (Fig. 43.7a, b) [4, 5].

Careful selection of the approach on anorectal malformations reconstruction cannot be stressed enough. A purely posterior sagittal approach only in those patients with high rectum can pose dangerous. First, the dissection travels deep into the pelvis often requiring a coccygectomy in order to reach the peritoneal reflection. Second, if the rectum in high, the bladder can be easily confused with the rectum and leading to misidentification and injury to the urinary tract.

Once the indication of laparoscopy is made with the help of the lateral view of the high-pressure distal colostogram, a limited posterior sagittal incision can be beneficial. Some authors advocate not performing any incision or dissection of the sphincter mechanism. They perform a straight pull-through placing a trocar in the perineum without opening the muscles [6]. Normally, the malformations that require laparoscopy are high, which also correlate with a poor sphincter complex development, spinal cord and sacral issues, and weak pelvic musculature. These factors taken together can result in rectal prolapse [3]. With the help of a limited posterior sagittal incision, the rectum is anchored to the edges of the sphincter complex minimizing the risk of rectal prolapse [4]. Another advantage of the mini-posterior sagittal incision is that the center of the sphincter mechanism and the angle the muscles take as they merge into the levators are clearly identified. This also allows for a safer trajectory into the pelvis [7]. Overall, the morbidity of a mini-posterior sagittal incision is low and the benefits are remarkable.

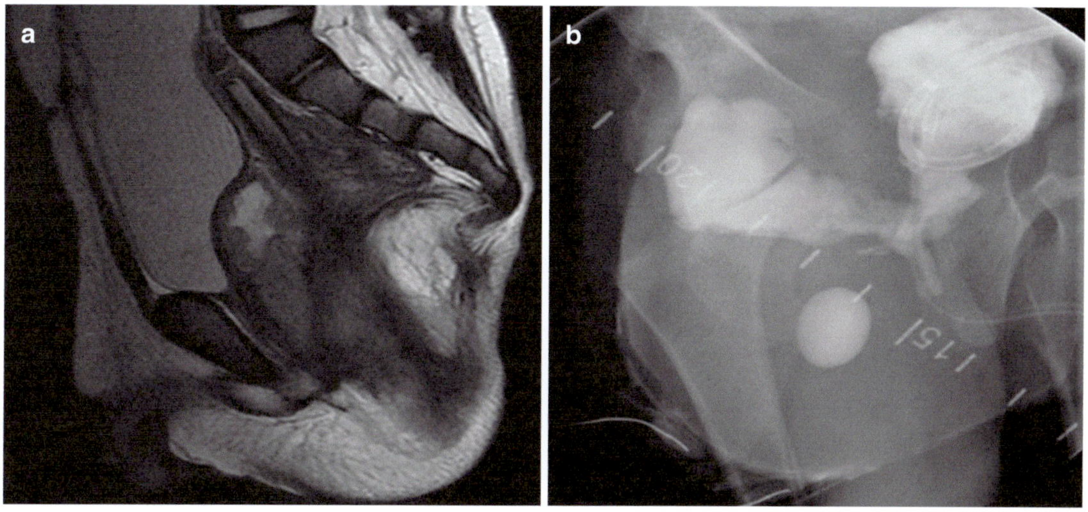

Fig. 43.7 (**a**) MRI demonstrating large ROOF emanating from the prostate. (**b**) VCUG demonstrating filling of the ROOF with contrast

References

1. Bischoff A, Levitt MA, Peña A. Update on the management of anorectal malformations. Pediatr Surg Int. 2013;29:899–904.
2. Georgeson K. Laparoscopic-assisted anorectal pull-through. Semin Pediatr Surg. 2007;16:266–9.
3. Bischoff A, Martinez-Leo B, Peña A. Laparoscopic approach in the management of anorectal malformations. Pediatr Surg Int. 2015;31:431–7.
4. Bischoff A, Levitt MA, Peña A. Laparoscopy and its use in the repair of anorectal malformations. J Pediatr Surg. 2011;46:1609–17.
5. Alam S, Lawal TA, Peña A, Sheldon C, Levitt MA. Acquired posterior urethral diverticulum following surgery for anorectal malformations. J Pediatr Surg. 2011;46:1231–5.
6. Wang C, Diao M, Li L, Liu S, Chen Z, Li X, Cheng W. Laparoscopic dissection and division of distal fistula in boys with rectourethral fistula. J Surg Res. 2017;211:147–53.
7. Srimurthy KR, Ramesh S, Shankar G, Narenda BM. Technical modifications of laparoscopically assisted anorectal pull-through for anorectal malformations. J Laparoendosc Adv Surg Tech A. 2008;18:340–3.

Laparoscopic Management of Acute Appendicitis

44

Philipp Szavay

44.1 Introduction

Over the last 10–15 years, the management of appendicitis in childhood has changed with regard to diagnosis and therapy. From the first report of conventional appendectomy in 1894 for decades, appendectomy through an incision as described by McBurney [1] has been the gold standard in surgical treatment of (suspected) acute appendicitis. With the implementation of ultrasound, scoring systems to facilitate the surgical indication and minimal invasive techniques for surgery since the 1980s, nowadays ranging from conventional laparoscopy to single-site surgery the surgical treatment of appendicitis has been undergoing significant advances. The aim is to propose practical clinical guidelines for the current gold standard of laparoscopic appendectomy.

44.2 Current Status and General Aspects of Laparoscopic Appendectomy

Meanwhile advantages of laparoscopic appendectomy are widely acknowledged as well as accepted. Compared to open surgical procedures [1], the rate of wound infections is lower, cosmesis is superior, while the length of hospitalization is shorter, and postoperative pain is less, respectively [2–6]. A nationwide survey from Germany reported the current status of laparoscopic appendectomy [7]. In 71 out of 98 pediatric surgical institutions, appendectomy is performed laparoscopically; however still only 56 institutions considered it to be their standard approach. In 90% a three-trocar technique was preferred, while 10% of surgeons used a single-incision laparoscopic approach. In 93% of pediatric surgical institutions, a single-shot antibiotic therapy was administered perioperatively. In those institutions where laparoscopic appendectomy was considered to be the standard approach, during regular working hours in 87%, the procedure was carried out as a training procedure with a resident or fellow, respectively, operating. This number decreased to 63% during on-call times. In conclusion this report could show that laparoscopic appendectomy is the standard for surgical therapy of acute appendicitis.

44.3 Preoperative Preparation

Informed consent is obtained from all patients or their parents, respectively, prior to surgery. General anesthesia with muscle relaxation is provided. A Foley catheter is inserted in order to control urinary drainage as well as providing an empty bladder during laparoscopy for improved

P. Szavay (✉)
Department of Pediatric Surgery, Lucerne Children's Hospital, Lucerne, Switzerland
e-mail: philipp.szavay@luks.ch

C. Esposito et al. (eds.), *ESPES Manual of Pediatric Minimally Invasive Surgery*,
https://doi.org/10.1007/978-3-030-00964-9_44

working space and view. Perioperative single-shot antibiotic therapy with cefuroxime and metronidazole is administered according to the weight of the patient. The patient is prepped and placed according to local standards and following the rules of asepsis.

44.4 Positioning and Ergonomics

The patient is placed in supine position. According to the specific operating theater specification and set-up, respectively, the monitor is positioned on the right side of the patient in order to provide the surgeon with a view in direction to the operating field. Additional monitors are placed meaningfully around the patient to facilitate view for the assistant surgeon, scrub nurses, anesthetists, and others, respectively. Surgeon's position is on the left side of the patient, while the assistant surgeon driving the camera is standing on the same side, with both the surgeons looking in direction to the patient's right side. The scrub nurse is standing across at the patient's right side.

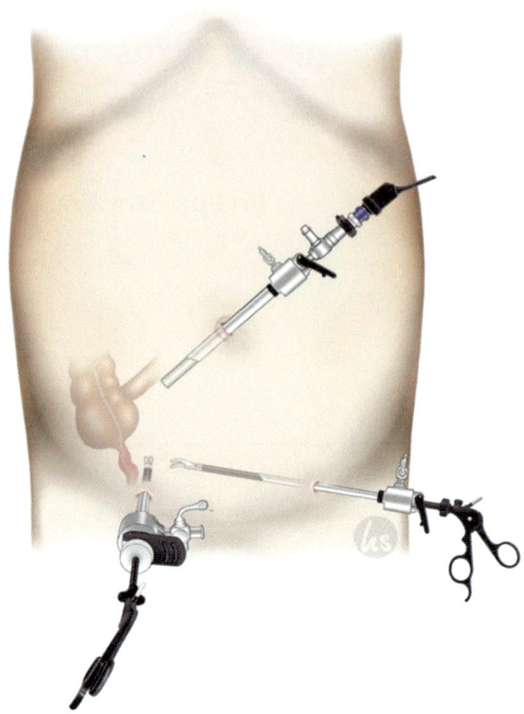

Fig. 44.1 Trocar sites for conventional laparoscopic appendectomy

44.5 Instrumentation

The conventional approach for laparoscopic appendectomy is a three-trocar access to the abdomen, with one 5 or 10 mm trocar, respectively, at the umbilicus as for a 5 mm camera, as well as two 5 mm working ports in the lower abdomen. Those can be either placed symmetrically at the "bikini-line" thus suprapubic lateral in the right and the left lower quadrant, respectively, or asymmetrically with one trocar in the midline. As in general triangulation should be the goal with respect to the appendix (see Fig. 44.1).

44.6 Technique

Surgical steps of laparoscopic appendectomy are defined as identification of the (inflamed) appendix, dissection of the mesoappendix, resection of the appendix, and recovery of the appendix from the abdominal cavity. Before removing the trocars, other pathology should be ruled out, such as Meckel's diverticulum or ovarian pathology.

For dissecting the mesoappendix, different techniques and according techniques are suitable. Those comprise the use of either monopolar or bipolar dissection, but also harmonic or vessel sealing devices in order to control the vessel supply of the appendix safely. However the latter are more expensive and mostly disposable devices. Ligation of the appendix and care for the appendicular stump may be achieved by using pre-provided loops, such as PDS® endoloops, clips, or stapling devices [8]. In our hands, monopolar and bipolar dissection with the use of PDS® endoloops has proved to be safe and cost-effective. However there is some evidence, that in case of complicated appendicitis, the use of an endostapler offers advantages with regard to postoperative abscess formation and reoperation [6]. The appendix might be recovered through the umbilical trocar when a 10 mm trocar is used for this purpose. This offers the ability to change with the 5 mm optic to one of the working ports, while the 10 mm trocar then allows recovering the appendix without contaminating the abdominal wall or trocar site, respectively. In case the appendix will not fit in, the use of a recovery bag either provided by a manufacturer or using a finger from a surgeon's glove is reasonable.

Other techniques regarding the surgical approach are summarized with the so-called single-site or single-incision laparoscopic surgery, respectively, aiming to approach the abdomen through just one single trocar most preferable at the site of the umbilicus. For this different acronyms have been implemented. See Table 44.1.

Meanwhile the established and used techniques are variant and include laparoscopically assisted techniques, where the appendix is pulled out through the umbilical trocar site to be dissected and removed outside the abdomen. In contrary the true laparoscopic single-trocar techniques accomplish the complete procedure intracorporally. Therefore a variety of single-use, disposable trocar systems are available; however reusable trocars exist too. A weight-adapted approach is possible with the use of such trocars for a large variety of indications in pediatric laparoscopy. See Fig. 44.2.

A simplified technique using surgical gloves as a "port", with the single digits functioning as gate for instruments and camera respectively has been described. In comparing the different techniques of single-trocar laparoscopic surgery, multiple publications report no clear advantages for this technique nor for any other technique. The question whether to operate openly or laparoscopically for acute appendicitis has been overcome by rather raising the issue of conventional three-port laparoscopy versus single-trocar surgery. With

Table 44.1 Acronyms for single-trocar techniques for laparoscopy

Acronym	Meaning
LESS	Laparoendoscopic single-site surgery
SILA	Single-incision laparoscopic appendectomy
SILS™	Single-incision laparoscopic surgery
SIPES	Single-incision pediatric endosurgery

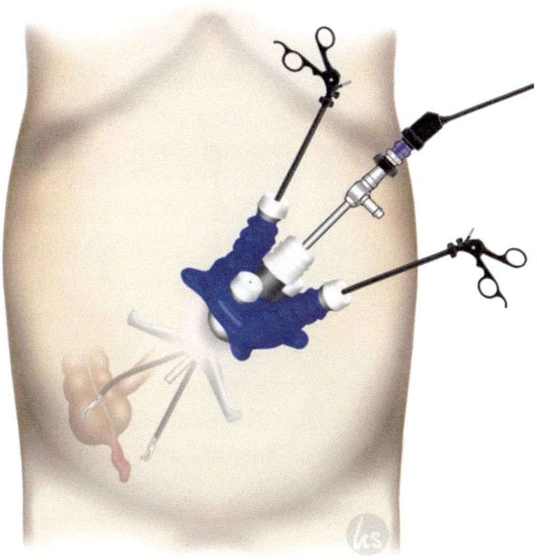

Fig. 44.2 Example of reusable single-site trocar for laparoscopic appendectomy

the use of a single-trocar approach, it seems at least that none of the advantages which have been achieved with laparoscopy seem to be at risk to be compromised. There might be differences with regard to cosmesis; however there is still a lack of evidence whether there is superior approach in terms of patient's satisfaction. A criterion for decision-making on which devices and material should be used is cost efficiency, which obviously is an issue with disposable trocar systems.

In patients with perforated appendicitis, it could be shown that with the achievements of laparoscopic surgery as well as of the improvement in technical skills even in the case of abscess formation, early laparoscopic appendectomy is not just possible but shows no differences regarding recurrence of an abscess, complications, length of hospital stay, and costs, respectively, compared to patients undergoing a so-called interval appendectomy following antibiotic treatment.

Irrigation of the surgical site (locally—thus avoiding spillage to other abdominal quadrants) and suctioning are appropriate measures to control local inflammation intraoperatively. The use of drainages should be avoided. They do not offer any additional advantage [6].

44.7 Postoperative Care

Antibiotic treatment is administered according to local guidelines, however, and may be adapted with regard to intraoperative findings. Oral feeding may be allowed up to 6 h after surgery, however again, and need to be adapted to the intraoperative assessment of inflammation, peritonitis, and paralysis of the bowel, respectively. Analgetics for postoperative pain control should be administered with a low treshold and in general following international recommendations such as the WHO "Treatment Guidelines on Pain" which should be adapted for local requirements and specifities. Patients with uncomplicated appendicitis can usually be discharged 1–3 days after surgery.

44.8 Discussion

It took 99 years from McBurney's report on open appendectomy [1] to the first laparoscopic appendectomy by Semm in 1983 [9]. Another 8 years later, Valla reported a first series on laparoscopic appendectomy in children [10]. Meanwhile laparoscopic appendectomy has evolved to become the gold standard for the surgical therapy of acute appendicitis in children [7, 11–16]. Laparoscopic appendectomy has been proven to be effective, safe, associated with a low complication rate and on the same hand offering low morbidity due to the surgical trauma, while providing superior cosmesis, fast recovery and quick return to daily and social activities. Laparoscopic appendectomy has been also shown to be the treatment of choice in case of complicated appendicitis; however it is considered to be equally effective as interval appendectomy [3–5, 12]. As a side effect, laparoscopy for suspected appendicitis offers the possibility to rule out other surgical diseases in the abdomen such as ovarian pathology, Meckel's diverticulum, other bowel-related inflammatory affections, or even helminthiasis. See Fig. 44.3.

Thus, laparoscopy for suspected appendicitis offers diagnostic as well as therapeutic options even in case the appendix is not affected.

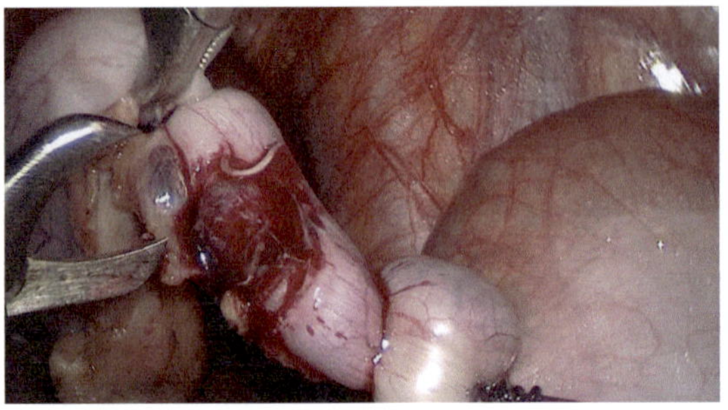

Fig. 44.3 Dissection of appendix, revealing oxyures responsible for appendicitis

In conclusion laparoscopic appendectomy is not only the gold standard for suspected acute and complicated appendicitis but should be considered as the true technique of choice for surgical treatment of appendicitis in children [4, 7, 16]. The question whether to operate openly or laparoscopically has been resolved in favor of laparoscopy, and the question whether to operate on with conventional or single-trocar laparoscopic surgery depends on personal as well as from local preferences [17–19].

References

1. McBurney C. The incision made in the abdominal wall in cases of appendicitis, with a description of a new method of operating. Ann Surg. 1894;20:38–43.
2. Chandler NM, Danielson PD. Single-incision laparoscopic appendectomy vs multiport laparoscopic appendectomy in children: a retrospective comparison. J Pediatr Surg. 2010;45:2186–90.
3. St Peter SD, Sharp SW, Holcomb GW III, Ostlie DJ. An evidence-based definition for perforated appendicitis derived from a prospective randomized trial. J Pediatr Surg. 2008;43:2242–5.
4. Holcomb GW III, St Peter SD. Current management of complicated appendicitis in children. Eur J Pediatr Surg. 2012;22:207–12.
5. St Peter SD, Aguayo P, Fraser JD, Keckler SJ, Sharp SW, Leys CM, Murphy JP, Snyder CL, Sharp RJ, Andrews WS, Holcomb GW 3rd, Ostlie DJ. Initial laparoscopic appendectomy versus initial nonoperative management and interval appendectomy for perforated appendicitis with abscess: a prospective, randomized trial. J Pediatr Surg. 2010;45:236–40.
6. St Peter SD, Snyder CL. Operative management of appendicitis. Semin Pediatr Surg. 2016;25(4):208–11.
7. Dingemann J, Metzelder M, Szavay P. Current status of laparoscopic appendectomy in children. A

nationwide survey in Germany. Eur J Pediatr Surg. 2013;23(3):226–33.
8. Escolino M, Becmeur F, Saxena A, Till H, Holcomb GW III, Esposito C. Endoloop versus endostapler: what is the best option for appendiceal stump closure in children with complicated appendicitis? Results of a multicentric international survey. Surg Endosc. 2018;32(8):3570–5.
9. Semm K. Endoscopic appendectomy. Endoscopy. 1983;15:59–64.
10. Valla JS, Limonne B, Valla V, Montupet P, Daoud N, Grinda A, Chavrier Y. Laparoscopic appendectomy in children: report of 465 cases. Surg Laparosc Endosc. 1991;1(3):166–72.
11. Ure BM, Spangenberger W, Hebebrand D, Eypasch EP, Troidl H. Laparoscopic surgery in children and adolescents with suspected appendicitis: results of medical technology assessment. Eur J Pediatr Surg. 1992;2:336–40.
12. Blakely ML, Williams R, Dassinger MS, Eubanks JW III, Fischer P, Huang EY, Paton E, Culbreath B, Hester A, Streck C, Hixson SD, Langham MR Jr. Early vs interval appendectomy for children with perforated appendicitis. Arch Surg. 2011;146:660–5.
13. Aziz O, Athanasiou T, Tekkis PP, Purkayastha S, Haddow J, Malinovski V, Paraskeva P, Darzi A. Laparoscopic versus open appendectomy in children: a meta-analysis. Ann Surg. 2006;243:17–27.
14. Esposito C, Borzi P, Valla JS, Mekki M, Nouri A, Becmeur F, Allal H, Settimi A, Shier F, Sabin MG, Mastroianni L. Laparoscopic versus open appendectomy in children: a retrospective comparative study of 2,332 cases. World J Surg. 2007;31:750–5.
15. Alkhoury F, Burnweit C, Malvezzi L, Knight C, Diana J, Pasaron R, Mora J, Nazarey P, Aserlind A, Stylianos S. A prospective study of safety and satisfaction with same-day discharge after laparoscopic appendectomy for acute appendicitis. J Pediatr Surg. 2012;47:313–6.
16. Iqbal CW, Ostlie DJ. The minimally invasive approach to appendectomy: is less better? Eur J Pediatr Surg. 2012;22:201–16.
17. Szavay P, Luithle T, Nagel C, Fuchs J. Weight adapted surgical approach for laparoendoscopic single-site surgery in pediatric patients using low-cost reusable instrumentation: a prospective analysis. J Laparoendosc Adv Surg Tech A. 2013;23(3):281–6.
18. Hayashi M, Asakuma M, Komeda K, Miyamoto Y, Hirokawa F, Tanigawa N. Effectiveness of a surgical glove port for single port surgery. World J Surg. 2010;34:2487–9.
19. St Peter SD, Adibe OO, Juang D, Sharp SW, Garey CL, Laituri CA, Murphy JP, Andrews WS, Sharp RJ, Snyder CL, Holcomb GW III, Ostlie DJ. Single incision versus standard 3-port laparoscopic appendectomy: a prospective randomized trial. Ann Surg. 2011;254:586–90.

45 Laparoscopic Cecostomy for Constipation and Incontinence

François Becmeur and C. Klipfel

45.1 Introduction

Antegrade colonic enema (ACE) has proved effective for children with chronic and severe constipation and in the treatment of fecal incontinence. The indications are applied as soon as all medical therapies have failed [1].

In case of constipation, it may be a slow transit constipation or a refractory constipation secondary to cystic fibrosis.

In case of continence deficiency, it may be due to high anorectal anomalies, sacral agenesis, Currarino triad/syndrome, spina bifida, and other consequences of any pelvic surgery as a huge sacrococcygeal teratoma.

The principle of antegrade colonic irrigation for stool evacuation is ancient [2]. Initial surgical technique to access the colon has been described in 1990 by Malone and Ransley [3]. ACE was performed using catheterization of the exteriorized appendix. During the three last decades, several modifications of the initial technique have been reported. There are three main techniques allowing access to the colon: appendix, a tubularized segment of bowel, and various percutaneous devices such as button (Chait Trapdoor button or those used after percutaneous endoscopic gastrostomy such as a Mic-Key low-profile button) [4–7].

We propose to describe the laparoscopic insertion of antegrade continent enema catheter [8–10]. Then we will describe the alternatives. Actually, there are many different options.

45.2 Preoperative Preparation

At the beginning of our experience, the preparation included one or two enemas with serum saline (500 mL–1 L) the day before surgery. But more recently most patients do not receive any specific preparation before surgery, although they are encouraged to continue their current laxative regime. We decide wether or not to do a preoperative specific preparation depending on the level of retention of feces.

Nevertheless, in all cases, a single-dose intravenous metronidazole is administered as we start the procedure.

45.3 Positioning

The patient is lying in a dorsal decubitus. Monitor is placed on the right side of the patient as for a laparoscopic appendectomy. The surgeon is on the left side in front of the left iliac fossa. The assistant is on his right side and the scrub nurse on the left.

F. Becmeur (✉)
Pediatric Surgery Unit, University of Strasbourg, Hôpital de Hautepierre, Strasbourg, France
e-mail: francois.becmeur@chru-strasbourg.fr

C. Klipfel
Pediatric Surgery Unit, Service de Chirurgie Infantile, University of Strasbourg, Hôpital de Hautepierre, Strasbourg, France

C. Esposito et al. (eds.), *ESPES Manual of Pediatric Minimally Invasive Surgery*,
https://doi.org/10.1007/978-3-030-00964-9_45

45.4 Instrumentation

Colonoscope was used in our first cases to check the introduction of the trapdoor button into the cecum (Fig. 45.1). It is still used by several teams [11]. But colonic gas due to endoscopic insufflation may enlarge the size of the colon and makes laparoscopy difficult. It is rarely needed; it increases operative time and makes the procedure more painful due to the colonic inflation of gas, as well.

We need a 5-mm 0° telescope and one 3-mm operative trocar. Sometimes an additional 3-mm operative trocar is required.

A 3-mm atraumatic forceps and a 3-mm needle holder are needed.

45.5 Technique

An open laparoscopy is performed with a 5-mm 0° telescope through the umbilicus, and an additional operative trocar is placed in the left lower quadrant for cecostomy and in the right lower quadrant in case of sigmoidostomy. An 8-mmHg carbon dioxide pressure insufflation is used. Laparoscopy allows the selection of the site for cecostomy by looking at the place where the cecum can be hung to the anterior abdominal parietal wall. At the same time, the surgeon decides the correct site to place the button on the abdomen, low enough to be under the belt line but not too low and far enough from the iliac crest. Two U stitches according to the Georgeson [12] procedure for gastrostomy are used to anchor and secure the bowel to the abdomen wall. Those transparietal stitches are to be tightened outside not directly on the skin but on a little compress and removed quickly, 5 days later, in order to avoid any scar. They grasp the colon; they pass through the entire bowel wall avoiding the mucosa when possible. Generally we use Ethilon 2-0 depending on the size of the child. A long needle is then inserted into the Chait trapdoor button (Cook Medical, Bloomington, IL) [8].

A no. 11 blade is pulled through the abdominal wall to prepare the entry of the button. The needle introduced in the button, which is rigidified by this way (Figs. 45.2 and 45.3), is pushed through the parietal abdominal wall and straight into the bowel into a part of tenia coli. The needle covered by the button is then guided by laparoscopy, up to the right flexure. It is important to be sure the needle is then getting forward in the bowel lumen and will not jab and cross out the opposite wall of the colon.

Previously, when preparing the needle and the button outside, some drops of sterile oil are

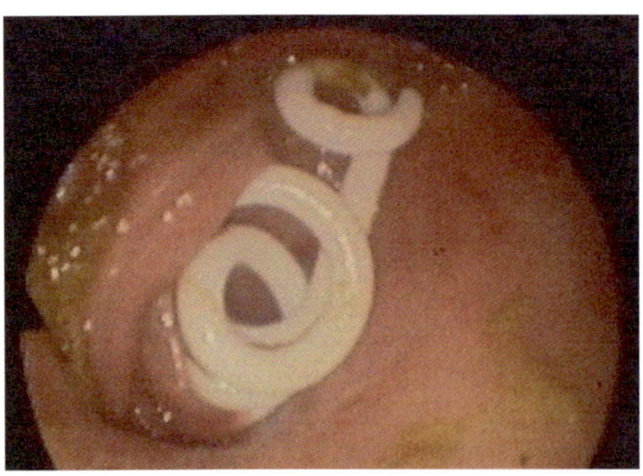

Fig. 45.1 Colonoscopic view of the button. At the beginning of our experience, we thought it was important to check the good position and perfect rollout of the Chait button

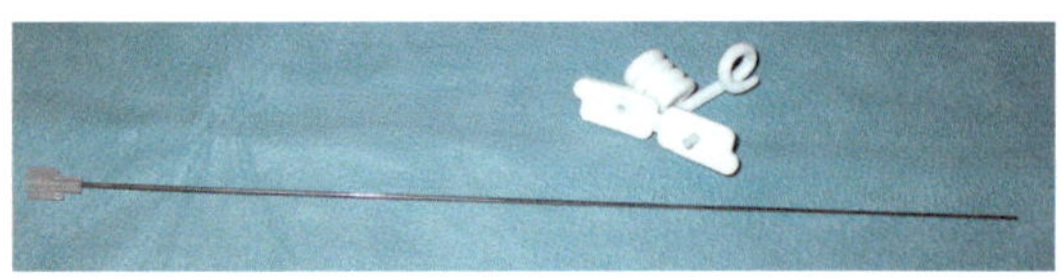

Fig. 45.2 The Chait button and the needle

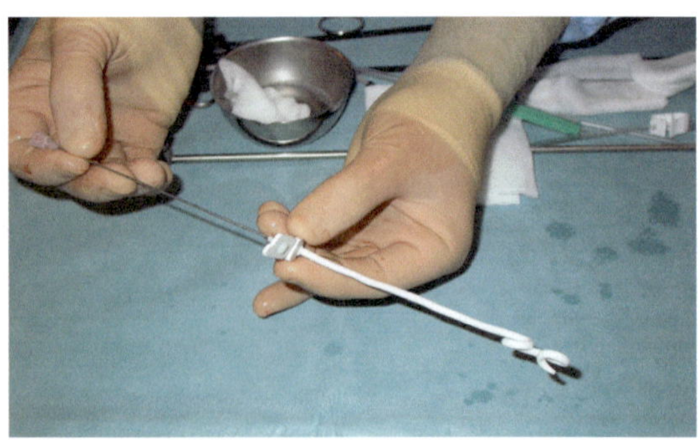

Fig. 45.3 The button is rigidified and rolled out thanks to the needle

injected inside the button to allow an easy withdrawal of the needle, allowing the button retraction and returning to its initial spring shape, when it reaches the bowel lumen.

45.6 Postoperative Care

The U stitches are removed early in the fifth postoperative day to avoid any scar due to the suture. Daily irrigation by using small amount of saline solution may be used to maintain tube patency [11]. But in our experience, it is not required. The button placement may be done in a day-care surgery.

Parents and child are trained on the care and use of the cecostomy tube, a few weeks after surgery, when pain disappears during mobilization of the button. During this consultation, the first antegrade enema is given by the nursing staff so that the parents and the patient can be educated in the use of the device and care surrounding the skin [13]. The saline solution has to be warm enough and the irrigation slow enough to avoid any bowel spasm. The child is sitting on the toilets; the saline solution bag is hanging above the level of the child not too high to get a slow and gentle irrigation. Pocket video games are useful to divert the patient during this half an hour antegrade enema. For young patients, the advice is to perform irrigation at the end of the day, wearing a diaper for the night following the irrigation.

45.7 Result

The average length for surgery is about half an hour. We started our experience in 2002. We did not have any intraoperative complication. If the button becomes unnecessary, it may be removed during a consultation. If it has to be changed due to a normal use 1 year later, a new button is replaced under hypnosis. Indeed, it may be frightening to see a long needle covered by the stretched button coming into the abdomen. Very rarely, we observed accidental tube dislodgement. More often patients may have granulation tissue and leaks that may lead to a wound infection. These complications are linked to inadequate care of the cecostomy site and insufficient irrigation with stool impaction in the cecum.

45.8 Discussion

Appendicostomy has been first proposed to allow ACE. The technique, as originally described [3, 4], involves removing the appendix and placing it in a reversed orientation (anisoperistaltism) within a submucosal tunnel within the cecum creating a Mitrofanoff-like, non-refluxing channel that can be catheterized. Many technical modifications were described: use of a no reversed continent appendicostomy and use of tubularized cecum or ileum when the appendix was not available. The advantages of these techniques are not a main asset to avoid stool leakage through the stoma. That is why the very easy and safe modified Chait procedure has to be offered first.

Actually, several complications were described with appendicostomy as stomal stenosis or occlusion requiring a redo procedure or dilation. Leakage from appendicostomy is frequent [1]. Some authors proposed to leave a Chait button in the appendix to avoid leaks and self-catheterization [14]. Indeed, it may be impossible for the patients to catheterize the appendix by themselves. False passage during cannulation of appendix was described. Stoma prolapse, bleeding from stoma edges, and granulation tissue were noticed. Most of these disadvantages may be avoided with a percutaneous cecostomy using a button as a Chait or Mic-Key [7, 15].

Main problems related to the Chait button are similar to those described with gastrostomy buttons: catheter dislodgement, hypertrophic granulation tissue, and mechanical failure of the catheter that has to be removed and changed. Granulation tissue has to be treated with silver nitrate. And generally, this granulation tissue is secondary to a leakage due to fecal impaction facing the button. The rhythm of enemas has to be modified.

When we began our experience, we used endoscopy and laparoscopy [7, 11] to be sure to place the Chait button in a proper manner. But it appeared to be unnecessary and more complicated: patients needed a washout to get a satisfactory bowel preparation. Colonoscopy was an issue during laparoscopy. The colon increased in size due to gas insufflation during endoscopy. It was often necessary to empty the colon from gas.

A question remains about the site of the button in the colon: is it necessary to perform irrigations of the entire colon or is it enough to irrigate the sigmoid [7]. The major area of dysfunction is the left rather than the right colon. This discussion implies particularly on patients with terminal constipation.

References

1. Kim J, Beasley SW, Moate K. Appendicostomy stomas and antegrade colonic irrigation after laparoscopic antegrade continence enema. J Laparoendosc Adv Surg Tech A. 2006;16:400–3.
2. Cataldo PA. History of stomas. In: Mac Keigan JM, Cataldo PA, editors. Intestinal stomas. Principles, techniques and management. St Louis: Quality Medical Publishing; 1993. p. 3–37.
3. Malone PS, Ransley PG, Kiely EM. Preliminary report: the antegrade continence enema. Lancet. 1990;336:1217–8.
4. Curry JI, Osborne A, Malone PS. How to achieve a successful Malone antegrade continence enema. J Pediatr Surg. 1998;33:138–41.
5. Chait PG, Shandling B, Richards HF. The cecostomy button. J Pediatr Surg. 1997;32:849–51.
6. Gauderer MWL. Percutaneous endoscopic gastrostomy. 20 years later: a historical perspective. J Pediatr Surg. 2001;36:217–9.
7. Gauderer MWL, DeCou JM, Boyle JT. Sigmoid irrigation tube for the management of chronic evacuation disorders. J Pediatr Surg. 2002;37:348–51.
8. Becmeur F, Demarche M, Lacreuse I, Molinaro F, Kauffmann I, Moog R, Donnars F, Rebeuh J. Cecostomy button for antegrade enemas: survey of 29 patients. J Pediatr Surg. 2008;43:1853–7.
9. Koyfman S, Swartz K, Goldstein AM, Staller K. Laparoscopic-assisted percutaneous endoscopic cecostomy (LAPEC) in children and young adults. J Gastrointest Surg. 2017;21:676–83.
10. Yamout SZ, Glick PL, Lee YH, Yacobucco DV, Lau ST, Escobar MA, Caty MG. Initial experience with laparoscopic Chait trapdoor cecostomy catheter placement for the management of fecal incontinence in children: outcomes and lessons learned. Pediatr Surg Int. 2009;25:1081–5.
11. Rodriguez L, Flores A, Gilchrist BF, Goldstein AM. Laparoscopic-assisted percutaneous endoscopic cecostomy in children with defecation disorders. Gastrointest Endosc. 2011;73:98–102.
12. Georgeson KE. Laparoscopic fundoplication and gastrostomy. Semin Lap Surg. 1998;5:25–30.
13. Holbrook C, Tsang T. Laparoscopic insertion of antegrade continence enema catheter: a technique enabling early postoperative usage. Surg Laparosc Endosc Percutan Tech. 2012;22:58–60.
14. Stanton MP, Shin YM, Hutson JM. Laparoscopic placement of the Chait cecostomy device via appendicostomy. J Pediatr Surg. 2002;37:1766–7.
15. Peeraully MR, Lopes J, Wright A, Davies BW, Stewart RJ, Singh S, More BB. Experience of the MACE procedure at a regional pediatric surgical unit: a 15-year retrospective review. Eur J Pediatr Surg. 2014;24:113–6.

Laparoscopic Management of Persistent Complete Rectal Prolapse in Children

46

Cindy Gomes Ferreira, François Becmeur, and Paul Philippe

46.1 Introduction

Rectal prolapse (RP) is a herniation of the rectum through the anal canal. The prolapse may involve only the mucosa (*partial* or *mucosal prolapse*) or all the layers of the rectum (*complete* or *full-thickness prolapse*, also called *procidentia*). Mucosal rectal prolapse presents as radial folds protruding less than 2 cm from the junction with the anal skin. Complete rectal prolapse is characterised by circular folds of the mucosa protruding usually more than 2 cm [1, 2]. If the rectal wall has prolapsed but does not protrude through the anus, it is called an *occult* (*internal*) *rectal prolapse* or a *rectal intussusception*. *Rectocele* (protrusion of the anterior rectal wall) and/or *enterocele* (interposition of intestine into the prolapsed mass along the Douglas pouch, compressing the rectum) may be associated with complete persistent RP [3].

RP occurs at the extremes of age. In the paediatric population, RP is usually diagnosed prior to the age of 4 years with an equal sex distribution [1, 2]. Important anatomical considerations are thought to be related with high incidence in early childhood: the low position and vertical course of the rectum, the straight surface of the sacrum and the flatter coccyx, the increased mobility of the sigmoid colon, the poor levator ani muscular support, the loose attachment of the rectal mucosa to the muscularis and the absence of Houston's valves [1, 2]. The incidence of RP is low in late childhood and early adulthood to increase again after the age of 40, women being six times more affected. In this population, RP is primarily due to pelvic muscular weakness related with childbirth and advancing age [1].

Children presenting RP and older than 4 years usually have a predisposing condition. These older patients usually present recurrent or persistent RP and tend to require surgical repair more often, while RP is usually a self-limiting condition that resolves spontaneously in younger patients [2].

46.2 Preoperative Workout

The diagnosis of RP is mostly clinical. RP should be considered a symptom of an underlying condition rather than a distinct disease entity. The preoperative workout has to search for a possible underlying condition that may predispose to RP. The paediatrician should start a conservative treatment directed by the associated condition before referring to the surgical team [1, 2]. Many unrelated conditions predispose to RP:

C. Gomes Ferreira (✉) · P. Philippe
Service de Chirurgie Pédiatrique, Kannerklinik, Centre Hospitalier de Luxembourg, Luxembourg, Luxembourg
e-mail: gomes.cindy@chl.lu

F. Becmeur
Service de Chirurgie Infantile, Hôpital de Hautepierre, University of Strasbourg, Strasbourg, France

C. Esposito et al. (eds.), *ESPES Manual of Pediatric Minimally Invasive Surgery*,
https://doi.org/10.1007/978-3-030-00964-9_46

- Increased intra-abdominal pressure caused by straining due to chronic constipation, toilet training, protracted coughing or vomiting and chronic straining during micturition (including infravesical obstruction or neurogenic bladder dysfunction). Constipation is the most common associated diagnosis in developed countries [1].
- Acute or chronic diarrhoea caused by bacterial infection, alimentary allergies and/or malabsorption syndromes such as coeliac disease or pancreatic insufficiency [1].
- Parasitic and neoplastic disease that may provide a leading point for intussusception, thus prolapsing the rectum [1].
- Malnutrition is a major predisposing factor due to the disappearance of the ischiorectal fat and resulting in decreased perirectal support. In developing countries, malnutrition and parasitic and diarrheal diseases are the most common risk factors for RP [1, 2].
- Cystic fibrosis used to be considered a common condition associated with RP. Many reports recommended a systematic sweat test to be performed on any child presenting RP (not only those with recurrent RP, but even those with a single episode). Since the development of newborn screening for cystic fibrosis, it is nowadays recommended to do a sweat chloride test in patients with recurrent RP or without an identifiable underlying condition [2].
- Pelvic floor weakness because of neurological disorders affecting the pelvic musculature enervation (myelomeningocele) or following pelvic surgery (correction of anorectal malformation, Hirschsprung's disease) [1, 2, 4, 5].
- Behavioural and psychiatric disorders or the medication to treat them are suggested to be a strong risk factor contributing to RP, as well as for complications and recurrences following surgical treatment [2, 6].
- Miscellaneous: Ehlers-Danlos syndrome, congenital hypothyroidism, extensive burns or suction trauma, etc. [1, 2].

Conservative treatment, regardless of the underlying diagnosis, consists in a combination of treatments including not only stool softeners or laxatives but also behavioural and psychological care targeting increased adherence to medication regimens, increased dietary fibre and clear fluids and increased cooperation with avoidance of prolonged straining and also physical therapy emphasising effective toileting postures, pelvic floor relaxation and evacuation mechanics [1, 2, 6].

If RP is persistent despite a well-conducted medical treatment for at least 6 months, surgical treatment should be considered. In older cooperative patients, dynamic defecography is very useful and advisable before surgery to help identify evacuatory pelvic floor disorders (measurement of the anorectal angle, presence of rectocele or enterocele, sigmoid intussusception) [3].

46.3 Surgical Management of RP

Surgical treatment may be required for recurrent rectal prolapse refractory to conservative measures [1, 2, 4–15]. Numerous surgical treatments are available in the surgeon's armamentarium not only to respond to the surgeon's habits and surgical preferences but also to be adjustable to the anatomical findings of each patient. The aim of each surgical treatment is to control prolapse, restore continence and prevent constipation or impaired evacuation, with an acceptable recurrence and morbidity rate. No surgical treatment has proven its superiority in the paediatric population due to the limited patient numbers, and therefore there is a significant controversy regarding its surgical treatment [4–15].

In paediatric literature, the operative procedures are classified as "less invasive", including injection sclerotherapy, anal encircling (Thiersch procedure), transanal suture rectosacropexy (Ekhorn's procedure) and "more invasive" abdominal or perineal procedures. Perineal operations (Delorme's procedure, perineal rectosigmoidectomy or Altemeier's procedure, stapled transanal rectal resection) are rarely described in children. In adults, perineal procedures are associated with higher recurrence rate [16, 17].

Abdominal surgery involves rectal dissection and fixation aiming to reduce RP. Several techniques or fixation variations are in use. In this chapter, we will emphasise on the laparoscopic transabdominal approach, very popular in adult surgery, gaining more and more acceptance in the paediatric population.

46.4 Preoperative Care

Bowel preparation with enemas and PED solutions are used to insure more working space in the narrow pelvis [7, 8, 11–14], though some authors do not [15]. A bladder catheter can be placed for the time of surgery. Intravenous antibiotic prophylaxis with second-generation cephalosporin and/or metronidazole is recommended. Surgery is performed under general endotracheal anaesthesia after written consent of the patient and the parents. Before induction of general anaesthesia, some surgeons ask the patient to strain out their prolapse to easily access rectosigmoid redundancy and laxity of the pelvic floor [13].

46.5 Theatre Setting Up and Instrumentation

The patient is placed in supine Trendelenburg position. The surgeon and scrub nurse stand on the right side of the patient, while the camera holder stays on the left side. The laparoscopic monitor is placed at the end of the table near the patient's feet.

For the optical port inserted through the umbilicus, depending on the necessity to introduce a mesh or not, either a 5 or a 10 mm port can be used. We recommend a 5 mm 30° scope. For the working ports, 3 or 5 mm ports can be used depending on the patient's size and the surgeon's preference. We use two to three working ports: the first two ports are inserted on the midclavicular line at the level of the umbilicus or slightly above; if needed for retraction, a third working port is inserted in the right lower quadrant. This third working port can also be suitable to do some suturing with better ergonomics for the surgeon during the procedure. The pneumoperitoneum is created at a pressure of 10–12 mmHg. To do dissection using 3 mm ports, a simple electrocautery is sufficient. When using 5mm ports, bipolar or harmonic instruments are used to devide peritoneum and proceed with Douglas pouch resection.

If a mesh is used, either polypropylene mesh [4, 11–13, 18] or polyester fibre mesh [15] can be inserted. In adult literature, there is no evidence of less complication rate by using biological meshes compared to synthetic meshes [17].

46.6 Surgical Techniques

The aim of all laparoscopic abdominal procedure is to reduce rectal mobility and include rectosacral fixation using a suture or mesh. An inherent step in all rectopexies is the full mobilisation of the rectum, but this step may lead to autonomic nerve lesion and the subsequent postoperative dysmotility and impaired evacuation. Thus, some authors believe that extensive posterolateral mobilisation of the rectum may cause new onset or worsening of postoperative constipation [15–18]. All types of abdominal procedure can be associated with a sigmoid resection in case of redundant sigmoid and history of intractable constipation.

We will describe laparoscopic suture rectopexy (LSR), laparoscopic posterior mesh rectopexy (LPMR) and laparoscopic ventral mesh rectopexy (LVMR). All three procedures start with evaluation of the local anatomy: assessment of the redundancy of the rectosigmoid colon, evaluation of the deepness of the Douglas pouch (see Fig. 46.1) and assessment of the laxity of the pelvic floor [12, 13, 15].

To do rectal dissection, the assistant retracts the rectosigmoid ventrally and to the left to expose the peritoneal reflection on the right side of the mesorectum. The right ureter is visualised on its crossing over the iliac vessels. The peritoneum is divided from the sacral promontory down to the deep Douglas pouch and the pelvic floor. Care is taken not to injure the hypogastric nerves at the pelvic inlet. The peritoneum of the deep Douglas pouch can be

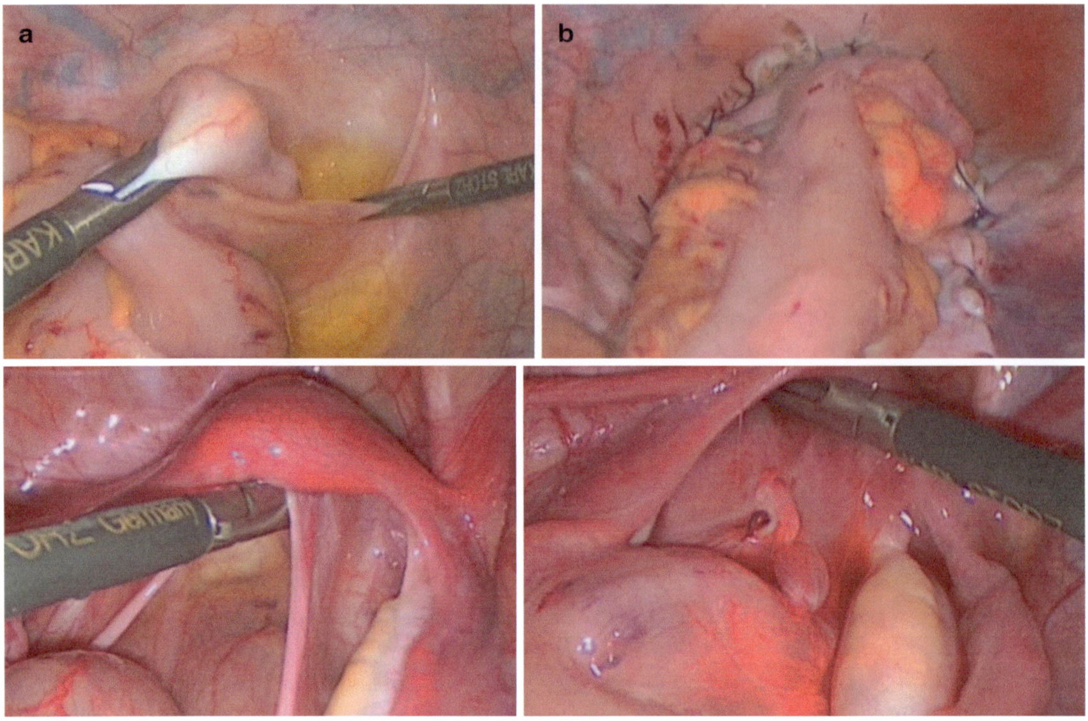

Fig. 46.1 Laparoscopic view of the deep Douglas pouch before surgical treatment (**a**) and after Douglas resection and reconstruction of the neo-Douglas pouch (**b**). Examples of the intraoperative view in a boy (1) and a girl (2)

resected in order to create a neo-Douglas pouch that will be elevated (in order to reduce the depth of the Douglas pouch) (see Fig. 46.1). The adhesions thus created by the obliteration of the deep rectal pouch will reinforce the pelvic floor and potentially decrease the risk of enterocele. The peritoneum can also be divided along the left side of the mesorectum in case of full rectal mobilisation, after having visualised the left ureter. Rectal mobilisation is possible after retrorectal blunt dissection from the promontory down to the pelvic floor through the rectosacral bloodless plane. Transsection of the lateral rectal ligaments is no longer recommended in any surgical technique.

46.6.1 Laparoscopic Suture Rectopexy

Laparoscopic suture rectopexy (LSR) involves a thorough mobilisation of the rectum and its upward and straight fixation to the sacrum (see Fig. 46.2). The postoperative fibrosis tends to keep the rectum fixed and in an elevated position [7–11, 13, 14].

After having mobilised the rectum circumferentially, the assistant pulls the rectum cranially relatively tautly, and the rectum is fixed to the sacral promontory: non-absorbable sutures fix the lateral rectal wall on both sides on the rectum to the periosteum of the promontory [7, 8]. Some authors prefer to do a unilateral peritoneal window and fix the rectum to the sacral promontory only on the right side [9, 10, 13, 14]. A pair of stitches is then disposed below to avoid excessive tension before closing the peritoneum with absorbable sutures. Attempts to limit the perirectal mobilisation, avoiding completely retrorectal dissection, have shown a non-acceptable recurrence rate [11].

In this technique, the rectum is in a straight position in the pelvis. Redundant sigmoid colon should be resected to avoid kinking of the sigmoid over the rigid rectosigmoid junction and/or sigmoid volvulus.

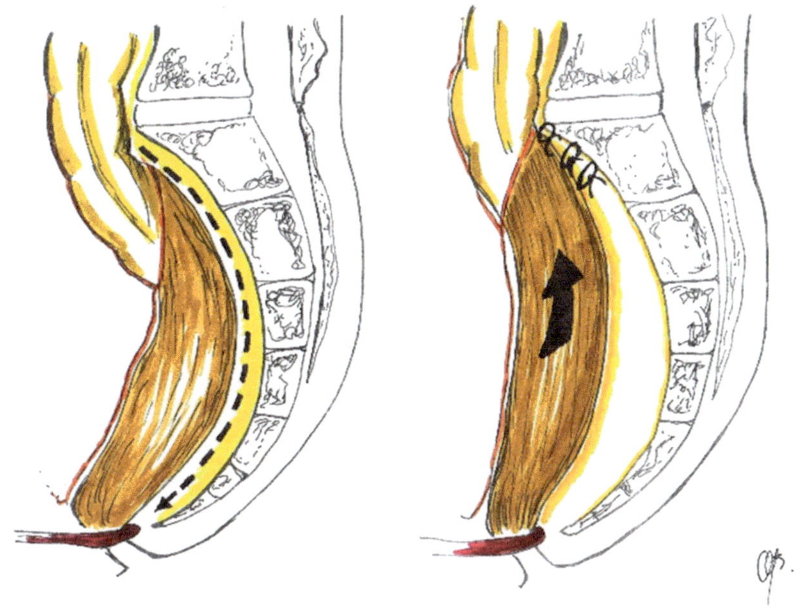

Fig. 46.2 Schema of LSR figuring the retrorectal dissection from the promontory down to the pelvic floor and the elevation of the rectum after LSR

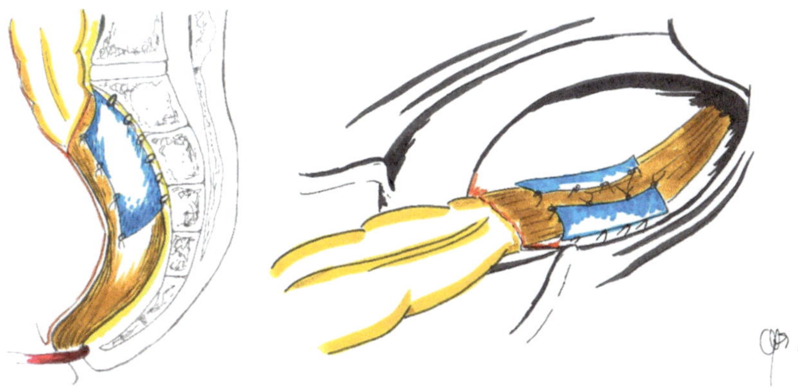

Fig. 46.3 Schema of LPMR according to Wells' procedure

46.6.2 Laparoscopic Posterior Mesh Rectopexy

Posterior mesh rectopexy was first described by Wells (see Fig. 46.3). After complete rectal mobilisation, a mesh is inserted between the sacrum and the rectum. This mesh is fixed and wrapped around the rectum about 270° leaving a small non-covered surface on the anterior wall of the rectum. The mesh is then sutured to the periosteum of the sacral promontory with non-absorbable sutures. Like for the other techniques, the peritoneum is closed to minimise the risk of adherence of small bowel to the mesh. The strong fibrous reaction between the sacrum and the rectum restores the normal anorectal angle.

46.6.3 Laparoscopic Ventral Mesh Rectopexy

LVMR is inspired from the Orr-Loygue open procedure that suspends the rectum to the sacral promontory with bilateral nylon stripes. In the technique as we report it [15], after complete rectal mobilisation and resection of the Douglas pouch, a large tailored inverted y-shaped strip of mesh is fixed to the anterior wall of the rectum with non-absorbable sutures and suspended to the sacral promontory with no traction after reduction of the prolapse. Vaginal fornix fixation to the same mesh can be done in case of important enterocele. The ventral covering of the rectum by a mesh may also treat associated rectocele.

In LVMR it is essential to close the lateral borders of the incised peritoneum over the mesh to avoid any later small bowel adhesion or internal hernia, reconstruct the neo-Douglas pouch and limit (vaginal) mesh erosion.

46.7 Postoperative Care

Standard post-surgery care is initiated. Feeding is resumed as tolerated immediately after surgery. Antibiotics are maintained for two days if a mesh was used. Excessive straining after surgery should be avoided with the help of diet and if needed stool softeners or laxatives for a limited time. In older patients, thrombose prophylaxis should be discussed as for all pelvic surgery. There is a trend to reduce hospital stay with some reports of outpatient surgery for the LSR technique [10], but most authors prefer to maintain hospitalisation until first spontaneous defecation. Discharge is allowed when the patient is apyretic, free of significant pain, walks, eats and smiles.

Follow-up will focus on dietary, life style management, avoidance of constipation and initiation of good defecation practices, often in a multicenter setting. Recurrence often occurs in the first months after surgery but may appear even after a couple of years, so that follow-up should be programmed until adulthood.

46.8 Discussion

With more than 100 different surgical techniques, the treatment of rectal prolapse is challenging. In the adult population, with a much larger number of surgical patients, there is no consensus as to which operation should be used in any given clinical situation [17]. With the scarce number of surgical patients in the paediatric population, the controversy is even bigger.

Furthermore, the physiopathology of PR is different in childhood and adulthood, so that adult surgical procedures must be adapted to the underlying conditions and anatomical findings of our little patients:

For example, for PR after pull-through for anorectal malformations, the recto-perineal junction is "artificial" with no presence of lateral rectal ligaments and an unfamiliar rectal innervation. Most patients don't have the luxury to have a redundant rectosigmoid, and the recto-anal path goes straight down the pelvis. In this population, continence, impaired evacuation and constipation are very important issues that cannot be worsened dealing with secondary complete and persistent RP. Numerous technical tricks have been advocated to reduce RP after laparoscopic-assisted anorectal pull-through (LAARP): colic washout of the distal loop to evacuate meconium and have less distension of the rectum during dissection to reduce the risk of redundancy during dissection [5], limited dissection of the rectosigmoid to have a precise length enough to be brought down without excessive redundancy [5], limited peritoneal pression for laparoscopic exposure after recto-perineal anastomosis to limit tension on the descended colon and application of an anchoring stitch with one absorbable suture to track the rectum to the presacral periosteum after recto-perineal anastomosis [5]. This last trick highlighted by Leung et al. [5] managed to significantly reduce the occurrence of RP and reduce soiling in a large series of LAARP. The team of Graz [4] also reported an interesting case report of laparoscopic Wells' procedure done for a secondary RP after LAARP in a 4-year-old patient: this technique is very interesting in this patient as it achieves a physiological anorectal angle, helping postoperative continence and evacuation, but may worsen constipation because of the extensive dissection. It is the only report of a laparoscopic Wells' procedure in paediatric literature, even if this technique was very popular in the UK open approach and is largely used with laparoscopy in the adult population. Another simplified technique for LPMR with good functional results is described by Shalaby et al. [12] consisting in a uniateral right peritoneal incision, retrorectal blunt dissection and rectosacral posterior fixation with a tailored small mesh without wrapping the rectum as described by Wells. In this simplified technique, the redundant sigmoid is also fixed to the peritoneum on the left quadrant, avoiding kinking without sigmoid resection [12, 13].

In case of RP associated with rectocele or a rare case of enterocele, a LVMR could be the right tool in the surgical armamentarium to reduce RP, correcting the middle pelvic compartment. As limited paediatric literature exists for this technique, should LVMR be generalised to every child presenting a deep Douglas pouch or would another technique combined with Douglas resection be beneficial?

Ventral mesh rectopexy is often associated to the Ripstein's procedure which consists in an anterior rectal sling aiming to restore the posterior curve of the rectum. As this procedure can cause narrowing of the rectum and stricture during child growth, it is not popular in the paediatric surgical societies. Paediatric reports of LVMR are scarce. We recently published a retrospective study of a modified Orr-Loygue technique [15] with promising results considering post-operative constipation and recurrence rate, but the data was limited. In this report, we described a circumferentiel rectal dissection before mesh rectosacropexy without any tension. Retrorectal complete mobilisation was achieved with blunt dissection without any use of electrocautery in this very sensitive region. The large anterior mesh was designed to spread evenly the tension on the fixation sutures and leave the rectum sufficiently mobile. In this study, the resection of the redundant Douglas pouch was also described to reinforce the pelvic floor. In adult literature, LVMR is popular since the description by D'Hoore et al. [18]. In this novel technique, LVMR is done avoiding any posterolateral rectal mobilisation to minimise the risk of autonomic neural damage. A long strip of mesh is placed with no traction in the ventral part of the distal rectum with associated vaginal fornix fixation and Douglas pouch resection, to reinforce the rectovaginal septum. The anterior position of the mesh allows permanent support for the neo-Douglas pouch, which is elevated above the mesh. This technique limiting functional side effects is widespread in the adult laparoscopic societies [16, 17]. A similar technique was described in the paediatric population by Randall et al. [11]. They describe a LVMR without posterior rectal dissection with high recurrence rate. In this report, there is no notice of an extended dissection of the Douglas pouch down to the pelvic floor, nor of the resection of the redundant Douglas pouch, that could explain the recurrences. Nevertheless, ventral meshes for rectopexy in adult female population are reluctantly placed before having completed their family desire, as there is concern about the potential reduction of fecundity due to postoperative pelvic adherences, the possible luxation of mesh during pregnancy and the decreased elasticity of the rectovaginal septum with potential risk for foetal safety and significant maternal obstetric trauma during vaginal delivery [16]. A recent retrospective study by Hogan et al. [16] showed no adverse impact on maternal pelvic floor or on the outcome of pregnancy and delivery after ventral mesh application. Other mesh-related complications are described in literature as infection, vaginal mesh erosion/fistulation, intrarectal mesh migration and rectal stricture. Adult literature recognised risk factors for developing these complications [17] being smoking, use of steroids, poorly regulated diabetes, pelvic hematoma, history of pelvic irradiation or pelvic surgery and the use of polyester mesh. Therefore, biological meshes have recently been used for RP correction. In theory, this graft could decrease complications as chronic infections and erosion but may also lead to higher recurrence rate with partial resolution of the material. No evidence for superiority of biological mesh use has been reported so far in adults [16, 17] where biological grafts are recommended in young patients, especially women of reproductive age, diabetics, smokers, patients with history of pelvic radiation or surgery, inflammatory bowel disease and in case of intraoperative breach of the rectum or vagina [17].

As the use of grafts in the paediatric population should remain an exception, LSR is still a largely used surgical technique with recurrence and complication rates that are well described in literature [7–11, 13–14]. To have the best results with this technique, it seems mandatory to realise a laparoscopic full posterior mobilisation before realising rectopexy. Additionally, a possibly associated redundant rectosigmoid should be managed on the same operative time.

Hence, with the improving skills in laparoscopy and the always changing technic devices, the paediatric surgeon cannot be stubborn and confine under a unique surgical technique as every RP in children is different with different underlying conditions and anatomical findings.

46.9 Conclusion

Even if rectal prolapse has been well described in the *Hippocratic Corpus*, its underlying physiopathology and treatment still generate much interest. Nowadays, the surgeon can choose a technique in a large surgical armamentarium that is constantly increasing. We hope that this chapter could open your mind to the different possibilities that laparoscopy offers to deal with this relatively common condition in children.

References

1. Sialakas C, Vottler TP, Andersen JM. Rectal prolapse in pediatrics. Clin Pediatr (Phila). 1999;38(2):63–72.
2. Cares K, El-Baba M. Rectal prolapse in children: significance and management. Curr Gastroenterol Rep. 2016;18(5):22.
3. Zhang SC, Wang WL, Liu X. Defecography used as a screening entry for identifying evacuatory pelvic floor disorders in childhood constipation. Clin Imaging. 2014;38(2):115.121.
4. Elhaddad A, Amerstorfer EE, Singer G, Huber-Zeyringer A, Till H. Laparoscopic posterior rectopexy (Well's procedure) for full-thickness rectal prolapse following laparoscopic repair of an anorectal malformation: a case report. Int J Surg Case Rep. 2018;42:187–90.
5. Leung JL, Chung PHY, Tam PKH, Wong KKY. Application of anchoring stitch prevents rectal prolapse in laparoscopic assisted anorectal pullthrough. J Pediatr Surg. 2016;51(12):2113–6.
6. Hill SR, Ehrlich PF, Felt B, Dore-Stites D, Erickson K, Teitelbaum DH. Rectal prolapse in older children associated with behavioral and psychiatric disorders. Pediatr Surg Int. 2015;31(8):719–24.
7. Koivusalo AI, Pakarinen MP, Rintala RJ. Laparoscopic rectopexy in the treatment of persisting rectal prolapse in children. A preliminary report. Surg Endosc. 2006;20(6):960–3.
8. Koivusalo AI, Pakarinen MP, Rintala RJ. Rectopexy for pediatric rectal prolapse: good outcomes but not without postoperative problems. Pediatr Surg Int. 2014;30(8):839–45.
9. Laituri CA, Garey CL, Fraser JD, Aguayo P, Ostlie DJ, St Peter SD, Snyder CL. 15-Year experience in the treatment of rectal prolapse in children. J Pediatr Surg. 2010;45(8):1607–9.
10. Potter DD, Bruny JL, Allshouse MJ, Narkewicz MR, Soden JS, Patrick DA. Laparoscopic suture rectopexy for full-thickness anorectal prolapse in children: an effective outpatient procedure. J Pediatr Surg. 2010;45(10):2103–7.
11. Randall J, Gallagher H, Jaffray B. Laparoscopic rectopexy for external prolapse in children. J Pediatr Surg. 2014;49(9):1413–5.
12. Shalaby R, Ismail M, Abdelaziz M, Ibrahem R, Hefny K, Yehya A, Abdelghany E. Laparoscopic mesh rectopexy for complete rectal prolapse in children: a new simplified technique. Pediatr Surg Int. 2010;26(8):807–13.
13. Ismail M, Gabr K, Shalaby R. Laparoscopic management of persistent complete rectal prolapse in children. J Pediatr Surg. 2010;45(3):533–9.
14. Awad K, El Debeiky M, AbouZeid A, Albaghdady A, Hassan T, Abdelhay S. Laparoscopic suture rectopexy for persistent rectal prolapse in children: is it a safe and effective first-line intervention? J Laparoendosc Adv Surg Tech A. 2016;26(4):324–7.
15. Gomes Ferreira C, Schneider A, Philippe P, Lacreuse I, Becmeur F. Laparoscopic modified Orr-Loygue mesh rectopexy for rectal prolapse in children. J Pediatr Surg. 2015;50(2):353–5.

16. Hogan AM, Tejedor P, Lindsey I, Jones O, Hompes R, Gorissen KJ, Cunningham C. Pregnancy after laparoscopic ventral mesh rectopexy: implication and outcomes. Colorectal Dis. 2017;19(9):O345–9.
17. Van Iersel JJ, Paulides TJ, Verheijen PM, Lumley JW, Broeders IA, Consten EC. Current status of laparoscopic and robotic ventral mesh rectopexy for external and internal rectal prolapse. World J Gastroenterol. 2016;22(21):4977–87.
18. D'Hoore A, Penninckx F. Laparoscopic central recto(colpo)pexy for rectal prolapse: surgical technique and outcome for 109 patients. Surg Endosc. 2006;20(12):1919–23.

47 Minimal-Access Colorectal Surgery in Pediatric Age

G. Mattioli, M. C. Y. Wong, and M. G. Faticato

47.1 Introduction

Colorectal surgery includes total colectomy, segmental colectomy, ileocecal resection, and ileorectal anastomosis with or without pouch.

Subtotal colectomy or total colectomy is indicated in patients with moderate-severe ulcerative colitis (UC) refractory to medical therapy, colon Crohn's disease (CD), familial adenomatous polyposis (FAP), and total colonic Hirschsprung disease (HD).

Segmental colectomy includes left hemicolectomy, right hemicolectomy, and ileocecal resection. They are indicated in patients with segmental inflammatory bowel disease (IBD) like CD, colon duplications, other cystic abdominal masses, complicated ileocecal intussusception, and complicated appendicitis with peritonitis.

Ileorectal anastomosis with or without pouch represents the reconstructive phase following a subtotal proctocolectomy in patients with UC; ileoanal anastomosis could be the reconstructive phase following a proctocolectomy in patients with CD, FAP, or total colonic HD.

HD and IBD represent the main indication for colorectal surgery in pediatric population. The incidence of Hirschsprung disease is approximately 1:5000 live births with male preponderance [1]. IBD are increasing in pediatric population. The incidence of pediatric onset UC is 1–4 of 100,000/year in most North American and European regions [2, 3]. The incidence of CD in children is 2.5–11.4 per 100,000, with an estimated prevalence of 58/100,000 [2, 4].

In our experience, the surgical pathway in children with UC includes first subtotal colectomy with ileostomy, then, after at least 3 months, subtotal proctectomy and ileorectal anastomosis (straight or with pouch) with protective ileostomy, followed by recanalization within 2 months.

In this chapter, we describe laparoscopic total and segmental colectomy, laparoscopic proctectomy, and restorative J-pouch ileorectal (ileoanal) anastomosis.

47.2 Preoperative Preparation

All patients and their parents have to sign a specifically formulated informed consent before the procedure. In case of elective surgery, fast track surgical organization is planned: no fasting or colon cleaning is suggested in the days before the operation. Patient hospital admission is organized in the same day of the operation.

Preoperative intravenous antibiotics are administered at least 30 min before the incision. In patients who are under antibiotic therapy, the preoperative prophylaxis is not indicated.

G. Mattioli (✉) · M. C. Y. Wong · M. G. Faticato
Pediatric Surgery Unit, IRCCS Giannina Gaslini Institute, DINOGMI, University of Genoa, Genoa, Italy
e-mail: girolamomattioli@gaslini.org

C. Esposito et al. (eds.), *ESPES Manual of Pediatric Minimally Invasive Surgery*,
https://doi.org/10.1007/978-3-030-00964-9_47

The surgical procedures are performed under general anesthesia. A nasogastric tube is positioned to decompress the stomach. A urinary bladder catheter is placed.

47.2.1 Laparoscopic Subtotal/Total Colectomy

47.2.1.1 Positioning

The patient is placed in supine Trendelenburg position with left side up (Fig. 47.1). As the operating bed tilt changes during the procedure to keep the small bowel far from the colon, the patient must be well secured.

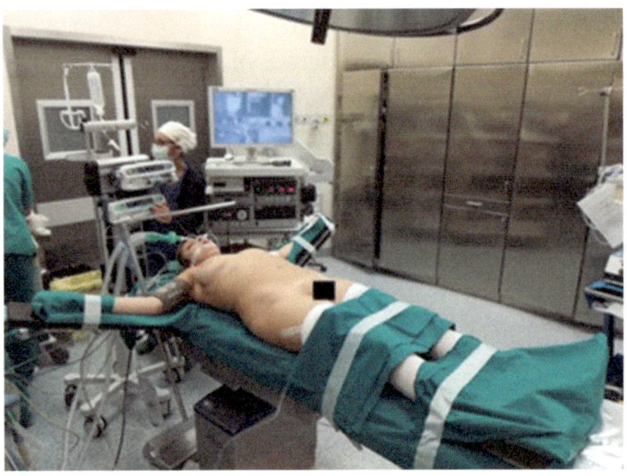

Fig. 47.1 Patient in supine Trendelenburg position with left side up, well secured to the bed, as during the operation it is moved

Skin preparation is performed, and the operative field is prepared from nipples to suprapubic line, in order to include the whole abdomen. The video monitor is positioned on the left side of the patient toward the shoulder. The surgeon and assistant will shift position during the procedure. At the beginning of the operation, they stand on the right side of the bed, with scrub nurse on the opposite side, as the colectomy starts from the sigmoid region and continues along the descending colon (Fig. 47.2). When the colon dissection arrives to the transverse segment, surgeons switch position, standing on the left side of the bed with scrub nurse on the right side, and the patient is put in anti-Trendelenburg position. A quality controlled time-out checklist is always performed before incision to avoid the risk of incomplete compliance.

47.2.1.2 Instrumentation

Two 12 mm ports and two 5 mm ports are used. The second port must be of 12 mm in diameter as the intracorporeal linear stapling device has to be inserted.

The laparoscopic instrumentation consists of a 10 mm 30° scope, two 5 mm graspers, one 5 mm sealing/dividing forceps (high frequency or harmonic), one 5 mm suction device, and one 12 mm intracorporeal linear stapling device.

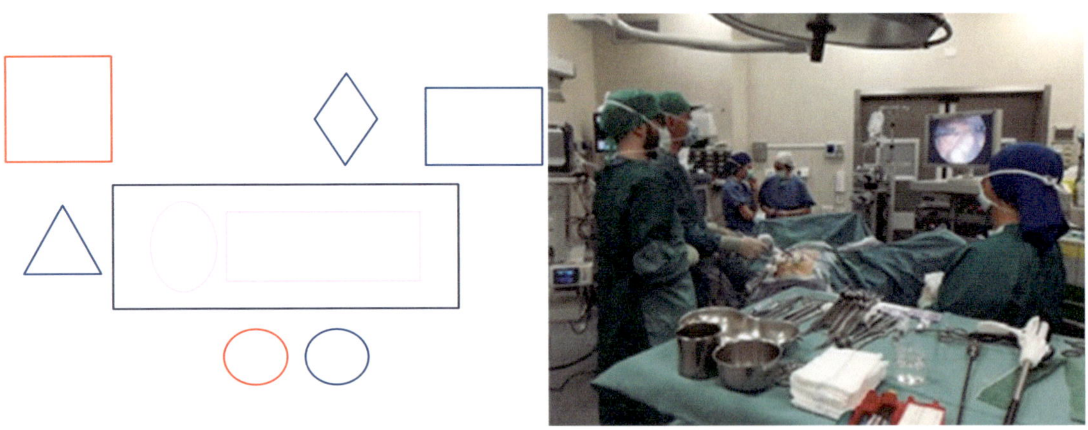

Fig. 47.2 Team position at the beginning of the colectomy: red ring is the first surgeon, blue ring is the assistant surgeon, rumble is the scrub nurse, triangle is the anesthetist, red square is the video monitor, and blue rectangle is the scrub table

47.2.1.3 Technique

The first 12 mm port is placed in the umbilicus. Intra-abdominal pressure of 12–15 mmHg is used to create the pneumoperitoneum. Other three ports are inserted: one 5 mm in the right hypochondrium, one 5 mm in the left flank region, and one 12 mm in the right iliac region, where the ileostomy will be fashioned (Fig. 47.3). A fifth port could be added in the epigastric region, if necessary.

The colonic mobilization starts at the sigmoid region: a window through the sigmoid mesocolon is performed with sealing/dividing forceps. The window is widened distally until the peritoneal reflection in the pelvis, and sigmoid colon is dissected with intracorporeal linear stapling device, leaving a rectal stump close to the peritoneal fold (Fig. 47.4). The colon is progressively mobilized from left to right, and the mesocolon is dissected using sealing/divider forceps, staying close to the colon wall in order to avoid adjacent structures injuries. The left lateral peritoneal attachment of the colon to the abdominal wall is dissected until the splenic flexure. The gastrocolic ligament is opened with access to the lesser sac, and the transverse colon can now be mobilized, staying close to the colon wall. Surgeons change position, and they now stand on the left side of the bed, with scrub nurse on the opposite side, and the bed is placed in a reverse Trendelenburg, in order to let the small bowel move toward the pelvis. The transverse colon mobilization continues until the hepatic flexure (Fig. 47.5). In this step, it is mandatory to pay attention to duodenum, biliary tract, and cava vein during the dissection. Next, the cecum and terminal ileum are mobilized, incising the right lateral peritoneal attachment of the colon to the abdominal wall using sealing/divider forceps.

Once the colon is completely mobilized, it is extracted from the right iliac region trocar, extending the incision (Fig. 47.6). A terminal

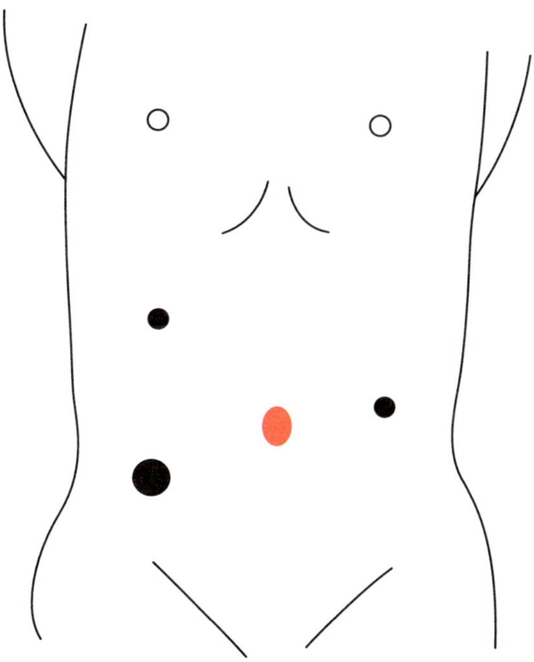

Fig. 47.3 Position of port sites in laparoscopic colectomy. Red point, 12 mm scope port; black points, 5 mm ports in the right hypochondrium and in the left flank region and 12 mm in the right iliac region

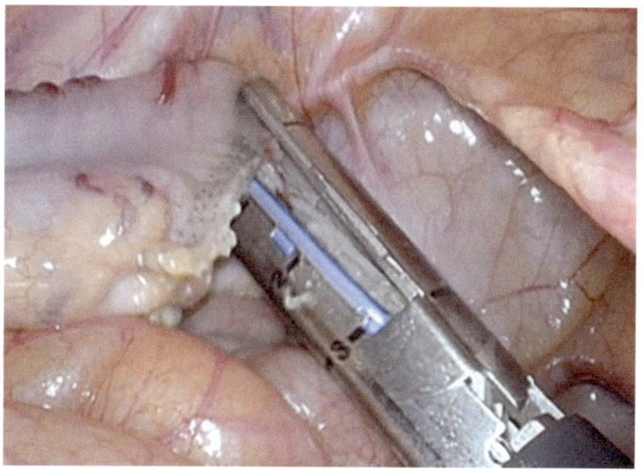

Fig. 47.4 After bilateral ureteral identification, the sigmoid colon is resected with intracorporeal linear stapling device, staying close and proximally to the peritoneal fold

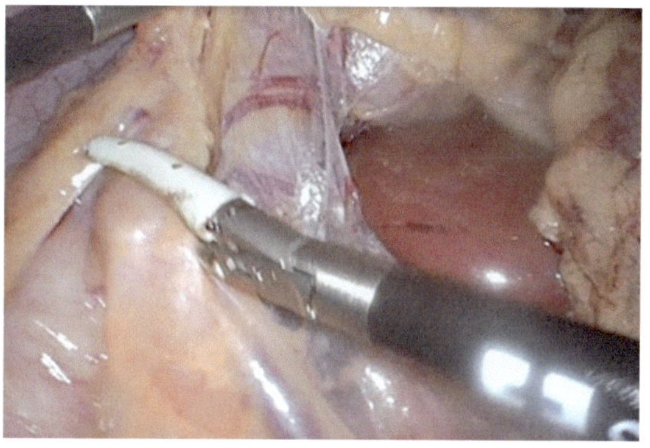

Fig. 47.5 The colonic mobilization continues in the right colon. In this step, it is mandatory to pay attention to duodenum, biliary tract, and cava vein during the dissection

ileostomy is constructed, taking care not to twist the ileal mesenteric vessel. The ports are removed and the port sites are closed with fascial and skin stitches.

47.2.2 Laparoscopic Subtotal Proctectomy with Restorative J-Pouch Ileorectal Anastomosis or Ileoanal Anastomosis Without Pouch

47.2.2.1 Positioning

The patient is placed in supine position with spread legs, with a slight Trendelenburg (Fig. 47.7). Skin preparation is performed, and the operative field is prepared from nipples to the superior half of the legs, in order to include the whole abdomen and to have access to the perineum, facilitating the transanorectal stapled anastomosis.

The video monitor is positioned toward the feet of the patient. The surgeon and scrub nurse stand on the left side of the bed and assistant surgeons on the opposite side (Fig. 47.8). A quality controlled time-out checklist is always performed before incision to avoid the risk of incomplete compliance.

47.2.2.2 Instrumentation

One 12 mm port, one single incision soft access device with three port systems, and two 5 mm ports are used. The laparoscopic instrumentation

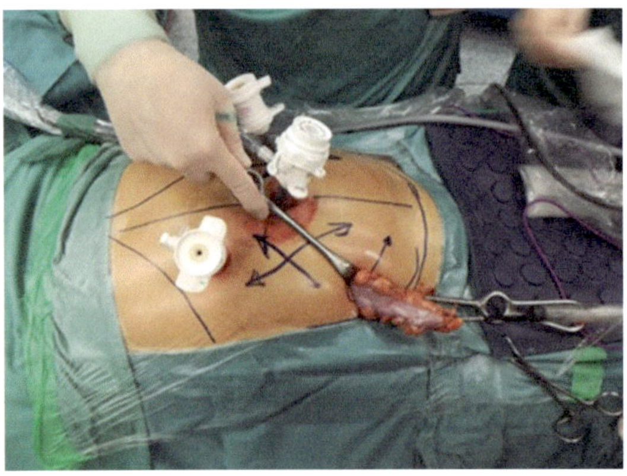

Fig. 47.6 The colon is extracted extending the right iliac region port incision, where the protective ileostomy will be fashioned

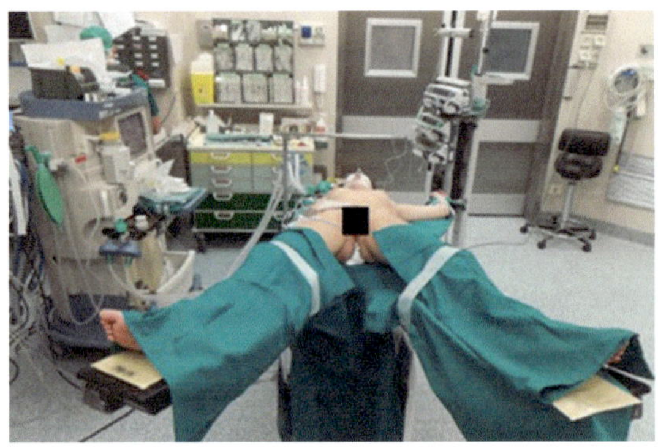

Fig. 47.7 Patient in supine Trendelenburg position with spread legs, well secured to the bed

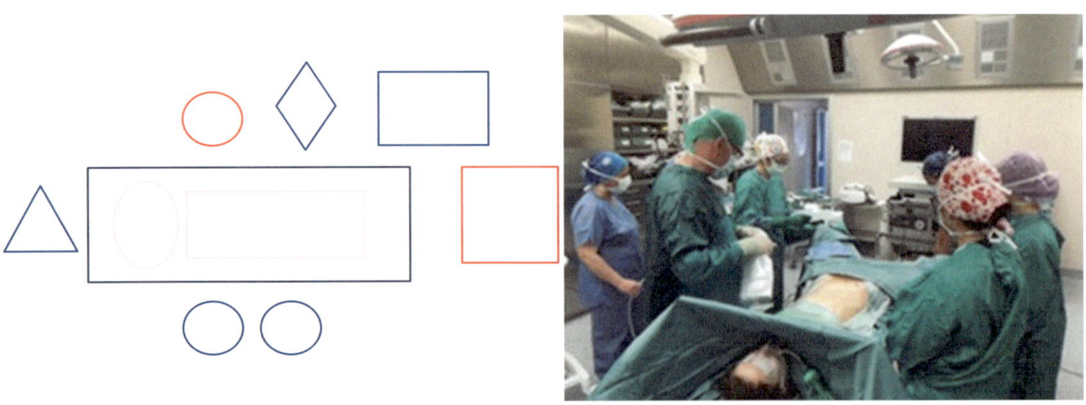

Fig. 47.8 Team position during laparoscopic subtotal proctectomy and restorative J-pouch ileorectal anastomosis: red ring is the first surgeon, blue ring is the assistant surgeon, rumble is the scrub nurse, triangle is the anesthetist, red square is the video monitor, and blue rectangle is the scrub table

consists of a 10 mm 30° scope, two 5 mm graspers, one 5 mm sealing/dividing forceps, one 5 mm suction, one 12 mm intracorporeal linear stapling device, and one circular stapling device.

47.2.2.3 Technique

The first 12 mm port is placed in the umbilicus. Intra-abdominal pressure of 9–12 mmHg is used to create the pneumoperitoneum in order to see the ileostomy from inside. The laparoscopy is stopped and the terminal ileostomy is detached from the abdomen.

The terminal part of the ileostomy is dissected and a 3 cm J-pouch is created extracorporeally. To construct the J-pouch, the ileum is bent on itself and fixed with stay sutures. A small incision is created in the apex of the folded ileum, and a linear stapling device is inserted with one arm in each limb (Fig. 47.9). The stapling device is locked and fired and the pouch is created. The anvil of the circular stapling device is inserted in the enterostomy, and a purse-string suture is fashioned around it (Fig. 47.10).

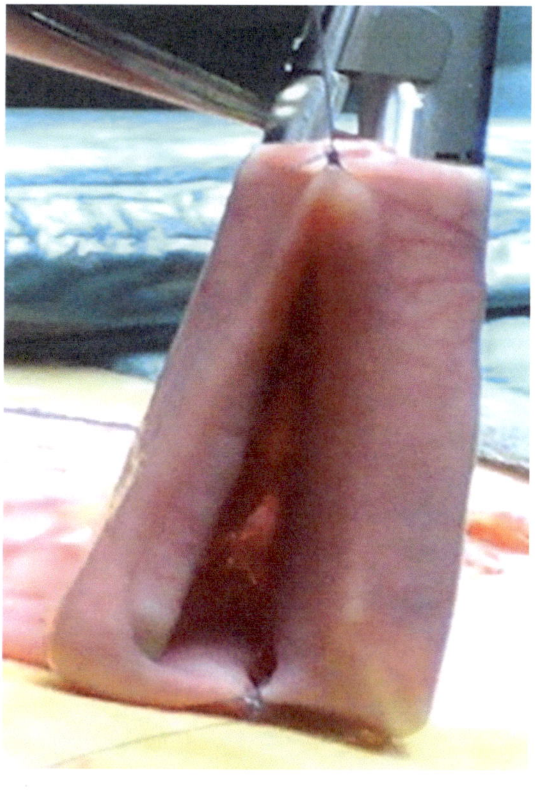

Fig. 47.9 The linear stapling device is inserted with one arm in each limb, it is fired, and the 3 cm pouch is created

It is important to assure the amount of pouch mobility: the J-pouch apex should reach the pubis bone. If necessary, the surgeon can incise the mesenteric peritoneum in order to earn some centimeters and to reduce the vascular compression.

The J-pouch is now pushed inside the abdomen, and the single incision soft access device with three port systems is placed through the ileostomy site. The pneumoperitoneum is recreated, and other two 5 mm ports are inserted: one in the left lumbar region and one in the right hypochondrium (Fig. 47.11).

The rectum is dissected down to the obturator level taking care not to damage adjacent structures such as nerves, vessels, vagina (in females), and bladder neck (in males). The rectal dissection is facilitated by a rigid rectal probe, which is moved by an assistant surgeon. The rectal stump is closed with linear stapling device. The blunt portion of the circular stapling device is inserted through the anus, the spike and the anvil are connected, and the circular stapling device is fired, creating the ileorectal anastomosis (Fig. 47.12).

The anastomosis is checked and the pneumoperitoneum is evacuated. Ports are removed and the port sites are closed with fascial and skin stitches. Protective ileostomy is fashioned in the right iliac region. In case of CD, the surgeon performs a straight ileo-sigmoid anastomosis without pouch.

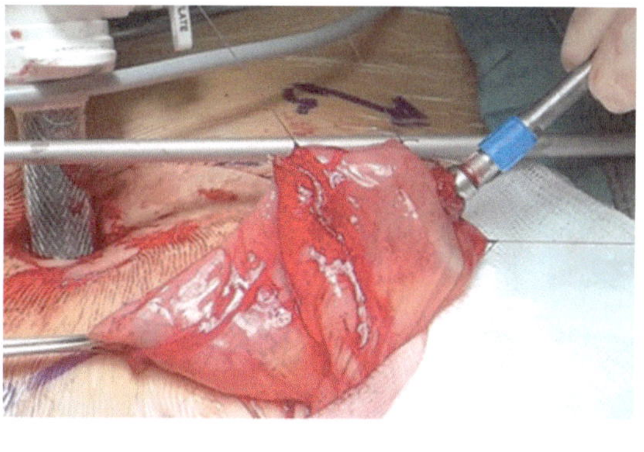

Fig. 47.10 The anvil of the circular stapling device is put in the created J-pouch, and a purse-string suture is fashioned around it

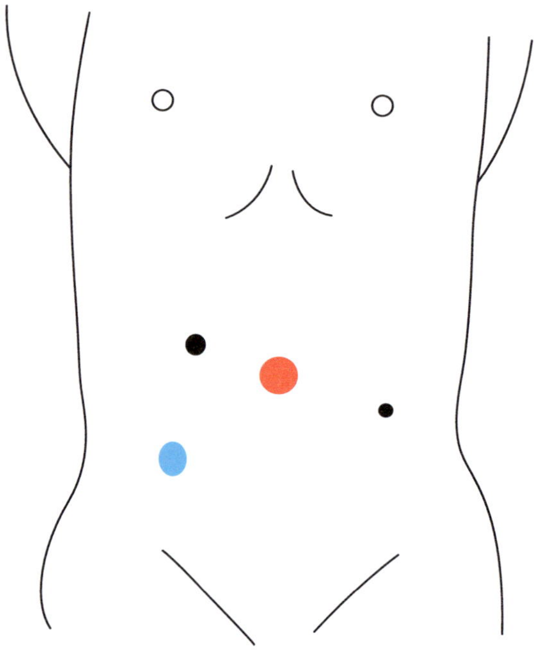

Fig. 47.11 Position of port sites in laparoscopic proctectomy and ileorectal anastomosis. Red point, 12 mm scope port; black points, 5 mm ports in the right hypochondrium and in the left flank region; blue point, single incision soft access device with three port systems in the right iliac region

47.2.3 Laparoscopic Right Colon Resection

47.2.3.1 Positioning

The patient is placed in supine position, with the right side up. The patient must be secured to the operating bed. Skin preparation is performed, and the operative field is prepared from nipples to suprapubic line, in order to include the whole abdomen.

The video monitor is positioned on the right side of the patient toward the feet. The surgeon, the assistant surgeon, and the scrub nurse stand on the left side of the bed (Fig. 47.13).

A quality controlled time-out checklist is always performed before incision to avoid the risk of incomplete compliance.

47.2.3.2 Instrumentation

Two 12 mm ports and one 5 mm port are used.

The laparoscopic instrumentation consists of a 10 mm 30° scope, two 5 mm graspers, one 5 mm sealing/dividing forceps, one 5 mm suction, one 12 mm intracorporeal linear stapling device, and one 5 mm needle holder.

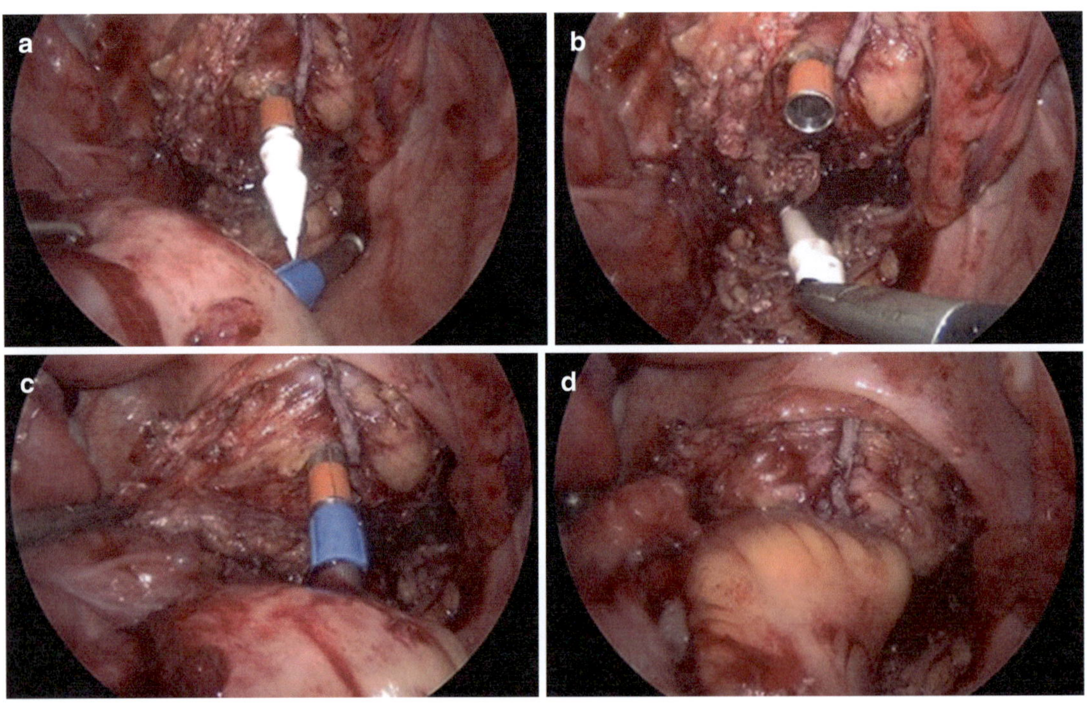

Fig. 47.12 Circular stapling device. (**a**) the blunt portion is inserted through the anus; (**b** and **c**) the spike and the anvil are connected; (**d**) the circular stapling device is fired, and the ileorectal anastomosis is created

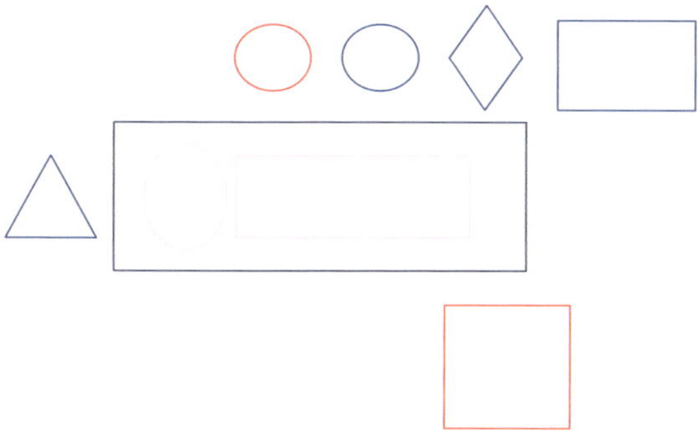

Fig. 47.13 Team position. Red ring is the first surgeon, blue ring is the assistant surgeon, rumble is the scrub nurse, triangle is the anesthetist, red square is the video monitor, and blue rectangle is the scrub table

47.2.3.3 Technique

The first 12 mm port is placed in the umbilicus. Intra-abdominal pressure of 12–15 mmHg is used to create the pneumoperitoneum. Other two ports are inserted: one 12 mm in the suprapubic region and one 5 mm in the right iliac region (Fig. 47.14).

The first step consists in detecting the extent of ileocecal disease and determining the extent of the resection. If the ascending colon is not involved, a limited ileocecal resection is sufficient; otherwise, a right colon resection is preferred.

The right lateral peritoneal attachments are mobilized by sharp dissection, as it is an avascular plane. The mesocolon is dissected with sealing/dividing forceps for the extent of the resection, paying attention to stay close to the bowel wall. The terminal ileum is divided using intracorporeal linear stapling device. Once the distal resection margin is reached, the colon is divided with intracorporeal linear stapling device.

The surgeon can decide to perform the anastomosis intra or extracorporeally. The anastomosis can be performed as end-to-end or side-to-side using linear stapling device.

If the anastomosis is performed extracorporeally, the two ends of bowel are brought out through the extended incision of the right iliac region port, the anastomosis is hand sewn, the mesenteric window is closed, and the bowel is pushed again inside the abdomen.

If the anastomosis is performed intracorporeally, the proximal and distal ends are overlapped

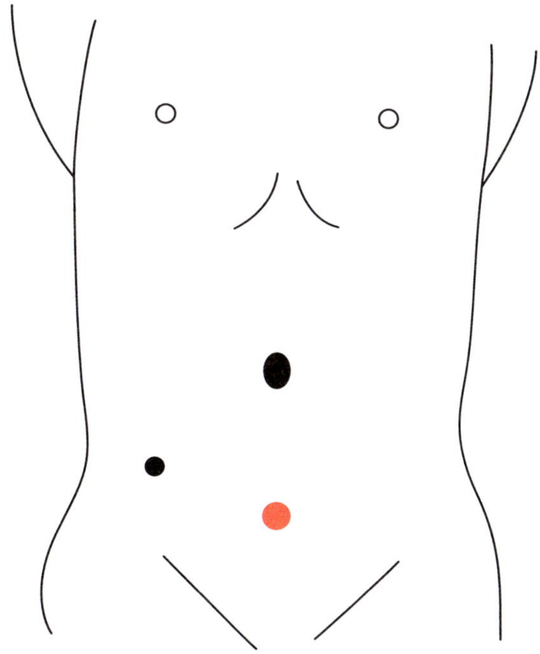

Fig. 47.14 Position of port sites in ileocecal resection/right hemicolectomy. Red point, 12 mm scope port; black points, 5 mm port in the right iliac region and 12 mm in the umbilicus

for 5–6 cm, and stay sutures are placed to align and stabilize the bowel. Small enterotomies are made in each limb at the proximal end of the overlap. Each arm of the intracorporeal linear stapling device is placed in each bowel limb. The stapling device is locked and fired, and the side-to-side isoperistaltic anastomosis is created. The resultant enterotomy is closed with running suture or interrupted stitches. The mesenteric window is closed. The ileocecal specimen is extracted, enlarging the right iliac region port. The pneumoperitoneum is evacuated, the ports are removed, and the port sites are closed with fascial and skin stitches. Protective ileostomy can be fashioned if necessary.

47.3 Postoperative Care

In the postoperative period, the patients can keep a normal decubitus. Nasogastric tube is removed at the end of the operation. The urinary catheter is left in place until opioid analgesics are used.

Otherwise, the urinary catheter can be removed after 24 h.

Oral feeding can restart when ileostomy output starts. Antibiotic prophylaxis is continued for 24 h after surgery. The analgesic therapy is managed by a specialized team which follows the patient daily.

All patients are discharged when bowel function returns and no complication occurs. No shower is admitted for 1 week after surgery. Parents are instructed on how to treat ileostomy by a specialized stoma care team.

47.4 Results

Between January 2006 and December 2017, a total of 135 laparoscopic procedures were performed in 79 patients with IBD. Diagnoses included 52 UC, 24 CD, and 3 IBD undetermined. Indications to surgery for patients with UC were mostly represented by hemorrhagic colitis with failure of medical treatment.

Fifty-eight colectomies, 6 right colon resections, 9 ileocecal resections, 50 laparoscopic J-pouch ileorectal restorative anastomoses, and 12 laparoscopic straight ileo-sigmoid anastomoses were performed.

In 54 patients, laparoscopic colectomy was associated to a protective temporary ileostomy, while 4 patients underwent J-pouch ileorectal anastomosis in the same stage procedure.

Two patients required conversion to open surgery due to the extremely difficult mobilization and manipulation of the inflamed and fragile small bowel.

47.5 Tips and Tricks

Division of mesocolon can be performed by several methods, depending on surgeon's preference, degree of inflammation, and thickening of mesocolon. If the patient has been under steroid therapy, the tissue can be friable, and the risk of bleeding is higher, so it is important to pay attention during the mesocolon dissection.

The surgeon must stay close to the bowel wall during dissection, in order to avoid adjacent structures injury.

In case of intracorporeal anastomosis, during the running suture, the surgeon is helped by placing a stay suture at the bottom of the suture line in order to gain counter tension. Sometimes the surgeon can add some separate stitches over the running suture in order to be sure of the anastomosis.

When an ileorectal anastomosis is performed, it is advisable to use the largest circular stapler which goes inside the anus.

Protective ileostomy is generally suggested in case of restorative ileorectal J-pouch anastomoses.

In general, ileostomy can be fashioned as protection or in case of dehiscence symptoms, but in pediatric population, it is preferable to avoid the ileostomy, when possible, for psychological reasons.

47.6 Discussion

IBD are increasing in pediatric population. The risk of surgery at the age of 30 for patients with onset of CD in childhood is 48 ± 5% compared with 14 ± 2% for patients with adult-onset CD [5]. Childhood-onset UC is extensive in 60–80% of all cases, twice as often as in adults [6]. Because disease extent has been associated with disease severity, it is not surprising that pediatric-onset UC has a worse disease course, with a 30–40% colectomy rate at 10 years, as compared with 20% in adults [6]. For these reasons, also colorectal operations are increased in number in the last decades.

The application of minimally invasive surgical (MIS) techniques in the pediatric population has exponentially increased in the last 30 years. In recent years surgeons have moved from conventional laparotomy to minimally invasive laparoscopic approach also in IBD.

For IBD, total or segmental colectomy shows results that overlap and/or overcome those of conventional open surgery [7]. In our experience, ileostomy is usually performed after colectomy.

A meta-analysis demonstrated that, though basing on a very few good-quality studies, pouch procedures should be preferred in UC in order to achieve better survival and functional outcome [8]. Although pouch needs frequent endoscopic follow-up and a relatively high incidence of pouchitis (reported in up to 50% of patients), pouch procedures represent at the moment the gold standard for reconstruction after colectomy in children with IBD.

In case of ileocecal resection, although some authors suggest to perform the "safer" extracorporeal anastomoses due to the inflamed and fragile bowel [9, 10], both alternatives have proved to be safe and effective in experienced hands and are now used worldwide in CD [11].

Single incision soft access device has been adopted to contain the trauma of abdominal wall and to improve the outcome of the patients both in terms of reduced pain, shorter postoperative stay, earlier recovery of normal bowel functions, and improved cosmetic appearance [11].

In our experience, MIS has shown optimal results in terms of short-term and long-term results, and, when possible, it is suggested [11–14].

References

1. Suita S, Taguchi T, Ieiri S, Nakatsuji T. Hirschsprung's disease in Japan: analysis of 3852 patients based on a nationwide survey in 30 years. J Pediatr Surg. 2005;40(1):197–201; discussion 201–2.
2. Benchimol EI, Fortinsky KJ, Gozdyra P, Van den Heuvel M, Van Limbergen J, Griffiths AM. Epidemiology of pediatric inflammatory bowel disease: a systematic review of international trends. Inflamm Bowel Dis. 2011;17:423–39.
3. Henderson P, Hansen R, Cameron FL, Gerasimidis K, Rogers P, Bisset WM, Reynish EL, Drummond HE, Anderson NH, Van Limbergen J, Russell RK, Satsangi J, Wilson DC. Rising incidence of pediatric inflammatory bowel disease in Scotland. Inflamm Bowel Dis. 2012;18:999–1005.
4. Kappelman MD, Rifas-Shiman SL, Kleinman K, Ollendorf D, Bousvaros A, Grand RJ, Finkelstein JA. The prevalence and geographic distribution of Crohn's disease and ulcerative colitis in the United States. Clin Gastroenterol Hepatol. 2007;5:1424–9.
5. Pigneur B, Seksik P, Viola S, Viala J, Beaugerie L, Girardet JP, Ruemmele FM, Cosnes J. Natural history of Crohn's disease: comparison between childhood- and adult-onset disease. Inflamm Bowel Dis. 2010;16:953–61.
6. Van Limbergen J, Russell RK, Drummond HE, Aldhous MC, Round NK, Nimmo ER, Smith L, Gillett PM, McGrogan P, Weaver LT, Bisset WM, Mahdi G, Arnott ID, Satsangi J, Wilson DC. Definition of phenotypic characteristics of childhood-onset inflammatory bowel disease. Gastroenterology. 2008;135:1114–22.
7. Gerstle JT, Kim PC, Langer JC, Diamond IR. Outcomes after laparoscopic surgery in children with inflammatory bowel disease. Surg Endosc. 2010;24:2796–802.
8. Tilney HS, Constantinides V, Ioannides AS, Tekkis PP, Darzi AW, Haddad MJ. Pouch-anal anastomosis vs straight ileoanal anastomosis in pediatric patients: a meta-analysis. J Pediatr Surg. 2006;41:1799–808.
9. Simon T, Orangio G, Ambroze W, Schertzer M, Armstrong D. Laparoscopic-assisted bowel resection in pediatric/adolescent inflammatory bowel disease: laparoscopic bowel resection in children. Dis Colon Rectum. 2003;46:1325–31.
10. Bonnard A, Fouquet V, Berrebi D, Hugot JP, Belarbi N, Bruneau B, Aigrain Y, de Lagausie P. Crohn's disease in children. Preliminary experience with a laparoscopic approach. Eur J Pediatr Surg. 2006;16(2):90–3.
11. Mattioli G, Guida E, Pini-Prato A, Avanzini S, Rossi V, Barabino A, Coran AG, Jasonni V. Technical considerations in children undergoing laparoscopic ileal-J-pouch anorectal anastomosis for ulcerative colitis. Pediatr Surg Int. 2012;28(4):351–6.
12. Pini-Prato A, Faticato MG, Barabino A, Arrigo S, Gandullia P, Mazzola C, Disma N, Montobbio G, Mattioli G. Minimally invasive surgery for paediatric inflammatory bowel disease: personal experience and literature review. World J Gastroenterol. 2015;21(40):11312–20.
13. Mattioli G, Pini-Prato A, Barabino A, Gandullia P, Avanzini S, Guida E, Rossi V, Pio L, Disma N, Mameli L, Mirta DR, Montobbio G, Jasonni V. Laparoscopic approach for children with inflammatory bowel diseases. Pediatr Surg Int. 2011;27(8):839–46.
14. Mattioli G, Pini Prato A, Razore B, Leonelli L, Pio L, Avanzini S, Boscarelli A, Barabino P, Disma NM, Zanaboni C, Garzi A, Martigli SP, Buffi NM, Rosati U, Petralia P. Da Vinci robotic surgery in a pediatric hospital. J Laparoendosc Adv Surg Tech A. 2017;27(5):539–45.

Part IV

Urology

Laparoscopic and Retroperitoneoscopic Nephrectomy

48

Ciro Esposito, Maria Escolino, Alessandro Settimi, Fulvia Del Conte, Alessandra Farina, Giovanni Esposito, Mariapina Cerulo, Agnese Roberti, and Jean Stephane Valla

48.1 Introduction

Nephrectomy using MIS was described in pediatric surgery at the beginning of the 1990s [1]. Nephrectomy is probably the most popular urologic indication for the video surgical procedure in children. There are mainly three ways to approach the kidney in MIS: laparoscopy and retroperitoneoscopy, which are the most used techniques adopted in children, and the prone posterior approach adopted rarely by some authors [2–5]. In this chapter the authors will show the main aspects of laparoscopic and retroperitoneoscopic approach.

48.2 Preoperative Preparation

All patients and their parents have to sign a specifically formulated informed consent before the procedure. A Foley catheter is positioned in the bladder before surgery.

C. Esposito (✉) · M. Escolino · A. Settimi
F. Del Conte · A. Farina · G. Esposito · M. Cerulo
A. Roberti
Pediatric Surgery Unit, Department of Translational Medical Sciences (DISMET), University of Naples "Federico II", Naples, Italy
e-mail: ciroespo@unina.it

J. S. Valla
Pediatric Surgery Unit, CHU Lenval, Nice, France

48.3 Positioning

The surgeon's choice to perform laparoscopic or retroperitoneoscopic nephrectomy was based on the indication for surgery, body habitus, and a previous renal or abdominal surgery [6–8]. All the procedures are performed under general anesthesia with the patients positioned in lateral decubitus for retroperitoneoscopy and in semi-lateral decubitus for laparoscopy (Figs. 48.1 and 48.2). We use always a 10 mm optic because we always used the optic orifice to remove the kidney (Fig. 48.3). In laparoscopy we used a 30° optic; a 0° optic was always adopted in retroperitoneoscopy. In retroperitoneoscopy we always use three trocars because operative chamber is small. In laparoscopy we use three trocars, but sometime we use a fourth trocar to retract the liver or on the left side to retract the spleen or the loops. In general the trocars adopted are of 5 mm in diameter because we need to use during the procedure a clip applier for vessel control, a sealing device, or a peanut. The trocars are positioned in triangulation with the optic to have a better ergonomy.

48.4 Instrumentation

In general we need few instruments to perform MIS nephrectomy: a couple of atraumatic fenestrated forceps to manage tissues, a curve dissector to isolate hilar vessels, a hook cautery to perform

C. Esposito et al. (eds.), *ESPES Manual of Pediatric Minimally Invasive Surgery*,
https://doi.org/10.1007/978-3-030-00964-9_48

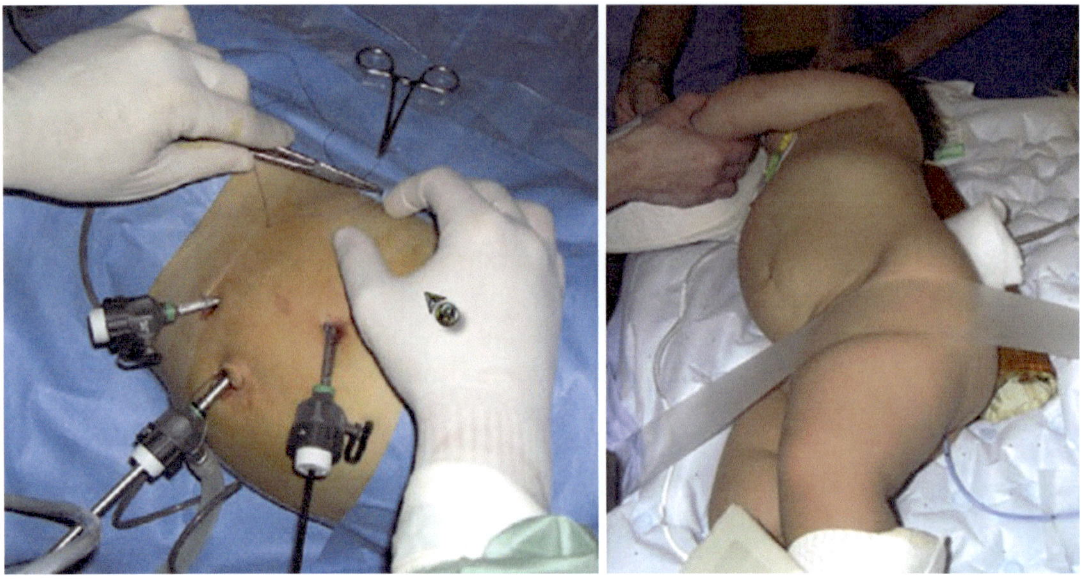

Fig. 48.1 Patient's position and trocar placement for laparoscopic nephrectomy

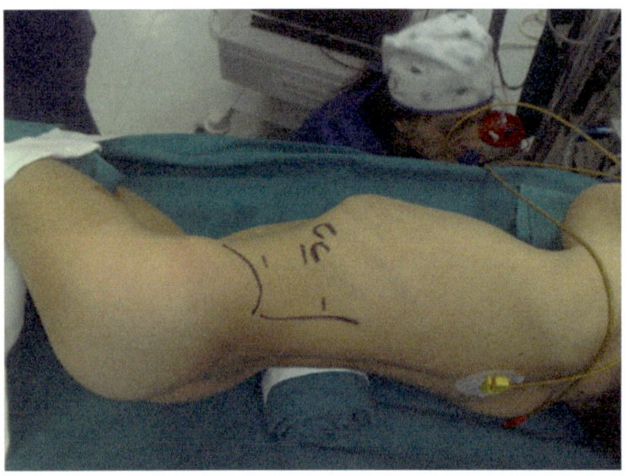

Fig. 48.2 Patient's position for retroperitoneoscopic nephrectomy

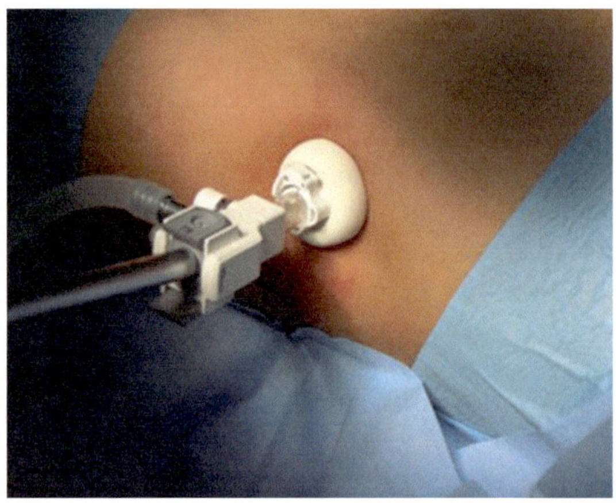

Fig. 48.3 In case of retroperitoneoscopic nephrectomy, it is preferable to use a balloon trocar for the optic to avoid gas leak around the cannula

dissection, and a scissors to cut. A needle holder is rarely adopted for this procedure.

To perform hilar vessels control, we used 5 mm titanium clips, or in the last 10 years, hemostatic devices as Starion MLS3 or Ultracision or Ligasure can be useful to perform a faster and safer dissection and to seal vessels. A peanut can be adopted sometimes for dissection. It is safe to prepare a suction aspiration device and put it on the bench because it can be useful in case of bleeding. In general no endobag is necessary to remove the kidney that is removed to the trocar orifice; an endobag can be necessary only in case of kidney infection or for oncological indication (Figs. 48.4 and 48.5).

48.5 Technique

In laparoscopy, thanks to the semi-lateral decubitus, the loops slide down, and you have only to detach the colon before opening the Gerota fas-

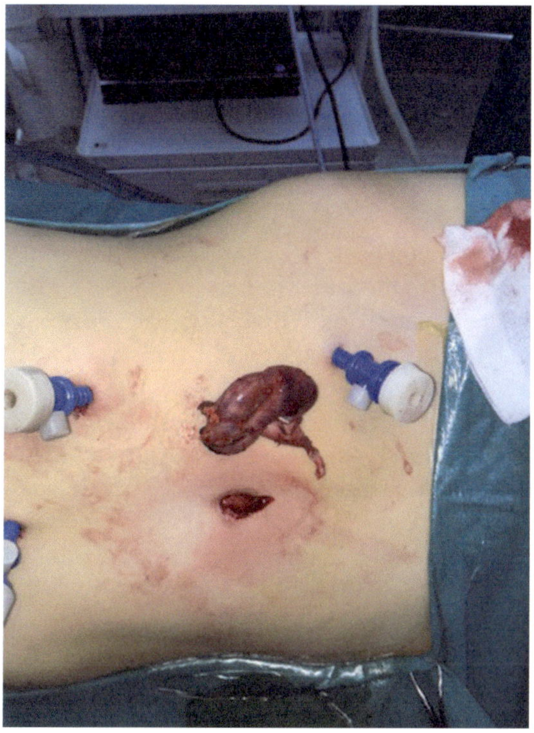

Fig. 48.4 Laparoscopic nephrectomy: at the end of procedure, the kidney is removed through the umbilical orifice

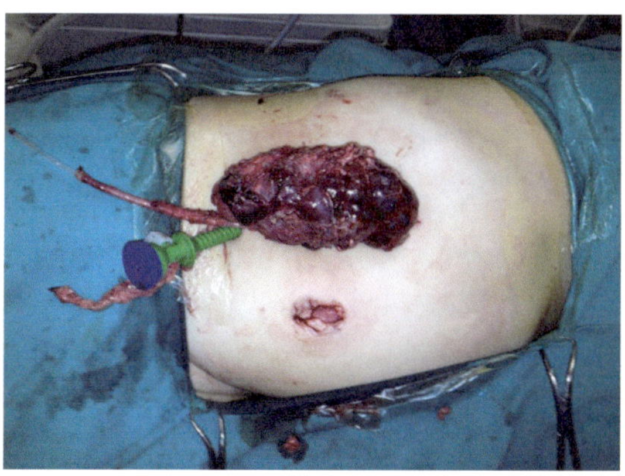

Fig. 48.5 Laparoscopic nephrectomy: also big kidney can be removed easily through the umbilical orifice

cia and to isolate the kidney. Another alternative can be to pass trans-meso, but above all in older children, it can be difficult due to fat tissue in the mesocolon, and in addition you are at risk of creating an injury to mesocolon vessels; for this reason the majority of authors prefer to detach the colon.

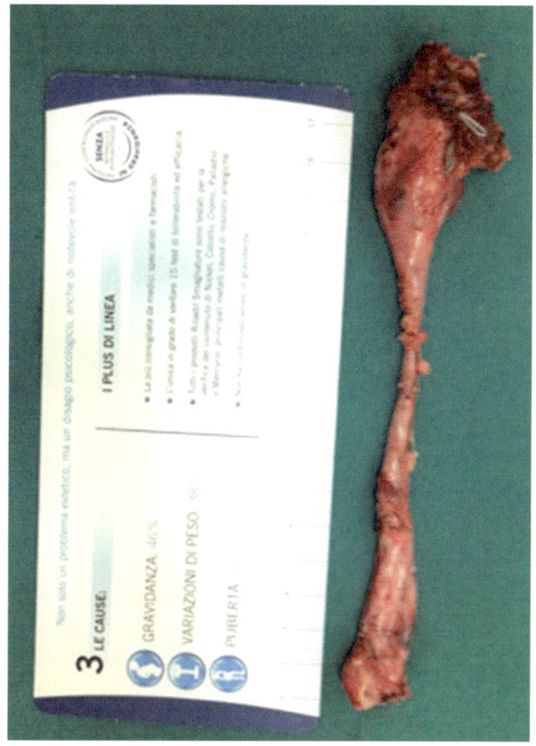

Fig. 48.6 Laparoscopic nephrectomy: if the indication for nephrectomy is VUR, you have to remove the kidney and all the ureter

You can do it using hook cautery or in a faster way using sealing device. After opening the Gerota fascia, the ureter is isolated, it is followed upward arriving to the kidney, hilar vessels are isolated separately, and then they have to be clipped and sectioned. Another alternative is to seal the vessels using sealing device. Then the kidney is separated from posterior attachment, and the ureter is isolated arriving near the bladder, if the indication for nephrectomy is reflux (as happens in the majority of cases). In case of VUR as indication, you have to remove all the ureter arriving near the bladder, and you have to ligate it preferably using an endoloop (Fig. 48.6). If the indication is not VUR, you can leave the ureter open.

In laparoscopy the kidney is always removed through the trocar orifice at umbilical level.

In retroperitoneoscopy, it is preferable to use a 10 mm balloon trocar for the optic because you have to remove the kidney through this orifice and because you have to avoid gas leak around the

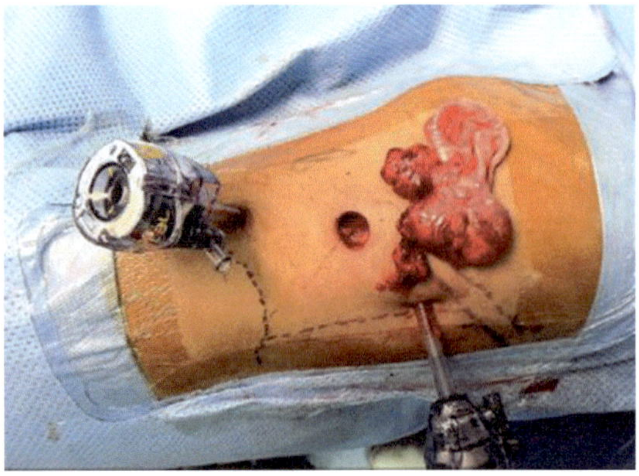

Fig. 48.7 Retroperitoneoscopic nephrectomy: the kidney is removed through the optic orifice

cannula; then two 5 mm trocars are used in triangulation (Figs. 48.3 and 48.7). After entering in retroperitoneal space, the Gerota fascia is opened. A key point of the technique is to leave the kidney attached to the roof; in this way it is easier to isolate hilar vessels that appear perpendicular. As in laparoscopy, you have to clip or to seal them and then section them, and then the kidney is separated from its attachments. The ureter is isolated as down as possible. The main disadvantage of retroperitoneoscopy is that it is not possible to isolate the ureter arriving near the bladder as in laparoscopy. This is a problem because if the indication is VUR, you can leave a long ureteral stump with the risk to have a postoperative reflux with UTI and the risk to have a second procedure to remove the stump.

In retroperitoneoscopy the kidney is removed through the optic orifice.

No drainages are necessary for both techniques.

48.6 Postoperative Care

Patients start oral feeding few hours after surgery. Analgesic requirement is rarely necessary, in general only paracetamol the evening of the procedure. A short antibiotic therapy is given for a couple of days. Patients are discharged from hospital on day 1 or 2. Postoperative controls are scheduled at POD7 and POD31, and then the controls change according to the indication for surgery.

48.7 Results

Analyzing the international literature, the conversion rate in laparoscopic nephrectomy is near 0, and in retroperitoneoscopy, it is a little bit higher above all at the beginning of experience due to a peritoneal opening during dissection. As for operative time, it is shorter using laparoscopy varying from 30 to 130 min (average 47 min), while in retroperitoneoscopy the length of surgery is a little bit longer, and it varies from 60 to 150 min (average 80 min).

Analyzing the length of surgery, the duration of surgery in laparoscopy was statistically shorter than in retroperitoneoscopy ($p < 0.001$). In addition the use of new hemostatic devices for dissection shortened significantly the time of surgery compared with the use of monopolar coagulation to perform dissection.

As for complications, the complication rate is lower than 5%. In laparoscopy reported mainly are bleeding from hilar vessels or infectious complication when the indication for nephrectomy is xanthogranulomatous pyelonephritis. In retroperitoneoscopy, over these two kinds of complications, the main complication represented is the peritoneal perforations during dissection or the symptomatic long refluxing ureteral stump after RN that required a redo surgery to remove it.

Complication rate was statistically significant higher after RN compared to LN (10.4% vs. 2.9%, $\chi 2 = 0.05$). The hospital stay was similar for both approaches; as for the need of drugs, it was minimal for both techniques.

48.8 Tips and Tricks

As for laparoscopy, the position of the patient in lateral decubitus is a crucial point for the success of the procedure; in this way the loops slide down, and you have an excellent view of the renal loggia. To perform a nephroureterectomy is fundamental to detach the colon; in this way you can easily isolate the kidney and the full ureter arriving near the bladder. Four trocars can be necessary above all on the right side to retract the liver but sometimes also on the left side.

For sure, using sealing device for dissection, it makes the procedure bleeding-free, faster, and safer.

As for the management of hilar vessels, also if sealing devices have a FDA approval to seal vessels of 5–7 mm in diameter, we think that is safer to close hilar vessels using clips.

It is important to remember that if you use clips to close vessels, it is forbidden to use monopolar scissors or sealing devices to cut between clips, because you risk having the clips detach immediately or in the postoperative period.

At the end of the procedure, it is not necessary to reattach the colon to the colonic loggia.

As for retroperitoneoscopy, before starting this procedure, it is mandatory to well master the technique of creation of retroperitoneal space because this is the main problem of retroperitoneoscopic route. As for the technique itself, after creating the retroperitoneal chamber, the retroperitoneoscopic nephrectomy is easier in particular for the isolation of hilar vessels, and you have no problems deriving from the presence of intestinal loops as happens in laparoscopy.

On the contrary in retroperitoneoscopy, it is impossible to isolate the lower part of the ureter; for this reason when you perform a retroperitoneoscopic nephrectomy, you leave at least 5 cm of the ureter attached to the bladder.

For this reason if the indication for nephrectomy is VUR, it is mandatory to perform nephrectomy via laparoscopy. As for the dimension of the kidney, it doesn't matter because also huge kidney can be removed through optic orifice in particular in laparoscopy (Fig. 48.5). In conclusion, we think that both ways are excellent approaches to perform nephrectomy, but there are no doubts that laparoscopic nephrectomy is easier, faster, and with a lower complication rate compared to retroperitoneoscopy.

48.9 Discussion

Nephrectomy is the most common urological procedure performed in pediatric patients using MIS, and it can be considered the gold standard procedure for kidney removal in children in case of benign diseases [6–8]. However, there is a strong debate among pediatric surgeons and pediatric urologists if it is preferable to approach the kidney in MIS using laparoscopy or retroperitoneoscopy [9, 10].

While retroperitoneoscopy meets all the criteria of open renal surgery avoiding opening the peritoneum to reach the kidney, it is technically more difficult due to the creation of a not existing operative chamber [11, 12]. In addition the retroperitoneal space is too small, and you can use few trocars that are difficult to move. As for laparoscopy, you work in a well-known and large space; you can use more trocars, but to approach the kidney, you have to mobilize the colon or to open the mesocolon [13]. As for the techniques to adopt to perform nephrectomy using MIS, we critically analyzed our 20 years of experience doing some considerations [14]. In our opinion, LN is easier and faster to perform compared to RN. Analyzing our experience, it seems that laparoscopy is statistically significantly faster than retroperitoneoscopy; instead, the length of hospital stay and the need for drugs in postoperative period is similar for both approaches [14, 15].

As for the indication for surgery, according with the reports of the international literature, we think that MIS nephrectomy has to be used only for benign diseases. Otherwise for kidney malignancy, you have to discuss the indication with pediatric oncologists to evaluate the pros and cons of MIS technique [7, 14]. Retroperitoneoscopy to perform nephrectomy presents some contraindications: first of all it is extremely difficult to perform a RN if the patients had a previous renal surgery or a renal infectious disease as xanthogranulomatosis pyelonephritis because in both cases there are too many adhesions in retroperitoneal space and it is impossible to create the working space [7, 14].

On the basis of our experience, we think that in case of reflux nephropathy it is mandatory to perform a LN rather than a RN, because this approach permits to perform a complete ureterectomy near the bladder dome, avoiding to leave a residual distal ureteral stump [3, 14]. In laparoscopy you can remove almost the entire length of the ureter arriving near to the bladder base leaving only 3–5 mm of the distal ureter, compared to a 5 cm stump that you usually leave in retroperitoneoscopy [2, 11, 14].

Also in case of ectopic pelvic kidneys, laparoscopy is preferable to retroperitoneoscopy.

As for technical point of view, we think that LN is technically easier than RN even if for the hilar vessels control probably RN is better because vessels are perpendicular to the roof of the field and it is quite easy to isolate and to cut them [8, 14]. In the last 10 years, we have started to use the new hemostatic devices (Starion, Ligasure, Ultracision) to perform advanced MIS procedures, and we used these devices also for renal surgery. Even if this devices are expensive and not strictly necessary to perform a standard nephrectomy, they are very useful to perform dissection because they eliminate the risk of bleeding, and they permit to perform a surgery significantly faster compared with the dissection performed using monopolar coagulation [5, 7, 14]. Otherwise in case of renal infections or in case of previous renal or abdominal surgery, hemostatic devices are essential to perform a safe surgery and to reduce complications [14]. As for the technical point of view, even if in laparoscopy it is easy to join the kidney, in our experience, we prefer, as the majority of authors, to detach the colon and to reach the kidney, but also trans-meso approach is quite easy to perform [9, 10, 14]. At the beginning of the experience, we reattached the colon to the lateral abdominal wall, but after the first 20–30 cases, we noted that this fixation was not strictly necessary; for this reason in the last 70–80 LN, we did not refix the colon with the same results for the patient. In general the dissection of the ureter, of the kidney, and of the hilar vessels is easy to perform; however, in case of previous kidney infections or in case of xanthogranulomatosis pyelonephritis, the dissection phase is very complicated because there is not a true plan of dissection between the kidney and the surrounding tissues [7, 14]. As for the postoperative course, it was similar for both approaches; the need of drugs was minimal, and children started liquid diet few hours after surgery and full oral intake in the evening or maximum the following day. Also the average hospital stay was about 2–3 days even if it is possible to perform this kind of procedure in a day-hospital setting. We never leave a drainage after MIS nephrectomy except in case of kidney infections. As for the number of trocars, in the majority of patients, it is possible to perform a nephrectomy using three trocars; a fourth trocar may be used in case of a difficult dissection due to adhesions or in case of a huge liver on the right side. As for the learning curve period, we think that it is longer for RN than for LN [1, 14]. In RN the longer learning curve is due to the fact that at the beginning, it is not so easy to create the retroperitoneal chamber and to well position the three trocars; the second difficult point in RN is the risk to open the peritoneum during dissection as happened in two cases at the beginning of our experience [6, 13, 14]. In case of a small peritoneal opening, you can continue the procedure in retroperitoneoscopy adding a third trocar or a Veress needle to close the hole; in case of a large hole, it is preferable to convert RN into LN. However, we think that for both approaches, it is useful to have a mentorship period with an expert tutor for three to five cases for LN and for about ten cases for RN. As for the kidney retrieval, we always removed the kidney through the optic orifice; for this reason we always used a 10 mm optic. In general with training it is quite easy to remove the kidney, and it is not necessary to use an endobag except in case of kidney infection.

On the basis of our 20 years of experience in pediatric nephrectomy using MIS, we believe that video surgical nephrectomy is an intriguing surgery to perform, and we clearly prefer to perform a nephrectomy using laparoscopy rather than retroperitoneoscopy because LN is easier, faster, and safer compared to RN [14]. In the recent years, we performed practically all the nephrectomies using laparoscopy leaving the indication to adopt RN only for the rare cases of MKDK.

References

1. Borzi PA. A comparison of the lateral and posterior retroperitoneoscopic approach for complete and partial nephroureterectomy in children. BJU Int. 2001;87:517–20.
2. You D, Hong S, Lee C, Kim KS. Feasibility and safety of laparoscopic ablative renal surgery in infants: comparative study with children. J Urol. 2012;188(4):1330–4.
3. Mulholland TL, Kropp BP, Wong C. Laparoscopic renal surgery in infants 10 kg or less. J Endourol. 2005;19:397–400.
4. Esposito C, Valla JS, Yeung CK. Videosurgery in pediatric urology. Surg Endosc. 2004;18:1559–64.
5. Hammad FT, Upadhyay V. Indications for nephrectomy in children: what has changed? J Pediatr Urol. 2006;2(5):430–5.
6. Mattioli G, Pini-Prato A, Costanzo S. Nephrectomy for multicystic dysplastic kidney and renal hypodysplasia in children: where do we stand? Pediatr Surg Int. 2010;26:523–8.
7. McDougall EM, Clayman RV. Laparoscopic nephrectomy for benign disease: comparison of the transperitoneal and retroperitoneal approaches. J Endourol. 1996;10:45–9.
8. Varlet F, Petit T, Leclair MD, Lardy H, Geiss S, Becmeur F, Ravasse P, Rod J, de Lambert G, Braik K, Lardellier-Reynaud F, Lopez M. Laparoscopic treatment of renal cancer in children: a multicentric study and review of oncologic and surgical complications. J Pediatr Urol. 2014;10(3):500–5.
9. Dindo D, Demartines N, Clavien PA. Classification of surgical complications. A new proposal with evaluation in a cohort of 6336 patients and results of a survey. Ann Surg. 2004;240:205–13.
10. Kim C, McKay K, Docimo SG. Laparoscopic nephrectomy in children: systematic review of transperitoneal and retroperitoneal approaches. Urology. 2009;73:280–4.
11. Baez JJ, Luna CM, Mesples GF, Arias AJ, Courel JM. Laparoscopic transperitoneal and retroperitoneal nephrectomies in children: a change of practice. J Laparoendsc Adv Surg Tech A. 2010;20(1):81–5.
12. Lorenzo Gomez MF, Gonzalez R. Laparoscopic nephrectomy in children: the transperitoneal vs the retroperitoneal approach. Arch Esp Urol. 2003;56(4):401–13.
13. Valla JS. Retroperitoneoscopic surgery in children. Semin Pediatr Surg. 2007;16(4):270–7.
14. Esposito C, Escolino M, Corcione F, Draghici IM, Savanelli A, Castagnetti M, Turrà F, Cerulo M, Farina A, Settimi A. Twenty-year experience with laparoscopic and retroperitoneoscopic nephrectomy in children: considerations and details of technique. Surg Endosc. 2016;30(5):2114–8.
15. Esposito C, Iaquinto M, Escolino M, Farina A, La Manna A, Savanelli A, Settimi A, Di Mezza A. Is retroperitoneoscopic renal ablative surgery easier and safer using a new hemostatic device compared with clips and monopolar coagulation? A comparative study. Minerva Urol Nefrol. 2014;66(2):101–5.

Laparoscopic Partial Nephrectomy

49

Philipp Szavay, Fulvia Del Conte, Marco Severino, Maria Escolino, and Ciro Esposito

49.1 Introduction

Duplication of the renal system is one of the most common congenital anomalies of the urinary tract. The majority of these anomalies remains clinically silent. A smaller number of them become evident as a consequence of hydronephrosis, vesicoureteral reflux (VUR), or incontinence. Recently, antenatal diagnosis permits to identify many urologic anomalies, including different variants of ureteral duplications, which are clinically asymptomatic. A duplex renal system often has one moiety that is either poor or nonfunctioning. In these cases, there is an indication to remove surgically the nonfunctioning moiety.

The surgical management of children with renal duplication depends on a variety of factors such as parenchymal function of each unit and the presence or absence of other associated anatomic anomalies and pathologies, such as ectopic ureterocele or vesicoureteral reflux.

Actually, different surgical approach can be used to treat the diseased kidney as a posterior retroperitoneal, a lateral retroperitoneal, and a transperitoneal approach [1–3]. Basically, a posterior retroperitoneal approach is suitable for isolated heminephrectomy without the need for extensive mobilization and excision of a dilated megaureter in younger children (<5 years). In comparison, a lateral retroperitoneal approach (RHN), with greater working space, is indicated for extensive distal ureteral manipulation, as heminephrectomy in older children, heminephroureterectomy, or excision of low-lying kidneys. Instead, for duplex systems with nonfunctioning unit and complicated ureteroceles, a one-stage procedure including ureterocelectomy, reimplantation of the lower part ureter, and bladder base repair would be best treated by a transperitoneal approach (THN) [1]. In this chapter we will only deal with the THN; RHN will be dealt with in another chapter.

49.2 Preoperative Preparation

Preoperative examinations should focus on the anatomical malformations of the whole urinary tract and their functional implications.

Investigations have to include ultrasonography and DMSA scintiscan, if necessary intravenous pyelography (IVP) or even a magnetic resonance (MR) urogram.

In some cases, cystoscopy may help to understand the anatomy.

P. Szavay
Department of Pediatric Surgery, Lucerne Children's Hospital, Lucerne, Switzerland

F. Del Conte · M. Severino · M. Escolino
C. Esposito (✉)
Pediatric Surgery Unit, Department of Translational Medical Sciences (DISMET), University of Naples "Federico II", Naples, Italy
e-mail: ciroespo@unina.it

C. Esposito et al. (eds.), *ESPES Manual of Pediatric Minimally Invasive Surgery*,
https://doi.org/10.1007/978-3-030-00964-9_49

An intestinal preparation with simethicone, enema, and liquid diet is desirable especially in young children.

Preoperative antibiotic prophylaxis should be administered either with a broad-spectrum medication or according to the child's specific urine testing.

All patients and their parents have to sign a specifically formulated informed consent before the procedure.

Patients received a general anesthesia. A Foley catheter is positioned in the bladder before surgery.

49.3 Positioning

For THN the patient should be placed in a semilateral position close to the edge of the operating table with the ipsilateral side elevated. The surgeon and assistant stand on the contralateral.

side, facing the pathology and the monitor in a straight line. This approach utilizes gravity for retraction of the colon, allows clear dissection of the ureters even down to the bladder level, and facilitates a safe access to the renal pedicle (Fig.49.1).

We use always a 10 mm optic 30° because we always used the optic orifice to remove the kidney moiety. In laparoscopy we use three trocars, but above all on the right side, we use a fourth trocar to retract the liver or on the left side to retract the

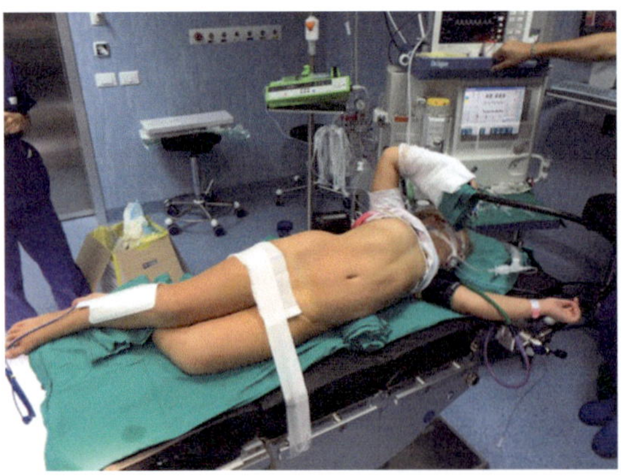

Fig. 49.1 Semi-lateral decubitus and crew's position for laparoscopic nephrectomy

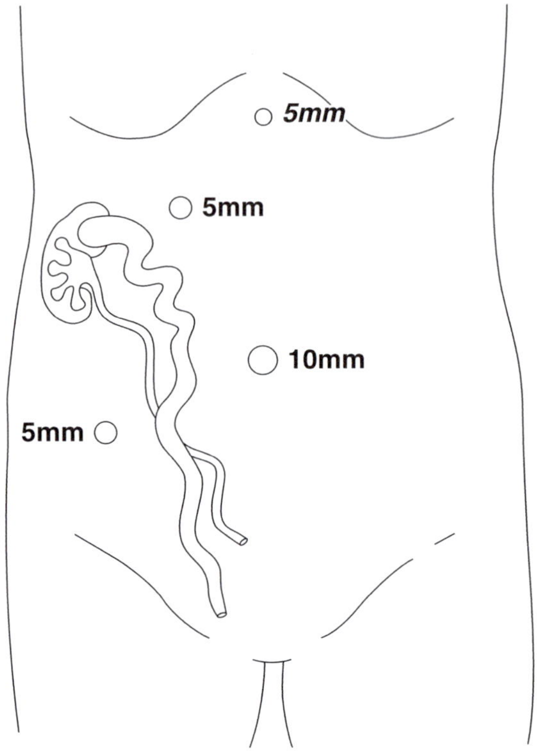

Fig. 49.2 Trocar position for a right laparoscopic nephrectomy

spleen or the loops. In general the trocars adopted are of 5 mm in diameter because we need to use during the procedure a clip applier for vessel control, a sealing device, or a peanut. The trocars are positioned in triangulation with the optic to have a better ergonomy (Fig. 49.2): periumbilical for the optic and upper quadrant and lower quadrant (always ipsilateral to the diseased kidney) for the instruments.

49.4 Instrumentation

Generally we start performing a cystoscopy to place a stent into normal ureter moiety to use it as guide. In this step we need an operative cystoscope.

Then for laparoscopic procedure, we use a couple of atraumatic fenestrated forceps to manage tissues, a curve dissector to isolate vessels, a hook cautery to perform dissection, and scissors to cut. Usually we adopt an endoloop to close the distal ureter. A needle holder is rarely adopted for this procedure. To perform hilar vessel control, we used 5 mm titanium clips, or in the last 10 years, hemostatic devices Starion MLS3 or Ultracision or Ligasure can be useful to perform a faster and safer dissection. A peanut can be adopted sometimes for dissection. It is safe to prepare a suction aspiration device, and put it on the bench because it can be useful in case of bleeding. In general no endobag is necessary to remove the renal moiety that is removed to the trocar orifice; an endobag can be necessary only in case of infected kidney.

49.5 Technique

The technique is divided into two phases: cystoscopy and laparoscopy.

Cystoscopy is performed to place a stent in the ureter of the unaffected pole; this will be your guide during laparoscopy step to identify and to avoid damaging the ureter of the normal moiety (Fig. 49.3).

In laparoscopy, thanks to the semilateral decubitus, the loops slide down, and you have only to detach the colon before opening the Gerota fascia and to isolate the kidney. Another alternative can be to pass trans-meso, but above all in older children, it can be difficult due to fat tissue in the meso and to the risk to create an injury to meso-vessels; for this reason the majority of author prefer to detach the colon. You can do it using hook cautery or in a faster way using sealing device. After opening the Gerota fascia, the ureter of the affected pole is identified and isolated, it is followed upward arriving to the kidney, hilar vessels of the affected moiety are isolated separately, and then they have to be clipped and sectioned. Another alternative is to seal the vessels using sealing device. Now a demarcation line designed by devascularization will be visible and the affected moiety removed easily with sealing device. Then the affected pole is separated from posterior attachment, and the ureter is isolated arriving near the bladder. If vesicoureteral reflux is present (as happens in the majority of cases), you have to remove as much ureter as possible arriving near the bladder, and you have to ligate, preferably using an endoloop, the distal part of the ureter. If the indication is not VUR, you can leave the ureter open. In laparoscopy, the resected moiety and the ureter are removed through the trocar orifice at umbilical level.

A drainage can be placed to check possible urinary leakage in the postoperative period.

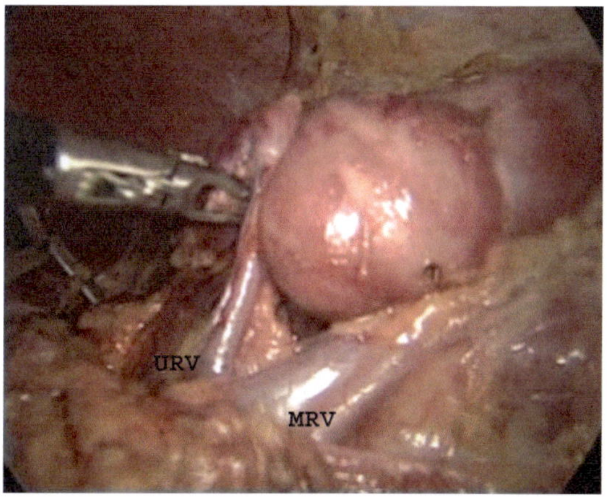

Fig. 49.3 Laparoscopy permits a clear identification of upper renal vessels (UPV) and main renal vessels (MRV)

49.6 Postoperative Care

Patients start oral feeding few hours after surgery. Analgesic requirement is rarely necessary; in general we give only paracetamol the evening of the procedure. A short antibiotic therapy is given for a couple of days. Patients are discharged from hospital on day 2 or 3. Postoperative controls are scheduled at POD7 and POD31, and then the controls change according to the indication for surgery, and an echo-color Doppler (ECD) renal ultrasounds is performed 1 month and 1 year after surgery.

49.7 Results

The median duration of surgery is generally 1 h. The conversion rate in laparoscopic partial nephrectomy, if it is performed by expert hands, is near 0.

In general, there was no intraoperative bleeding.

The indication for surgery is generally recurrent UTIs (secondary to VUR and associated with an ureterocele), loss of kidney moiety function, and ectopic ureter causing incontinence.

A recent multicenter study [4] recorded 10/52 (19.2%) complications (4 urinomas, 2 recurrent UTIs in symptomatic ureteral stumps, 4 prolonged urinary leakages), classified as grade II complications according to Clavien–Dindo grading system [5], but no conversion to open surgery nor intraoperative complications was recorded. The patients with prolonged urinary leakage were managed conservatively, leaving the bladder catheter and the drainage in situ until the complete resolution of the leakage (max 10 days). In a patient who underwent upper heminephrectomy, the urinary leakage was discovered intraoperatively, and methylene blue was injected to the stent introduced through the normal ureter to identify the leak and to close it with a couple of stitch. The remaining complications (four urinomas and two recurrent UTIs in symptomatic refluxing ureteral stumps) resolved spontaneously or after antibiotic therapy, without the need of a new surgical procedure.

ECD renal ultrasounds were normal in all patients, either 1 month or 1 year after surgery (Fig. 49.4).

Postoperative DMSA scan demonstrated no loss of function of the residual kidney moiety (mean value 37.8%) compared to before surgery (mean value 38.1%) in all operated children.

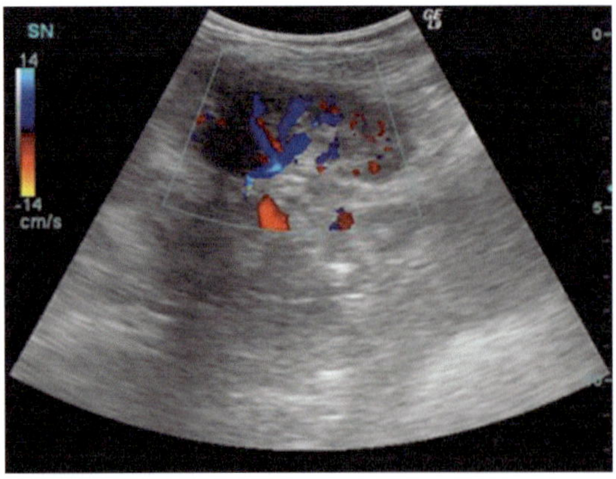

Fig. 49.4 ECD exam show a normal vascularization of normal moiety in the postoperative period

Analyzing the papers reporting results of LPN in children published in the last 10 years [6–8], a 0% conversion rate was reported in all the analyzed papers. The median operative time varied between 90 and 198 min. The complication rate varied between 7.4 and 52.9%.

49.8 Tips and Tricks

It is mandatory before starting laparoscopy to perform a cystoscopy to place a stent in the normal ureter to avoid damaging it during the procedure.

As for laparoscopy, the position of the patient in lateral decubitus is a crucial point for the success of the procedure; in this way the loops slide down, and you have an excellent view of the renal loggia. To perform a partial nephroureterectomy is fundamental to detach the colon; in this way you can isolate easily the kidney and the full ureter arriving near the bladder.

A fourth trocar can be necessary above all on the right side to retract the liver but sometimes also on the left side; the need of a fourth trocar depends on the spleen size and on the surgeon's preference. Probably at the beginning of experience, it is better to use always four trocars on both sides to have an adequate exposure of the operative field.

A useful expedient in our experience is to check the integrity of the parenchymal resection edge by injection of methylene blue dye into the ureteral catheter positioned preoperatively into the ureter of the normal functioning moiety. In this way, we can check that the normal functioning kidney moiety has not been opened during the resection of the nonfunctioning moiety. We also recommend to leave a drain in the abdominal cavity for at least 24–48 h after surgery to check an eventual leakage.

Finally, we think that another important recommendation is to always perform distal ureterectomy to the level of the bladder hiatus and to ligate the ureteric stump in patients with reflexive systems to avoid postoperative symptoms associated with recurrent UTIs.

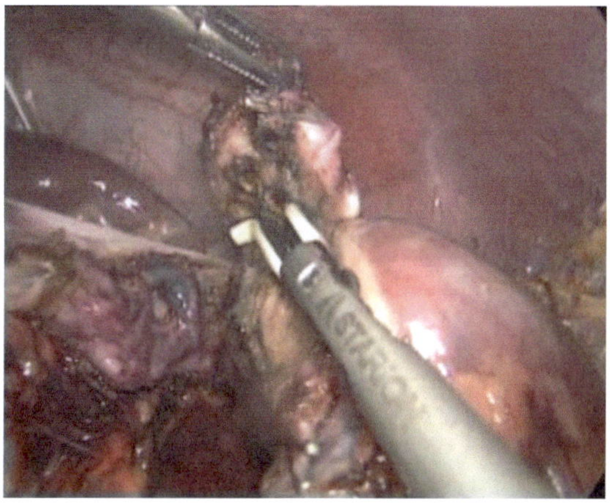

Fig. 49.5 New hemostatic devices permit the parenchymal section without any bleeding

For sure, using sealing device for dissection makes procedure bleeding-free, faster, and safer (Fig. 49.5).

As for the management of hilar vessels, also if sealing devices have a FDA approval to seal vessels of 5–7 mm in diameter, we think that it is safer to close hilar vessels with clips.

It is important to remember that if you use clips to close vessels, it is forbidden to use monopolar scissors or sealing devices to cut between clips, because you risk having the clips detach immediately or in the postoperative period.

At the end of the procedure, it is not necessary to reattach de colon to the colonic loggia.

49.9 Discussion

Advanced laparoscopic procedures in pediatric urological surgery have gained wide acceptance in the last two decades [9, 10]. Some advanced laparoscopic procedures in pediatric urology are now facilitated by the use of the advanced technologies available on the market as HD cameras, miniaturized instruments, and in particular special hemostatic devices [11]. Excluding oncological indications, the main indication for partial nephrectomy in children is to remove a nonfunctioning upper or lower pole secondary to complicated duplex anomalies of the kidney [7]. Laparoscopic partial nephrectomy is technically more demanding than laparoscopic nephrectomy [12]. In particular during the resection of the nonfunctioning moiety, there exists a risk to damage the vascularization of the residual kidney, and there is a risk of urine leakage at the level of the parenchymal resection or at the level of the residual ureteral stump [7].

After the first description of laparoscopic partial nephrectomy in children by Jordan and Winslow more than 25 years ago in 1993 [13], this procedure has gained wider acceptance compared to the open approach, thanks to the reported advantages of decreased hospital stay, lower analgesic requirements, and cosmesis [14]. This procedure can be carried out through either a retroperitoneal or transperitoneal approach [10]. Also if there is no evidence in the international literature about which technique between laparoscopy and retroperitoneoscopy is the best to adopt to perform LPN, analyzing the international literature, it seems that retroperitoneoscopy has a higher rate of conversion and a higher number of major complications compared to LPN [15].

The most frequent complications occurred in our experience in LPN were urinomas and prolonged leakages that are related to urine leakage at the level of the parenchymal resection or of the residual ureteral stump. This leakage could be due to residual excretive structures of an incompletely resected kidney moiety or to the opening of the normal functioning kidney moiety. Probably on the basis of our experience, it seems that the prolonged leakage can be due also to an excessive peritoneal secretion due to the fact that the colon is mobilized to better expose the kidney and ureter. In addition, we recorded two cases of recurrent UTIs due to symptomatic residual ureteric stumps.

The use of laparoscopy to perform PN has the main benefit of a good overall exposure of the anatomy of the kidney and its vasculature; in particular, it is extremely easy to identify the vascularization of the nonfunctioning kidney, thanks to the use of a 30° optic (Fig. 49.6). In addition, during the dissection of the dilated ureter, in male infant, it is very important to identify and save the gonadal vessels that cross the ureter in particular on the left side.

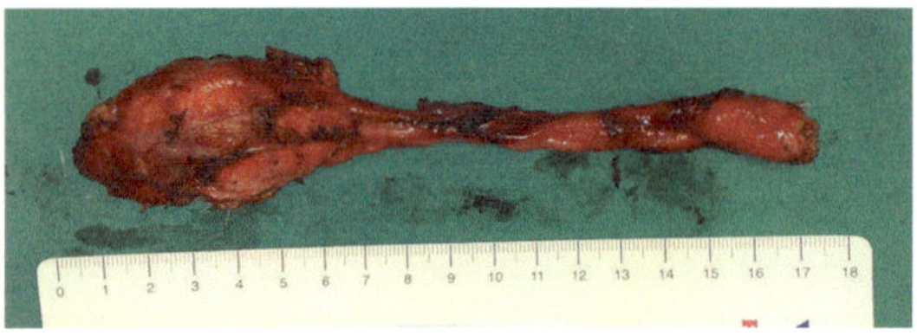

Fig. 49.6 At the end of procedure, the nonfunctioning moiety with the ureter is removed through the umbilicus

In conclusion we think that laparoscopic partial nephrectomy is easier than retroperitoneoscopic PN, but it still remains a challenging procedure performed only in pediatric centers with high experience in MIS.

In our mind, the principal advantages of laparoscopy are the complete and clear view of all urinary tract, the possibility to remove all the ureter near the bladder dome and to have a very good view of renal hilar vessels. Although the median operative time was higher than 90 min, generally we recorded no conversions nor intraoperative complications.

References

1. Borzi PA, Yeung CK. Selective approach for transperitoneal and extraperitoneal endoscopic nephrectomy in children. J Urol. 2004;171:814–6.
2. Jordan GH, Winslow DH. Laparoendoscopic upper pole partial nephrectomy with ureterectomy. J Urol. 1993;150:940–3.
3. Esposito C, Varlet F, Patkowski D, Castagnetti M, Escolino M, Draghici IM, Settimi A, Savanelli A, Till H. Laparoscopic partial nephrectomy in duplex kidneys in infants and children: results of an European multicentric survey. Surg Endosc. 2015;29(12):3469–76.
4. Esposito C, Miyano G, Caione P, Escolino M, Chiarenza F, Riccipetitoni G, Yamataka A, Cerulo M, Savanelli A, Settimi A, Valla JS. Retroperitoneoscopic heminephrectomy in duplex kidney in infants and children: results of a multicentric survey. J Laparoendosc Adv Surg Tech A. 2015;25(10):864–9.
5. Wang DS, Bird VG, Cooper CS, et al. Laparoscopic upper pole heminephrectomy for ectopic ureter: initial experience. Can J Urol. 2004;11:2141–5.
6. Dindo D, Demartines N, Clavien PA. Classification of surgical complications. A new proposal with evaluation in a cohort of 6336 patients and results of a survey. Ann Surg. 2004;240:205–13.
7. Piaggio L, Franc-Guimond J, Figueroa TE, Barthold JS, Gonzalez J. Comparison of laparoscopic and open partial nephrectomy for duplication anomalies in children. J Urol. 2006;175:2269–73.
8. Singh R, Wagener S, Chandran H. Laparoscopic management and outcomes in non-functioning moieties of duplex kidneys in children. J Pediatr Urol. 2010;6:66–9.
9. Schneider A, Ripepi M, Geiss S. Laparoscopic transperitoneal partial nephrectomy in children under 2 years old: a single-centre experience. J Pediatr Urol. 2010;6(2):166–70.
10. Janetschek G, Seibold J, Radmayr C, Bartsch G. Laparoscopic heminephroureterectomy in pediatric patients. J Urol. 1997;158:1928–30.
11. El-Ghoneimi A, Valla JS, Steyaert H, Aigrain Y. Laparoscopicrenal surgery via a retroperitoneal approach in children. J Urol. 1998;160:1138–41.
12. Elashry OM, Wolf JS Jr, Rayala HJ, McDougall EM, Clayman RV. Recent advances in laparoscopic partial nephrectomy: comparative study of electrosurgical snare electrode and ultrasound dissection. J Endourol. 1997;11:15–22.
13. Yao D, Poppas DP. A clinical series of laparoscopic nephrectomy, nephroureterectomy and heminephroureterectomy in the pediatric population. J Urol. 2000;163:1531–5.
14. Robinson BC, Snow BW, Cartwright PC, DeVries CR, Hamilton BD, Anderson JB. Comparison of laparoscopic versus open partial nephrectomy in a pediatric series. J Urol. 2003;169:638–40.
15. Esposito C, Escolino M, Miyano G, Caione P, Chiarenza F, Riccipetitoni G, Yamataka A, Savanelli A, Settimi A, Varlet F, Patkowski D, Cerulo M, Castagnetti M, Till H, Marotta R, La Manna A, Valla JS. A comparison between laparoscopic and retroperitoneoscopic approach for partial nephrectomy in children with duplex kidney: a multicentric survey. World J Urol. 2016;34(7):939–48.

MIS Management of Duplex Kidneys

50

M. Asimakidou and I. Mushtaq

50.1 Introduction

Duplex kidneys are present in 0.7–4% of the population [1]. The true incidence may be higher because in the pre-ultrasound era, these kidneys would escape diagnosis and would be discovered incidentally in later childhood or adulthood. Today with the widespread use of antenatal scanning, the vast majority of these kidneys are diagnosed prenatally. However, not all duplex kidneys will require surgical intervention. Occasionally one of the two moieties will be affected by either obstruction or reflux and often with an associated reduction in function. When the moiety is non-functioning, then it will often require removal, and in the majority of cases, it is the upper moiety that is affected.

Traditionally these renal moieties have been removed by an open procedure through a lumbar or anterior extraperitoneal approach. More recently laparoscopic surgery through a transperitoneal or retroperitoneoscopic approach is perhaps more popular [2–4].

In this chapter we describe the retroperitoneoscopic approach for partial nephrectomy which, once mastered, gives an excellent aesthetic result and a fast postoperative recovery.

M. Asimakidou · I. Mushtaq (✉)
Department of Paediatric Urology, Great Ormond Street Hospital for Children, London, UK
e-mail: imran.mushtaq@gosh.nhs.uk

50.2 Preoperative Preparation

Informed consent is obtained from those with parental responsibility ideally a few days before the procedure in the pre-assessment clinic. The patient can be admitted to the hospital on the day of the procedure and is marked on the affected side. All patients receive on induction a dose of intravenous co-amoxiclav or other appropriate antibiotic if there are positive preoperative urine cultures. A urinary catheter can be placed at the beginning of the procedure according to local practice.

50.3 Positioning

The patient is positioned fully prone with the affected side close to the edge of the operating table. Care is taken to place pressure paddings under the chest and hips to allow the abdomen to be free for respiration. Once the patient is secured in place and before draping the spinous processes, iliac crest and the 11th and 12th ribs are marked (Fig. 50.1). Some surgeons at this stage would prefer to position the patient in a semi-prone position with the affected side slightly tilted upward. In this case the patient is placed with the non-affected side closer to the edge of the operating table.

C. Esposito et al. (eds.), *ESPES Manual of Pediatric Minimally Invasive Surgery*,
https://doi.org/10.1007/978-3-030-00964-9_50

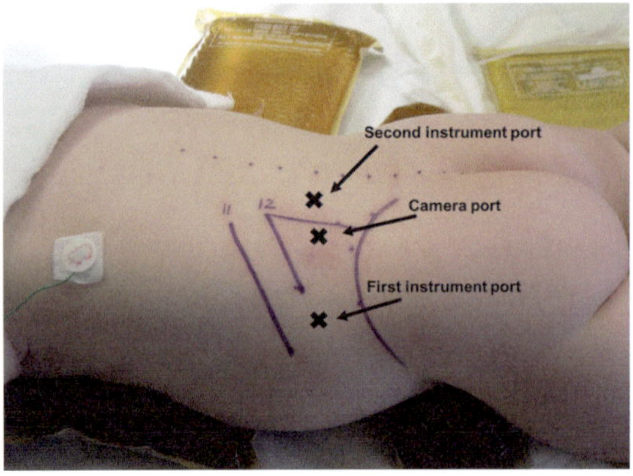

Fig. 50.1 Positioning and marking of the patient

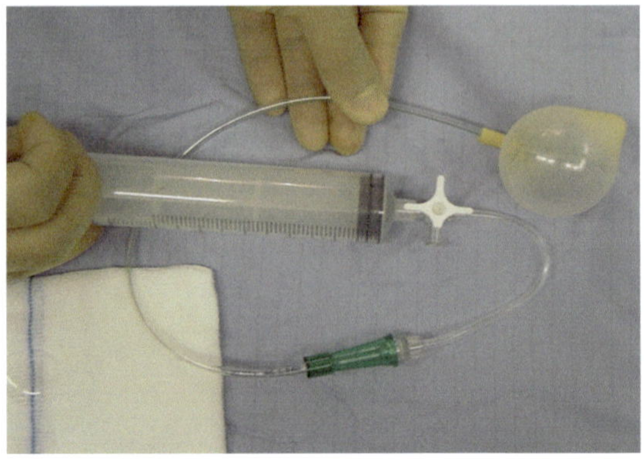

Fig. 50.2 Custom made balloon for the creation of retroperitoneal space

50.4 Instrumentation

A single 5 mm incision is used in order to access the retroperitoneal space around the kidney. This first incision is placed midway between the 12th rib and the iliac crest at the lateral border of the sacrospinalis muscle. The muscles are cut down to the level of the retroperitoneum, and the initial working space is created with the use of a home-made balloon or gauze swab (Fig. 50.2). The balloon is inserted in the retroperitoneal space, and 80–120 mL of the air is instilled in the balloon in order to create the working space for the nephrectomy [5, 6]. The camera port is then inserted, and insufflation is maintained with a flow of 2 L/min and an insufflation pressure of 12–15 mmHg. A 5 mm instrument port is inserted under direct vision laterally to the camera port between the 11th rib and the iliac crest (Fig. 50.3). A third port could be placed if needed under direct vision more medially in order to achieve triangulation. A 5 mm 30-degree laparoscope is best suited to this surgery as it will allow for an enhanced view of the renal structures over the posterior surface of the kidney.

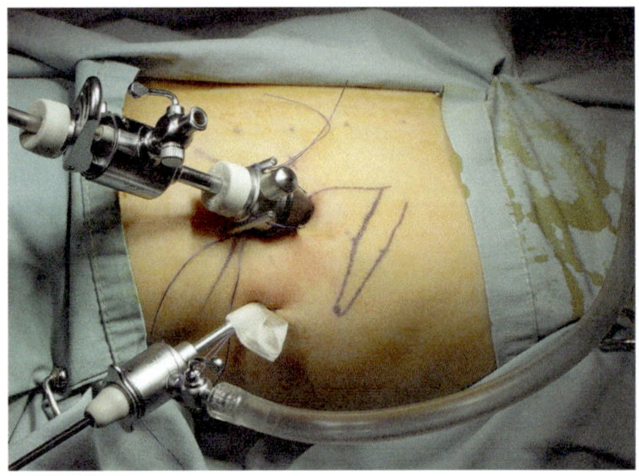

Fig. 50.3 Positioning of the ports. In most of the cases, it is feasible to proceed with the utilization of only two ports

50.5 Technique

The kidney is identified, and the Gerota's fascia is incised in a cruciate manner. The perinephric fat is dissected in a blunt manner using monopolar diathermy in order to expose the posterolateral surface of the kidney. Dissection is then carried out toward the medial part of the kidney with an aim to expose the hilar vessels which will readily come into view (Fig. 50.4). It is important always to confirm the duplex anatomy of the kidney before proceeding to dissection and division of the vessels. The vessels to the affected pole are identified and ligated/divided in accordance with the operating surgeons' preference (Harmonic scalpel, Ligasure, endoclips, suture) (Fig. 50.5). This maneuver will create a line of demarcation between the upper and the lower moieties of the kidney, which will aid the subsequent excision (Fig. 50.6). At this point care must be taken to identify possible anomalous vessels to the affected moiety, particularly on the anterior aspect and divide them. This is seen more frequently when removing an affected upper pole, where there can also be short vessels coming from the lower pole very close to the parenchymal

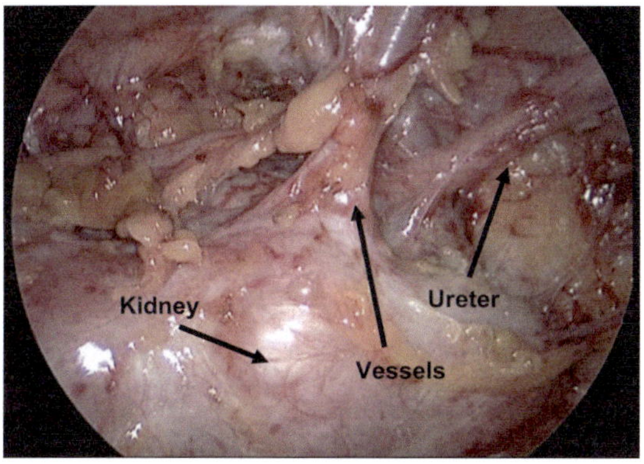

Fig. 50.4 Intraoperative picture after the dissection around the kidney and the vessels

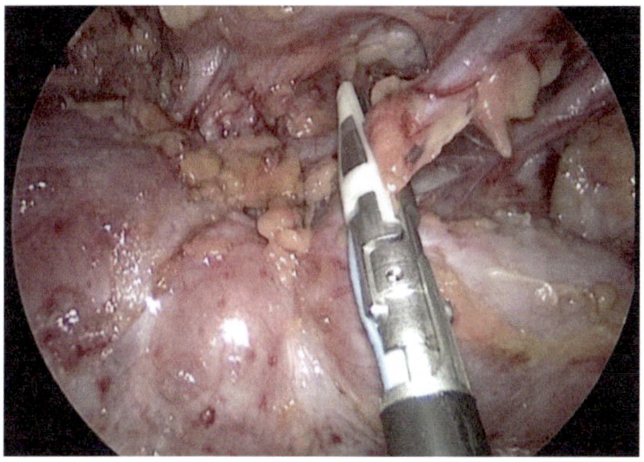

Fig. 50.5 Intraoperative picture. The vessels leading to the affected moiety are ligated

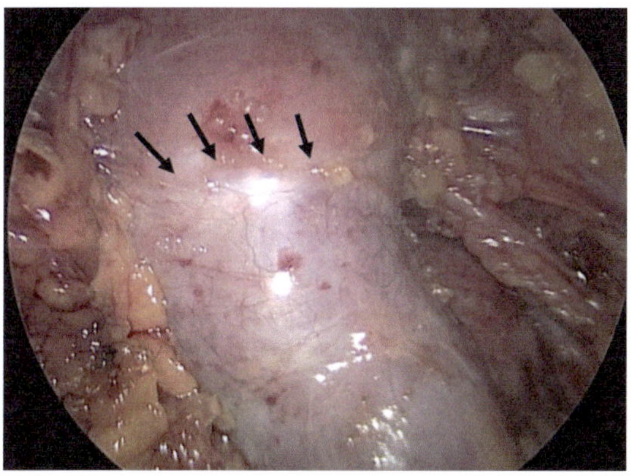

Fig. 50.6 Intraoperative picture. Demarcation zone (arrows) is evident after the ligation of the vessels to the affected moiety

junction of the upper and lower poles. Once all appropriate vessels are ligated, the affected ureter should be divided in a short distance (2 cm) from the renal pelvis. The proximal divided ureter can be used to rotate the affected moiety laterally in order to expose additional vessels at the anterior surface of the kidney. If the ureter to be excised is associated with reflux, then it should be ligated as far distally as safely as possible. If there is no reflux present, it is safe to leave the ureter without ligation. The affected moiety is excised with the use of diathermy hook or Ligasure/Harmonic scalpel. In cases where the specimen is relatively small, it can be retrieved directly through the port site. For larger specimens an endopouch is used for retrieval. At the end of the procedure, all port sites are approximated with 4/0 Vicryl, and the skin is closed with tissue glue.

50.6 Postoperative Care

Postoperatively the patient is returned to the ward. Oral feeds are commenced on the same day, and IV antibiotics are administered for the first 48 h after surgery. It is common for the patient to have some pyrexia in the first 24 h after surgery, probably related to the spillage of urine.

If a urethral catheter has been placed, it is removed after 48 h or once the patient can mobilize to the bathroom. Regular paracetamol is used for the first 48–72 h with the addition of ibuprofen if required (if not contraindicated).

50.7 Results

The surgery normally lasts for 90–120 min depending on the status of the kidney. Preoperative pyelonephritis might create local scarring and hence lengthen the kidney dissection phase. Most of the patients will be discharged on the second or third postoperative day. Rarely patients are kept for an extra day, and these are usually older children with slower recovery. Patients can return to their regular activities 7 days after the surgery. Follow-up is arranged 3 months after the procedure with a repeat ultrasound scan of the kidneys. If this is satisfactory, then a further ultrasound is performed at 12 months after surgery, with the addition of a nuclear scan (MAG3/DMSA) at the same time.

50.8 Tips and Tricks

In young children the space between the ribs and the iliac crest is limited. Bending the patient's spine toward the normal side will create a larger distance on the affected side. This is usually achieved by moving the patient's legs away from the affected side on the operative table.

Creating the initial retroperitoneal space outside the Gerota's fascia is crucial. This space is avascular, and the initial dissection would be blood free. In order to achieve that, the surgeon should dissect the muscles with a small clip. While gradually dissecting through the muscle layers, two separate "gives" should be felt. After that the tip of the clip is just at the working space that needs expansion. The balloon is inserted and inflated slowly. Lubricating gel on the surface of the balloon can facilitate creation of the space.

After the creation of the working space and the insertion of the ports, the Gerota's fascia is opened. It is very important to create a cruciate opening. This way the fascia will retract away from the operative field providing maximal view and operative space.

During the procedure the diathermy should be used liberally. The working space is limited and even small amount of bleeding could obstruct good vision. Furthermore, even when bleeding is controlled, the blood that has infiltrated the tissues would absorb light and hinder optimal vision.

50.9 Discussion

Laparoscopic techniques are gaining increased popularity, and in experienced hands, complication rates are now similar to the open procedures. Minimally invasive techniques require time for the learning curve to plateau. Retroperitoneoscopic approach is deemed more challenging due to the reversed anatomy (posterior view of the kidney) and the limited working space. In this context familiarity with the approach and often exposure to the procedure are required to minimize complication rates [4].

In total nephrectomy the complication rate between the transperitoneal and the retroperitoneoscopic approach is similar. However, the retroperitoneoscopic approach offers the invaluable advantage of leaving the peritoneal space intact [2, 7]. In partial nephrectomy the current literature is rather conflicting. A recent study has reported that the complication rate might be higher with the retroperitoneoscopic approach. Additionally, in the same study, the postoperative course was found longer for the retroperitoneoscopic approach [8]. These findings were consistent with previous smaller studies that reported higher complication rates in the retroperitoneoscopic group [2]. Most of these complications are classified as grade II or III according to the Clavien-Dindo classification [8].

Taking a closer look at the specific complications of the technique, these could be divided into intraoperative, immediate postoperative, and long term. During the initial dissection, the peritoneum could be inadvertently opened, and the procedure may need to be converted to open. Similarly, if intraoperative bleeding occurs and it is difficult to control, then conversion is required. The limited space in the retroperitoneoscopic approach makes even small amount of bleeding quite challenging. Conversion rates are between 2.5 and 18% [9]. In transperitoneal laparoscopic partial nephrectomy, the conversion rates are lower, between 0 and 4% [2]. Despite that even in our early experience, we encounter no conversions [3].

The most common immediate postoperative complication is a local collection, in most cases a urinoma. The urinoma occurs due to leak from the remaining moiety and is usually initially managed with the insertion of a urethral catheter. Some urinomas though will require percutaneous drainage. The incidence of urinomas in retroperitoneoscopic partial nephrectomy ranges between 2.5 and 13.5% [9]. In laparoscopic transperitoneal approach, the incidence of complications due to urinary leak seems to be negligible or to occur in lower rates [2, 3].

The long-term complications could include recurrent urine infections due to the refluxing ureteric stump (ureteric stump syndrome), asymptomatic cyst formation (27–48%), and loss of function to the remaining moiety (2.5–9%) [9–11]. The ureteric stump can become problematic in the postoperative period in cases of refluxing ureter, and as such some surgeons prefer to utilize the transperitoneal approach over the retroperitoneoscopic as it can provide better access to the very distal ureter [12, 13]. The formation of an asymptomatic cyst is a rather common finding, and it has been related with the technique used, especially the use of endoloop [14]. Recent data suggest that the technique used to resect the parenchyma does not collate with the formation of these cysts and other reasons should be sought [11].

Retroperitoneoscopic partial nephrectomy is feasible and safe in the pediatric population. Despite some data suggesting a higher complication rate, we believe that the increased experience in centers which use the retroperitoneoscopic approach routinely for other surgeries could obviate this difference. The advantages of a more direct approach to the kidney and the vascular pedicle, combined with minimal risk to the adjacent intraabdominal organs and an intact peritoneal cavity, make it an attractive approach to master.

References

1. Didier RA, Chow JS, Kwatra NS, Retik AB, Lebowitz RL. The duplicated collecting system of the urinary tract: embryology, imaging appearances and clinical considerations. Pediatr Radiol. 2017;47(11):1526–38.
2. Antoniou D, Karetsos C. Laparoscopy or retroperitoneoscopy: which is the best approach in pediatric urology? Transl Pediatr. 2016;5(2):205–13.
3. Mushtaq I, Haleblian G. Laparoscopic heminephrectomy in infants and children: first 54 cases. J Pediatr Urol. 2007;3(2):100–3.
4. Cerulo M, Escolino M, Turrà F, Roberti A, Farina A, Esposito C. Benefits of retroperitoneoscopic surgery in pediatric. Urology. 2018;16:1–5.
5. Gaur DG. Retroperitoneoscopy: the balloon technique. Ann R Coll Surg Engl. 1994;76(4):259–63.
6. Gaur DD, Gopichand M, Dubey M, Jhunjhunwala V. Mini-access for retroperitoneal laparoscopy. J Laparoendosc Adv Surg Tech A. 2002;12(5):313–5.
7. Gundeti MS, Patel Y, Duffy PG, Cuckow PM, Wilcox DT, Mushtaq I. An initial experience of 100 paediatric laparoscopic nephrectomies with transperitoneal or posterior prone retroperitoneoscopic approach. Pediatr Surg Int. 2007;23(8):795–9.
8. Esposito C, Escolino M, Castagnetti M, Savanelli A, Manna AL, Farina A, et al. Retroperitoneal and laparoscopic heminephrectomy in duplex kidney in infants and children. Transl Pediatr. 2016;5(4):245–50.
9. Jayram G, Roberts J, Hernandez A, Heloury Y, Manoharan S, Godbole P, et al. Outcomes and fate of the remnant moiety following laparoscopic heminephrectomy for duplex kidney: a multicenter review. J Pediatr Urol. 2011;7(3):272–5.
10. Joyeux L, Lacreuse I, Schneider A, Moog R, Borgnon J, Lopez M, et al. Long-term functional renal outcomes after retroperitoneoscopic upper pole heminephrectomy for duplex kidney in children: a multicenter cohort study. Surg Endosc Other Interv Tech. 2017;31(3):1241–9.
11. Esposito C, Escolino M, Troncoso Solar B, Iacona R, Esposito R, Settimi A, et al. Diagnosis and long-term outcome of renal cysts after laparoscopic partial nephrectomy in children. BJU Int. 2017;119(5):761–6.
12. Escolino M, Farina A, Turrà F, Cerulo M, Esposito R, Savanelli A, et al. Evaluation and outcome of the distal ureteral stump after nephro-ureterectomy in children. A comparison between laparoscopy and retroperitoneoscopy. J Pediatr Urol. 2016;12(2):1193.e1–19.e8.
13. Esposito C, Escolino M, Corcione F, Draghici IM, Savanelli A, Castagnetti M, et al. Twenty-year experience with laparoscopic and retroperitoneoscopic nephrectomy in children: considerations and details of technique. Surg Endosc Other Interv Tech. 2016;30(5):2114–8.
14. Hiorns MP, Mazrani W, Mushtaq I, McHugh K. Follow-up imaging after laparoscopic heminephrectomy in children. Pediatr Radiol. 2008;38(7):762–5.

51 Laparoscopic Management of Intrinsic Ureteropelvic Junction Obstruction (UPJO)

Philipp Szavay

51.1 Introduction

Ureteropelvic junction obstruction (UPJO) is the most common cause of hydronephrosis in infants and children. Since Anderson and Hynes described their technique of open dismembered pyeloplasty through a retroperitoneal approach, this has been considered the gold standard in surgical care for UPJO. When in 1995 Peters reported on the first pediatric laparoscopic pyeloplasty, a new era for laparoscopy in pediatric urology began. For the first time reconstructive surgery on the upper urinary tract was hereby implemented. Meanwhile pyeloplasty in children either by a laparoscopic or a retroperitoneoscopic approach has become an established technique to operate on UPJO in infants and children. The aim is to propose practical clinical guidelines for the current gold standard of laparoscopic dismembered pyeloplasty.

51.2 Current Status and General Aspects of Laparoscopic Dismembered Pyeloplasty

Meanwhile advantages of laparoscopic upper urinary tract surgery in children and infants are widely acknowledged as well as accepted. Compared to the former gold standard of open pyeloplasty [1], the minimally invasive approach offers a superior cosmesis, while functional results proofed to be at least equal both in children and infants. The length of hospitalization could be decreased, and there might be additional advantages such as less postoperative pain (nn). Apart from those issues, laparoscopic dismembered pyeloplasty offers superior visualization of the anatomy, accurate anastomotic suturing, and thus precise reconstruction of the UPJ which promises good functional results. Therefore laparoscopic transperitoneal dismembered pyeloplasty can be considered as the gold standard for surgical treatment of intrinsic UPJO.

51.3 Indications for Surgery of Intrinsic UPJO

Intrinsic UPJO is defined as a defect of the smooth muscle of the ureter, consecutively leading to an obstruction of the UPJ. Indication for surgery is given when:

- Differential renal function (DRF) of the affected side below 40%
- Decrease of DRF, documented in more than just one examination, such as a renal scintigram or a MRI, respectively
- Relevant urodynamic obstruction in renal scintigram or MRI, respectively
- Recurrent urinary tract infection (UTI) and/or pyelonephritis

P. Szavay (✉)
Department of Pediatric Surgery, Lucerne Children's Hospital, Lucerne, Switzerland
e-mail: philipp.szavay@luks.ch

C. Esposito et al. (eds.), *ESPES Manual of Pediatric Minimally Invasive Surgery*,
https://doi.org/10.1007/978-3-030-00964-9_51

- Subjective patient complaints, such as flank pain
- Special anatomical condition such as horseshoe kidney along with obstruction

The aim of surgery is to maintain DRF and to improve urinary drainage.

51.4 Preoperative Diagnostic Work-Up

Preoperative diagnostic work-up includes:

- Ultrasound
- Diuretic renal scintigram
- MRI

To indicate an intravenous pyelography is meanwhile obsolete and should be restricted to very rare and complex indications only.

51.5 Preoperative Preparation

Informed consent is obtained from all patients or their parents, respectively, prior to surgery. General anesthesia with muscle relaxation is provided. A Foley catheter is inserted in order to control urinary drainage as well as provide an empty bladder during laparoscopy for improved working space and view. Perioperative single-shot antibiotic therapy is administered according to the weight of the patient and to local preferences, respectively. The patient is prepped and placed according to local standards and following the rules of asepsis.

51.6 Positioning and Ergonomics

The patient is placed in supine position. The flank of the affected side to operate on is slightly elevated with a gel pad or similar. According to the specific operating theater specification and setup, respectively, the screen is positioned on the side of the patient who will be operated on in order to provide the surgeon with a view in direction to the operating field. Additional monitors are placed meaningfully around the patient to facilitate view for the assistant surgeon, scrub nurses, anesthetists, and others, respectively. To provide an ergonomic posture for the surgeon, the monitors may be positioned rather low, so that the surgeon is more looking downward such as in an open procedure. Surgeon's position is on the opposite side of the patient, while the assistant surgeon driving the camera is standing or rather seated on the same side, with both the surgeons looking in direction to the side of the operating field. The scrub nurse is standing across at the patient's opposite side.

51.7 Instrumentation

The conventional approach for laparoscopic pyeloplasty is a three-trocar access to the abdomen, with one 5 mm trocar at the umbilicus as for a 5 mm scope, as well as 2–3 mm working ports in the upper and lower abdomen of the affected side, respectively. As in general triangulation should be the goal with respect to the renal pelvis to operate on (see Fig. 51.1).

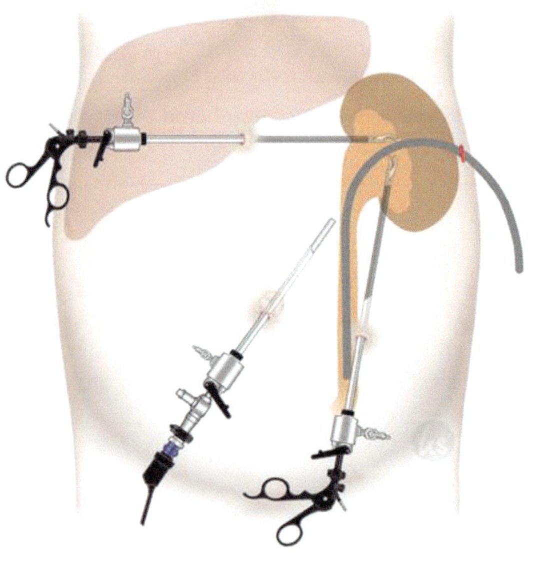

Fig. 51.1 Trocar sites for laparoscopic transperitoneal pyeloplasty (left-sided)

51.8 Technique

Surgical steps of laparoscopic transperitoneal pyeloplasty are defined as gaining access to the affected kidney, either through a retro-colonic or a trans-mesocolic access to Gerota's fascia. Following the incision of the fascia as well as of the fatty capsule of the kidney, a blunt/sharp dissection leading to the pyelon is carried out. When the pyelon becomes visible and is identified a direct attempt should be made to grasp it and then further dissect it out, again using a blunt and/or sharp technique with electrocautery, scissors, harmonic or similar devices respectively. When the renal pelvis has been sufficiently exposed, thus the UPJ has also been dissected out, two transabdominal hitching sutures will help to expose the pyelon in order to perform the resection of the UPJ. Those should be placed with care, safely sparing the renal hilar vessels, and the caudal one placed behind the UPJ, so the resection of the UPJ can be carried out in front of the hitching suture (see Fig. 51.2).

Following the resection of the UPJ, the ureter now is incised but not cut completely at a level safe below the UPJ and then spatulated on his lateral aspect in order to provide a sufficient length of ureteral wall for achieving a wide side-to-side anastomosis (see Fig. 51.3).

The idea behind leaving the resected part of the pyelon, UPJ, and proximal ureter, respectively, in place and not cutting them off completely is that this tissue may provide as a "handlebar" during the following suturing process to achieve the anastomosis (see Fig. 51.4). Thus the ureteral tissue does not have to be grabbed and compromised by instrument manipulation. A side-to-side anastomosis is then carried out, starting with the back side. The anastomosis can be performed with either a single interrupted technique or a running suture as well. The single interrupted sutures will offer more safety in achieving a watertight anastomosis and may be more tissue-sparing as well. The running suture may allow a rather time-saving technique however requires constantly the application of tension to the thread in order to avoid loosening which might be the cause for urinary leakage later. Meanwhile

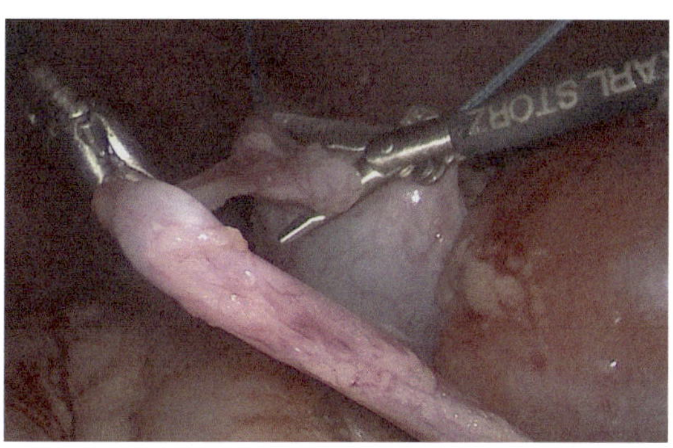

Fig. 51.2 Resection of UPJ, facilitated through two transabdominal hitching sutures

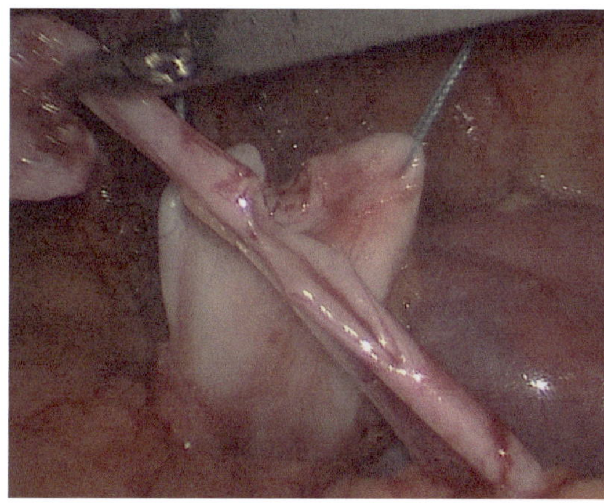

Fig. 51.3 Aspect of the incised and spatulated ureter

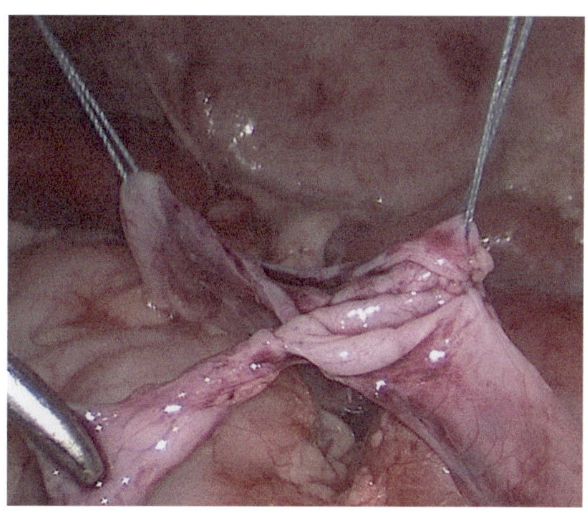

Fig. 51.4 Using the resected part of the UPJ as a "handlebar" to drive the tissue during suturing

barbed sutures are available down to metric sizes of 4/0 that may facilitate performing a running suture in this setting. Otherwise we prefer to use braided sutures in sizes of 6/0 for infants and 5/0 for older patients. An inverting technique of suturing is recommended to avoid any suturing material to be exposed to intraluminal as this might cause crystallization at the thread with consecutive bacterial colonization. After completion of the back side, the patency of the anastomosis should be checked, before continuing the anastomosis of the front side (see Fig. 51.5).

When the front side of the anastomosis has been completed in the same fashion (see Fig. 51.6), the remaining open pyelon can be closed again using a running suture or "Z-type" single interrupted sutures. The final aspect should be confirming a wide side-to-side anastomosis with a newly created patent UPJ.

There is some ongoing discussion whether to stent the anastomosis and what kind of stent to use. We prefer using a transabdominal, trans-anastomotic stent technique. A 6-8 F stent is brought into the abdomen using a curved (custom-made) spear and then brought through the open pyelon and through an identified calyx, respectively, while puncturing the renal parenchyma brought out again through the abdominal wall laterally. The tip of the catheter is then pulled into the abdomen and finally is then introduced into the distal ureter. This allows an atraumatic technique that does not require a second general anesthesia to remove the stent like with the use of any kind of double-J stents (see Fig. 51.7).

Other techniques include double-J stents, percutaneous nephrostomy stents, and others.

Following the completion of the pyeloplasty, the hitching sutures are removed, the kidney is repositioned, and the eventually mobilized bowel

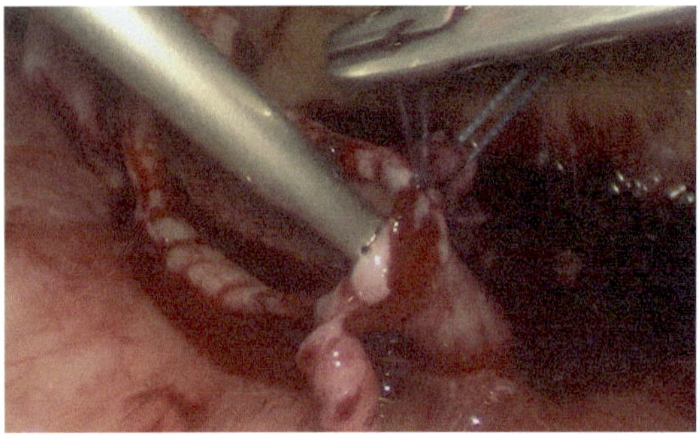

Fig. 51.5 Checking the patency of the anastomosis after completion of the back wall

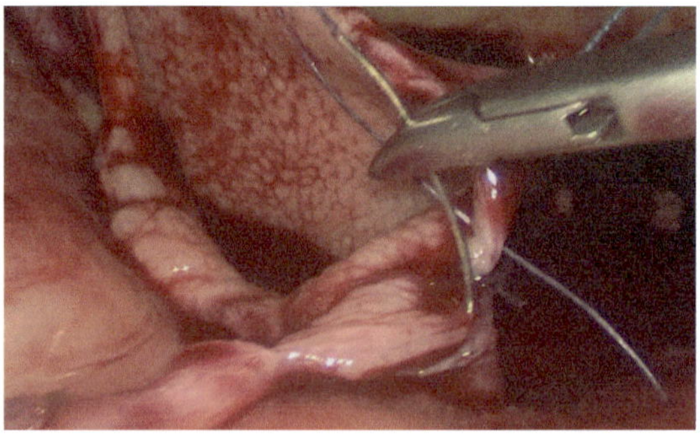

Fig. 51.6 Single interrupted suture of the front side anastomosis, using the resected UPJ as a "handlebar"

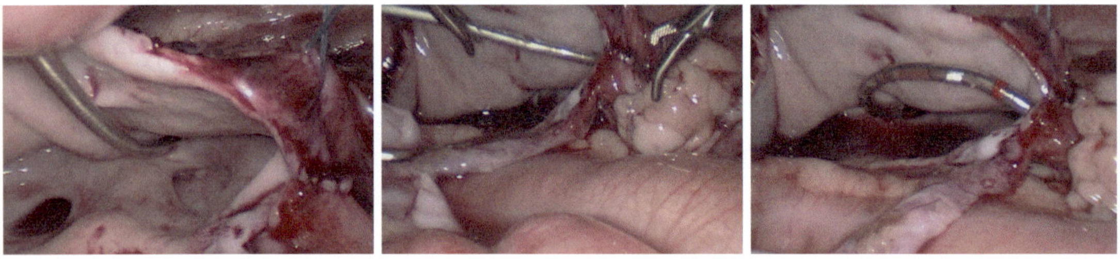

Fig. 51.7 Placement of a transabdominal, trans-anastomotic ureteral stent [2]

is brought back to its original position. In a regular case, an additional drainage will not be required. The specimen of the resected pyelon and UPJ, respectively, is removed from the abdomen along with one of the working ports.

51.9 Postoperative Care

Antibiotic treatment is administered according to local guidelines; however, it may be adapted with regard to intraoperative findings. Oral feeding may be allowed the same day. The use of analgesics for postoperative pain control should be liberal and in general following international recommendations such as the WHO "Treatment Guidelines on Pain," adapted to local requirements and guidelines. Patients can be discharged theoretically on day 1 or 2, respectively; however we tend to leave the trans-anastomotic stent for 7 days while the patient stays in the hospital. The question whether to put a stent in and if so how long those should stay remains to the preference of the surgeon as there is so far no evidence in favor for one of the mentioned methods.

51.10 Discussion

Laparoscopic dismembered pyeloplasty has evolved to become the gold standard for the surgical treatment of intrinsic UPJO since a surgical first in 1995 by Craig Peters [1]. It has been proven to be safe, effective, and associated with a low complication rate with excellent functional results [3–10]. This is obviously also true for recurrent UPJO [11, 12]. Laparoscopic dismembered pyeloplasty on the same hand offers low morbidity due to the reduced surgical trauma, superior cosmesis, fast recovery, and quick return to daily and social activities. It has been therefore surpassed open pyeloplasty in many centers as the gold standard surgical management for UPJO.

Compared to open surgery, there have been implications coming along with minimally invasive approach techniques. The most remarkable one is probably the less reduction of the renal pelvis as compared to the original technique described by Anderson and Hynes. However different authors considered a less reductive resection of the renal pelvis not to be determinative in terms of the functional result [13, 14]. Whether to use running or single interrupted sutures, respectively, remains to the preference of the surgeon. There might be some higher surgical efficiency with the running suture method [15]. One striking advantage of transperitoneal laparoscopic pyeloplasty is that the approach is a standard procedure for many indications in both pediatric surgery and urology. In addition it is applicable also for children below 1 year of age. There is sufficient evidence in literature that also in infants laparoscopic dismembered pyeloplasty has been proven to be a safe procedure providing the same functional outcomes as the open approach [16–18]. In comparing laparoscopic multiport pyeloplasty with single-site approaches such as the trans-umbilical approach, it could be demonstrated that although the cosmetic result with the single-site approach is satisfactory, the multiport access did affect the shape of the umbilicus; thus the cosmetic result was considered to be better [19]. Multiple studies were aiming to describe differences in between open, laparoscopic, and robotic pyeloplasties, respectively [20, 21]. All of those demonstrate that patients undergoing robotic-assisted laparoscopic pyeloplasty had a shorter hospital stay and less request of pain medication; however, there could be no difference shown in the success rates for open, laparoscopic, and robotic-assisted laparoscopic pyeloplasty, respectively. In conclusion and with regard to a higher cost associated with robotic pyeloplasty thus making it less available to the majority of patient population, laparoscopic pyeloplasty considered to be equally effective as all other available techniques should be considered as the true technique of choice for surgical treatment of intrinsic UPJO in children and infants.

References

1. Peters CA, Schlussel RN, Retik AB. Pediatric laparoscopic dismembered pyeloplasty. J Urol. 1995;153(6):1962–5.
2. Obermayr F, Luithle T, Fuchs J. Laparoscopically guided external transanastomotic stenting in dismembered pyeloplasty: a safe technique. Urology. 2015;86(1):200–4.
3. Peters CA. Laparoscopy in pediatric urology. Curr Opin Urol. 2004;14(2):67–73.
4. Symons SJ, Bhirud PS, Jain V, Shetty AS, Desai MR. Laparoscopic pyeloplasty: our new gold standard. J Endourol. 2009;23(3):463–7.
5. Chacko JK, Piaggio LA, Neheman A, González R. Pediatric laparoscopic pyeloplasty: lessons learned from the first 52 cases. J Endourol. 2009;23(8):1307–11.
6. Szavay PO, Luithle T, Seitz G, Warmann SW, Haber P, Fuchs J. Functional outcome after laparoscopic dismembered pyeloplasty in children. J Pediatr Urol. 2010;6(4):359–63.
7. Juliano RV, Mendonça RR, Meyer F, Rubinstein M, Lasmar MT, Korkes F, Tavares A, Pompeo AC, Tobias-Machado M. Long-term outcome of laparoscopic pyeloplasty: multicentric comparative study of techniques and accesses. J Laparoendosc Adv Surg Tech A. 2011;21(5):399–403.
8. Piaggio LA, Corbetta JP, Weller S, Dingevan RA, Duran V, Ruiz J, Lopez JC. Comparative, prospective, case-control study of open versus laparoscopic pyeloplasty in children with ureteropelvic junction obstruction: long-term results. Front Pediatr. 2017;5:10.
9. Gatti JM, Amstutz SP, Bowlin PR, Stephany HA, Murphy JP. Laparoscopic vs open pyeloplasty in children: results of a randomized, prospective, controlled trial. J Urol. 2017;197(3 Pt 1):792–7.
10. Penn HA, Gatti JM, Hoestje SM, DeMarco RT, Snyder CL, Murphy JP. Laparoscopic versus open pyeloplasty in children: preliminary report of a prospective randomized trial. J Urol. 2010;184(2):690–5.
11. Abdel-Karim AM, Fahmy A, Moussa A, Rashad H, Elbadry M, Badawy H, Hammady A. Laparoscopic pyeloplasty versus open pyeloplasty for recurrent ureteropelvic junction obstruction in children. J Pediatr Urol. 2016;12(6):401.e1–401.
12. Moscardi PR, Barbosa JA, Andrade HS, Mello MF, Cezarino BN, Oliveira LM, Srougi M, Dénes FT, Lopes RI. Reoperative laparoscopic ureteropelvic junction obstruction repair in children: safety and efficacy of the technique. J Urol. 2017;197(3 Pt 1):798–804.
13. Morsi HA, Mursi K, Abdelaziz AY, Elsheemy MS, Salah M, Eissa MA. Renal pelvis reduction during dismembered pyeloplasty: is it necessary? J Pediatr Urol. 2013;9(3):303–6.
14. Reismann M, Gratz KF, Metzelder M, Ure B, Glüer S. Excision of the dilated pelvis is not necessary in laparoscopic dismembered pyeloplasty. Eur J Pediatr Surg. 2008;18(1):19–21.
15. Shao P, Qin C, Ju X, Meng X, Li J, Lv Q, Zhang W, Xu Z, Yin C. Comparison of two different suture methods in laparoscopic dismembered pyeloplasty. Urol Int. 2011;87(3):304–8.
16. Fuchs J, Luithle T, Warmann SW, Haber P, Blumenstock G, Szavay P. Laparoscopic surgery on the upper urinary tract in children below one year of age—technical aspects and functional outcome. J Urol. 2009;182(4):1561–8.
17. García-Aparicio L, Blazquez-Gomez E, Martin O, Manzanares A, García-Smith N, Bejarano M, Rodo J, Ribó JM. Anderson-hynes pyeloplasty in patients less than 12 months old. Is the laparoscopic approach safe and feasible? J Endourol. 2014;28(8):906–8.
18. Turner RM, Fox JA, Tomaszewski JJ, Schneck FX, Docimo SG, Ost MC. Laparoscopic pyeloplasty for ureteropelvic junction obstruction in infants. J Urol. 2013;189(4):1503–7.
19. Liu D, Zhou H, Ma L, Xie H, Tao T, Cao H, Zhou X, Luo X, Chen S. Transumbilical multi-port laparoscopic pyeloplasty versus transumbilical single-site laparoscopic pyeloplasty for ureteropelvic junction obstruction in children: a retrospectively comparative study. J Pediatr Urol. 2017;13(6):618.e1–5.
20. Chan YY, Durbin-Johnson B, Sturm RM, Kurzrock EA. Outcomes after pediatric open, laparoscopic, and robotic pyeloplasty at academic institutions. J Pediatr Urol. 2017;13(1):49.e1–6.
21. Song SH, Lee C, Jung J, Kim SJ, Park S, Park H, Kim KS. Comparative study of pediatric open pyeloplasty, laparoscopy-assisted extracorporeal pyeloplasty, and robot-assisted laparoscopic pyeloplasty. PLoS One. 2017;12(4):e0175026.

52 Laparoscopic Management of Extrinsic Ureteropelvic Junction Obstruction (UPJO) by Crossing Vessels

Salvatore Fabio Chiarenza and Cosimo Bleve

52.1 Introduction

Open or laparoscopic dismembered pyeloplasty (DP) is the gold standard procedure to treat UPJO since the procedure was first described by Anderson and Hynes (AHDP) in 1949 [1]. UPJO may be caused by intrinsic disorganization or by extrinsic compression from crossing vessels (CV); extrinsic causes often present symptomatically in older children. The association between UPJ obstruction and extrinsic aetiology by lower pole CV was first described by Von Rokitansky in 1842 [2]. UPJO due to CV, frequently observed in adults, is a rare condition in neonates and has a slight incidence in older children. An alternative approach to pure extrinsic UPJO was first described by Hellström [3] always in 1949; it involved displacing the lower pole vessels cranially and then anchoring them to the anterior pelvic wall using vascular adventitial sutures. Chapman [4] further modified this technique by securing a more superior position of the lower pole vessels within a wrap of the anterior redundant pelvic wall without the need for vascular adventitial sutures. This technique has since been described in children as an alternative to open DP, with the largest series reported in 1999 by Pesce [5]. Aberrant vessels usually cause intermittent UPJO. These cases present a normal perinatal history, followed by the subsequent onset of clinical signs and symptoms, often influenced by the child's hydration status, characterized by intermittent hydronephrosis on imaging and normal kidney function. The CV typically cross over the UPJ to perfuse the lower pole of the affected kidney. Currently, there are no definitive imaging techniques or intraoperative procedures available to confirm the aetiology of UPJO. As noted by Schneider [6], frequently one encounters anatomic variability in the relationship between the renal pelvis and the lower pole vessels. Some authors have proposed DP to exclude intrinsic associated anomalies; others, in order to minimize technical difficulties and improve outcomes, have described simpler procedures that do not involve pyeloureteral anastomosis. We describe in this chapter the paediatric laparoscopic vascular hitch (LVH), a mini-invasive approach to UPJO by CV, suggesting a simple and uncomplicated intraoperative test, DT, to confirm the relief of the obstruction. This technique gives excellent results in our hands.

52.2 Preoperative Diagnosis and Preparation

A preoperative diagnosis of extrinsic UPJO was based on complete medical history and a specific imaging examination. All patients with

S. F. Chiarenza (✉) · C. Bleve
Department of Pediatric Surgery and Pediatric Minimally Invasive Surgery and New Technologies, San Bortolo Hospital, Vicenza, Italy
e-mail: fabio.chiarenza@aulss8.veneto.it

C. Esposito et al. (eds.), *ESPES Manual of Pediatric Minimally Invasive Surgery*,
https://doi.org/10.1007/978-3-030-00964-9_52

UPJO undergo, respectively, ultrasonography/Doppler scan and MAG3renogram, reserving functional magnetic resonance urography (fMRU) in case of suspected extrinsic obstruction (Fig. 52.1a–c). Suspicion of CV was based on a normal perinatal history with absence/non-significative renal pelvis dilation at prenatal ultrasound (as in our series), a late presentation with intermittent symptoms (vomiting, flank pain or renal colic), marked hydronephrosis at the time of pain with primarily extrarenal dilatation and an obstructed pattern on a diuretic MAG3renogram. Surgical indications included two or more of the following conditions: presence of clinical symptoms, obstruction on diuretic renogram (99mTc-MAG3), decrease on relative renal function, clear or suspected image of polar vessels on fMRU and worsening of intermittent hydronephrosis on follow-up. The patients are hospitalized 24 h before surgery and started with liquid diet and bowel cleansing with laxative and enemas to obtain bowel deflation and facilitate laparoscopic approach. All patients and their parents have to sign a specifically formulated informed consent before the procedure. Patients received a general anaesthesia and antibiotic prophylaxis with i.v. amoxicillin-clavulanic acid or cephalosporin.

52.3 Positioning

Considering the renal anatomy (aberrant polar vessel anteriorly to the renal pelvis), it is preferable a transperitoneal approach because this provides better anterior access to the renal pelvis and easier anterior CV hitching. In operatory theatre, patient is placed in a semilateral position (45°) at the edge of the surgical table. A bladder catheter and nasogastric tube are positioned before starting the procedure. The monitor is placed behind the patient. Surgeon's position is in front of the abdomen of the patient with the assistant on his left/right trying to obtain for the surgical team the best possible ergonomy for the shoulders. The scrub nurse is on the side of the surgeon (on the right) (Fig. 52.2a, b).

52.4 Instrumentation

After an umbilical open approach, a 5 or 10 mm optical port is inserted (according to weight and age of the patient), and then an optical laparoscope is introduced to explore the abdominal cavity; usually a 30° scope is preferable to better visualize the different angulation of the operative field. Two other 3 mm working ports are then

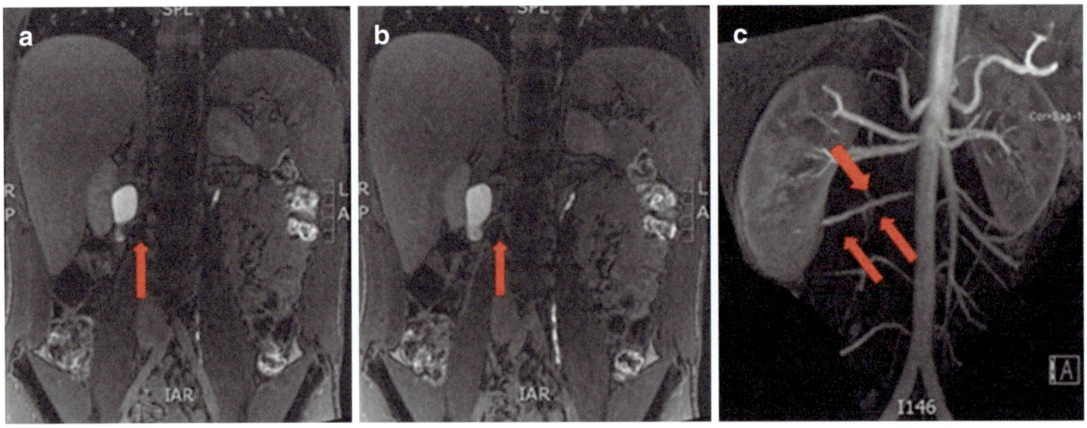

Fig. 52.1 (**a**, **b**) MRI showing the aberrant vessel crossing the right renal pelvis; (**c**), three-dimensional reconstruction

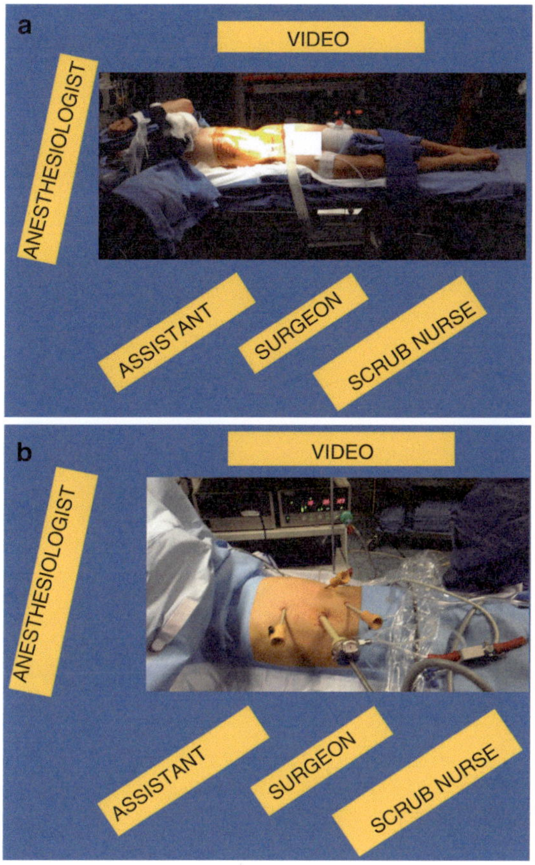

Fig. 52.2 (**a**, **b**) Team position and trocars position

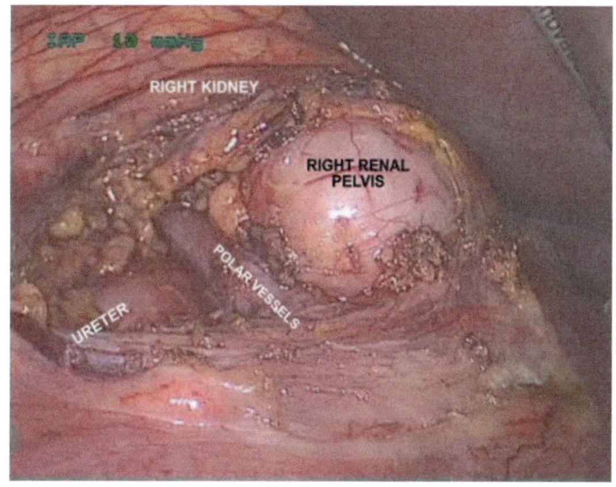

Fig. 52.3 Exposure of the right dilated pelvis, UPJ, ureter and lower aberrant CV

placed, one in the epigastrium and one in the ipsilateral iliac fossa at the midclavicular line, to allow an ideal triangulation during dissection of the CV and completion of the pelvic wrap. Sometimes could be useful to use a third 3 mm lateral operative port to move the colon or to suspend the aberrant vessels. Pneumoperitoneum is induced by insufflating CO2 at the minimal pressure to obtain an acceptable operative space (pressure varies from 5 to 10 mmHg).

52.5 Technique

The technique consisted in exposure of the lower aberrant CV via the transperitoneal approach without ipsilateral colon mobilization. This is usually obtained on the left side through a window in the mesocolon, while on the right side, by working just on the upper side of the colonic flexure that is freed (Fig. 52.3). Once the dilatation is identified and CV are visualized, we proceed with their dissection and mobilization off the UPJ or the proximal ureter. Diuretic test is then performed administering a bolus of normal saline (20 mL/kg IV) before complete vessel mobilization followed by furosemide (1 mg/kg IV) after complete mobilization (Fig. 52.4a, b). Full mobility of the UPJ is confirmed by moving freely the upper and lower portions of the anterior pelvis wall just behind the CV as a shoeshine (shoeshine manoeuvre). The UPJ is then carefully inspected for any intrinsic visible stenosis (significant narrowing). To be sure of a pure extrinsic obstruction, the CV must be temporarily transposed and the surgeon must observe the peristalsis associated with the easy urine passage across the junction and, finally, deflation of the pelvis. Once the test is successfully completed, the cranially displaced lower pole CV are then positioned away from the UPJ by performing a loose wrap of the anterior pelvic wall around these vessels using 3-4/0 polydioxanone or alternative polyglactin sutures (pyelo-pyelic sleeve). Two/three interrupted sutures may be necessary to achieve an adequate tunnel within the anterior pelvic wall (Fig. 52.5a, b). One possible tip is to pass the first suture transparietally, stabilizing and fixing

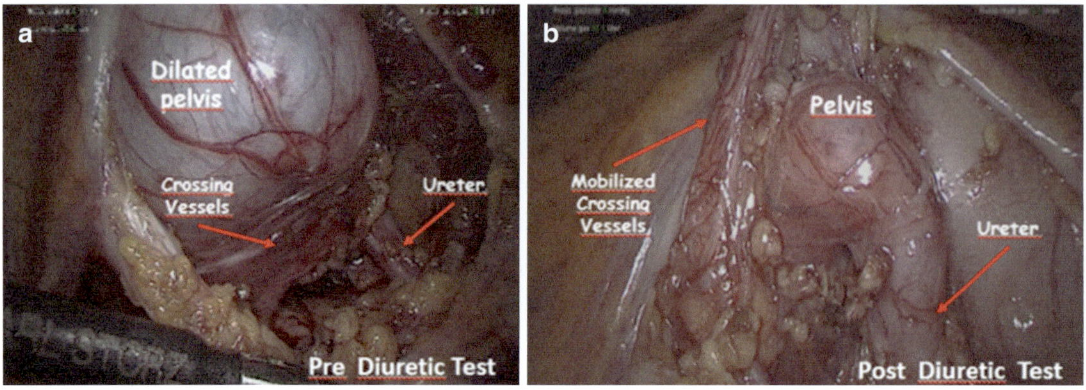

Fig. 52.4 (**a**) Pre-diuretic test; (**b**) post-diuretic test

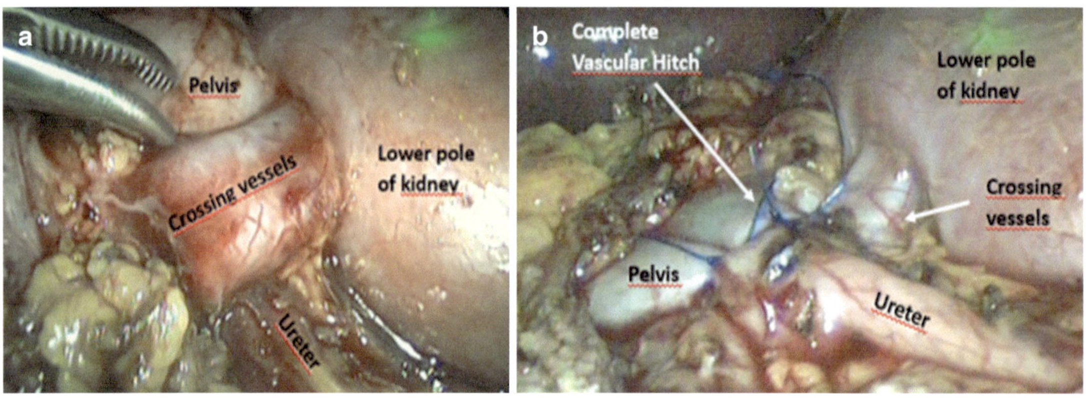

Fig. 52.5 (**a**) Wrap of the anterior pelvic wall around these vessels; (**b**) vascular hitch

the vascular bundle into the pelvic tunnel to assist the remaining suture. At the end of the procedure is very important to check the floppiness of the wrap and the absence of ischemia of the lower pole of the kidney. No double J stent or abdominal drain is required.

52.6 Postoperative Care

In the postoperative period, the patient can keep a normal decubitus.

A full oral feeding intake can start few hours after surgery. The analgesic requirement (paracetamol every 6–8 h) is generally limited to the first 24 postoperative hours. All patients are discharged on the second or maximum on the third postoperative day.

52.7 Results

Laparoscopic vascular relocation was feasible in all cases without open conversion. The median operative time was 95 min (range 45–125 min). The mean hospital stay was 3 days (range 2–4 days).

All patients underwent intraoperative DT in the first stages of laparoscopy, which showed reduction of hydronephrosis after the complete mobilization of the vessels in 45 children. We did not report intraoperative neither postoperative complications in our series of an 11-year period.

All patients had clinical evaluation and a renal US at 1–6 months, and diuretic renogram at 6 months following surgery. Follow-up (range 12–132 months) showed complete resolution of symptoms (pain, haematuria) and decrease in hydronephrosis grade. Although none of the children displayed significant improvement in relative renal function, all of them showed improved drainage on 99mTc-MAG3 renogram and became unobstructed. One had recurrent symptoms of flank pain associated with recurrent pelvic dilatation 18 months after surgery. She underwent successful laparoscopic-AHDP 2 years after the original LVH procedure.

52.8 Tips and Tricks

During laparoscopy, each case must be carefully evaluated regarding the presence and position of CV, appearance of the UPJ, ureter course and DT response of the dilated pelvis after vessel displacement. The main criteria to apply VH were the following: (I) hydronephrosis with the presence of obstructing lower pole CV, (II) normal UPJ on inspection and (III) DT response with emptying of the dilated pelvis after vessel displacement in order to confirm release of the obstruction and to exclude intrinsic UPJ anomalies. We divided our patients into two groups on the basis of anatomical relationships between CV, renal pelvis, UPJ and the ureter according to Schneider's classification [6].

These are the AHDP group with the vessels placed in front of the UPJ which present a really intrinsic stenosis (Schneider's second type) and the LVH group (45 patients), in which the vessels cross inferiorly the UPJ, resulting in variable ureteral kinking (defined as a ureteral curl or bend around the polar vessels similar to a swan neck ureter), observing intraoperatively peristalsis and demonstrating the absence of intrinsic UPJO (Schneider's third type). In particular, the very low incidence of relapse suggests that intraoperative DT must be done correctly in every suspected extrinsic UPJO (after CV transposition) to exclude associated intrinsic obstruction.

52.9 Discussion

Usually UPJO is caused by the presence of an aperistaltic dysplastic segment of the UPJ. Besides this intrinsic aetiology, extrinsic factors, as aberrant lower pole CV, may be the causative factor. Although there are no studies to date, crossing the UPJ by an aberrant vessel may be the most common extrinsic cause of UPJO above all in older children. CV are thought to cause from 40% to over 50% of extrinsic UPJO in adults; they are more often ventrally located than dorsally to the UPJ. These CV are usually normal morphologic vessels of the lower pole segment, which can be divided into additional renal arteries arising from the aorta and accessory renal segment, which can be divided into additional renal arteries arising from the aorta and accessory renal arteries arising from branches of the aorta. The controversy regarding the functional significance of vessels crossing at the UPJ is not a new one, although the debate has been resurrected in recent years because of improved detection due to the advent of advanced imaging techniques such as CT scan and fMRU.

The CV incidence in the aetiology of UPJO in children has been reported to range from 11 to 15% but was as high as 58% in a series of older children with symptomatic UPJO and a history of normal antenatal renal ultrasonography.

Open AHDP is the gold standard procedure to treat UPJO in children, but laparoscopic approach has shown similar outcomes. Laparoscopic pyeloureteral anastomosis in small children remains a challenging task, although robotic pyeloplasty in the last year has been felt to be technically easier. Although some authors have proposed AHDP to exclude intrinsic associated anomalies, an alternative approach to pure extrinsic UPJO is laparoscopic vascular transposition. In literature, there are few published series of laparoscopic relocation of lower pole CV in children with extrinsic UPJO. The most recent series reported by Schneider [6] and Miranda [7] with a successful outcome in up to 95% [8] and by Chiarenza-Bleve, successful in 97% of patients, provided a careful selection of candidates [9]. Meng and Stoller (in 2003) were the first authors reporting vascular relocation using the Hellström technique via laparoscopic approach. They reported this procedure in nine adults, with resolution in all cases. These authors observed that the herniation and subsequent ureteral kinking were responsible for the obstruction and stated that changing the geometry may be enough to alleviate the obstacle [10]. Another important condition is the existence of several anatomic variations as studied by Sampaio [11]. These double vascular bundles form a vascular window and could facilitate a UPJ prolapse with increasing obstruction. Vascular compression in these cases is not in the UPJ but in the proximal ureter. Therefore, the junction is certainly healthy, and correcting the herniation is all that is needed [6, 8]. This observation is supported by histological analysis of the UPJ and CV. Normal muscle density was found and suggests an inherently different UPJ configuration between intrinsic and extrinsic obstruction. Only patients with pure extrinsic UPJO can be treated with this procedure, so any associated intrinsic UPJ abnormality must be ruled out. Some authors, as Janetschek, have recommended that the UPJ should always be explored by a longitudinal incision in order to rule out such associated intrinsic anomalies, which they report in up to 33% of their patients [12]. Some reports analysed the histology of resected UPJ tissue and have showed evidence of intrinsic fibrosis and inflammation in cases where CV was thought to be the aetiology of the obstruction. Lower pole vessels may predispose the UPJ to the narrowing that favours infection or inflammatory episodes or that causes tension and ischemia, thus resulting in fibrosis and stenosis of the urothelium. The presence of this UPJ fibrosis could be one cause of hypothetical failure of the VH procedure [6–13], even though there is no evidence to suggest that the fibrosis is progressive. In addition, electron microscopy studies of extrinsically obstructed UPJ tissue demonstrate no significant structural changes in muscle or collagen content or in nerve distribution, immunohistochemically, when compared to normal controls. Conversely, intrinsically obstructed tissue showed thinning of muscle fascicles with dense collagenous deposits when compared with controls. Careful selection of patients is essential to maintain a high success rate with LVH procedure; it is based on three criteria: preoperative patient selection, accurate diagnostic studies and performance of intraoperative DT to confirm extrinsic obstruction. Preoperatory various imaging modalities have been used, but none have an accuracy of 100% in the diagnosis of pure extrinsic UPJO by CV. Therefore, we believe that an accurate clinical history remains the basis for correct selection. No patients had history of prenatal hydronephrosis. They all presented with intermittent colicky flank pain, sometimes associated with vomiting or haematuria. All showed marked hydronephrosis with a dilated pelvis but relatively mild calyceal dilatation when they were symptomatic that resolved shortly after they became asymptomatic. Godbole [13] reported success with a similar procedure in 12/13 patients with a median age of 10 years; Esposito C, Chiarenza S.F. and Bleve C. et al. were successful in all 51 patients [14]. On our experience, we believe that a success rate >90% may be achieved with LVH procedure, but that close cooperation between surgeon and anaesthesiologists is required to perform the intraoperative diuretic test correctly. The saline bolus needs to be timed so that the renal pelvis is well dilated prior to vessel dissection and mobilization, and with IV furosemide administration, the operator will observe rapid emptying of the bloated renal pelvis, followed by normal ureteral peristalsis and urine passage. If UPJ has intrinsic abnormalities, pelvic dilatation remains even after furosemide administration. The test is crucial because it allows to discriminate a variability of cases that can occur, related to the location of the abnormal vessels and their relations with the ureter and UPJ, the size of the vessels, the presence of hydronephrosis with sufficient tissue to consent the VH (index of the presence of an obstruction), the size of the junction and the presence of ureteral peristalsis. Some authors have suggested the use of pelvic distension with saline by direct puncture of the pelvis or an intraoperative pelvic pressure measurement with laparoscopic visualization prior to ureteral dissection inserting percutaneously into the renal pelvis a needle evaluating the ureteral opening pressure with a column device before and after the procedure was completed [6, 7]. One of the great advantages of the LVH procedure is to preserve the UPJ integrity, eliminating the risk of leakage or urinoma and preserving the physiologic pyeloureteral motility and ureteral peristalsis; in addition operative time is shorter. In several cases, it was possible to observe the pyeloureteral peristalsis after the vessel mobilization. LVH is also particularly indicated and recommended in patients with symptomatic hydronephrosis due to CV in particular anatomic condition as horseshoe kidney. In these cases the UPJ anatomy is disadvantageous to a resection/re-anastomosis between the ureter and renal pelvis [15]. As for the technical point of view, in our mind laparoscopy is the procedure of choice to perform this procedure, but it is important that surgeons have a strong experience. We recommend careful patient selection based on preoperative clinical and radiologic findings that are diagnostic of extrinsic UPJO, combined with intraoperative DT, to confirm the appropriate selection of corrective procedure.

References

1. Anderson JC, Hynes W. Retrocaval ureter; a case diagnosed pre-operatively and treated successfully by a plastic operation. Br J Urol. 1949;21:209–14.
2. Von Rokitansky CF. Handbuch der Pathologischen Anatomie. Vienna: Braumüller und Seidel; 1842.
3. Hellström J, Giertz G, Lindblom K. Pathogenesis and treatment of hydronephrosis. In: Presented at VIII Congreso de la Sociedad International de Urologia, Paris, France; 1949.
4. Chapman TL. Urology in outline. Edinburgh, London: Churchill Livingstone; 1959. p. 82.
5. Pesce C, Campobasso P, Costa L, Battaglino F, Musi L. Ureterovascular hydronephrosis in children: is pyeloplasty always necessary? Eur Urol. 1999;36:71–4.
6. Schneider A, Gomes Ferreira C, Delay C, Lacreuse I, Moog R, Becmeur F. Lower pole vessels in children with pelviureteric junction obstruction: laparoscopic vascular hitch or dismembered pyeloplasty? J Pediatr Urol. 2013;9:419–23.
7. Miranda ML, Pereira LH, Cavalaro MA, Carvalho Pegolo P, De Oliveira-Filho AG, Murray Bustorff-Silva J. Laparoscopic transposition of lower pole crossing vessels (vascular hitch) in children with pelviureteric junction obstruction: how to be sure of the success of the procedure? J Laparoendosc Adv Surg Tech A. 2015;25:847–51.
8. Gundeti MS, Reynolds WS, Duffy PG, et al. Further experience with the vascular hitch (laparoscopic transposition of lower pole crossing vessels): an alternate treatment for pediatric ureterovascular ureteropelvic junction obstruction. J Urol. 2008;180:1832–6; discussion 1836.
9. Chiarenza SF, Bleve C, Fasoli L, et al. Ureteropelvic junction obstruction in children by polar vessels. Is laparoscopic vascular hitching procedure a good solution? Single center experience on 35 consecutive patients. J Pediatr Surg. 2016;51:310–4.
10. Meng MV, Stoller ML. Hellström technique revisited: laparoscopic management of ureteropelvic junction obstruction. Urology. 2003;62:404–8; discussion 408–9.
11. Sampaio FJ. The dilemma of the crossing vessel at the ureteropelvic junction: precise anatomic study. J Endourol. 1996;10:411–5.
12. Janetschek G, Peschel R, Franscher F. Laparoscopic pyeloplasty. Urol Clin North Am. 2000;27:695e704.
13. Godbole P, Mushtaq I, Wilcox DT, et al. Laparoscopic transposition of lower pole vessels—the 'vascular hitch': an alternative to dismembered pyeloplasty for pelvi-ureteric junction obstruction in children. J Pediatr Urol. 2006;2:285–9.
14. Esposito C, Bleve C, Escolino M, Caione P, Gerocarni Nappo S, Farina A, Caprio MG, Cerulo M, La Manna A, Chiarenza SF. Laparoscopic transposition of lower pole crossing vessels (vascular hitch) in children with pelviureteric junction obstruction. Transl Pediatr. 2016;5(4):256–61.
15. Bleve C, Bucci V, Conighi ML, Battaglino F, Costa L, Fasoli L, Zolpi E, Chiarenza SF. Horseshoe kidney and uretero-pelvic-junction obstruction in a pediatric patient. Laparoscopic vascular hitch: a valid alternative to dismembered pyeloplasty? Pediatr Med Chir. 2017;39(4):178. https://doi.org/10.4081/pmc.2017.178.

Laparoscopic Approach to Urinary Stones

53

Lorenzo Masieri

53.1 Introduction

Pediatric urolithiasis is one of the important renal disorders encountered in clinical practice. It is uncommon in developed countries with a prevalence of 1–5% [1].

The management of urinary tract calculi has changed in the past two decades, mainly due to the improvement and efficacy of pediatric endourology instruments and lithotripsy techniques. However, a substantial proportion of pediatric cases still need surgery. A surgical approach is required not only for failed endourologic or extracorporeal shock wave/percutaneous lithotripsy but also as a first choice in patients with anatomic considerations that preclude the use of these minimally invasive modalities. Classical open procedures such as pyelotomy, nephrotomy, and ureterotomy have been reported as reproducible by minimal access surgery [2].

We describe in this chapter the pediatric pure laparoscopic and laparoscopic robot-assisted approach to pediatric urolithiasis.

L. Masieri (✉)
Pediatric Urology Unit, Meyer Children Hospital, University of Florence, Florence, Italy
e-mail: lorenzo.masieri@meyer.it

53.2 Preoperative Preparation

Patient selection: renal pelvic stones >1 cm diameter and ureteric stones >1 cm diameter or smaller refractive to extracorporeal lithotripsy.

All patients' parents have to sign a specifically formulated informed consent before the procedure. Patients received a general anesthesia and antibiotic prophylaxis with i.v. cefalosporine.

53.3 Positioning

The patient is placed in a slight flank position with the ipsilateral side rotated approximately 60° to the table. The ipsilateral arm is positioned near the head, and the patient was secured to the bed with two bands across chest and legs. The surgeon and the assistant are standing on the same side.

53.4 Instrumentation

In pure laparoscopic approach, we used 5 mm trocars, with a dedicated set of instruments as a monopolar scissor, a fenestrated atraumatic forceps, a grasper ad a bipolar Maryland, and a 5 mm 30° optical trocar.

Robotic approach allows easier maneuvering and better ergonomy for the surgeon. We used three-arm configuration system with the same

C. Esposito et al. (eds.), *ESPES Manual of Pediatric Minimally Invasive Surgery*,
https://doi.org/10.1007/978-3-030-00964-9_53

instruments used in laparoscopy and the same positioning of the patient. We used da Vinci Xi or Si robotic system with 8 mm trocars.

53.5 Technique

53.5.1 Pyelotomy Technique

The camera trocar is positioned trans-umbilically, and pneumoperitoneum is established and maintained at 10 mmHg throughout the procedure.

After the abdomen is insufflated, two 5 mm ports are usually placed under vision in order to achieve an optimal triangulation of instruments at the anatomic target.

A third 5 mm port is usually placed at the level of the umbilicus in the posterior axillary line to aid in renal pelvis retraction. In case of Robotic assisted laparoscopic procedure we normally use three 8 mm trocars for the camera and the Two robotic arms and a 5 mm trocar for the assistant. Trocar positioning, after the umbilical access for the camera, can change according to the abdomen surface and patient's age and has the aim to obtain the best triangolation and manueverability of robotic arms.

The line of Toldt is incised with electrocautery and the colon is reflected medially. The ureter is identified high in the retroperitoneum and followed toward the pelvis.

The Gerota's fascia is opened longitudinally, and the renal pelvis is freed from adjacent structures via blunt dissection.

The renal pelvis is incised along the major diameter of the stone (Fig. 53.1). A Maryland grasper is used to remove stones from the pelvis.

If the stones are too large for the port site, they are placed in a laparoscopic sac and removed via the umbilical port site by extending the umbilical incision (Fig. 53.2).

In case of multiple and small stones in a calyx, a flexible ureteroscopic or cystoscopic instrument can be used to reach and remove them.

The pelvis is closed with a 6-0 poliglecaprone 25 (Monocryl®) running suture cut to 12–15 cm

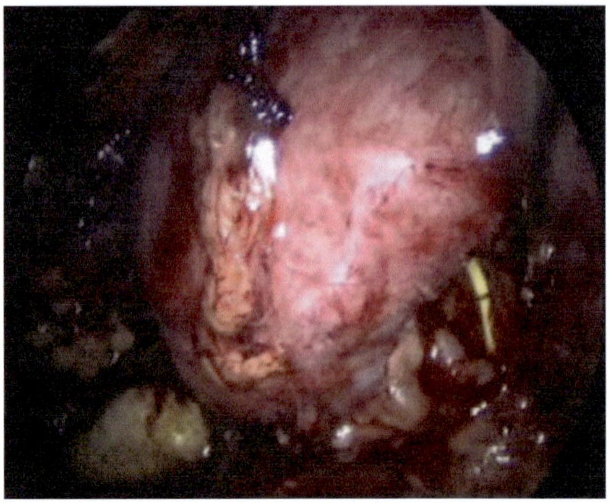

Fig. 53.1 The renal pelvis is incised along the major diameter of the stone

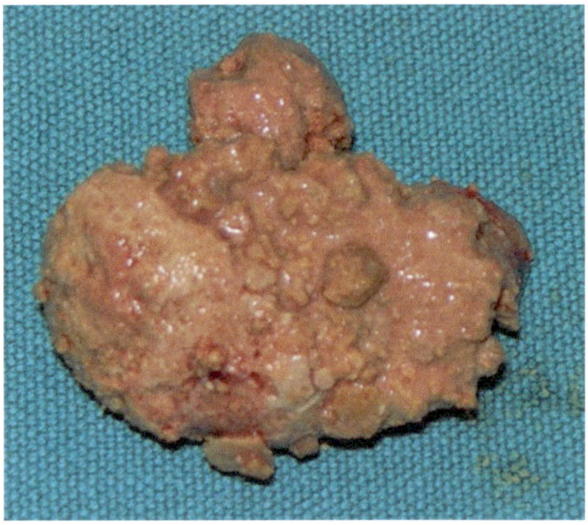

Fig. 53.2 The stone is extracted from the umbilicus using a laparoscopic bag

in length and introduced through the 5 mm port (Fig. 53.3). The knots are tied intracorporeally and placed outside the lumen.

53.5.2 Ureterolithotomy Technique

After trocars positioning, the ureter is identified and isolated on a vessel loop. An atraumatic grasp is positioned proximal to the stone to avoid the slippage of the stone into the proximal dilated ureter. The ureter is incised longitudinally and the procedure is carried out as described for renal pyelotomy.

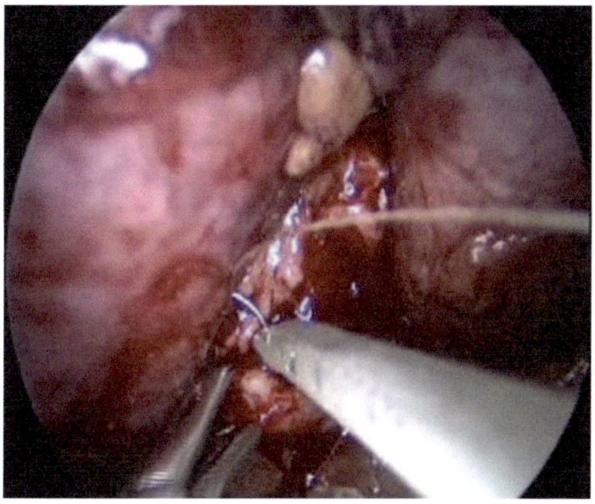

Fig. 53.3 The pelvis is closed using a running suture

We usually position a ureteral double J stent according to antegrade technique [3] introducing the wire and the stent through one of the 5 mm trocars or percutaneously.

A Penrose drain is left near to the anastomosis and brought out through the lower quadrant port. The abdominal cavity is inspected and the trocars are removed under direct vision.

We closed trocar sites at the fascial level except for the site where the Penrose drain exits. Trocar skin incisions were closed with a subcuticular absorbable suture.

53.6 Postoperative Care

In the postoperative period, the patients can restart full oral feeding few hours after surgery. For the first 24–58 h e.v. antibiotic therapy and liquids are somministrated. Bladder catheter is usually removed in the first or second postoperative day if the urine is clear and there is no fever.

The analgesic protocol (Paracetamol 15 mg/kg every 6 h and Toradol 1 mg/kg) is generally limited to the first 24 postoperative hours. The bladder catheter is removed on postoperative day 1 or 2. The day after the removal of the catheter, if no increase output was observed, the drain can be removed, and the child is discharged from the hospital.

The patients are recommended to rest at home for 3–4 days and to get adequate hydration and regular micturition.

The double J stent is removed under a brief general anesthesia 2 weeks after the operation by cystoscopy.

53.7 Results

A total of 11 procedures were performed: 8 pielolitothomy (3 robot-assisted, 5 pure laparoscopic) and 2 upper and 1 lower robot-assisted ureterotomy.

The average length of surgery is about 120 (range 110–140) minutes for pure laparoscopic procedures and 70 (range 60–110) minutes for laparoscopic robot-assisted procedures. We did not report intraoperative neither postoperative complications in our series with a mean follow-up of 19 months (range 3–26 months).

Follow-up is carried out by renal ultrasonography at 1 and 3 months after surgery.

53.8 Discussion

Pediatric urinary tract calculi, although relatively uncommon in comparison to adult stone disease, pose a significant challenge in view of the smaller size of the urinary tract and a greater risk of stone recurrence, due to higher incidence of metabolic causes and longer risk period, especially in the presence of residual calculi.

Despite the advances in stone treatment technology (SWL, PNL, and RIRS), data show an increased requirement for open procedures in pediatric urolithiasis (up to 17%) as compared to adults [4].

The reasons are due to lack of experience in younger patients and smaller size of ureter, frequent anatomic abnormalities associated, higher rate of complications, and lack of suitable instrumentations.

Shock wave lithotripsy (SWL) is not so effective in stones greater than 1.5 cm and stones with cystine components. Performing

PCNL in children is on debate regarding parenchymal damage and the associated effects on renal function, radiation exposure with fluoroscopy, and the risks of major complications as sepsis and bleeding. Ureteroscopy is not considered a primary option for managing of upper tract stones in children due to concern for complications as ureteral ischemia, perforation, stricture formation, and development of vesicoureteral reflux as a result of dilatation of small caliber ureteral orifices [5].

Laparoscopy and robotic-assisted laparoscopy have been utilized successfully in adults for treatment of calculi. Small series utilizing these techniques in children have only recently been described and showed safe and effective alternative to open stone surgery [2, 6].

In our experience transperitoneal laparoscopic pielolitothomy or ureterotomy is safe and feasible in management of selected patients, especially when endoscopic treatment failed or is not possible. We believe that is feasible and it introduces a novel approach for managing kidney stones in pediatric population. However, more future studies should be designed, especially in lower age range. In conclusion, to treat stones in children is crucial to have all the equipment available, to combine different approaches. Experience on adult patient is a key point to offer the best treatment to our patients. Pure laparoscopic or robot assisted approaches should be considered for large urinary tract stones.

References

1. López M, Hoppe B. History, epidemiology and regional diversities of urolithiasis. Pediatr Nephrol. 2010;25(1):49–59.
2. Casale P, Grady RW, Joyner BD, Zeltser IS, Kuo RL, Mitchell ME. Transperitoneal laparoscopic pyelolithotomy after failed percutaneous access in the pediatric patient. J Urol. 2004;172(2):680–3; discussion 683.
3. Minervini A, Siena G, Masieri L, Lapini A, Serni S, Carini M. Antegrade stenting in laparoscopic pyeloplasty: feasibility of the technique and time required for stent insertion. Surg Endosc Other Interv Tech. 2009;23(8):1831–4.
4. Agrawal V, Bajaj J, Acharya H, Chanchalani R, Raina VK, Sharma D. Laparoscopic management of pediatric renal and ureteric stones. J Pediatr Urol. 2013;9(2):230–3. https://doi.org/10.1016/j.jpurol.2012.03.001.
5. Soltani MH, Simforoosh N, Nouralizadeh A, Sotoudeh M, Mollakoochakian MJ, Shemshaki HR. Laparoscopic pyelolithotomy in children less than two years old with large renal stones: initial series. Urol J. 2016;13(5):2837–40.
6. Lee RS, Passerotti CC, Cendron M, Estrada CR, Borer JG, Peters CA. Early results of robot assisted laparoscopic lithotomy in adolescents. J Urol. 2007;177:2306–9.

54 Vesicoureteric Reflux (VUR): Laparoscopic Lich-Gregoir Repair

Aurélien Scalabre, Sophie Vermersch, and François Varlet

54.1 Introduction

Vesicoureteric reflux (VUR) is defined as a permanent or intermittent intrusion of bladder urine into the upper urinary tract due to a defective ureterovesical junction. The pathophysiology of VUR remains unclear, but there is a general consensus that intrarenal reflux of infected urine can cause renal damage (reflux nephropathy). VUR can be the result of a morphological abnormality at the level of the vesicoureteric junction (primary malformative VUR) or secondary to lower urinary tract dysfunction. Primary malformative VUR can be diagnosed prenatally when associated with urinary tract dilatation. It is more frequent in boys, and the regression rate is low. VUR secondary to lower urinary tract dysfunction is more common. It usually occurs in girls with poor bladder and bowel function. Its resolution rate is high with education regarding good micturition and medical treatment against constipation. There is currently no consensus regarding indications for surgery in children with VUR [1, 2]. However, decreasing renal function on isotope studies and repeated pyelonephritis despite sufficient hydration, voiding micturition education and antibioprophylaxis are strong arguments for surgical treatment.

Different techniques are available for the surgical treatment of VUR. The Cohen technique described in 1969 is often considered the gold standard [3]. Minimally invasive surgery techniques were recently developed in order to reduce postoperative pain, avoid postoperativc haematuria and shorten hospitalization. They include endoscopic treatment, pneumovesicoscopic reimplantation and laparoscopic reimplantation.

The Lich-Gregoir technique is an extravesical ureteral reimplantation described by Lich et al. in 1962 and Gregoir and Van Regemorter in 1964 [4, 5], more recently adapted for laparoscopic approach [6]. This technique is often used for unilateral reflux, but concerns regarding the risk of postoperative urinary retention have limited its indications for bilateral cases [7]. Nevertheless, bilateral reimplantation is possible as laparoscopy allows an easy approach to the posterior bladder wall with a limited dissection sparing bladder innervation [8, 9].

54.2 Preoperative Preparation

Renal isotope study, ultrasonographic scanning and micturating cystography are realized before treatment. Micturating cystography is the standard method to identify and grade VUR in children with recurrent febrile urinary tract infections. Indications

A. Scalabre (✉) · S. Vermersch · F. Varlet
Pediatric Surgery Unit, University Hospital of Saint Etienne, Saint-Etienne, France
e-mail: aurelien.scalabre@chu-st-etienne.fr

C. Esposito et al. (eds.), *ESPES Manual of Pediatric Minimally Invasive Surgery*,
https://doi.org/10.1007/978-3-030-00964-9_54

for surgery are discussed upon the results of a renal ultrasonography and isotope studies. The different techniques available for the treatment of VUR and their potential complications are explained to the patients and their parents before surgery. A bacteriologic urine exam is performed a few days before surgery to ensure that urine is sterile.

54.3 Anaesthesia

General endotracheal anaesthesia is complemented by caudal anaesthesia. A broad-spectrum antibiotic is routinely administered intravenously on induction of general anaesthesia.

54.4 Initial Cystoscopy

A cystoscopy may be performed initially if bladder control is required, especially in children with a duplex system, to assess the location of the ureteral orifices and to check the anatomy. In children with asymmetric bilateral VUR, endoscopic treatment of a contralateral low-grade reflux can be performed before the unilateral Lich-Gregoir procedure.

54.5 Positioning

The patient is placed in a supine position with the arms lying along the body (Fig. 54.1). The surgeon stands at the head of the patient, and the assistant and the nurse on one side, usually opposite to the refluxing ureter (Fig. 54.2). The video column is placed at the feet of the patient (Fig. 54.3). When the child is too tall, the surgeon

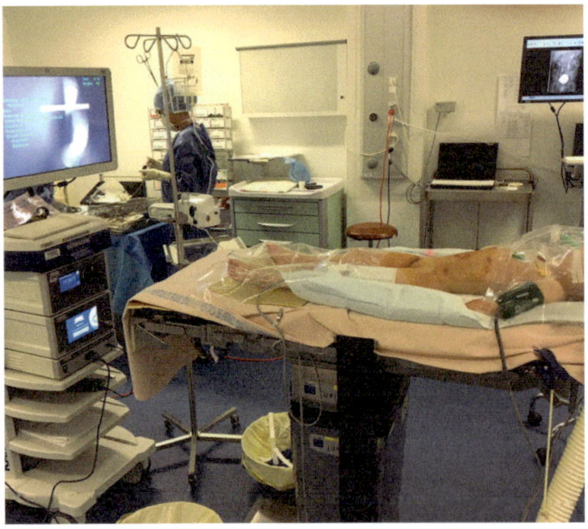

Fig. 54.1 Positioning of the patient and video column

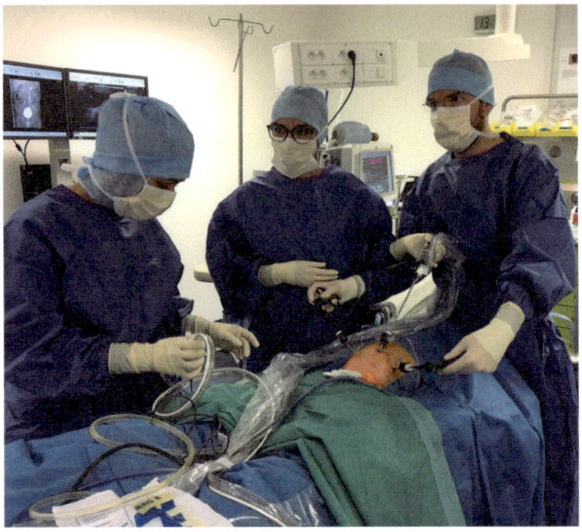

Fig. 54.2 Team position. The head of the patient is close from the edge of the table

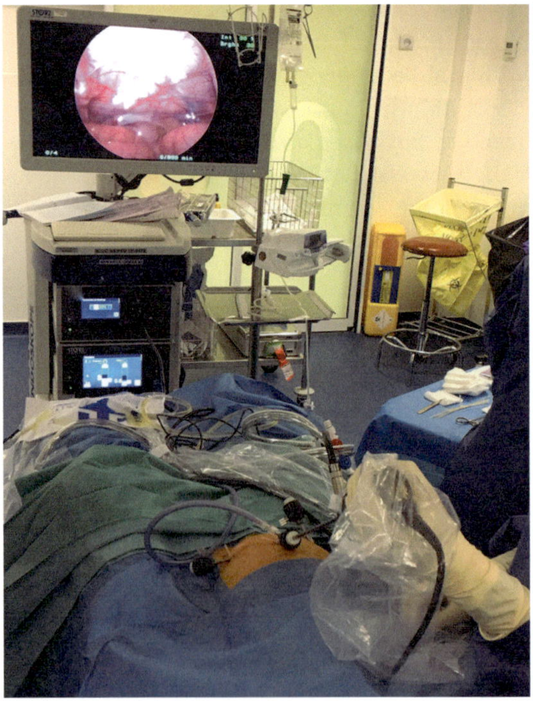

Fig. 54.3 The video column is placed at the feet of the patient. The surgeon, the telescope, the bladder and the monitor form a straight line

must stand laterally, on the right side for the left ureter and on the left side for the right ureter.

54.6 Instrumentation

After preparation of the abdominal wall, a bladder catheter is placed. It must be accessible during the procedure. A 5 mm 30° telescope and 3 mm instruments are used: blunt graspers, bipolar forceps, hook, needle holder and scissors.

54.7 Technique

A transperitoneal approach is used. A 5 mm port is inserted through a lateral or trans-umbilical incision under vision to avoid visceral damage. Two 3 mm trocars are inserted in the left and right flanks under direct vision. They are inserted at the umbilicus level in children before 2 years old and lower in older children.

54.7.1 Ureteral Dissection

The ureter is easily identified where it crosses the external iliac vessels. The peritoneum is opened down to the ureterovesical junction (Fig. 54.4(1)). To avoid excessive handling of the ureter, a large surgical loop is wrapped around it and used for manipulation (Fig. 54.5). In boys, the vas deferens is teased away from the ureter. In girls, the mesosalpinx is opened, and the ureter is pulled up between the bladder and the mesosalpinx. The ureter is mobilized to achieve sufficient freedom for a tension-free reimplantation. Dissection and coagulation must be minimal around the lower ureter to avoid bladder nerve damage, especially during bilateral procedures.

The bladder dome is suspended to the anterior abdominal wall with a transparietal stay suture in order to expose the posterior bladder wall and the ureterovesical junction (Fig. 54.4(2)).

54.7.2 Detrusorotomy and Exposure of the Bladder Mucosa

The bladder is filled with 50–100 mL saline serum. The direction and length of the muscular trench are outlined with the monopolar coagulation following Paquin's rule: the length of the submucosal tunnel should be at least five times the ureteric diameter.

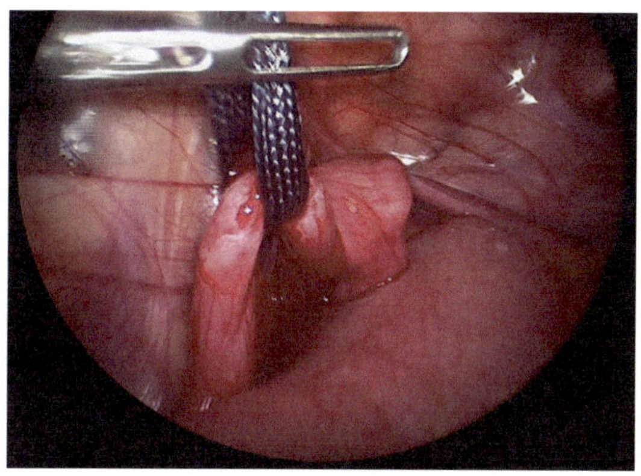

Fig. 54.5 The ureter is manipulated using a large surgical loop wrapped around it

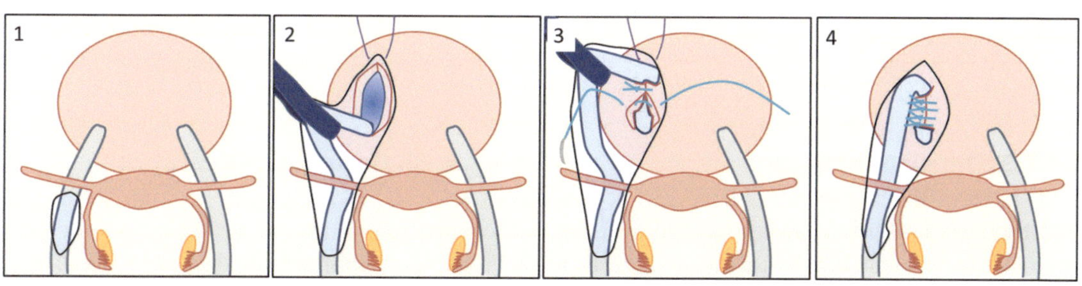

Fig. 54.4 (1) Opening of the peritoneum. (2) Detrusorotomy. (3) Detrusororrhaphy. (4) Finished reimplantation

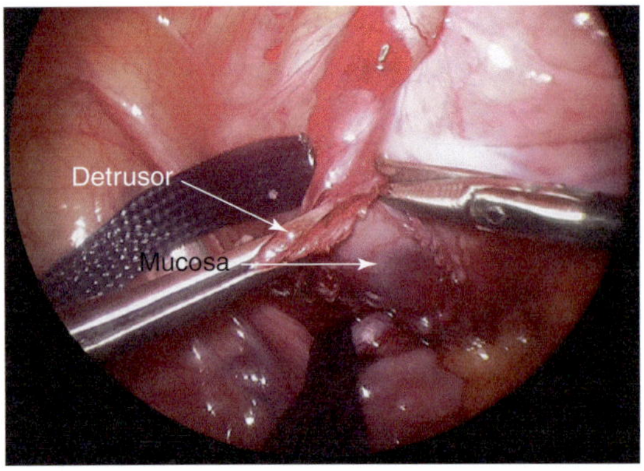

Fig. 54.6 Detrusorotomy

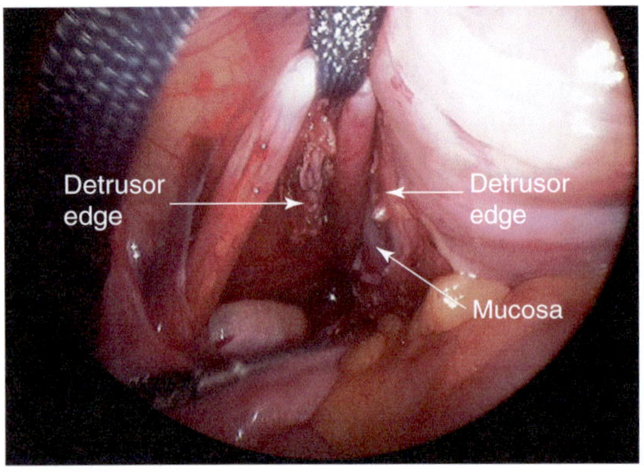

Fig. 54.7 The ureter is placed in position along the muscular trench

A second transparietal suspension is placed at the tip of the incision. The muscular fibres are coagulated and divided with scissors or monopolar hook to reach the bladder mucosa (Fig. 54.6). The trench is ended at the level of the terminal part of the ureter. In case of mucosal tear, the mucosa around the breach can be grasped and closed by an endoloop. If the tear is too large, the bladder should be emptied, and the mucosa can be closed by a running suture.

54.7.3 Detrusororrhaphy

The ureter is laid between the two edges of the muscular trench and kept in this position with a third transparietal stay suture through the surgical loop used for mobilization of the ureter

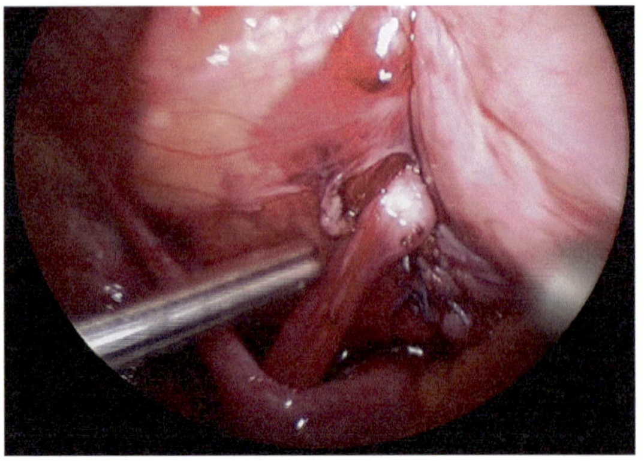

Fig. 54.8 Finished reimplantation

(Figs. 54.4(3) and 54.7). In case of ureteral duplication, both ureters are dissected and laid into the trench together.

The detrusor is then reapproximated over the ureter with four to five stitches of 3/0 or 4/0 sutures, either absorbable or not.

We usually start by the lower stitch. Special attention should be given to avoid narrowing the entry of the ureter into the trench. When all stitches are done, the transperitoneal suspensions are removed. The new ureteral entry in the bladder must be large enough to avoid ureteral obstruction (Fig. 54.4(4)). In case of excessive tension, the ureter is released proximally (Fig. 54.8).

54.7.4 Closure

Drainage is not mandatory. The trocars are removed, their orifices are stitched and the bladder catheter is removed. It is possible to leave 100–150 mL of saline serum in the bladder to allow a quick postoperative micturition before discharge in an outpatient setting.

54.7.5 Bilateral Reimplantation

The same procedure can be done on both sides with the same approach, with special attention to avoid excessive coagulation during dissection of the distal parts of the ureters (Fig. 54.9).

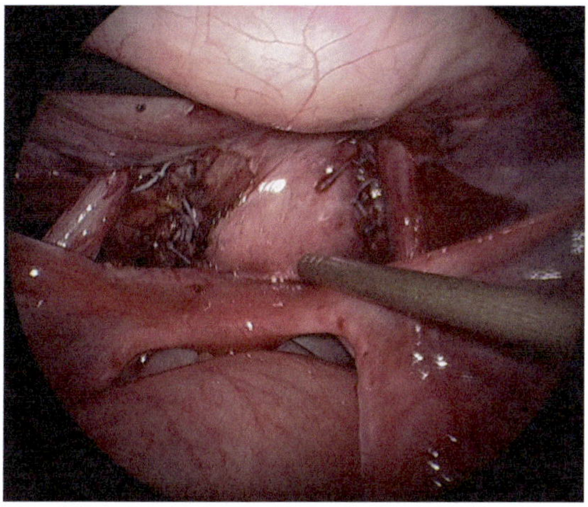

Fig. 54.9 Finished bilateral reimplantation in a girl

54.7.6 Postoperative Care

Unilateral reimplantation following this technique can be performed as day case, the patient being discharged after complete micturition. Only standard painkillers are needed. For bilateral reimplantations, we prefer to keep the patient hospitalized until the next day, as the risk of urinary retention is higher. The child is kept off school for 8 days with no sport for 1 month. An ultrasound scan is performed 1 month later. As for open surgery, micturating cystography is not routinely performed [10].

54.8 Results

We operated on 117 children (159 renal units) with this technique over the past 9 years. We performed 49 bilateral and 61 unilateral reimplantations. Fifteen patients had contralateral endoscopic sub-ureteral injection during the same procedure. Eight patients had Hutch diverticulum treated by doing a precautionary suture in the lower part of the bladder channel. Twenty-eight patients had VUR in the lower pole of a duplicated collecting system (DCS) including 5 bilateral VUR. The mean operative time was 96 min (±37.7 min) for unilateral reimplantation and 128 min (±46.1 min) for bilateral reimplantation. One-third of these procedures were performed by a resident or a registrar under supervision of an experienced surgeon.

In five cases, a mucosal perforation occurred during the detrusorotomy, treated immediately by an endoloop repair.

The mean hospital stay was 25.3 h (±6.3 h).

Two temporary urinary retentions occurred after bilateral reimplantation. A suprapubic catheter was placed under general anaesthesia and removed 10 days later with uneventful recovery. At the beginning of our experience, two patients needed reintervention for an uretero-peritoneal fistula 7 and 15 days after surgery. One was treated by Cohen procedure and one by ureteral suturing and insertion of a JJ stent.

We observed two VUR recurrences. They were both revealed by pyelonephritis recurrence and confirmed by VCUG. The resolution rate, in terms of no further febrile urinary tract infection, accounted for 98.3% (115/117 patients).

54.9 Tips and Tricks

The two ureteral perforations at the beginning of our experience made us slightly modify the surgical technique. We reviewed the surgery videos but did not find the traumatic cause for these perforations. We assume that possible causes were ischemia caused by excessive handling of the ureter, a burn with the monopolar hook dissection or an excessive closing of the detrusor trench. To avoid this complication, we opted to wrap a large surgical loop around the ureter for its manipulation and to limit the amount and duration of cautery. No more ureteral perforation occurred since we made this modification.

Suspension of the bladder by transparietal stay suture is a good way to obtain correct exposition without adding unnecessary trocars, and we regularly use this technique for other surgeries. Sometimes a second transparietal suspension allows a better exposure of the posterior wall of the bladder. We usually use a 24 or 26 mm needle that we straighten to easily go through the anterior abdominal wall.

To prevent postoperative urinary retention, the surgeon must be really careful not to use extensive monopolar cautery, especially on the lower part of the bladder wall.

In case of mucosal perforation, the mucosa can be closed immediately by grasping the whole tear and closing it with an endoloop.

It is also important to check that the final trench is not too obstructive after reimplantation. If the tunnel seems too tight, the closer stitch to the new ureteral entry must be removed.

All our laparoscopic interventions are video-recorded, which help in sharing our experience and techniques with students, residents and colleagues. We also review and criticize our procedures afterwards to improve our technique when we front complications.

54.10 Discussion

VUR management is controversial. There is no strong consensus about prophylactic antibiotic treatment, operative indications, age of surgery or follow-up management [1]. According to recommendations from the European Association of Urology and the American Urological Association, we decided to operate on children with VUR grade III or more, with renal dysfunction (DMSA < 40%) or renal scarring demonstrated on isotope renography, and children developing recurrent pyelonephritis despite optimal medical treatment.

The goal of any anti-reflux procedure is to restore anti-reflux mechanism of the ureterovesical junction. Open ureterovesical reimplantation by Cohen's procedure is often considered to be the gold standard for ureteral reimplantation, with a success rate over 98% [11]. However, the Lich-Gregoir technique is also associated with a high success rate with some advantages including lower pain, shorter recovery and hospital stay, with excellent cosmetic results [2, 8, 9, 12]. This technique avoids postoperative bladder spasms and adverse effects of bladder opening like haematuria. Furthermore, the ureteral meatus is still in its initial position, allowing easier endourology in the future if necessary.

The main issue with this approach is the 8–15% reported incidence of urinary retention after bilateral extravesical reimplantation by open approach [7]. This might be a result of neurovascular injury during wound handling and ureteral and bladder dissection. A nerve-sparing technique proposed by David in 2004 allows to reduce this complication (2% of transitory bladder retention) [6]. In 2012, Bayne et al. reported a cohort of patients undergoing extravesical ureteral reimplantation by laparoscopy with the Lich-Gregoir technique with a 6.5% incidence of urinary retention after bilateral reimplantation [13]. In our experience only two patients presented with a transitory bladder emptying difficulty after a bilateral reimplantation. Lateral dissection of the ureter and bladder should be limited to avoid damage to pelvic nerves [14], and we recommend a gentle and soft tissue dissection around the lower ureteral part with no extensive coagulation. In our opinion, no bladder catheter is needed during the postoperative period. In addition, faster recovery compared to open surgery allows discharge a few hours after surgery [8, 9, 15].

One of the most common operative complications in laparoscopic extravesical ureteral reimplantation is ureteral injury or obstruction (ischemia) owing to excessive handling of the ureter or excessive closure of the trench [16]. Lakshmanan and Kasturi in 2000 and 2012, respectively, reported 6.3% (3/47) and 0.6% (1/150) intra-abdominal urinary leak requiring drainage and bilateral pigtail stents for 2 months [17, 18]. Bayne et al. observed a 2.04% rate of ureteral leakage [13], and Esposito et al. showed a 1.33% of the same complication in open Cohen procedures [11]. We recommend a limited use of the monopolar coagulation and handling of the ureter by a surgical loop to avoid this complication. After more than 100 cases treated using a surgical loop, no more ureteral perforation occurred.

The results of laparoscopic Lich-Gregoir reimplantation are comparable with pneumovesicoscopic reimplantation [19, 20]. However, it is technically challenging to obtain a correct pneumovesicum with bladder sealing at the start of the procedure. Moreover, pneumovesicoscopic reimplantation requires postoperative drainage. On the other hand, the pneumovesicoscopic approach allows treatment of ureteroceles and Hutch diverticula, whereas only small diverticula can be treated by laparoscopy.

The open Lich-Gregoir technique for unilateral VUR is also done with good results as an outpatient procedure [12, 15]. Advantages of laparoscopy over open surgery in this context are a better bladder wall exposition and less scaring.

54.11 Conclusion

Laparoscopic extravesical ureteral reimplantation with the Lich-Gregoir technique is a safe and effective procedure for the treatment of VUR in children. Its results are comparable to open procedures. The technique results in reduced hospital stay and recovery period. It can be applied to unilateral VUR, bilateral VUR and duplex system. With cautious dissection, the risk of urinary retention following this procedure is low.

References

1. Peters CA, Skoog SJ, Arant BS, Copp HL, Elder JS, Hudson RG, et al. Summary of the AUA guideline on management of primary vesicoureteral reflux in children. J Urol. 2010;184(3):1134–44.
2. Hajiyev P, Burgu B. Contemporary management of vesicoureteral reflux. Eur Urol Focus. 2017;3(2–3):181–8.
3. Cohen MH, Rotner MB. A new method to create a submucosal ureteral tunnel. J Urol. 1969;102(5):567–8.
4. Lich R, Howerton LW, Davis LA. Ureteral reflux, its significance and correction. South Med J. 1962;55:633–5.
5. Gregoir W. [The surgical treatment of congenital vesico-ureteral reflux]. Acta Chir Belg. 1964;63:431–9.
6. David S, Kelly C, Poppas DP. Nerve sparing extravesical repair of bilateral vesicoureteral reflux: description of technique and evaluation of urinary retention. J Urol. 2004;172(4 Pt 2):1617–20.
7. Fung LC, McLorie GA, Jain U, Khoury AE, Churchill BM. Voiding efficiency after ureteral reimplantation: a comparison of extravesical and intravesical techniques. J Urol. 1995;153(6):1972–5.
8. Lopez M, Varlet F. Laparoscopic extravesical transperitoneal approach following the Lich-Gregoir technique in the treatment of vesicoureteral reflux in children. J Pediatr Surg. 2010;45(4):806–10.
9. Soulier V, Scalabre AL, Lopez M, Li C-Y, Thach S, Vermersch S, et al. Laparoscopic vesico-ureteral reimplantation with Lich-Gregoir approach in children: medium term results of 159 renal units in 117 children. World J Urol. 2017;35(11):1791–8.
10. Grossklaus DJ, Pope JC, Adams MC, Brock JW. Is postoperative cystography necessary after ureteral reimplantation? Urology. 2001;58(6):1041–5.
11. Esposito C, Escolino M, Lopez M, Farina A, Cerulo M, Savanelli A, et al. Surgical management of pediatric vesicoureteral reflux: a comparative study between endoscopic, laparoscopic, and open surgery. J Laparoendosc Adv Surg Tech A. 2016;26(7):574–80.
12. Palmer JS. Extravesical ureteral reimplantation: an outpatient procedure. J Urol. 2008;180(4 Suppl):1828–31.
13. Bayne AP, Shoss JM, Starke NR, Cisek LJ. Single-center experience with pediatric laparoscopic extravesical reimplantation: safe and effective in simple and complex anatomy. J Laparoendosc Adv Surg Tech A. 2012;22(1):102–6.
14. Casale P, Patel RP, Kolon TF. Nerve sparing robotic extravesical ureteral reimplantation. J Urol. 2008;179(5):1987–90.
15. Wicher C, Hadley D, Ludlow D, Oottamasathien S, Wallis MC, Devries C, et al. 250 consecutive unilateral extravesical ureteral reimplantations in an outpatient setting. J Urol. 2010;184(1):311–4.
16. Riquelme M, Lopez M, Landa S, Mejia F, Aranda A, Rodarte-Shade M, et al. Laparoscopic extravesical ureteral reimplantation (LEVUR): a multicenter experience with 95 cases. Eur J Pediatr Surg. 2013;23(2):143–7.
17. Lakshmanan Y, Fung LC. Laparoscopic extravesicular ureteral reimplantation for vesicoureteral reflux: recent technical advances. J Endourol. 2000;14(7):589–94.
18. Kasturi S, Sehgal SS, Christman MS, Lambert SM, Casale P. Prospective long-term analysis of nerve-sparing extravesical robotic-assisted laparoscopic ureteral reimplantation. Urology. 2012;79(3):680–3.
19. Yeung CK, Sihoe JDY, Borzi PA. Endoscopic cross-trigonal ureteral reimplantation under carbon dioxide bladder insufflation: a novel technique. J Endourol. 2005;19(3):295–9.
20. Valla JS, Steyaert H, Griffin SJ, Lauron J, Fragoso AC, Arnaud P, et al. Transvesicoscopic Cohen ureteric reimplantation for vesicoureteral reflux in children: a single-centre 5-year experience. J Pediatr Urol. 2009;5(6):466–71.

Vesicoureteral Reflux (VUR): Endoscopic Treatment

55

Hiroshi Murakami, Geoffrey J. Lane, and Atsuyuki Yamataka

55.1 Introduction

Vesicoureteral reflux (VUR) is one of the most common urologic morbidities in children, with an estimated prevalence of approximately 1% of the general pediatric population, but which can be as high as 30% in children with a history of febrile urinary tract infection (UTI) [1, 2]. The goals of treating a child with VUR are (1) to prevent recurring febrile UTI, (2) to prevent renal damage, and (3) to minimize/prevent adverse effects of treatment [3].

Management regimes incorporate a spectrum of philosophies and modalities ranging from observation with or without continuous antibiotic prophylaxis to active surgical intervention [3]. Essentially, the optimal treatment for VUR has yet to be established. Whether surgical intervention is indicated for treating children with persistent reflux, renal scarring, or recurrent febrile UTI is currently controversial because of the major change in treating VUR that followed Puri's first clinical report about an endoscopic procedure they called the STING method published in 1984 [4]. Since then, the STING method has been modified to improve VUR cure rates, for example, by introducing the hydrodistention implantation technique (HIT) [5] and double HIT [6].

Several tissue-augmenting substances have been used for subureteral injection, such as polytetrafluoroethylene, collagen, silicone, autologous chondrocytes, and Deflux® [7], followed by a succession of new substances; for example, in 2010, the preliminary results of a prospective multicenter study of a new substance "polyacrylate polyalcohol copolymer (PPC/Vantris®)" was published [8]. While Deflux® is still the most widely used bulking agent [9], recently, Deflux® treatment (DT) has been implicated as a potential cause of ureteral obstruction (UB).

Here, we describe a simple noninvasive technique we pioneered to identify post-DT UB and patients at risk for UB, especially late-onset UB.

55.2 Preoperative Preparation and Positioning

General anesthesia is induced and the trachea intubated. No other anesthesia is required. The patient is placed in the lithotomy position, prepared and draped, and single dose of an antibiotic is administered intravenously. Figure 55.1 shows the standard layout for left DT. The operating surgeon will stand on the patient's right side for left DT cases and between the patient's legs for right and bilateral DT cases.

H. Murakami · G. J. Lane · A. Yamataka (✉)
Department of Pediatric General and Urogenital Surgery, Juntendo University School of Medicine, Tokyo, Japan
e-mail: hmuraka@juntendo.ac.jp; yama@juntendo.ac.jp

C. Esposito et al. (eds.), *ESPES Manual of Pediatric Minimally Invasive Surgery*,
https://doi.org/10.1007/978-3-030-00964-9_55

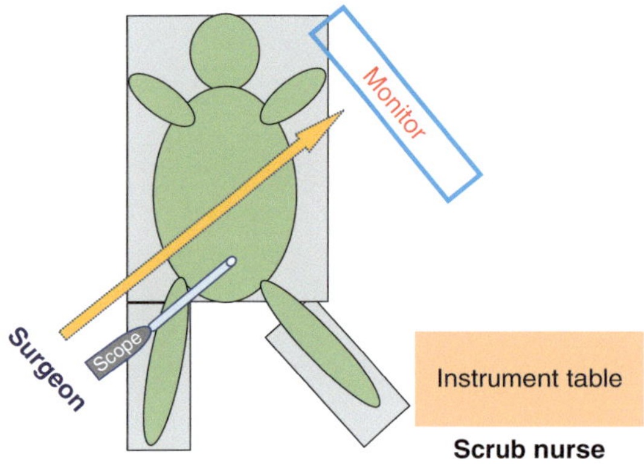

Fig. 55.1 Diagram of standard operating room layout. Figure shows the standard operating room layout for left DT. The operating surgeon will stand on the right side for left DT, and on the left side for right DT, and between the patient's legs for bilateral cases. The surgeon's direction of view and the orientation of the cystoscope are the same

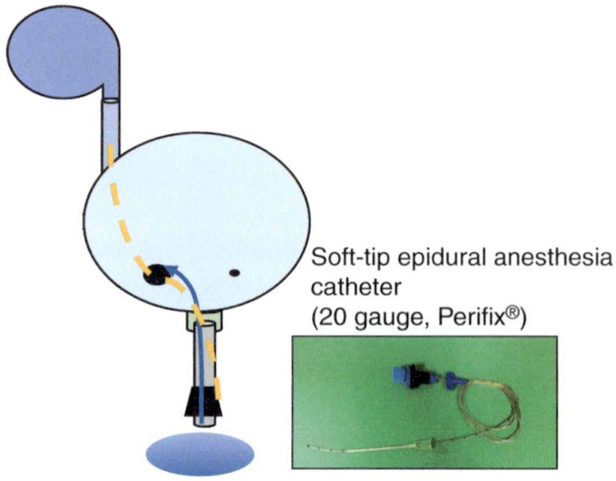

Fig. 55.2 Diagram of our epidural catheter technique. Our technique involves inserting an epidural catheter into the ureter on the Deflux®-treated side and injecting indigo carmine solution

55.3 Technique

We routinely use an 8.0 or 9.5 Fr pediatric cystoscope (Karl Storz, Inc., Tuttlingen, Germany) with an offset lens for injecting Deflux® because the offset lens permits direct passage of a 3.7 Fr needle in line with the ureter without needing to bend the Deflux® needle. After the bladder is filled to three quarter volume to permit visualization of the ureteric orifice, we insert a soft-tip epidural anesthesia catheter (20 gauge, Perifix®) (B. Braun, Melsungen AG, Germany) through a side channel of the cystoscope. Once the epidural catheter is inserted into the ureter, the cystoscope is withdrawn leaving the epidural catheter in the ureter and the urethra (Fig. 55.2). The cystoscope is then carefully reinserted into the urethra with the epidural catheter in situ, and a needle is inserted through the side channel of the cystoscope. After confirmation that the Deflux® needle is in the desired position, Deflux® is injected submucosally according to the original technique reported by O'Donnell [4]. Immediately after this, 1–3 mL of 20% indigo carmine solution is injected through the epidural catheter, and after observation to confirm dye flow from the treated ureteric orifice into the bladder, the epidural catheter is removed (Fig. 55.3).

In cases where no dye flow is observed after a minimum of 15 min, the epidural catheter is clamped but not removed because the patient is at risk for UB, and the patient is transferred back to the ward with the epidural catheter in situ. The epidural catheter is left overnight during which time dye may appear in the urine. If dye is observed the next day, the patient may be discharged, but if no dye is observed, an ultrasonographic (US) examination is performed to examine for significant hydronephrosis which we consider as pathognomic of UB. If there are no signs of UB on US, the epidural catheter is removed in the ward the next day. Renal and bladder US are planned for 3 weeks later at outpatient clinic follow-up.

55.4 Routine Postoperative Care

All patients are commenced on prophylactic antibiotics postoperatively which are discontinued after VUR is confirmed to be absent or downgraded to grade I (both of which we regard as being "cure" of VUR) on voiding cystourethrography performed routinely 1 month after DT. Routine outpatient visits for assessing blood biochemistry and urinalysis and renal and

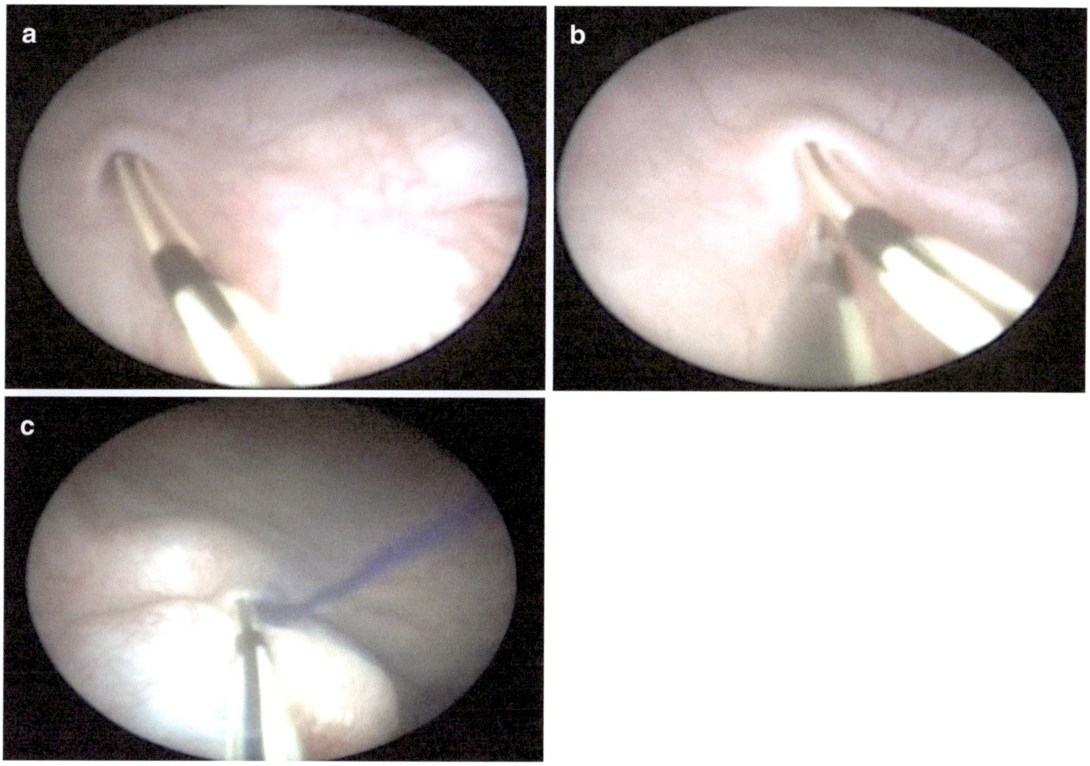

Fig. 55.3 Our epidural catheter technique being performed. Our epidural catheter technique. An epidural catheter is inserted into the ureter (**a**), then the Deflux® needle is inserted at the 6 o'clock position and Deflux® is injected (**b**). There is flow of dye from the treated ureteric orifice into the bladder (**c**)

bladder US are planned for 2 weeks and 3, 6, 12, and 24 months after DT to identify complications and late-onset UB.

55.5 Results

We treated 224 ureters with grades II to V VUR in 153 patients using our epidural catheter technique between 2011 and 2018. Of these, 92 were male and 61 were female; mean age at first DT is 4.4 years (range, 0.7–29.8). VUR severity in our series of 224 ureters was grade II in 38 (17.0%), grade III in 77 (34.4%), grade IV in 88 (39.3%), and grade V in 21 (9.4%). Mean operative time was 29.5 min (range, 9–45). Mean duration of postoperative follow-up was 4.1 years (range, 0.7–6.9).

The overall "cure" rate after the first DT was 57.6%, 79.9% after the second DT, and 82.6% after the third DT (Table 55.1a). The "cure" rate after the first DT for VUR grade II was 65.8%, 63.6% for grade III, 52.3% for grade IV, and 42.9% for grade V. The overall "cure" by the third DT for preoperative VUR grade II was 89.5%, 80.5% for grade III, 86.4% for grade IV, and 61.9% for grade V (Table 55.1b). The mean number of DT required to "cure" grade II was 1.13 times, 1.04 times for grade III, 1.19 times for grade IV, and 0.81 times for grade V.

Of the 224 ureters treated in this series, there were 6 (2.7%) with no dye flow after observing for 15 min. All were treated according to the protocol mentioned earlier (leaving the epidural catheter in situ overnight, reassessment for dye flow the next day, assessment for UB by US,

Table 55.1 Resolution of vesicoureteral reflux (VUR) per ureter after Deflux® treatment (DT) in our series

(a) "Cure" rates versus number of Deflux treatments (DT)

	After first DT	After second DT	After third DT
Overall "cure" rate	129/224 (57.6%)	179/224 (79.9%)	185/224 (82.6%)

(b) "Cure" rates versus grade of vesicoureteric reflux. *DT* Deflux treatment

VUR grade	After first DT	After second DT	After third DT	Overall "cure" rate after 3 DT
II	25/38 (65.8%)	25 + 9/38 (89.5%)	34 + 0/38 (89.5%)	34/38 (89.5%)
III	49/77 (63.6%)	49 + 8/77 (74.0%)	57 + 5/77 (80.5%)	62/77 (80.5%)
IV	46/88 (52.3%)	46 + 29/88 (85.2%)	75 + 1/88 (86.4%)	76/88 (86.4%)
V	9/21 (42.9%)	9 + 4/21 (61.9%)	13 + 0/21 (61.9%)	13/21 (61.9%)

"Cure" of VUR was defined as absence or downgrading to grade I on voiding cystourethrography

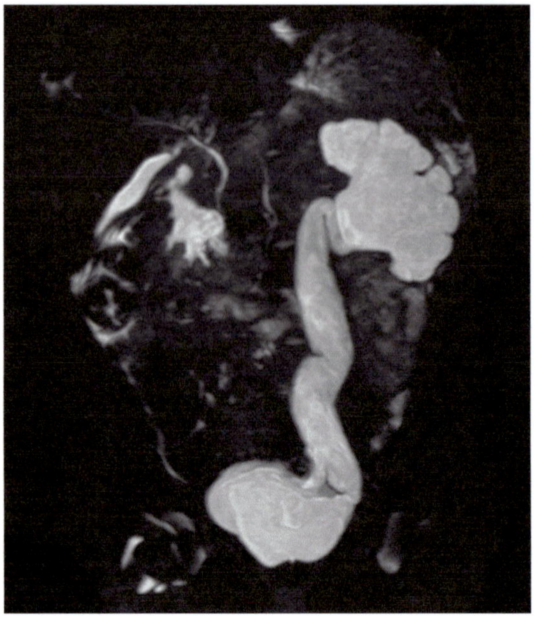

Fig. 55.4 Magnetic resonance urography appearance of ureteric obstruction after Deflux®. MR urography appearance of ureteric obstruction after Deflux® treatment without confirming passage of dye

repeat US at outpatient follow-up 3 weeks after DT). Of the six, two required surgical intervention. One case was a 10-year-old male whose epidural catheter was left in situ because there was no dye flow after 15 min of observation; however, when the epidural catheter was clamped, he developed flank pain and significant hydronephrosis was identified on US the next day, requiring insertion of a double J stent with complete resolution of pain and hydronephrosis. The stent was removed after 1 month. He has been pain-free with stable US findings since. The other case was a 1-year-old male in whom the epidural catheter was removed before confirming dye flow and required insertion of a double J stent because of gross hydronephrosis caused by Deflux® (Fig. 55.4). The stent is currently still in situ.

55.6 Discussion

Endoscopic treatment is now well accepted for treating VUR. The majority of parents clearly prefer endoscopic treatment over open surgery, and a growing number are likely to prefer it over chronic antibiotic prophylaxis [5]. Thus, the demand for DT is likely to increase, and the prevention of complications becomes a major issue.

While endoscopic treatment of VUR is a highly successful minimally invasive procedure with low rates of reported complications requiring surgical intervention, of the order of less than 1% [10], a recent study reported UB rates ranging from 0.7 to 7.6% [11], suggesting that identification of patients at risk for UB may be beneficial. A recently published report about late-onset UB, defined as newly developed or progressive hydronephrosis 8 weeks or more after Deflux® or Vantris® injection, found the rate of late UB after Deflux® or Vantris® injection was 1.9% and the mean time for onset of late UB was 13.4 months [12].

To date, we have not had any late-onset UB develop even though our mean follow-up (4.1 years) is longer than the mean time for late-onset UB to develop reported recently (1.1 years) [12]. We believe our catheter technique effectively identifies patients at risk for UB, both acute and late onset. If dye flow is delayed or absent, additional follow-up is enforced according to our protocol with early surgical intervention as required.

References

1. Kirsch A, Arlen A, Lackgren G. Current trends in dextranomer hyaluronic acid copolymer (Deflux) injection technique for endoscopic treatment of vesicoureteral reflux. Urology. 2014;84(2):462–8.
2. Skoog SJ, Peters CA, Arant BS Jr, Copp HL, Elder JS, Hudson RG, et al. Pediatric vesicoureteral reflux guidelines panel summary report: clinical practice guidelines for screening siblings of children with vesicoureteral reflux and neonates/infants with prenatal hydronephrosis. J Urol. 2010;184(3):1145–51.
3. Peters CA, Skoog SJ, Arant BS Jr, Copp HL, Elder JS, Hudson RG, et al. Summary of the AUA guideline on management of primary vesicoureteral reflux in children. J Urol. 2010;184(3):1134–44.
4. O'Donnell B, Puri P. Treatment of vesicoureteric reflux by endoscopic injection of Teflon. J Urol. 2002;167:1808–9.
5. Kirsch AJ, Perez-Brayfield M, Smith EA, Scherz HC. The modified Sting procedure to correct vesicoureteral reflux: improved results with submucosal implantation within the intramural ureter. J Urol. 2004;171(6):2413–6.
6. Cerwinka W, Scherz H, Kirsch AJ. Dynamic hydrodistention classification of the ureter and the double HIT method to correct vesicoureteral reflux. Arch Esp Urol. 2008;61:882–7.
7. Puri P, Pirker M, Mohanan N, Dawrant M, Dass L, Colhoun E. Subureteral dextranomer/hyaluronic acid injection as first line treatment in the management of high grade vesicoureteral reflux. J Urol. 2006;176:1856–9.
8. Ormaechea M, Ruiz E, Denes E, Gimenez F, Denes FT, Moldes J, et al. New tissue bulking agent (polyacrylate polyalcohol) for treating vesicoureteral reflux: preliminary results in children. J Urol. 2010;183(2): 714–7.
9. Warchol S, Krzemien G, Szmigielska A, Bombinski P, Toth K, Dudek-Warchol T. Endoscopic correction of vesicoureteral reflux in children using polyacrylate-polyalcohol copolymer (Vantris): 5-years of prospective follow-up. Cent European J Urol. 2017;70(3):314–9.
10. Romain J, Fourcade L, Centi J, Blanc P, Masselin MC, Lescure V, et al. Delayed-onset ureteral obstruction and calcification masquerading as renal colic following Deflux injection. Urology. 2016;94: 218–20.
11. Chung JM, Park CS, Lee SD. Postoperative ureteral obstruction after endoscopic treatment for vesicoureteral reflux. Korean J Urol. 2015;56(7):533–9.
12. Ben-Meir D, Bahouth Z, Halachmi S. Late-onset uretero-vesical junction obstruction following endoscopic injection of bulking material for the treatment of vesico-ureteral reflux. Urology. 2017;101:60–2.

56 Vesicoureteral Reflux (VUR): Pneumovesicoscopic Repair

Jean Stephane Valla, Agnese Roberti, Maria Escolino, and Ciro Esposito

56.1 Introduction

Vesicoureteral reflux (VUR) is one of the most important diseases in paediatric urology.

Most of the patients with VUR initially undergo conservative treatment options; however in patients with recurrent febrile infections despite antibiotic prophylaxis, surgical treatment should be warranted [1].

Interventional treatment modalities include endoscopic and open surgical correction techniques. Subureteric material injections have advantages of being minimally invasive and repeatable with reproducible results. However, the success rates with single injection are still far away from the open procedures, and the results become better with repeated injections. Several open techniques (with intravesical or extravesical approaches) have been described with universally high results, but these good results are obtained in consideration of an incision of the abdominal wall causing postoperative pain, bladder spasms, longer urinary diversion and prolonged hospital stay.

J. S. Valla
Pediatric Surgery Unit, CHU Lenval,
Nice, France

A. Roberti · M. Escolino · C. Esposito (✉)
Pediatric Surgery Unit, Department of Translational Medical Sciences (DISMET), University of Naples "Federico II", Naples, Italy
e-mail: maria.escolino@unina.it; ciroespo@unina.it

With the advances of laparoscopy in children for surgical correction of VUR, there was a decreasing of postoperative pain, a shortening of postoperative hospitalization and better cosmesis [2].

As for the open technique, the laparoscopic technique consists of two types of surgical approaches: laparoscopic extravesical transperitoneal approach (LETA) and laparoscopic intravesical technique or pneumovesicoscopic repair that require the creation of a pneumovesicum.

The goal of pneumovesicoscopy, also called pneumovesicum technique or transvesicoscopic access, is to reduce the morbidity associated with the classical abdominal and bladder wall incision while maintaining the same good results achieved by open surgery.

Initially, operative pneumovesicoscopy was performed to correct vesicoureteral reflux; however this technique is evolving and its application is gradually widening to other diseases like obstructive megaureter, ureterocele, bladder diverticulum, bladder lithiasis, incontinence (bladder neck surgery), etc.

The aim of this chapter is to describe the pneumovesicoscopic repair technique of VUR in paediatric patients.

56.2 Preoperative Preparation

The parents give their informed consent to the procedure. Children are prepared for surgery as

C. Esposito et al. (eds.), *ESPES Manual of Pediatric Minimally Invasive Surgery*,
https://doi.org/10.1007/978-3-030-00964-9_56

usual with or without bowel preparation, as the surgeon prefers.

A standard anaesthesia protocol is used after a premedication with midazolam: all children were mechanically ventilated after insertion of an appropriately sized endotracheal tube. Nitrous oxide is generally contraindicated to reduce bowel distension; a nasogastric tube is introduced for the same purpose.

Preoperative antibiotic dose is given according to the aetiology of urinary infections.

An intraoperative monitoring is performed with a pulse oximeter, non-invasive blood pressure monitor and an electrocardiogram; end-tidal carbon dioxide (ETCO2) was monitored through a capnogram.

56.3 Positioning

The patient is positioned supine with the legs separated apart for cystoscopy and bladder catheterization intraoperatively to create a working space for the pneumovesicum repair.

For small infants, the surgeon can stand and operate over the patient's head, whereas for older children, the surgeon usually stands on the patient's left side. The video column is placed between the patient's legs at the end of the table.

56.4 Instrumentation

To perform the pneumovesicoscopy is necessary:

1. Through the urethral catheter to insufflate the bladder with a gas (carbon dioxide) that allows to create a working space equal to the bladder capacity and to provide a clear intravesical vision, much better than the vision in a liquid-filled bladder.
2. To introduce in this distended natural cavity through suprapubic ports three trocars (3–5 mm), one median for the telescope and two lateral for operative instruments (hook electrocautery, diathermy hook, blunt grasper, endoscopic scissor); such a set-up provides 'a familiar forward intravesical view towards the trigone and the ureteric orifices that is similar to that obtained with an open bladder incision' [3].

56.5 Technique

The port placement is preceded by transurethral cystoscopy to allow placement of the first camera port under cystoscopic guidance. The bladder is first distended with saline and a 2-0 monofilament traction suture is passed percutaneously at the bladder dome under cystoscopic vision, through both the abdominal and bladder walls. This helps to keep the bladder wall from falling away when the first camera port site incision is made and during insertion of the cannula. A 5-mm Step port is then inserted under cystoscopic vision. A urethral catheter is then inserted to drain the bladder and start carbon dioxide insufflation to 10–12 mmHg pressure. The urethral catheter is used to occlude the internal urethral meatus to secure CO2 pneumovesicum, and it could also serve as an additional suction irrigation device during subsequent dissection and ureteric reimplantation [4]. A 5-mm 30-degree scope is used to provide intravesical vision. Two more 3–5 mm working ports are then inserted along the interspinous skin crease on either side of the lower lateral wall of the distended bladder under vesicoscopic guidance. A 3–4 cm long segment of an Fr 4 or 6 catheter is then inserted into the respective ureter as a stent to facilitate subsequent ureteral mobilization and dissection and secured with a 4-0 monofilament suture. Intravesical mobilization of the ureter, dissection of submucosal tunnel and a Cohen's type of ureteral reimplantation are then performed under endoscopic guidance, in a similar manner to the open procedure.

The ureter is mobilized by first circumscribing it around the ureteral orifice using hook electrocautery. With traction on the ureteric stent using a blunt grasper, the fibrovascular tissue surrounding the lower ureter can be seen and divided using fine 3-mm endoscopic scissors and diathermy hook, while preserving the main ureteric blood supply. Mobilization of the ureter is continued for 2.5–3 cm to the extravesical space (Figs. 56.1, 56.2, 56.3, 56.4, and 56.5).

Once adequate ureteral length is obtained, the muscular defect in the ureteral hiatus is repaired using 5-0 absorbable sutures, usually with an extracorporeal knot-tying technique. A submucosal tunnel is then created as in an open Cohen's procedure. Using a diathermy hook, a small incision is made over the future site of the new ureteral orifice, usually chosen to be just above the contralateral ureteral orifice. Dissection of the submucosal tunnel is then started from the medial aspect of the ipsilateral ureteral hiatus towards the new ureteral orifice, using a combination of endoscopic scissor dissection and diathermy hook for haemostasis. Once the submucosal tunnel dissection is completed, a fine grasper is passed and the mobilized ureter is gently drawn through the tunnel. Ureteroneocystostomy is performed under endoscopic guidance with intracorporeal suturing using

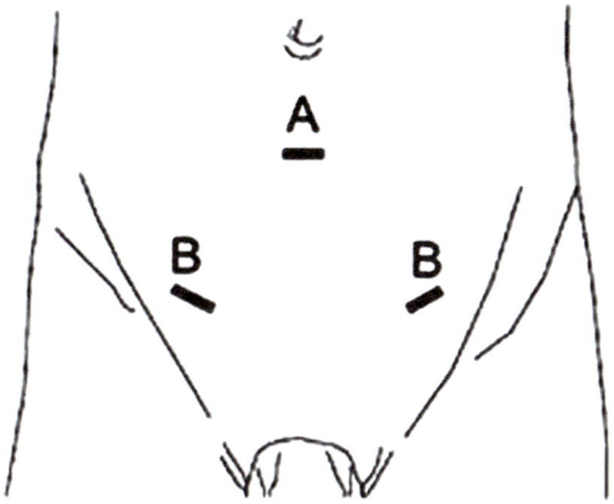

Fig. 56.1 First camera port site incision (A) and two more working ports (B-B)

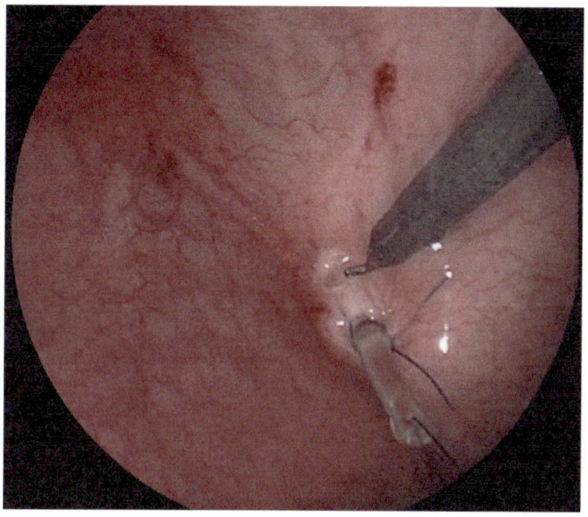

Fig. 56.3 The ureter is mobilized by first circumscribing it around the ureteral orifice using hook electrocautery

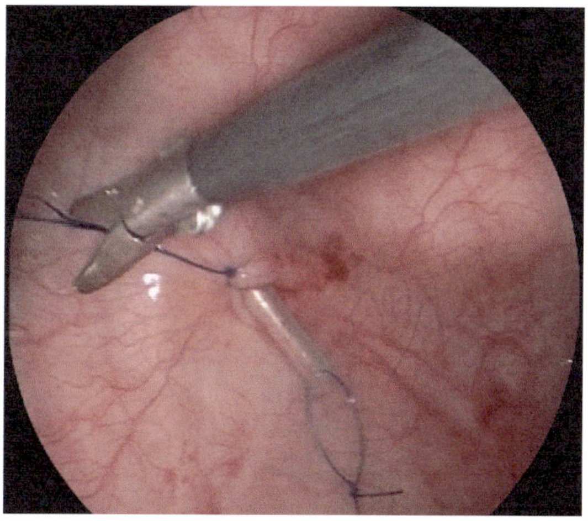

Fig. 56.2 A 3–4 cm long segment of an Fr 4 or 5 catheter is inserted into the ureter as a stent to facilitate subsequent ureteral mobilization and dissection and secured with a 4-0 monofilament suture

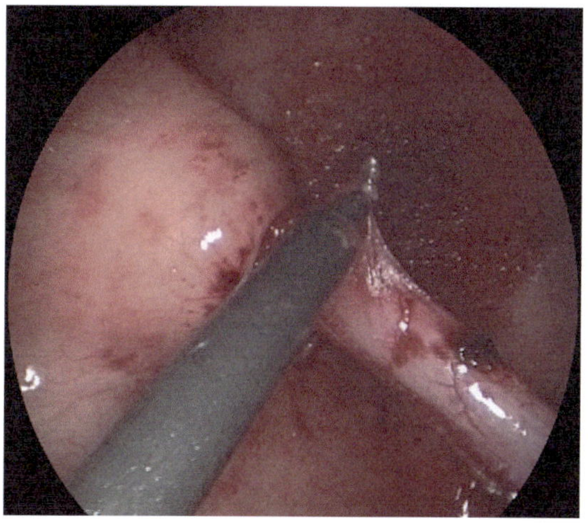

Fig. 56.4 With traction on the ureteric stent using a blunt grasper, the fibrovascular tissue surrounding the lower ureter can be seen and divided using fine 3-mm endoscopic scissors and diathermy hook, while preserving the main ureteric blood supply

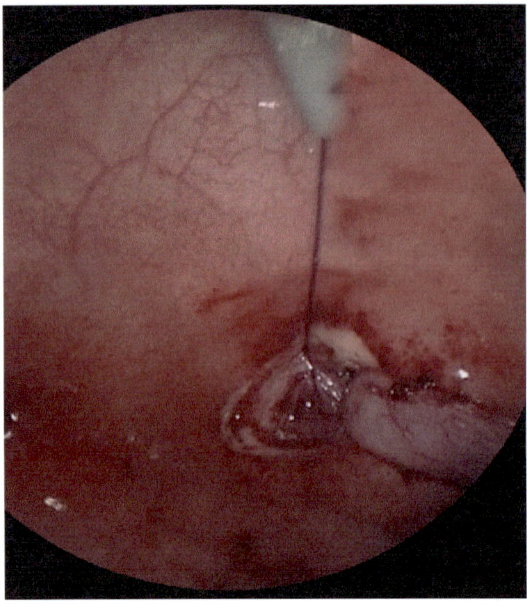

Fig. 56.5 Once adequate ureteral length is obtained, the muscular defect in the ureteral hiatus is repaired using 5-0 absorbable sutures, usually with an extracorporeal knot-tying technique

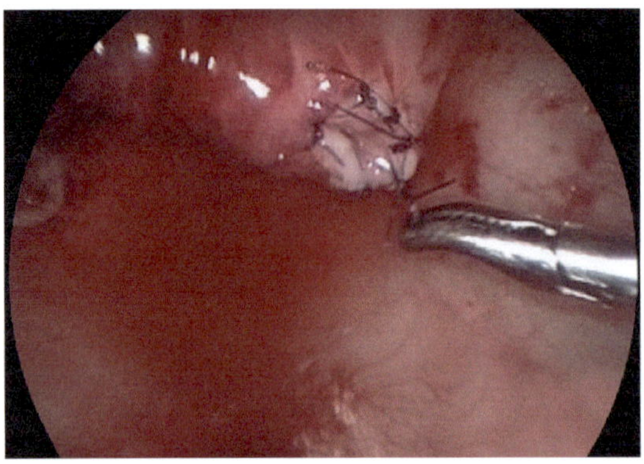

Fig. 56.6 Completed ureteroneocystostomy

interrupted 5-0 or 6-0 poliglecaprone or polydioxanone sutures (Fig. 56.6). A ureteral stent is not routinely used except for selected patients undergoing bilateral ureteral reimplantation or those with megaureters requiring tapering ureteroplasty [3]. The working ports are removed under endoscopic vision with evacuation of the pneumovesicum. The bladder-holding stitches are then tied. Each port site entry wound is then closed with a subcuticular monocryl suture [5–7].

56.6 Postoperative Care

In the postoperative period, the patients can keep a normal decubitus.

They can restart full oral feeding few hours after surgery. The analgesic requirement (paracetamol every 6 h) is generally limited to the first 24–48 postoperative hours.

It is necessary to monitor diuresis in the first 24 h with a bladder catheter to avoid a late diagnosis of ureteral obstruction or urinomas.

In case of drainage, the drain is removed at day 1 or day 2 post-op. An ultrasound is performed at 1 week and 1 month post-op.

The following annual controls (ultrasound, cystography and renal scintigraphy) are focused on the renal function and residual reflux.

56.7 Results

Several series of Cohen's pneumovesicoscopic reimplantation have been published since 10 years with good results [3–7]. Mean operative time for unilateral cases is 80–160 min and for bilateral cases is 130–180 min. Hospital stay is reported to be around 2 days. The success rate is varying between 91 and 97.6%. Conversion to open surgery is mostly due to port displacement and proximal migration of ureteral catheter. Ureteral stricture or obstruction may occur due to inappropriate handling and dissection of the distal ureter. Extraperitoneal extravasation or the urine leak is reported to occur due to inadequate closure of the bladder and improper ureterovesical anastomosis. Scrotal and suprapubic emphysema is related to the gas leakage to the subcutaneous tissue which always resolved spontaneously. In some occasions, inadvertent pneumoperitoneum treated by intraoperative intraumbilical Veress needle placement.

56.8 Tips and Tricks

- Port placement can be tricky; the specific problem of pneumovesicoscopy is, when introducing the ports, to go through two walls, firstly abdominal wall then the bladder wall, and during the procedure to avoid any dislodgment of the trocar out of the bladder. Suspending the bladder to the anterior abdominal wall and fixation of the trocar to the abdominal wall are of utmost importance.
- Of course filling the bladder with liquid offers a better counterpressure than with gas, and it can be an advantage because the bladder wall is particularly soft in children and can be distorted or pushed away by the trocar tip before being entered; but we changed for CO2 insufflation for two reasons: first blood oozing from the bladder port sites could cloud the cystoscopic fluid; second any liquid extravasation out of the bladder could occur and lead to collapse the bladder and poor visibility.
- During the postoperative period, the most feared complication is ureteral obstruction usually due to a too close dissection with monopolar hook (ischemia + burn): low power setting on the hook electrode and cautery away from the ureter are recommended.
- Of course as part of minimally invasive procedures, pneumovesicoscopic cure of vesicoureteral reflux is in competition with injection therapy using dextranomer/hyaluronic acid; however both techniques could be associated during the same procedure in case of bilateral disease (three cases in my experience): for example, low-grade reflux on one side and obstructive megaureter or ureterocele on the contralateral side; the "sting" realized during the cystoscopy allows to avoid bilateral reimplantation and to save time.

56.8.1 Limitations and Contraindications

- Related to the surgeon: all the vesicoscopic procedures are challenging. Expertise in intracorporeal suturing in confined spaces with fine 5-0 or 6-0 is essential; there is a tremendous learning curve; in short these procedures are still reserved to expert laparoscopic paediatric surgeons.
- Related to the patient: the major limiting factor is the bladder capacity. The smaller the bladder, the more reduced the working space. In the youngest patients of few months old, the decreased working space does make the procedure more technically demanding and may obviate the advantages of vesicoscopic repair. Hence this method seems difficult to apply under 1 year of age (or in bladder less than 100 mL). That explains why the use of robot, even if it seems theoretically a good solution, is not in fact the way to solve the problem [8].
- Another limiting factor is the bladder wall conditions: in case of markedly thickened or inflamed bladder wall, the procedure could be quite difficult. However previous failed injection therapy or previous intra- or extravesical surgery should not be considered a contraindication. This technique is also workable in augmented bladder.

56.9 Discussion

The laparoscopic approaches arose from the idea of combining minimal invasiveness of endoscopic treatments with the successful outcomes of open procedures. After the initial papers reporting the complexity and having no advantage of the procedure in children, new publications on this issue started to appear in the literature after 2000s.

The experience on Cohen's pneumovesicoscopic reimplantation is larger than the extraperitoneal technique. The allowance for bilateral reimplantation, reduced bladder trauma, absence of wide cystotomy and retraction of bladder wall may be counted as the benefits of this approach [4]. Besides these facts, it also allows intravesical repair of diverticula [9]. However, the operative field is smaller and intracorporeal suturing is more demanding. In a study of Kutikov et al., they noticed that complications mostly occurred in children who had small (<130 cm^3) bladder capacity and were younger than 2 years age [10]. Their observations showed that increasing intravesical pressures (>10 mmHg) were causing contractions; therefore they recommend to work under pressures between 6 and 8 mmHg. The effect of CO2 on the upper urinary tract was studied in sows, and pneumovesicum at a pressure of 10 mmHg for 2 h did not result in any demonstrable deleterious effect [11]. Canon et al. made one of the few comparative studies [6]. They showed in their retrospective study that the mean age was higher, the reflux grade was lesser, operative time was longer and narcotic analgesic need was lesser in vesicoscopic reimplantation group than the open group. Another smaller study also showed that financial cost-effectivity and hospital stay were favouring the laparoscopic technique [12]. Jayanthi with the largest experience in the literature recommended the low power cautery use, correct placement of ports and closure of port sites as Kutikov et al. also did. Kawauchi et al. compared 15 adults and 15 young patients and revealed no significant difference including the operative times, success and complication rates [13]. One study showed a decreased operative time with increasing experience [14].

In conclusion collected experiences helped to define the indications, advantages and disadvantages of laparoscopic approaches. For the present time, laparoscopy can be said to be reaching its goal about the high successful results with a minimally invasive nature. The only barrier on the way of widespread acceptance is the long operative times which will take some more time to be improved [2, 15].

References

1. Tekgül S, Riedmiller H, Hoebeke P, Kočvara R, Nijman RJ, Radmayr C, Stein R, Dogan HS, European Association of Urology. EAU guidelines on vesicoureteral reflux in children. Eur Urol. 2012;62(3):534–42. https://doi.org/10.1016/j.eururo.2012.05.059. Epub 2012 June 5. Review.
2. Hasan SD, Serdar T. Laparoscopic correction of vesicoureteral reflux in children: review of the current literature. Arch Esp Urol. 2014;67(8):660–72.
3. Yeung CK. Endoscopic cross trigonal ureteric reimplantation under carbon dioxide pneumovesicum. In: Bax KMA, Georgeson KE, Rothenberg SS, Valla JS, Yeung CK, editors. Endoscopic surgery infants and children. 2nd ed. New York: Springer; 2008. p. 730–5.
4. Valla JS, Steyaert H, Griffin SJ, et al. Transvesicoscopic Cohen ureteric reimplantation for vesicoureteral reflux in children: a single-centre 5-year experience. J Pediatr Urol. 2009;5(6):466–71.
5. Jayanthi V, Patel A. Vesicoscopic ureteral reimplantation: a minimally invasive technique for the definitive repair of vesicoureteral reflux. Adv Urol. 2008:973616.
6. Canon SJ, Jayanthi VR, Patel AS. Vesicoscopic cross-trigonal ureteral reimplantation: a minimally invasive option for repair of vesicoureteral reflux. J Urol. 2007;178(1):269–73; discussion 273.
7. Chung MS, Han SW, Jung HJ, Im YJ. Transvesicoscopic ureteral reimplantation in children with bilateral vesicoureteral reflux: surgical technique and results. J Laparoendosc Adv Surg Tech A. 2012;22:295–300.
8. Thakre AA, Bailly Y, Sun LW, et al. Is smaller workspace a limitation for robot performance in laparoscopy? J Urol. 2008;179:1142–3.
9. Badawy H, Eid A, Hassouna M, Elkarim AA, Elsalmy S. Pneumovesicoscopic diverticulectomy in children and adolescents: is open surgery still indicated? J Pediatr Urol. 2008;4(2):146–9.
10. Kutikov A, Guzzo TJ, Canter DJ, Casale P. Initial experience with laparoscopic transvesical ureteral reimplantation at the Children's Hospital of Philadelphia. J Urol. 2006;176(5):2222–5.
11. Xiang B, Liu JX, Sung HB, Yan B, Cheng W. The effect of CO2 pneumovesicum on upper urinary tract. J Pediatr Surg. 2010;45(9):1863–7.
12. Chung PH, Tang DY, Wong KK, Yip PK, Tam PK. Comparing open and pneumovesical approach for ureteric reimplantation in pediatric patients—a preliminary review. J Pediatr Surg. 2008;43(12):2246–9.
13. Kawauchi A, Naitoh Y, Soh J, Hirahara N, Okihara K, Miki T. Transvesical laparoscopic cross-trigonal ureteral reimplantation for correction of vesicoureteral reflux: initial experience and comparisons between adult and pediatric cases. J Endourol. 2009;23(11):1875–8.
14. Hong CH, Kim JH, Jung HJ, Im YJ, Won Han S. Single-surgeon experience with transvesicoscopic ureteral reimplantation in children with vesicoureteral reflux. Urology. 2011;77(6):1465–9.
15. Callaghan K, Gray E, Caldamone A, Ellsworth P. Factors involved in parental decision making for surgical correction of vesicoureteral reflux. J Urol. 2008;180(2):701–5; discussion 705–6.

57 Laparoscopic Decortication for Renal Cysts in Children

Mohamed Abouheba and Sameh Shehata

57.1 Introduction

The kidney is one of the commonest organs for cyst occurrence [1]. Causes are listed in Box 57.1 [2]. Autosomal dominant polycystic kidney disease (ADPKD) is the most common renal cystic disease in the United States [3]. On the other hand, simple renal cysts are comparatively rare in children and adolescents up to 18 years of age. Incidence ranges from 0.1 to 0.45% with a mean of 0.22% without sex predilection [4]. The incidence, however, rises with age reaching 20% and 50% at 40 and 60 years of age, respectively, with apparent male preponderance [5]. Despite originating within the nephron, simple renal cysts lose communication later and become excluded. They usually range from 1 to 10 cm in size, the majority being less than 2 cm [6]. They are usually oval or rounded, solitary or multiple, and unilateral or bilateral. Most cysts are unilocular and cortical in location and, rarely, medullary. They look glistening blue usually distorting renal contour. They are lined by a single layer of flattened or cuboidal epithelium and filled with a clear serous fluid. However, some may become septated and fibrosed or calcified from previous hemorrhage or infection [7].

Box 57.1 Classification of Renal Cysts [2]

Inheritable	Nonheritable
• Autosomal recessive (infantile) polycystic kidney disease • Autosomal dominant (adult) polycystic kidney disease • Juvenile nephronophthisis and medullary cystic disease complex • Juvenile nephronophthisis (autosomal recessive) • Medullary cystic disease (autosomal dominant) • Congenital nephrosis (familial nephrotic syndrome) (autosomal recessive) • Familial hypoplastic glomerulocystic disease (autosomal dominant) • Multiple malformation syndromes with renal cysts (e.g., tuberous sclerosis, von Hippel-Lindau disease)	• Multicystic kidney (multicystic dysplastic kidney) • Benign multilocular cyst (cystic nephroma) • Simple cysts • Medullary sponge kidney • Sporadic glomerulocystic kidney disease • Acquired renal cystic disease • Calyceal diverticulum (pyelogenic cyst)

Simple renal cysts are usually silent in children and, therefore, usually incidentally discovered. Rarely, huge cysts manifest as a flank pain, abdominal mass, or rupture into the pelvicalyceal system producing hematuria or compress the surrounding parenchyma leading to segmental ischemia and consequent hypertension or frank obstructive uropathy [8]. Their benign nature is easily ascertained if

M. Abouheba · S. Shehata (✉)
Division of Pediatric Surgery, Children's Hospital, Alexandria University, Alexandria, Egypt
e-mail: Sameh_Shehata@alexmed.edu.eg

C. Esposito et al. (eds.), *ESPES Manual of Pediatric Minimally Invasive Surgery*,
https://doi.org/10.1007/978-3-030-00964-9_57

Table 57.1 Modified Bosniak classification of adult renal cysts and recommended management [10]

Category	Description	Recommendation
Category I *Benign*	Simple benign cyst with (1) good through-transmission (i.e., acoustic enhancement), (2) no echoes within the cyst, (3) sharply marginated smooth wall	Follow-up Consider surgery if symptomatic
Category II *Benign*	Looks benign with some radiologic concerns, including septation, minimal calcification, and high density	Follow-up Consider surgery if symptomatic
Category II F *Likely benign*	Although calcification in wall of cyst may even be thicker and more nodular than in category II, the septa have minimal enhancement, especially those with calcium	Follow-up Consider surgery if symptomatic
Category III *Suspicious*	More complicated lesion that cannot confidently be distinguished from malignancy, having more calcification, more prominent septation of a thicker wall than a category II lesion	Surgical exploration Consider partial nephrectomy
Category IV *Malignant*	Clearly a malignant lesion with large cystic components, irregular margins; solid vascular elements	Radical nephrectomy

they meet certain U/S criteria: (a) round or oval shape, (b) no internal echoes, and (c) sharply demarcated wall with (d) acoustic enhancement behind [9]. Symptomatic cysts, clustered cysts, as well as failure to meet some of these criteria all raise suspicion of malignancy mandating further evaluation by CT, MRI, or even ultrasound-guided cyst aspiration for cytological examination [10].

Although management of symptomatic cysts is largely guided by CT criteria based on Bosniak classification in adults (Table 57.1) [11], the choice of the approach in children rather depends on patient factors and surgeons' preference [12]. Current options for simple renal cysts in children include decompression by percutaneous aspiration with or without sclerosis, open surgery, antegrade or retrograde endoscopic marsupialization, and laparoscopic decortication via transperitoneal or retroperitoneal approaches [13–16].

57.2 Preoperative Preparation

Before surgery, routine laboratory studies (complete blood picture, bleeding and coagulation profile, serum creatinine, and urine culture) should be done for all patients. In special scenarios, the patient should be consented for conversion to an open procedure or even nephrectomy should intraoperative complications arise (e.g., multiple renal cysts with hypertension or peripelvic cyst). If nephrectomy is a consideration, a contralateral functioning kidney should be secured during the preoperative workup.

A preoperative bowel preparation is beneficial in infants and children with stool softeners. A routine perioperative coverage with cephalosporin is enough but is rather guided by urinalysis and culture if indicated. After induction of anesthesia, the stomach and bladder are decompressed with a nasogastric tube and bladder catheter, respectively. If there is potential of transgressing the renal collecting system (e.g., peripelvic cysts), a ureteral stent is better placed at the beginning of the procedure for retrograde instillation of methylene blue to identify any inadvertent injury to the collecting system.

57.3 Positioning

The transperitoneal approach is ideal for anterior cysts, while the retroperitoneal approach is reserved for posterior cysts. For the transperitoneal approach, the patient is secured in the lateral oblique position with a back roll. The flank is opened by splinting the patient either over a roll under the contralateral costal margin in infants or by flexing the table in older children and adolescents. The axilla is well padded to avoid brachial plexus injury. The upper chest and thighs are secured to the bed with soft tape. For the retroperitoneal approach, the patient is secured in the frank lateral position. The flank is opened by splinting the patient over a lower chest roll. The lower arm rests on a board while the upper arm is flexed over the chest. The legs are well-padded taped to the table.

Box 57.2 Instruments for Laparoscopic Cyst Decortication

Instruments needed for laparoscopic decortication
• Cystoscopy set, if needed
• Direct vision access port (e.g., Visiport, US Surgical Corporation)
• Laparoscopic lens
• Two–three 10-/12-mm insufflating ports[a]
• Two 5-mm ports
• Laparoscopic instruments: scissors, graspers, and suction irrigator
• Laparoscopic ultrasound (if needed)
• Argon beam coagulator
• Retrieval bag
• 5-mm or 10-mm clip appliers[a]
• Oxidized cellulose
• Laparoscopic aspiration needle

[a]Depending on size of the child

57.4 Instrumentation

Before the procedure, ensure that the necessary equipment is open or readily available. Box 57.2 lists the equipment recommended for laparoscopic renal cyst decortication.

57.5 Technique

57.5.1 Trocar Placement

57.5.1.1 Transperitoneal Approach

Pneumoperitoneum is safer established by open method using a transumbilical insufflating 5-mm port under vision. All other ports are inserted under laparoscopic vision.

For left-sided cyst decortications, a 5-mm port is inserted below the umbilicus along the midclavicular line, and another 5-mm port is inserted along the midline in the linea alba midway between the xiphoid process and the umbilicus. For a right-sided procedure, a 5-mm upper midline is placed midway between the xiphoid and the umbilicus, and a 12-mm port is placed just below the level of the umbilicus at the right midclavicular line. An optional 3- or 5-mm port may be placed in the upper midline to facilitate retraction of the liver or spleen (Fig. 57.1).

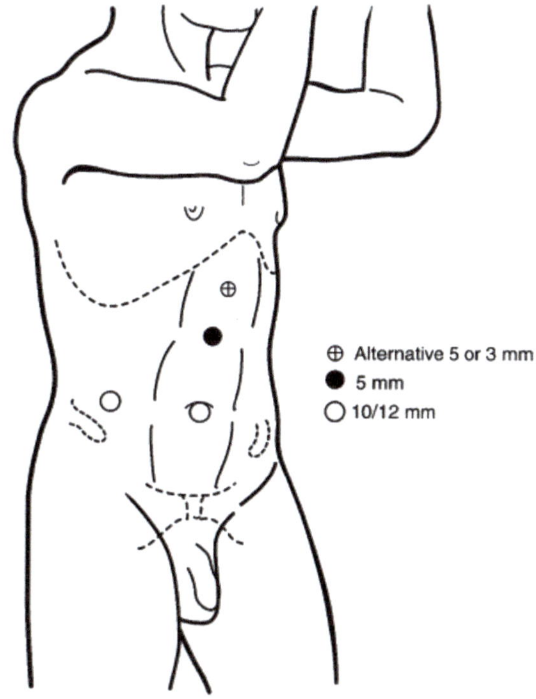

Fig. 57.1 Three ports are used for the transabdominal approach: the first 12-mm laparoscopic port is placed at the umbilicus, and the remaining ports are placed under laparoscopic vision as follows: a 12-mm port is placed just below the umbilicus along the midclavicular line, and a 5-mm port is placed in the midline between the xiphoid and the umbilicus (Reprinted with permission [15])

57.5.1.2 Retroperitoneal Approach

A 2-mm skin incision is made just at or posterior to the 12th rib at the superior lumbar triangle. A space is created by blunt finger dissection anterior to the psoas major and around Gerota's fascia to accommodate a balloon dilator. A trocar-mounted balloon or a modified Gaur balloon made of the middle finger of a latex surgeon's glove mounted on a 16F red rubber catheter is used to expand the retroperitoneal space to 500–800 cc. A 12-mm blunt-tipped cannula is placed at this site. A second 12-mm trocar is placed under laparoscopic vision along the anterior axillary line in line with the first trocar, taking care to avoid inadvertent injury to the peritoneum. A third 5-mm trocar is placed a few fingerbreadths posterior to the sec-

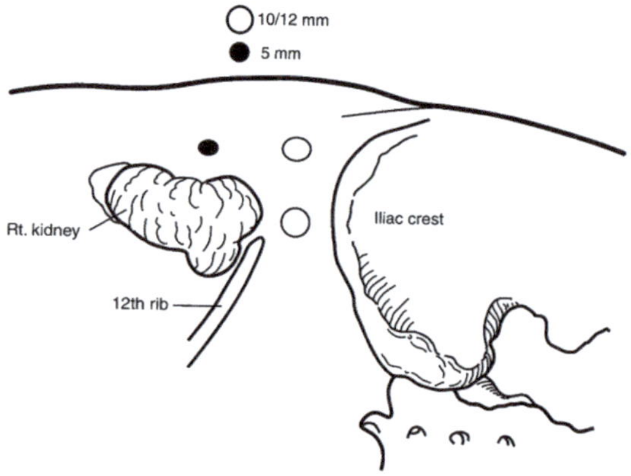

Fig. 57.2 In the retroperitoneal approach, a 12-mm blunt-tipped cannula is placed just at or posterior to the 12th rib at the superior lumbar triangle, and a second 12 mm trocar is placed in the anterior axillary line in line with the first trocar. This is placed under direct vision with care to avoid injury to the peritoneum, which can be swept medially as necessary. A third 5-mm trocar is placed a few finger breadths posterior (at the lateral border of the paraspinous muscles) under direct vision or superiorly above the 12-mm trocar in the anterior axillary line (Reprinted with permission [15])

ond trocar (at the lateral border of the paraspinous muscles) or superior to the 12-mm trocar in the anterior axillary line (Fig. 57.2).

57.5.2 Procedure

57.5.2.1 Transperitoneal Approach

After securing the trocars, the colonic white line of Toldt is incised from the splenic or hepatic flexures down to the iliac vessels, and the colon is reflected medially to expose the kidney. An extra 3- or 5-mm port may be needed to lift the liver (on the right side) or the spleen (on the left side). For full access, the splenicocolic and phrenicocolic ligaments are divided on the left side; and duodenum may be mobilized on the right side (Fig. 57.3).

The use of intraoperative ultrasonography via a laparoscopic transducer helps delineating cyst location, extension, and relation to renal vessels and collecting system at the hilum. It also helps exploring cyst interior septation, extension, calcification, and debris within raising suspicion of malignancy (vide supra).

For solitary cortical cysts, splitting the overlying Gerota's fascia provides direct access for simple unroofing. However, in case of complex, multiple, or peripelvic cysts, the kidney is better fully mobilized to expose the hilum.

For a solitary cyst, the perinephric fat overlying the cyst is dissected up to normal renal cortex (Fig. 57.4). Large tense cysts may be aspirated

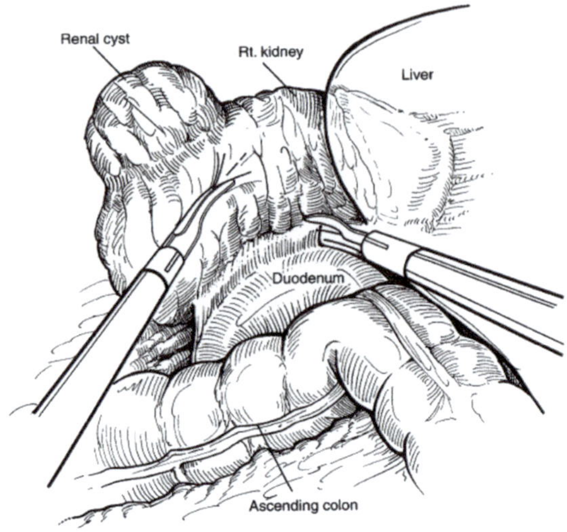

Fig. 57.3 On the right side, the colon is reflected medially, and a Kocher maneuver may be necessary to fully expose the kidney (Reprinted with permission [15])

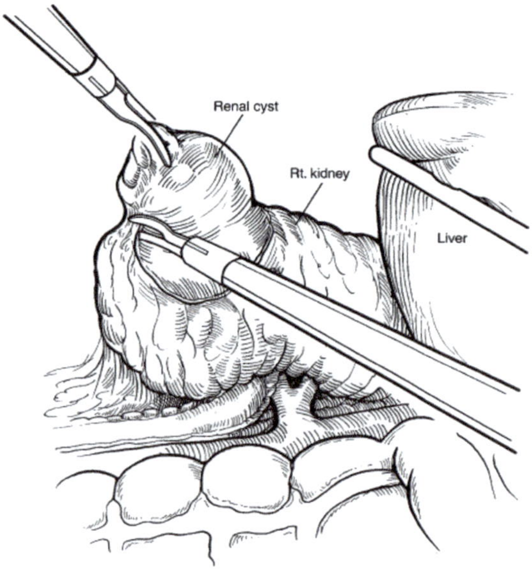

Fig. 57.4 The renal cyst can be identified through Gerota's fascia and the perinephric fat is mobilized until a rim of normal parenchyma is exposed (Reprinted with permission [15])

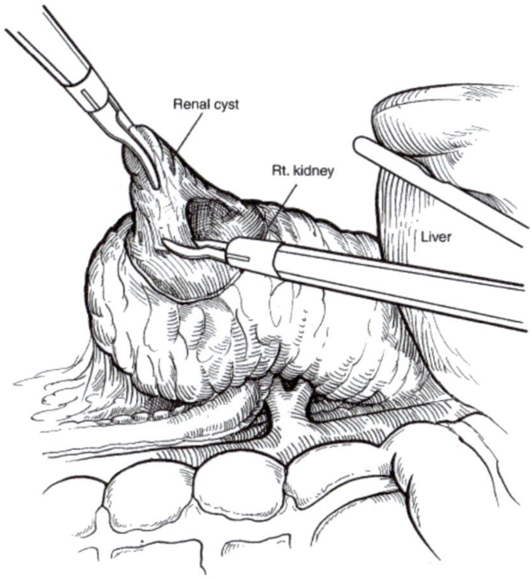

Fig. 57.5 The cyst wall is then grasped and electrocautery scissors used to excise the wall until it is flushed with the renal capsule (Reprinted with permission from [15])

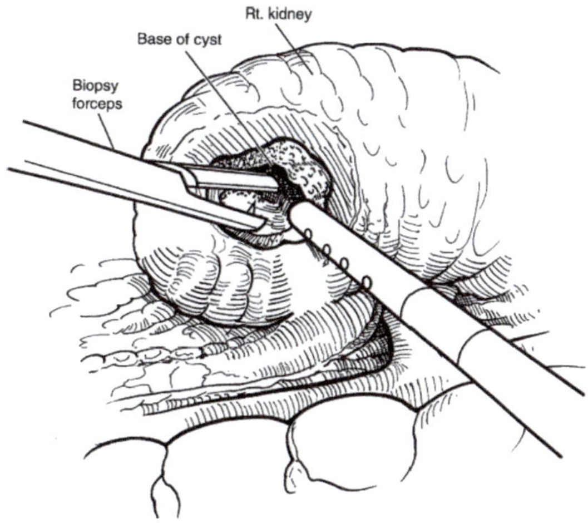

Fig. 57.6 The base of the cyst is inspected for suspicious nodules or irregularities that may be biopsied with cup biopsy forceps (Reprinted with permission [15])

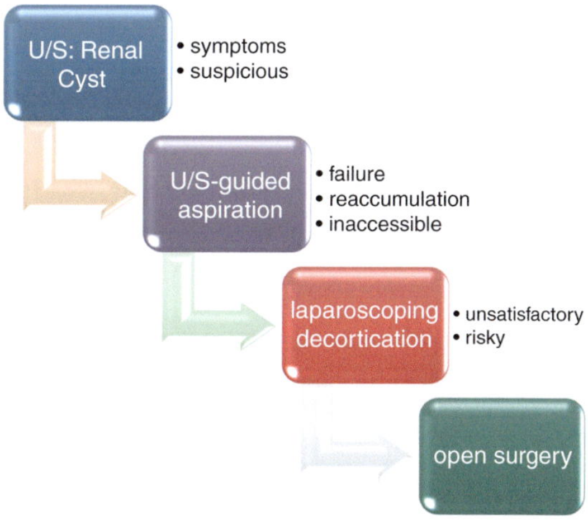

Fig. 57.7 Management algorithm of renal cysts in children [17]

for partial decompression using an appropriate spinal needle transcutaneously under laparoscopic vision. The now flaccid cyst wall is circumferentially resected flush with the renal capsule using low-energy laparoscopic scissors (Fig. 57.5) and sent for histopathological examination. Also, any suspicious nodules on the now exposed cyst floor are scooped with cup biopsy forceps (Fig. 57.6).

Any bleeding should be controlled with short buzzes of low-current monopolar electrocautery or argon beam coagulator. Avoid overuse of energy inside a large or deep cyst cavity to avoid collecting system injury.

Large cyst cavities are better plugged with perirenal fat to reabsorb cyst fluid preventing its reaccumulation or formally drained by a fine suction drain coming out through a lateral port.

Large deep intrarenal cysts pose a challenge for unroofing and may need intraoperative laparoscopic ultrasound transducer to localize them or even a preoperative percutaneous nephrostomy tube.

For peripelvic cysts, a ureteral catheter may be placed preoperatively to inject methylene blue to help distinguish the cyst from the collecting system. Electrocautery is particularly discouraged during their dissection at the hilum to avoid injuring the nearby vessels and collecting system.

For ADPKD, laparoscopic ultrasound may help locating deeper cysts (Fig. 57.7) puncturing many of them. Inaccessible cysts may just be aspirated.

57.5.2.2 Retroperitoneal Approach

The retroperitoneal approach is reserved for posterior and lower pole cysts in older children [18]. After securing the trocars, the peritoneum is swept medially exposing the psoas major where the Gerota's fascia is opened. Once the cyst is identified, it is tackled similarly to the transperitoneal approach.

57.6 Postoperative Care

Aim to start fluids the same night regardless of the approach. Once tolerated, a soft diet is started next morning and plan discharge. Remove the bladder catheter after ensuring a satisfactory urine output. Cephalosporin may be continued for 1–2 postoperative days unless otherwise indicated by urine culture. If, however, the patient develops ileus, feeding intolerance, fever, or abdominal distention, a urinoma or retroperitoneal hematoma should be suspected and is better drained under ultrasound guidance.

For urinomas, a Foley catheter is reinserted, and a percutaneous nephrostomy tube or ureteral stent placed. For retroperitoneal hematomas, observation and transfusion are usually sufficient, but rarely a renal arteriogram and transcatheter embolization are done for refractory hemorrhage.

57.7 Results

57.7.1 Simple Renal Cysts

Short-term follow-up reports 77–100% success rate as defined by resolution of symptoms and cysts (Table 57.2). The most comprehensive review done by Fahlenkamp et al. [24] in 4 different centers examining 139 laparoscopic cyst decortications at 4 centers reported only 5 complication categories: bleeding, open conversion, ileus, urinary fistula, and nerve paresthesia. The 4.5% overall complication rate compares favorably with the 32% rate reported for planned open cyst decortication [24].

Faith et al. [26] reported 45 patients who underwent laparoscopic decortication of symptomatic simple renal cysts with renal cyst wall excision and fulguration of the epithelial lining. Complex renal cysts were excluded. Of which, 24 (53.3%) had undergone previous cyst aspiration with injection of sclerosant material for ablation. The Wong-Baker pain scale was used to assess the preoperative and postoperative pain scores. Radiologic success was indicated as no recurrence on the most recent computed tomography scan. Of the 45 procedures, 44 were completed laparoscopically. One patient (1.8%) underwent open conversion because of excessive bleeding. The mean operative time was 89 min (range 48–170). Symptomatic success was achieved in 91.1% of patients, with a median follow-up of 52 months (range 3–132), and radiographic

Table 57.2 Outcome of laparoscopic decortication of simple renal cysts in various series [15]

Author	Pts	TP/RP	OR time (min)	Transf.	Conver.	Compl. (%)	LOS (day)	Conval. (week)	FU (months)	Success (%)
Rubenstein et al. [19]	10	9/1	147	10%	10%	20%	2.2	1	10	100
Guazzoni et al. [20]	20	TP	75	0%	0%	0%	2.2	1	3–6	100
Valdivia et al. [14]	13	TP	–	–	0%	–	–	–	0–12	–
Wada et al. [21]	13	TP	–	–	7.7%	7.7%	–	–	3	77
Ou et al. [22]	14	RP	78	–	–	7	4.2	1	8	100
Denis et al. [23]	10	8/2	92	–	10%	10%	5.4	–	8.3	100
Fahlenkamp et al. [24]	139	–	–	–	–	3.5%	–	–	–	–
Roberts et al. [25]	21	13/8	164	0%	0%	14%	1.9	–	15.8	95
Total	240	83/18	129	2.0% (1/51)	3.4% (3/87)	6.2% (14/227)	2.9	1	–	–

success was achieved in 95.5% of patients, with a median follow-up of 39 months (range 3–96) [26].

57.7.2 Complex Cysts

Literature is scarce on complex cysts in children. However, Santiago et al. [27] reviewed 35 patients with Bosniak II and III cysts who underwent laparoscopic cyst decortication. Among these patients, five (14.5%) had renal cell carcinoma, of whom four underwent immediate partial or radical nephrectomy and one patient underwent a delayed partial nephrectomy after pathologic confirmation. No recurrences were detected in this group of patients at a mean follow-up of 20 months [27].

Roberts et al. [25] also performed laparoscopic cyst decortication in eight patients with Bosniak class II/III cysts. One patient with a finding of a 0.8-cm focus of papillary renal cell carcinoma on permanent histopathological examination subsequently underwent an open radical nephrectomy with excision of the trocar site that was used for specimen extraction. With 60 months follow-up, no recurrence has been detected [25]. Warren et al. [28] reviewed the accuracy of the Bosniak classification and concluded that concordance between radiologic classification and malignancy is well established and accurate for class I and IV cysts, however, in the absence of large prospective studies, differentiating between class II and III cysts remains controversial [28]. Several groups reviewed by Warren utilized CT-guided biopsy of class II–III renal cyst to aid in their decision-making. Until longer follow-up and more patients are evaluated, laparoscopic cyst decortication for the intermediate cyst should be employed cautiously and selectively.

57.7.3 Peripelvic Cysts

Roberts et al. [25] reported the largest series to date of 11 peripelvic cysts who underwent laparoscopic decortication without any conversions, transfusions, or recurrences. However, prolonged urinary leakage and ileus was one yet serious complication. In contrast, both operative time was longer and mean blood loss was greater statistically for peripelvic cysts compared with simple cysts (164 vs. 233 min [$p = 0.003$], 98 vs. 182 mL [$p = 0.04$]).

57.7.4 Autosomal Dominant Polycystic Kidney Disease

Fewer series of ADPKD exist in children and have limitations regarding protocol and number of cysts excised (Table 57.3).

Table 57.3 Outcome of laparoscopic decortication of ADPKD in various series [15]

Author	Pts	TP/RP	EBL (mL)	OR time (min)	Transf.	Convers.	Compl.	LOS (day)	Recur.	F/U (month)	Pain relief
Elzinga et al. [29]	3	TP	–	–	–	–	–	–	–	–	–
Chehval and Neilsen [30]	3	TP	–	–	0	0	0	2.3	0	16.7	100% initial and F/U
Brown et al. [31]	8	TP	<150	164	0	0	0	<2	25%	12–28	85% initial, 50% F/U
Elashry et al.	2 (5 proc)	TP	85	207	0	0	0	2.4	0	9	100% initial and 6–22 months
Lifson et al. [32]	8 (11 proc)	10/1	116	137	9%	0	9%	2.2	–	28.6%(2/7)	11–65 71% at 6 months, 57% at 2 years
Lee et al. [33]	29	27/2	124	300	0	0	34	3.2	–	32	81% with a 50% pr
Dunn et al. [34]	15 (21 proc)	TP	88	330	0	0	33%	3.2	13.30%	26.4	86.7% initial, 73% at 2 years
Total	68 (80 proc)	77/3	112.6	226	4.2%	0%	16.7%	2.55	15.7%	–	–

Most current studies recommend extensive cyst decortication. Dunn et al. marsupialized an average 204 cysts/procedure aiming for better pain relief prolonging the mean operative time to 226 min. It is observed that initial complete pain relief on all patients may degrade later to partial relief on fewer patients on longer follow-up. Lifson et al. reported complete pain resolution in 71%, and 57% of seven patients who were pain-free at 6 months and 2 years, respectively. Dunn et al. also noted a reduction in pain in 73% of 15 patients at 2 years, with an average pain reduction of 62%.

Whether cyst decortications have ameliorated the natural history of ADPDK-related hypertension and renal impairment remains controversial. Dunn et al. [34] found no change in blood pressure in 40%, improvement in 20%, resolution in 7%, and worsening in 33% of 12 ADPDK patients who underwent extensive laparoscopic cyst decortication. Serum creatinine levels remained stable in 87% of patients.

57.8 Tips and Tricks

1. A trial of conservative management or percutaneous sclerotherapy for simple cysts can precede laparoscopic cyst decortication.
2. The laparoscopic management of complex renal cysts is controversial, and patient candidates for laparoscopic exploration and/or decortication require careful selection. For Bosniak II/III cysts, aspirated cyst fluid should be sent for cytology and samples of the cyst wall and base should be sent for histopathologic evaluation at the time of surgery.
3. Peripelvic cysts require careful dissection around the hilum and retrograde injection of methylene blue to rule out inadvertent injury to the collecting system.
4. Aggressive cyst decortication of as many surface and subsurface cysts as possible is advisable for ADPKD. Laparoscopic ultrasound will facilitate identification of accessible cysts.

57.9 Discussion

Asymptomatic renal cysts are usually an incidental finding in pediatric urology workup. Although mostly benign requiring only conservative treatment and regular follow-up, yet careful observation is necessary to filter suspicious ones for further imaging. Renal ultrasound, CT, and MRI in addition to guided aspiration for cytological examination are all valid tools in properly selected patients.

Percutaneous cyst aspiration with optional sclerotherapy can be offered as first-line therapy for simple symptomatic renal cysts that fail conservative medical management. However, complex cysts, ADPKD cysts, and peripelvic cysts may be best managed initially with formal open or laparoscopic decortication and proper tissue sampling for histopathological examination. Laparoscopic cyst decortication has been shown to be a safe, efficacious, and minimally invasive approach for treatment of renal cysts in experienced hands.

Long-term follow-up has confirmed that laparoscopic cyst decortication is an effective and durable treatment option for symptomatic simple renal cysts during long-term follow-up. It has the merit of minimal invasiveness, lower recurrence, and cost-effectiveness if compared to percutaneous cyst ablation, sclerotherapy, and open surgery. Hence, it should be offered as the first surgical option for symptomatic renal cysts in children. A suggested algorithm for renal cyst management in children is shown in Fig. 57.7.

References

1. Tada S, Yamagishi J, Kobayashi H, et al. The incidence of simple renal cyst by computed tomography. Clin Radiol. 1983;34:437–9.
2. Wein AJ, Kavoussi LR, Novick AC, et al. Campbell-Walsh urology. 11th ed; 2016. p. 2425–610. https://doi.org/10.1016/B978-1-4160-6911-9.00061-X.
3. Gabow P. Autosomal dominant polycystic kidney disease. N Engl J Med. 1993;329:332–42. https://doi.org/10.1056/NEJM199307293290508.

4. McHugh K, Stringer DA, Hebert D, Babiak CA. Simple renal cysts in children: diagnosis and follow-up with US. Radiology. 1991;178:383–5. https://doi.org/10.1148/radiology.178.2.1987597.
5. Laucks SPJ, McLachlan MS. Aging and simple cysts of the kidney. Br J Radiol. 1981;54:12–4. https://doi.org/10.1259/0007-1285-54-637-12.
6. Torres VE, Harris PC, Cystic diseases of Kidney. J Urol 2015;17:70–76.
7. Kissane JM, Smith MG. Pathology of infancy & childhood. St. Louis: Mosby; 1967.
8. Papanicolaou N, Pfister RC, Yoder IC. Spontaneous and traumatic rupture of renal cysts: diagnosis and outcome. Radiology. 1986;160:99–103. https://doi.org/10.1148/radiology.160.1.3715054.
9. Goldman S, Hartman D. The simple renal cysts. In: Pollack H, editor. Clinical urography. Philadelphia: Saunders; 1990. p. 1603.
10. Wallis MC, Lorenzo AJ, Farhat WA, et al. Risk assessment of incidentally detected complex renal cysts in children: potential role for a modification of the bosniak classification. Int Braz J Urol. 2009;35:115–6.
11. Bosniak MA. The current radiological approach to renal cysts. Radiology. 1986;158:1–10. https://doi.org/10.1148/radiology.158.1.3510019.
12. Karmazyn B, Tawadros A, Delaney LR, et al. Ultrasound classification of solitary renal cysts in children. J Pediatr Urol. 2015;11:149.e1–6. https://doi.org/10.1016/j.jpurol.2015.03.001.
13. Akinci D, Gumus B, Ozkan OS, et al. Single-session percutaneous ethanol sclerotherapy in simple renal cysts in children: long-term follow-up. Pediatr Radiol. 2005;35:155–8. https://doi.org/10.1007/s00247-004-1337-y.
14. Valdivia Uria JG, Abril Baquero G, Monzon Alebesque F, Lanchares Santamaria E. [Laparoscopic ablation of renal cysts]. Arch Esp Urol. 1994;47:246–52.
15. Lotan Y, Pearle MS, Cadeddu JA. Laparoscopic renal cyst decortication. In: Nakada SY, editor. Essential urologic laparoscopy: the complete clinical guide. Totowa: Humana Press; 2003. p. 59–78.
16. Esposito C, Escolino M, Troncoso Solar B, et al. Diagnosis and long-term outcome of renal cysts after laparoscopic partial nephrectomy in children. BJU Int. 2017;119:761–6. https://doi.org/10.1111/bju.13698.
17. Koh C, Cserni T, Hawkes R, et al. The management of symptomatic simple renal cysts in children. J Pediatr Surg Case Rep. 2018;28 https://doi.org/10.1016/j.epsc.2017.09.002.
18. Zafides B et al. Laparoscopic retroperitoneal decortication of a right renal cyst. J Endourol. 2016;30:A414–5. https://doi.org/10.1089/end.2016.29020.abstracts.
19. Rubenstein SC, Hulbert JC, Pharand D, et al. Laparoscopic ablation of symptomatic renal cysts. J Urol. 1993;150:1103–6.
20. Guazzoni G, Bellinzoni P, Montorsi F, et al. Laparoscopic unroofing of simple renal cysts. Urology. 1994;43:154–9. https://doi.org/10.1016/0090-4295(94)90035-3.
21. Wada T, Kamiryo Y, Tsuchida M, Kato M. Laparoscopic unroofing of a renal cyst. Hinyokika Kiyo. 1995;41:861–5. https://doi.org/10.1016/S0022-5347(17)37043-X.
22. Ou YC, Yang CR, Chang YY, et al. The clinical experience of gaseous retroperitoneoscopic and gasless retroperitoneoscopy-assisted unroofing of renal cyst. Zhonghua Yi Xue Za Zhi (Taipei). 1997;59:232–9.
23. Denis E, Nicolas F, Ben Rais N, et al. [Laparoscopic surgical treatment of simple cysts of the kidney]. Prog Urol. 1998;8:195–200.
24. Fahlenkamp D, Rassweiler J, Fornara P, et al. Complications of laparoscopic procedures in urology: experience with 2,407 procedures at 4 German centers. J Urol. 1999;162:765–71. https://doi.org/10.1097/00005392-199909010-00038.
25. Roberts WW, Bluebond-Langner R, Boyle KE, et al. Laparoscopic ablation of symptomatic parenchymal and peripelvic renal cysts. Urology. 2001;58:165–9. https://doi.org/10.1016/S0090-4295(01)01145-1.
26. Atug F, Burgess SV, Ruiz-Deya G, et al. Long-term durability of laparoscopic decortication of symptomatic renal cysts. Urology. 2006;68:272–5. https://doi.org/10.1016/j.urology.2006.03.009.
27. Santiago L, Yamaguchi R, Kaswick J, Bellman GC. Laparoscopic management of indeterminate renal cysts. Urology. 1998;52:379–83. https://doi.org/10.1016/S0090-4295(98)00213-1.
28. Warren KS, McFarlane J. The Bosniak classification of renal cystic masses. BJU Int. 2005;95:939–42.
29. Elzinga LW, Barry JM, Torres VE, et al. Cyst decompression surgery for autosomal dominant polycystic kidney disease. J Am Soc Nephrol. 1992;2:1219–26.
30. Chehval MJ, Neilsen C. Laparoscopic cyst decompression in polycystic kidney disease. J Endourol. 1995;9:281–2. https://doi.org/10.1089/end.1995.9.281.
31. Brown JA, Torres VE, King BF, Segura JW. Laparoscopic marsupialization of symptomatic polycystic kidney disease. J Urol. 1996;156:22–7. https://doi.org/10.1016/S0022-5347(01)65927-5.
32. Lifson BJ, Teichman JMH, Hulbert JC. Role and long-term results of laparoscopic decortication in solitary cystic and autosomal dominant polycystic kidney disease. J Urol. 1998;159:702–5. https://doi.org/10.1016/S0022-5347(01)63704-2.
33. Lee DI, Andreoni CR, Rehman J, et al. Laparoscopic cyst decortication in autosomal dominant polycystic kidney disease: impact on pain, hypertension, and renal function. J Endourol. 2003;17:345–54. https://doi.org/10.1089/089277903767923100.
34. Dunn MD, Portis AJ, Naughton C, et al. Laparoscopic cyst marsupialization in patients with autosomal dominant polycystic kidney disease. J Urol. 2001;165:1888–92.

58 Minimally Invasive Surgery Management of Urachal Pathology

A. A. Gusev, S. P. Yatzik, I. V. Kirgizov, and E. Yu. Dyakonova

58.1 Introduction

Urachal pathologies are mostly often found in newborns, and the frequency of its occurrence is rather high (according to some data, up to 30–50% of newborns have this or that urachal pathology). However considering the possible asymptomatic of some embodiments of this disease, as well as continuing to 1.5 years of overgrowing the duct, the incidence gradually decreases. Up to 95% of all urachal diseases are detected in childhood. This pathology is also diagnosed within adults, further less often, although with a frequency of up to 1:5000 and most of all according to autopsy data, since they cannot manifest themselves in any way throughout their life [1]. Meanwhile, there are sporadic cases of diagnosis in other studies (cystoscopy, cystography, ultrasound), as well as cases requiring surgical intervention (suppuration, diverticula, etc.) [2–6].

Urachus—the urinary duct, which connects the tip of the bladder with the umbilical cord, is a derivative of the intraperitoneal segment of the allantois and in the early stages of embryogenesis is a duct connecting the bladder to the extraembryonic allantoic part. By 5–7 months of intrauterine development, it is usually finally obliterated and becomes the middle vesicle-umbilical ligament. However, in some cases, the lumen of the urachus persists for the rest of life. It should also be noted that the immediate causes of disturbance of the obliteration of this duct are not clear yet. If the process of obliteration in the intrauterine period fails, then after the birth of the baby and falling of the umbilical cord, the duct (or part of it) remains open [7].

A. A. Gusev (✉) · S. P. Yatzik · I. V. Kirgizov
E. Yu. Dyakonova
Federal State Autonomous Institution "National Medical Research Center of Children's Health" of the Ministry of Health of the Russian Federation, Moscow, Russia
e-mail: DrGusev@yandex.ru

58.1.1 Classification

The development of urachus malformations is subdivided into four types depending on the imperforate degree: umbilical fistula, urachus cyst, bladder-navel fistula, and bladder diverticulum (Fig. 58.1).

The most common case is the non-obliterated umbilical urachal part or its cyst, formed after imperforate outer and inner parts of the embryonic bladder stroke. This is the "umbilical fistula" and "urachal cyst." Clinically, in umbilical fistula, the skin around is macerated and inflamed, and there are granulation and serous secretion. With probe exploring, a blindly terminating pocket is revealed in the direction of the bladder along the median line. Often, the umbilical fistula

C. Esposito et al. (eds.), *ESPES Manual of Pediatric Minimally Invasive Surgery*,
https://doi.org/10.1007/978-3-030-00964-9_58

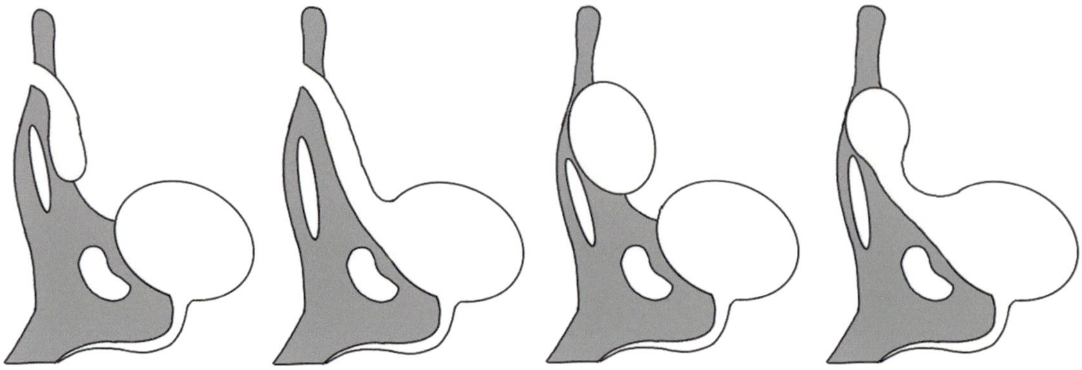

Fig. 58.1 Cysts type

may become infected and then joins purulent secretion. Urachal cyst may not manifest itself clinically until the moment of inflammation and is diagnosed exclusively when performing ultrasound or surgical interventions on the organs of the abdominal cavity. Depending on the location, paravesical, intermediate, and umbilical urachal cysts are distinguished. The urachal cyst can communicate with a narrow fistulous course with the navel, bladder, or simultaneously with both, and in this case, the symptoms of suppuration join the infection—there is pain, hyperemia of the skin over a tumorlike formation, fever, and inflammatory changes in clinical blood tests.

In the presence of a fistula of a festering cyst in the navel area, pus or pus mixed with blood is secreted from the fistula hole. With palpation of the anterior abdominal wall below the navel, the detachable amount is increased. When connecting festering urachal cysts with bladder, cystitis and pyuria occur. Also suppuration of the cyst can cause a phlegmon of the anterior abdominal wall, and a cyst rupture can lead to the emergence of diffuse peritonitis. The mechanism of formation and growth of cyst morphologists is explained by metaplasia of the transitional epithelium of the urachus in the cylindrical epithelium, which produces a serous fluid filling the lumen of the nonperforated portion of the embryonic duct, which leads to its expansion. Infection is also possible by hematogenous and lymphogenous or through the fistula way.

If the lower part of the urachal communicating with the bladder remains open, then the bladder diverticulum (apical diverticulum of the bladder) is diagnosed. The clinical picture will depend on its size, diameter of communication with the bladder; the inflammatory changes presence. Diverticulum also cannot clinically manifest itself and can be diagnosed accidentally during cystoscopy, cystography, or ultrasound exam. If the connection performed with a narrow hole, then emptying it is difficult, and residual urine will cause stretching and atony of the cystic walls, causing infection and the development of cystitis and diverticulitis. Dysuria, suprapubic pain appears. This pathology is best visualized with the cystography in a tight filling and/or at the height of the act of urination. The treatment of apical diverticulum of the bladder is only operative.

The least common is the functioning bladder-umbilical fistula. Clinically, the discharge of urine can be noted from the navel (drop by drop, but with a child's anxiety and the tension of the anterior abdominal wall—a flow). In the case of a complete fistula, the introduction of coloring agents (e.g., methylene blue or indigo carmine) helps in the diagnosis. Staining urine will indicate the communication of the fistula with the bladder. In the diagnosis of the fistula, X-ray fistulography and cystography are also performed [7].

58.1.2 Treatment

Conservative therapy for urachal malformations is possible only if there is an umbilical fistula (sinus). In all other cases (as well as in cases of ineffectiveness of conservative therapy), surgical treatment is performed. In the presence of an active inflammatory process, the acute exacerbation of the infection should be primarily reversed. If surgical treatment is performed during an acute inflammatory process, the likelihood of developing peritonitis and/or urosepsis is very high [8].

58.2 Open Surgery

(a) When the duct is completely open (functioning bladder-umbilical fistula)

The position of the patient "on the back" the bladder is firstly filled through the urethral catheter to facilitate the mobilization of the front wall. A probe or dye is injected into the bladder through the urachus. The lower midline incision (due to the high location of the children's bladder, the incision should be executed closer to the navel) or the lower cross section of the skin above the pubic symphysis is to be made further. Perform a complete extraperitoneal excision of the urachus all the way from the navel to the tip of the bladder. The defect of the wall of the bladder is eliminated by superimposing double-stranded sutures.

(b) In the umbilical fistula—a radical method of treatment is also the excision of the urachus along the entire length together with the umbilical part. However, in young children, it is primarily better to try conservative therapy because of possible independent obliteration of the fistula. Conservative therapy should be aimed at preventing and treating secondary infection.

(c) Urachal cyst

The treatment is exclusively surgical. Small (infected and uninfected) cysts should be removed simultaneously with the urachus right up to the bladder. Large ones can first drain through the abdominal wall. In the case of suppuration, the cyst surgery is performed in two stages: the first stage, the opening and drainage of the cysts and, the second, its radical removing with the urachus after decrease the inflammation.

(d) In the case of a diverticulum of the bladder

The treatment of apical diverticulum is focused on its complete excision throughout. The defect of the bladder wall around the entrance hole of the urachus is closed with a double-row suture.

58.3 Minimally Invasive Surgery Treatment of Urachal Malformations

Since surgical treatment is necessary in almost all cases of detection, in addition to the umbilical fistula, there are several options for accessing and locating trocars (from 3 to 4) for entering the abdominal cavity and for optimal visualization (Fig. 58.2). Some authors suggest installing trocars for instruments in one half of the abdominal cavity, part from both sides. Often a trocar for a video

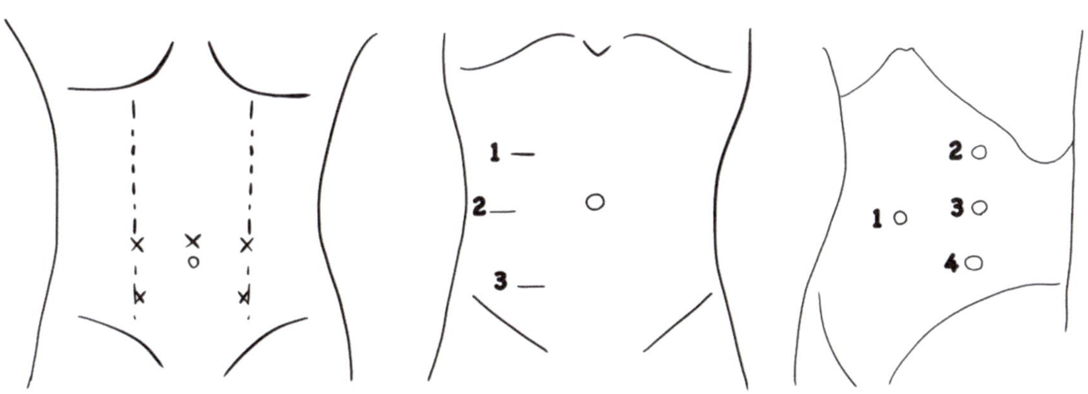

Fig. 58.2 Trocar placement

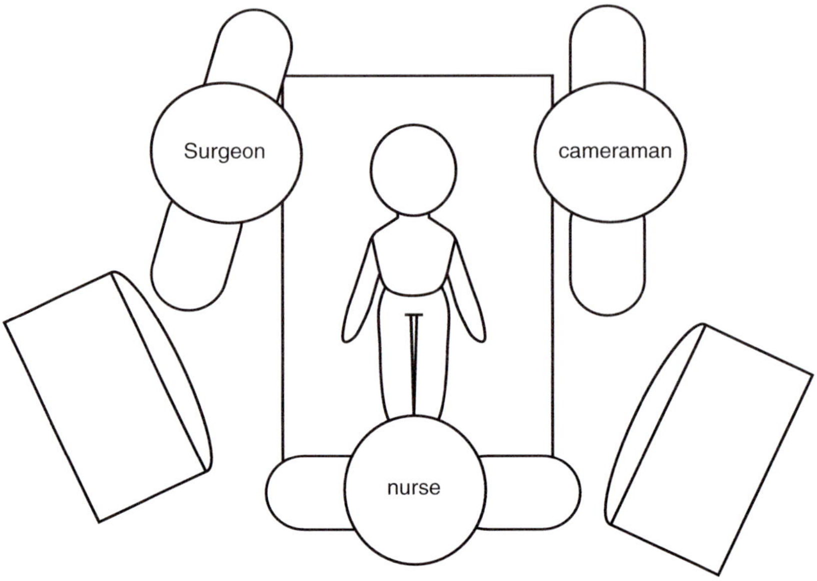

Fig. 58.3 Team position

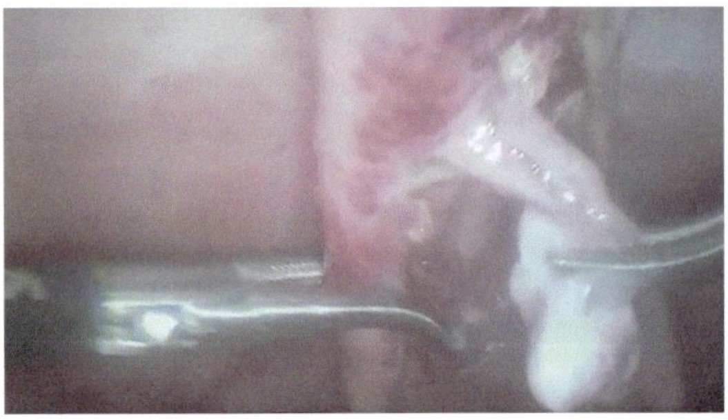

Fig. 58.4 Cyst's isolation and dissection

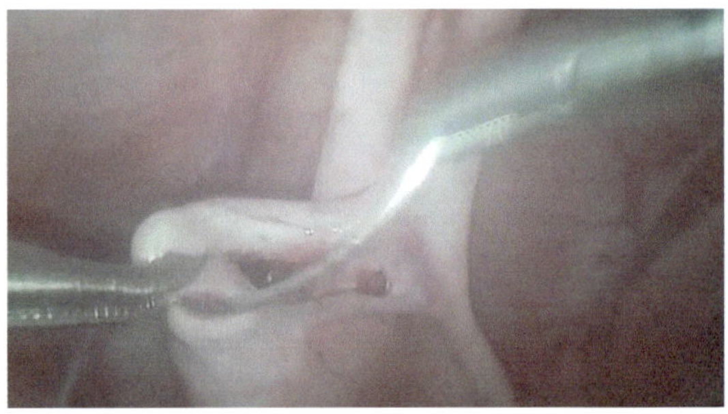

Fig. 58.5 Closure of the base of urachal cyst with a stitch

camera is placed in the navel area. However, a part of the authors (including in our experience) install it at 1–2 cm above the navel on the median line. Each of these techniques has the right to exist [9].

Direct surgical treatment is the maximum excision of the cyst itself and, accordingly, the ligament [10].

For an access to the abdominal cavity, we decided to use three trocars: one for the video camera and two for the instruments. A 5 mm trocar for video camera 30° was installed 2 cm above the navel on the median line, and the trocars for instruments—on the sides of the navel along the middle clavicular line—were also 5 mm. The layout of the staff is shown on Fig. 58.3 [11, 1].

When installing the camera and revision of the abdominal cavity below the umbilical ring, a

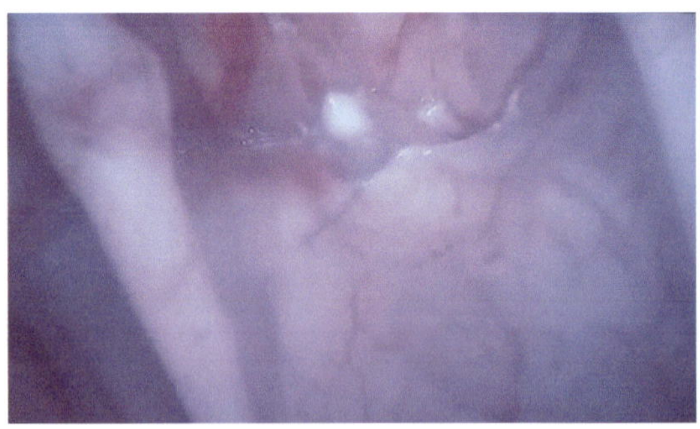

Fig. 58.6 Final aspect of the procedure

circular volume formation along the median line is revealed, and the body of the cyst is removed using coagulation (Fig. 58.4). After isolation and excision of the cyst, the median ligament is also isolated throughout the bladder and in the direction of the navel, stitched, coagulated, and cut (Figs. 58.5 and 58.6) [12].

58.4 Conclusion

Urachal malformations are fairly common anomaly in children. However, given the possibility of asymptomatic course of some variants of the disease, as well as the continuation of the imperforate flow until the age of 1–1.5 years, its rate is gradually reduced. The operation of choice for both uncomplicated and festering cysts should be considered as its radical excision along with the urinary duct. Minimally invasive surgical treatment should also be considered as a choice option for this pathology, since the laparoscopic access significantly reduces the volume of tissue traumatization, the duration of pain syndrome in the postoperative period, and the length of stay of the child in the hospital; apart from the cosmetic result of surgical treatment is qualitatively better [13–15].

References

1. Pedro PJ, Edgar V, Carlos R, Amilcar S. Urachal abscess clinically mimicking a malignancy. Clin Exp Pathol. 2013;4(1):154. https://doi.org/10.4172/2161-0681.1000154.
2. Ashley R, Inman B, Routh J, Rohlinger A, Husmann D, Kramer S. Urachal anomalies: a longitudinal study of urachal remnants in children and adults. J Urol. 2007;178:1615–8.
3. Castanheira de Oliveira M, Vila F, Versos R, et al. Laparoscopic treatment of urachal remnants. Actas Urol Esp. 2012;36:320–4.
4. Castillo OA, Vitagliano G, Olivares R, Sanchez-Salas R. Complete excision of urachal cyst by laparoscopic means: a new approach to an uncommon disorder. Arch Esp Urol. 2007;60:607–11.
5. Cutting CW, Hindley RG. Laparoscopic management of complicated urachal remnants. BJU Int. 2005;96:1417–21.
6. Ekwueme KC, Parr NJ. Infected urachal cyst in an adult: a case report and review of the literature. Cases J. 2009;2:6422.
7. Huang C, Luo C, Chao H, Chen H, Chu S. Urachal anomalies in children: experience at one institution. Chang Gung Med J. 2003;26:412–6.
8. Joung HJ, Han DY, Kwon W-A. Laparoscopic management of complicated urachal remnants. Chonnam Med J. 2013;49:43–7.
9. Kumar K, Mehenna D. Injury of urachal diverticulum due to laparoscope port: a case report, literature review and recommendations. J Med Cases. 2015;6(1):1–5.
10. Little D, Shah S, St Peter S, Calkins C, Murphy J, Gatti J, et al. Urachal anomalies in children: the vanishing relevance of the preoperative voiding cystourethrogram. J Pediatr Surg. 2005;40:1874–6.
11. Moore KL. The developing human: clinically oriented embryology. 2nd ed. Philadelphia: WB Saunders Company; 1977. p. 307–9.
12. Trondsen E, Reiertsen O, Rosseland A. Laparoscopic excision of urachal sinus. Eur J Surg. 1993;159:127–8.
13. Whitehead A, Arthur LG, Prasad R. Laparoscopic vs open excision of urachal remnants in children. J Surg. 2015;2(2):3.
14. Widni EE, Höllwarth ME, Haxhija EQ. The impact of preoperative ultrasound on correct diagnosis of urachal remnants in children. J Pediatr Surg. 2010;45:1433–7.
15. Yiee JH, Garcia N, Baker LA, Barber R, Snodgrass WT, Wilcox DT. A diagnostic algorithm for urachal anomalies. J Pediatr Urol. 2007;3:500–4.

59 Laparoscopic Resection of Wilms' Tumours

Marc-David Leclair

The Wilms' tumour (synonym: nephroblastoma) represents more than 90% of the paediatric renal tumours. Other possible aetiologies comprise clear cell sarcoma of the kidney (CCSK), malignant rhabdoid tumour of the kidney (MRTK), renal cell carcinoma (RCC), and congenital mesoblastic nephroma (CMN).

The hallmark of the SIOP-Renal Tumour Study Group strategy is based on preoperative chemotherapy (without preceding mandatory histological assessment), followed by surgery. This neoadjuvant chemotherapy strategy has been clearly associated with downstaging tumours, thereby sparing survivors the late effects of anthracycline and radiotherapy by 20% as compared to patients treated with primary surgery [1].

Consecutive SIOP protocols and trials have consistently considered open radical nephroureterectomy as the gold standard approach for treating WT. According to surgical guidelines, the procedure should be performed through a long transverse abdominal or thoraco-abdominal incision, to allow careful inspection of the abdominal cavity and liver, retroperitoneal lymph node sampling, and radical nephroureterectomy outside of the Gerota's fascia, including perirenal fat and sometimes the adrenal gland in monobloc resection.

With the development of a high level of expertise in laparoscopy in several paediatric surgery institutions, it became obvious during the last 15 years that some WT could be amenable to safe resection, following the same guidelines, using minimally invasive surgery. However, it should be kept in mind that WT carries an excellent oncological prognosis and that uncontrolled spreading of laparoscopic attempts at resections might jeopardise patients' survival through an increased risk of local relapse.

59.1 Indications

Achievement of complete microscopic resection represents a major stake in the treatment of Wilms' tumour, and the local stage remains a powerful independent prognostic factor. Hence, the indication for laparoscopy should be mostly grounded on the feasibility of a resection with the same safety margins as compared to open surgery. The SIOP-RTSG has provided a list of criteria, assessing the feasibility of safe laparoscopic radical nephroureterectomy. These criteria have been implemented in the recent SIOP-UMBRELLA protocol. The main philosophy is to exclude all tumours for which there may exists

M.-D. Leclair (✉)
Pediatric Surgery Department, NANTES University Children Hospital, Nantes, France
e-mail: mdleclair@chu-nantes.fr

C. Esposito et al. (eds.), *ESPES Manual of Pediatric Minimally Invasive Surgery*,
https://doi.org/10.1007/978-3-030-00964-9_59

a risk of microscopic incomplete resection or rupture, therefore requiring high toxicity adjuvant therapy such as radiotherapy and prolonged postoperative chemotherapy.

59.2 Indications for Laparoscopic Nephrectomy

1. Resection must adhere to oncological principles and include lymph node sampling.
2. Small, central tumours with rim of "normal" renal tissue.
3. The extraction of the specimen in a bag, without morcellation, through an adequate abdominal wall incision, is mandatory, not only to control the risk of dissemination but also to ensure adequate histopathological staging.
4. If a nephron-sparing surgery (NSS) is feasible, it should be preferred even if an open approach is needed.

59.3 Contraindications for Laparoscopic Nephrectomy

1. Tumour infiltrating extra renal structures or extended beyond the ipsilateral border of spinal column
2. Thrombus in the renal vein or vena cava
3. Peripheral location if NSS is not deemed feasible
4. Tumour without any response to chemotherapy due to the risk of tumour rupture
5. Little or no experience in laparoscopic nephrectomy (consider transfer to another unit or obtain more experienced help)

To the list of contraindications, it should probably be added any tumour with suspected fragility, for example, with subcapsular haemorrhage. Similarly, any tumour with suspicion of invasion of the liver capsule, colon, or abdominal wall should be excluded, predicting difficulties of resection with a risk of stage 3 which would be attributed to the laparoscopic technique until proven otherwise.

One major aspect is the understanding that lymph node sampling is extremely important to allow adequate staging of the disease. It has been shown that absence of LN sampling is associated with an increased risk of local relapse, as absence of diagnosis of LN metastases leads to understaging and under-treatment of the disease [2]. Therefore, the same rules of systematic inspection and sampling of retroperitoneal nodes should be followed with laparoscopy than open surgery. It is advisable that exclusively transperitoneal approach be considered when discussing MIS for Wilms' tumour resection; retroperitoneoscopic access, although theoretically feasible for radical nephrectomy of small tumours, hinders adequate LN sampling, total ureterectomy down to the ureterovesical junction, and most importantly impedes extraction of an intact specimen without morcellation for adequate staging analysis.

59.4 Technique

The patient is positioned in full or 3/4 lateral decubitus, to allow transperitoneal laparoscopic access. The video stack is placed in the back of the patient head, and surgeon stands at the front, his assistant on the same side at the level of the head for kidney dissection. Positions of the surgeon and his assistant will be switched for ureteric dissection. Markings for Pfannenstiel incision (to allow extraction of the specimen) are drawn when supine before positioning the patient.

Trocars placement (Fig. 59.1) follows the rules of transperitoneal access to kidney and adrenal gland surgery: three 5 mm ports are placed at equivalent distance of the ribs margin, leaving some space for a possible fourth port whenever necessary.

Optical trocar placement depends on the laparoscope used: umbilical position is suitable when using a 30° scope; if using a 0°, umbilical position might be too low and tangential to the bowel and requires placement along the edge of the rectus abdominis external sheath.

One of the instrument ports (usually in the iliac fossa) can be converted into a 10 mm trocar during the procedure, especially to allow the use

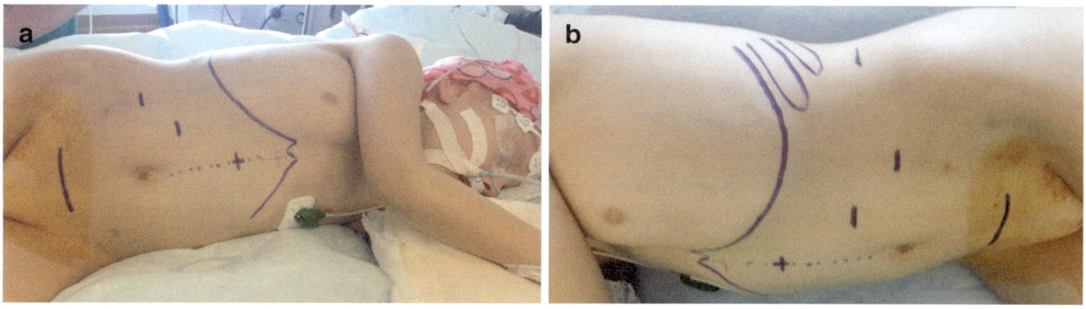

Fig. 59.1 Position of the trocars. (**a**) Front view of position for right nephrectomy. (**b**) Sagittal view for left nephrectomy (note the possibility of a fourth operating port posteriorly)

of large clips (10 mm hemolock clips, e.g., to allow safe control of a large vein in old children) and to allow introduction of a large bag before specimen extraction.

A fourth ancillary port may be necessary in different occasions: on the midline near the xiphoid to help maintaining liver retraction for right kidney tumours or posteriorly in the flank to assist kidney mobilisation and/or spleen retraction for left tumours.

59.5 Tactics and Strategy

The aim is to perform monobloc enlarged radical nephroureterectomy outside of the Gerota's fascia, with ureter ligation down at the level of the bladder. This implies exposition of the aorto-caval axis and ascending dissection along the inferior vena cava (IVC) or the aorta from the iliac vessels up to the renal pedicle. Complete resection with margins free of any microscopic residual disease is mandatory in WT; any microscopic residue requires intensive adjuvant treatment (radiation therapy and prolonged chemotherapy). General guidelines emphasise the need for ligation of the arterial vessels first, to avoid dangerous venous congestion and swelling of the tumour. It is however possible to perform primary division of the vein once the artery location has been ascertained hidden behind the vein, assuming arterial control will be greatly facilitated once the vein is divided. As a general rule, the renal artery should be controlled first whenever possible.

Right kidney tumour resection: main steps are listed below.

- Mobilisation of the right colon, including right colonic flexure and the cecum to provide access to the iliac vessels and the ureter.
- Dissection begins along the right edge of the right iliac vein and proceeds cranially along the IVC. Right gonadal vessels are usually unnecessarily divided twice, first when isolating the lower ureter and the iliac vein and then at their confluence in the IVC. Dissection continues cranially to expose the renal vein and proceeds upward to get control of the suprarenal IVC. Full external mobilisation of peritoneal attachment of the right liver is then necessary to allow adequate exposition of the upper pole of the kidney and the adrenal gland. An additional port may be necessary to maintain the liver.
- Mobilisation of the duodeno-pancreatic block, to allow access to the anterior IVC and the aorto-caval space. Control of the right renal artery should always be performed along the right aorta (as opposed to the right edge of the IVC).
- Once the renal pedicle has been controlled, mobilisation of the kidney is performed. Decision has to be made at the upper pole of the kidney whether excision should be extended to the right adrenal gland, according to preoperative imaging and intraoperative findings.
- Mobilisation of the upper pole should not hesitate to go through the diaphragmatic muscle

fibres if there is any suspicion of extension of the tumour beyond the limit of the Gerota's fascia. Similarly, mobilisation of the external and posterior aspects of the kidney can safely be performed through the thickness of the transverse and psoas most superficial fibres.
- Dissection of the ureter is followed down to the posterior bladder wall, trying to leave a stump as short as possible.
- Specimen must be placed in a bag with manipulations as limited as possible to avoid rupture or spillage and then extracted though a Pfannenstiel incision.

Left kidney tumour resection follows similar strategy with few tactical variants:

- The main anatomical landmark of the renal vein is the splenic vein. The spleen will be freed from its external peritoneal attachment. Lateral positioning of the child and gravity allow the spontaneous medial fall of the spleen, unveiling the posterior aspect of the pancreas tail. The splenic vein is then followed and usually leads to the left renal vein at its crossing the anterior aorta.
- The adrenal gland will be resected en bloc in the majority of left WT (as opposed to right tumours), as the left renal vein will often have to be ligated close to the IVC, therefore occluding the main adrenal venous flow.
- Following the left side of the aorta proximally, attention must be paid to move away from the adventitial plane and go laterally to the diaphragm left crus

59.6 Postoperative Care

Bladder catheter can be removed at the end of the procedure or left indwelling in case of postoperative IV administration of morphinic analgesia. Nasogastric tube can be removed at the end of surgery, and the patient kept nil by mouth for 12–24 h. Infiltration of scars with local anaesthetic or placement of catheter for postoperative continuous instillation of Naropin within the Pfannenstiel incision can be a useful adjunct.

59.7 Outcomes

Few series [3–6] have investigated the outcomes of laparoscopic WT resection, since its first description by RJ Duarte et al. in 2004. The same Brazilian group provide long-term update of their series [4], with limited complications and favourable oncological outcomes. Of note, they observed a rate of 8% microscopic residual disease, within a highly selected subgroup of tumours deemed amenable to complete resection. In the multicentric French experience [5], similar favourable outcomes were reported, without any case of tumour rupture, spillage, or microscopic residue.

One important question remains the actual proportion of WT safely amenable to laparoscopic resection. The Brazilian pioneer group reported that laparoscopy was performed in 40% of the newly diagnosed case during the study period. Similarly, we retrospectively assessed theoretical feasibility of MIS following SIOP-RTSG criteria among a series of 100 consecutive unscreened WT [7] and observed a similar figure of 38%. Although it is likely that more cases could be amenable to safe resection with laparoscopy, it remains crucial that initial experience with MIS be conducted following the SIOP-RTSG criteria. One must admit that theoretical benefits of minimally invasive surgery (cosmesis, postoperative comfort, fewer bowel adhesions) should not result in jeopardizing the excellent oncological outcome.

References

1. Pritchard-Jones K, Shannon R, Hutton C, Stevens S, Machin D, et al. Immediate nephrectomy versus preoperative chemotherapy in the management of nonmetastatic Wilms' tumour: results of a randomised trial (UKW3) by the UK Children's Cancer Study Group. Eur J Cancer. 2006;42(15):2554–62.
2. Shamberger RC, Guthrie KA, Ritchey ML, Haase GM, Takashima J, Beckwith JB, D'Angio GJ, Green DM, Breslow NE. Surgery-related factors and local recurrence of Wilms tumor in National Wilms Tumor Study 4. Ann Surg. 1999;229(2):292–7.
3. Duarte RJ, Dénes FT, Cristofani LM, Giron AM, Filho VO, Arap S. Laparoscopic nephrectomy for wilms tumor after chemotherapy: initial experience. J Urol. 2004;172(4 Pt 1):1438–40.

4. Duarte RJ, Cristofani LM, Filho VO, Srougi M, Dénes FT. Videolaparoscopic radical nephrectomy after chemotherapy in the treatment of Wilms' tumor: long-term results of a pioneer group. J Pediatr Urol. 2017;13:50e1–5.
5. Varlet F, Petit T, Leclair MD, Lardy H, Geiss S, Becmeur F, et al. Laparoscopic treatment of renal cancer in children: a multicentric study and review of oncologic and surgical complications. J Pediatr Urol. 2014;10:500e5.
6. Warmann SW, Godzinski J, van Tinteren H, Heij H, Powis M, Sandstedt B, et al. Minimally invasive nephrectomy for Wilms' tumor in children—data from SIOP 2001. Surgical Panel of the SIOP Renal Tumor Strategy Group. J Pediatr Surg. 2014;49:1544–8.
7. Héloury Y, Floret A, Pellier I, Renaudin-Autain K, Quere MP, Thebaud E, Leclair MD. Nephron sparing surgery for unilateral unscreened Wilms tumour: how often is it feasible ? In: 47th congress of the International Society of Paediatric Oncology, Cape Town, South Africa; 2015.

Laparoscopic Mitrofanoff Procedure

60

Alaa El-Ghoneimi, Matthieu Peycelon, and Annabel Paye-Jaouen

60.1 Introduction

The continent cystostomy technique was first described by Mitrofanoff in 1980 and originally applied to children with neurological disorders [1]. It consists in fashioning a catheterizable channel with a flap-valve continence mechanism, in order to be both continent to promote storage and accessible to allow emptying. This method allows an alternative procedure for patients with urethral disease (congenital or acquired after surgery: exstrophy-epispadias complex) or for those with neurological disabilities who are unable or unwilling to access the urethral meatus. Indications for the procedure are varied: it may be used as isolated procedure for clean intermittent catheterization (CIC) or associated with bladder augmentation and another bladder surgery.

The potential benefits of the laparoscopic approach include decreased postoperative pain, shorter hospital stay, and improved cosmesis [2]. In recent years, few published papers have reported their experience and transition from laparoscopic-assisted to fully laparoscopic Mitrofanoff and lastly with robotic-assisted procedures, with variable results in regard to efficacy and feasibility [3–8].

In this chapter, we will describe the Mitrofanoff procedure without bladder augmentation done by standard laparoscopic technique.

60.2 Preoperative Preparation

The most important preparation for these children is the education for CIC. Children are managed along with their parents by the educational team (specialized nurse, psychologist); the pediatric urologist confirms the indication when the family and the child are aware perfectly of all the details and the technique.

No specific diet or preparation for these children is needed. In cases of neurogenic bladder associated with bowel dysfunction, an evacuation enema is done the night before. Preoperative flash antibiotics are given routinely.

60.3 Positioning

The patient is placed in the supine position. A Foley catheter is inserted in the sterile field.

The patient is placed in a Trendelenburg position after the placement of trocars.

The surgeon is standing on the left side in elder children. In young children (under 6 years,

A. El-Ghoneimi (✉) · M. Peycelon · A. Paye-Jaouen
Department of Pediatric Urology, National Reference Center of Rare Urinary Malformations, MARVU, University Hospital Robert Debre, APHP, University Paris Diderot, Paris, France
e-mail: alaa.elghoneimi@aphp.fr

C. Esposito et al. (eds.), *ESPES Manual of Pediatric Minimally Invasive Surgery*,
https://doi.org/10.1007/978-3-030-00964-9_60

which is rare for this indication), the surgeon may stand behind the head of the patient.

60.4 Instrumentation

Trocars: 5 mm (reusable or single use)
Laparoscope: 5 mm, 30°
All standard laparoscopic instruments 5 mm: grasping atraumatic, scissors, needle holder
Coagulation devises: Monopolar hook, bipolar
3 mm instruments: One trocar, needle holder (see tips and tricks)

60.5 Technique

The procedure is done following the already described technique [7]. The procedure is performed using a transperitoneal four-port approach. A 30-degree down camera angle is optimal for viewing the appendix and the posterior wall of the bladder. A 5 mm laparoscopic camera port is placed on the Medline through an open technique, halfway between the umbilicus and xiphoid. Three additional ports are placed in the right and left hypochondrium and right lower quadrant (Fig. 60.1).

The appendix is harvested, using bipolar coagulation, with preservation of the vascular supply and ligated at its base, by 2-0 Vicryl (polyglactin 910) using laparoscopic intracorporeal free-hand knot-tying technique; the base is left intact with the cecum.

Attention is then turned to the implantation of the appendix into the bladder. The bladder is filled to keep it distended. Using a monopolar hook, a 5 cm vertical seromuscular incision is created along the posterior wall of the bladder, down to the mucosa (Fig. 60.2).

A trial with two forceps is carried out to position the appendix in the most suitable way between the posterior wall of the full bladder and the umbilicus. A decision is taken according to the best suitable way either the base or the tip of the appendix to be sutured to the bladder. Mobilization of the appendix mesentery is done with care to keep the mesentery wide without twisting.

In most of our cases, the base of the appendix was chosen for the bladder anastomosis. The proximal 10 mm of the appendix are excised and then spatulated over 1 cm by sharp scissors without coagulation.

A small cystostomy is created at the caudal apex of the detrusor muscle trough: the bladder mucosa is incised approximately 1 cm in length. Appendicovesical anastomosis is then performed circumferentially with two running sutures (5-0 PDS polydioxanone, 3/8 circle needle). The first caudal suture between the appendix and the bladder mucosa also includes the detrusor muscle to fix the caudal part of the anastomosis and stabilize the anastomotic line during suturing (Fig. 60.3). After completing the anastomosis, the appendix is placed in the newly prepared

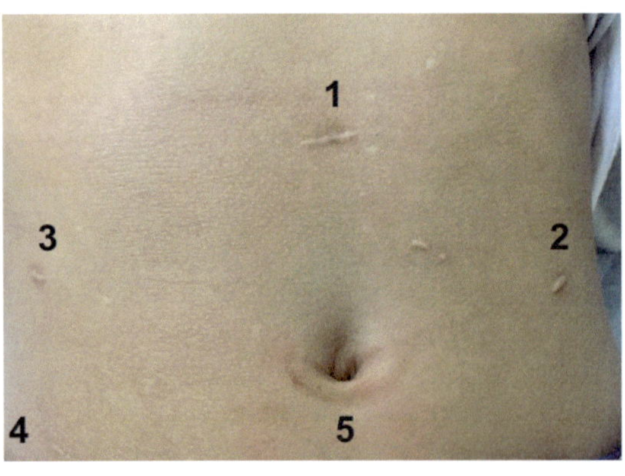

Fig. 60.1 Trocars placement and 1-year postoperative aspect: 5 mm camera (1), 5 mm operating trocars (2, 3, 4), umbilicus stoma aspect

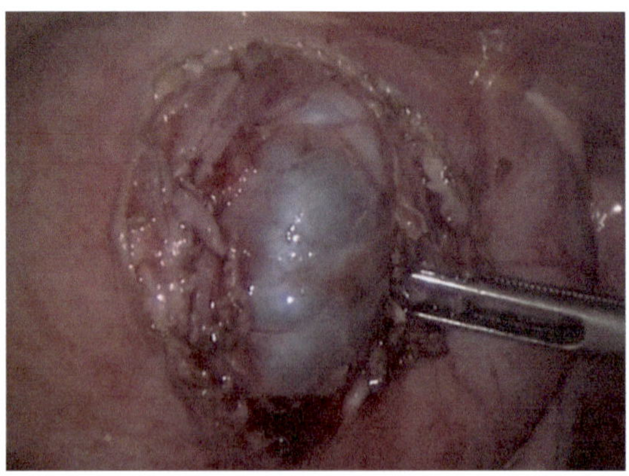

Fig. 60.2 Posterior wall detrusotomy

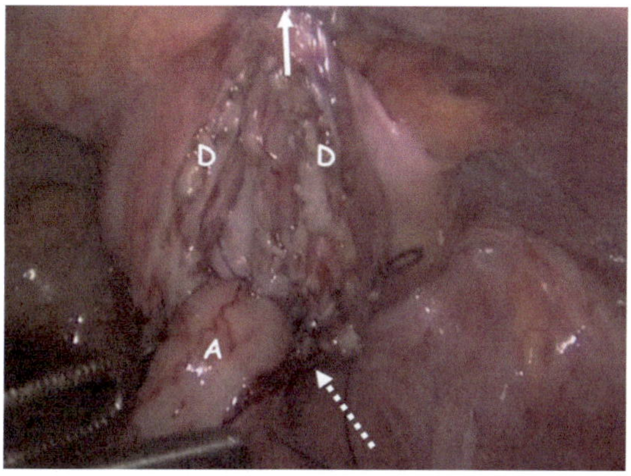

Fig. 60.3 The base of the appendix is anastomosed to the caudal end of the tunnel (interrupted arrow). The cranial end is retracted by a traction suture to facilitate the anastomosis (full arrow). *D* detrusor

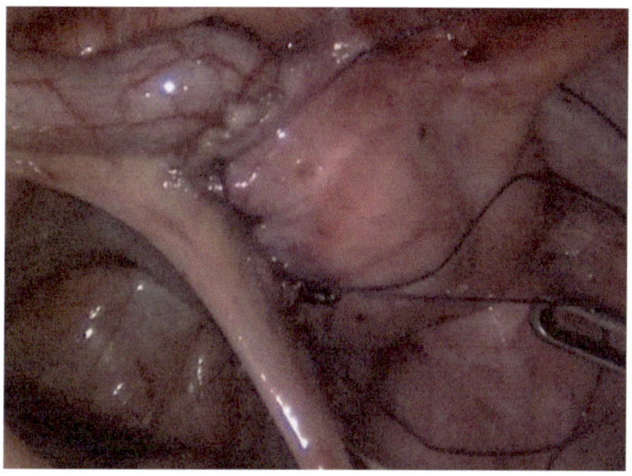

Fig. 60.4 The mesentery of the appendix is sutured to the pelvis peritoneum to avoid internal hernia

detrusor muscle trough, and the seromuscular layer of the bladder is closed over the appendix. To avoid compression of the mesentery, the sutures are done through the mesentery under laparoscopic vision, using interrupted 4-0 Vicryl, thus creating an antireflux mechanism. The window between the appendix and the peritoneum was closed to avoid internal hernia (only feasible in case of wide mesentery) (Fig. 60.4).

Care is taken to ensure absence of twisting or tension on the appendiceal mesentery. The tip of the appendix is brought up to the umbilicus (Fig. 60.5). Any extra length of the appendix is excised to obtain a straight channel without kinking. The appendix is then spatulated and anastomosed to the

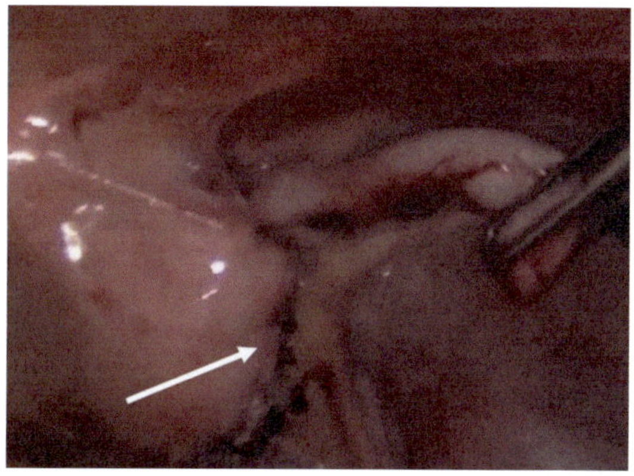

Fig. 60.5 The final aspect of the extra-mucosal tunnel, the appendix is extracted through the umbilicus

umbilicus using interrupted 5-0 PDS. Careful sharp dissection without coagulation is done to free the umbilical flap without ischemia of the skin. Neither the appendix nor the bladder is fixed to the abdominal wall.

The tightness of the bladder anastomosis is tested by bladder filling. Continence and ease of catheterization are checked and confirmed intraoperatively, after which a feeding tube (CH12) is inserted through the appendiceal conduit into the bladder, secured to the periumbilical skin with a suture and left indwelling for 2 weeks. The bladder is also drained by an indwelling urethral catheter. No abdominal drains are left.

60.6 Postoperative Care

Standard intravenous analgesics are given according to pain management protocol. No locoregional anesthesia (epidural catheter were used in our experience).

The child is discharged when no further need for IV analgesics.

The Mitrofanoff catheter was removed after 15 days, and CIC was then started. The initial training was done on outpatient clinic bases.

60.7 Results

Feasibility: The rate of conversion to open surgery is quite low (0–20%) and reported at the beginning of experience. The main reasons for conversion to an open procedure are:

1. Tearing of the bladder mucosa: this happens either during the creation of the tunnel, in the begining of our experience using the Hook harmonic scalpel, or during suturing.
2. The appendix is unsuitable for diversion: either by extensive dissection of the mesentery or more exceptionally the inadequate size.

The median operative time and hospital stay: In published series, the reported mean operative time is variable between 3 and 6 h. In our own experience, the median operative time is 4 h. No patient had anastomotic leakage. The reported median hospital stay is between 3 and 6 days, depending on the associated morbidity and other surgeries [4, 7, 8].

60.7.1 Early Complications

We did not observe any anastomotic leak, probably due to the efficient urine drainage by two catheters for 15 days.

60.7.2 Med- and Long-Term Complications

1. Stenosis: Stenosis may develop either at the stoma level or at the bladder level. In our experience we did not observe this complication. We believe that stenosis is an ischemia complication either from the skin flap or the appendix. Careful dissection of the appendix, without excessive coagulation, is certainly an important factor to prevent ischemia. Handling the skin flaps with care without excessive coagulation and mobilization is also an important factor.
2. Continence: Continent stoma is a challenging result and must be achieved for these patients. The rate of reported of incontinent stoma is still high.

In our initial experience, after a median follow-up of 18 months, none had stoma stenosis, and self-catheterization was easy.

Seven patients were continent; five experienced urinary leakage from the urethra and/or stoma. Stomal leak was observed within the first postoperative month. Three patients with stomal urinary leakage were successfully managed by Deflux (dextranomer-based implants) injection in the catheterizable channel. Two patients required an open revision of the appendicovesical anastomosis. The bladder access was easy with no adhesions on the anterior wall of the bladder. The patient with both stomal and urethral urinary leakage also required the implantation of an artificial urinary sphincter 1.5 years after the Mitrofanoff procedure. The other patients never underwent additional surgery (bladder or urinary tract) since the initial operation. Among the three converted patients, one was lost to follow-up, another has been augmented 3 years after the Mitrofanoff, and the third is doing well. In our current experience with additional ten cases (unpublished data), our incontinent stoma rate is 20%.

60.8 Tips and Tricks

For the last cases of the series (after the publication), some modifications were done because of the high rate of conversion due to early opening of the mucosa (harmonic hook) or difficult anastomosis.

1. Five millimeter trocars were used to change the 5 mm, 30° laparoscope position from the left to right subcostal area to better visualize the anastomosis.
2. 3 mm trocar: to optimize fine suturing during the anastomosis, we prefer 3 mm needle holder, so during the anastomosis, we insert a 3 mm trocar inside the 5 mm trocar to allow the temporary use of 3 mm instrument.
3. Use thread to measure exactly the length of the tunnel.
4. The anastomosis was suspended at its two ends during suturing. Transabdominal traction

suture of the bladder was inserted for better exposure of the anastomosis (hitch stitch) and to stabilize the anastomotic line during suturing (Fig. 60.2).

5. A monopolar hook was used to cut the detrusor muscle fibers, to avoid an incidental opening of the mucosa.
6. The window between the appendix and the peritoneum was closed to avoid internal hernia (only feasible in case of wide mesentery) (Fig. 60.4).

60.9 Discussion

The laparoscopic Mitrofanoff approach, although challenging, replicates the open surgical approach. We have already shown its feasibility and the need for further refinement to improve efficacy, for the management of patients with significant bladder dysfunction [7].

The optimal approach for lower urinary tract reconstruction is currently still to be defined. The conventional approach to a pediatric reconstructive procedure is open surgery using either a lower midline or Pfannenstiel incision. In recent years, several investigators have successfully incorporated laparoscopic and robotic-assisted approaches to reconstruct the lower urinary tract. Intracorporeal suturing is a technically demanding task that requires a significant amount of experience and surgical skill specifically when the suturing is located in the pelvic area.

These reports generally involve laparoscopic-assisted surgery that allows for mobilization of bowel segments, such as a high cecum, commonly seen in patients with myelomeningocele, followed by technically demanding reconstruction procedures by open surgery via a small incision. Chung et al. [2] reported 31 consecutive patients who underwent laparoscopic-assisted reconstructive surgery for continent stomas (antegrade continence enema or Mitrofanoff). Laparoscopy was used for lysis of adhesions, mobilization of colon, and/or harvesting the appendix. Jordan and Winslow [9] described a laparoscopic-assisted appendicovesicostomy: the appendix and right hemicolon were mobilized laparoscopically, and the appendicovesical anastomosis was completed through a Pfannenstiel incision.

The first laparoscopic application of the Mitrofanoff principle was reported by Strand et al. [10], who did a nephrectomy and creation of a cutaneous ureterovesicostomy using a transperitoneal laparoscopic approach.

Hsu and Shortliffe [8] performed the first fully LMA in an 11-year-old girl.

Two groups have published their preliminary experience of LMA in children [4, 5]. These series demonstrate the safety and feasibility of the procedure, using either the anterior or the posterior approach.

Since then, further reports have appeared in the pediatric literature describing appendicovesicostomy using the da Vinci robotic system [11–13], laparoscopic ileocystoplasty, robotically assisted laparoscopic ileocystoplasty, and Mitrofanoff appendicovesicostomy.

Certainly, the anastomosis is a difficult step especially as it is carried out on the most posterior and deepest part of the tunnel. The use of a robotic system is likely to make appendicovesical anastomosis easier and decrease the operative time.

The Chicago group of Gundeti reported the first case of complete intracorporeal robotic-assisted LMA with augmentation ileocystoplasty in a pediatric patient, and his group recently reported their experience in eight children with an anterior extravesical approach for isolated appendicovesicostomy and in 12 children with intravesical posterior bladder approach when concomitant enterocystoplasty was done [13].

To date, outcomes seem at least equal to those of traditional open approaches. In our experience, the laparoscopic approach was feasible in cases after previous abdominal surgery.

Among the potential benefits of a laparoscopic approach in young patients is decreased adhesion formation. Although follow-up is too short to comment on the impact of adhesion prevention in this series, there is ample evidence in the literature to suggest that long-term morbidity or future surgical complications related to abdominal adhesions should be minimal.

Beyond simply avoiding a large abdominal incision, thereby reducing postoperative pain and shortening the convalescent period, we believe that laparoscopy avoids the large dissection of the bladder necessary for its mobilization in open surgery. We found this of particular interest in this special group of patients, where the indication for future bladder augmentation was not excluded. In our current practice, we discuss bladder augmentation only in cases with prior treatment by CIC and anticholinergics. The laparoscopic approach in these patients does not need any bladder mobilization and leaves the anterior bladder wall free for any future bladder surgery.

We have chosen for the same reason to anastomose the appendix on the posterior wall of the bladder, to keep its anterior wall free for any further surgery. This choice was probably the source of difficulty to achieve the appendicovesical anastomosis. The depth of the field made suturing a challenging step. This difficulty was the reason for conversion in three cases. Our modification of the suturing step, by keeping a traction suture on each end of the anastomosis, allowed us to complete successfully the recent cases.

Badawy et al. [4] described their experience with successful fully laparoscopic approach. They did their first case doing the posterior wall anastomosis but changed to anterior wall anastomosis to ease the laparoscopic approach. We still believe that the anterior wall anastomosis is not the optimal anastomosis for an isolated Mitrofanoff procedure as it may reduce the potential benefits of the laparoscopic approach.

We have chosen not to use the umbilical site for the laparoscope trocar but to use a separate incision away from the umbilicus. This has added an extra incision, which may be considered as a reduction in cosmetic advantage. Nevertheless, we believe that the stoma site (umbilicus in our experience) should be kept only for the stoma anastomosis to avoid any skin trauma during the procedure. The choice of stoma site between umbilical and right iliac fossa is a question of surgeon's preferences as in open surgery.

However, choosing to perform a purely laparoscopic approach to lower urinary tract surgery in pediatric patients is uncommon, given the steep learning curve. In our experience the anastomosis remained the most difficult part of the surgery in spite of our large experience in reconstructive laparoscopic surgery.

In our early experience, we had the major complication of incontinent stoma in 5 patients (33%). In the paper by Leslie et al. [14], at least one subsequent surgical revision was performed in 39% of patients. Indications for surgical revision included stoma stenosis (at skin level) in 17% of patients, stricture in 8%, incontinence in 10%, and prolapse in 4%. This incontinence is poorly tolerated by the patients and their families as its management in daily life is complicated, thus reducing dramatically the benefits of the surgery for the patient. We have looked carefully at the details of the procedures for these children (recorded movies). One of them did not have fixation of the caudal end of the anastomosis to the detrusor muscle; probably the traction of the appendix to the umbilicus mobilized the appendix and significantly reduced the submucosal tunnel. For isolated stomal leakage, initial management with dextranomer/hyaluronic acid injection is favored, which is often successful with one or more treatments. Three patients had improved continence after Deflux injection associated with anticholinergics. Nevertheless, two children acquired a continent stoma after surgical revision. During redo surgery, it was clear that the tunnel was inexistent [15]. In our current practice for open surgery, we do not fix the bladder to the abdominal wall, and maybe the lack of this fixation together with the absence of fixation of the anastomosed appendix to the detrusor resulted in excessive traction on the appendix and shortening of the antireflux tunnel.

In the reported series with excellent results (100% continent stoma), these are bladders with high compliance and not hyperactive, such as prune belly bladders [13].

In other published series, the stoma continence rate is higher than in our series. Nguyen et al. [12] have reported nine patients fully done by robotic. In their series 2 of 9 (22%) had incontinent stoma and needed bladder augmentation in 1.

Gundeti et al. [8] reported the functional and perioperative outcomes of a multi-institutional cohort of pediatric patients who underwent robotic-assisted laparoscopic Mitrofanoff. This 5 North American centers' study included 88 children (17% had concomitant bladder augmentation, and 39% had bladder neck surgery). The 3-month rate of stoma incontinence was 15%. Mitrofanoff only procedure was done in 33 patients in 320 min (248–360).

To improve the efficacy of the antireflux mechanism, we suggest the following parameters: (a) suture the anastomotic line not only to the mucosa but also to the detrusor muscle to avoid excessive traction on the bladder mucosa; (b) suture the bladder to the abdominal wall, if the surgeon observes excessive traction; and (c) if it is possible according to the mesentery axes, the choice of the apex of the appendix for the bladder anastomosis would be easier to incorporate on the tunnel than the base of the appendix.

A limitation of the published studies is that they were carried out in a small number of children with different pathology and it could not be compared to an age-matched group of children with comparable bladder pathology. Moreover, in a life-lasting conduit, short-term follow-up reports are far behind reality especially for continence rate and stoma stenosis. In fact, the indication for this procedure in children without bladder augmentation is rare, and the learning curve is long because of the technical challenges.

References

1. Mitrofanoff P. Trans-appendicular continent cystostomy in the management of the neurogenic bladder. Chir Pediatr. 1980;21:297–305.
2. Chung SY, Meldrum K, Docimo SG. Laparoscopic assisted reconstructive surgery: a 7-year experience. J Urol. 2004;171:372–5.
3. Weller S, Bortagaray JI, Corbetta JP, Corro RJ, Durán V, Sager C, et al. Laparoscopic Mitrofanoff procedure using single "U-stitch" anastomosis: a way to make it simple. J Pediatr Urol. 2013;9:432–6.
4. Badawy H, Eid A, Dawood W, Hanno A. Safety and feasibility of laparoscopic appendicovesicostomy in children. J Pediatr Urol. 2013;9:427–31.
5. Nerli RB, Reddy M, Devraju S, Prabha V, Hiremath MB, Jali S. Laparoscopic Mitrofanoff appendicovesicostomy: our experience in children. Indian J Urol. 2012;28:28–31.
6. Casale P, Feng WC, Grady RW, Joyner BD, Lee RS, Mitchell ME. Intracorporeal laparoscopic appendicovesicostomy: a case report of a novel approach. J Urol. 2004;171:1899.
7. Blanc T, Muller C, Pons M, Pashootan P, Paye-Jaouen A, El Ghoneimi A. Laparoscopic Mitrofanoff procedure in children: critical analysis of difficulties and benefits. J Pediatr Urol. 2015;11(1):28.e1–8.
8. Gundeti MS, Petravick ME, Pariser JJ, Pearce SM, Anderson BB, Grimsby GM, Akhavan A, Dangle PP, Shukla AR, Lendvay TS, Cannon GM Jr, Gargollo PC. A multi-institutional study of perioperative and functional outcomes for pediatric robotic-assisted laparoscopic Mitrofanoff appendicovesicostomy. J Pediatr Urol. 2016;12(6):386.e1–5. https://doi.org/10.1016/j.jpurol.2016.05.031. Epub 2016 Jun 15.
9. Jordan GH, Winslow BH. Laparoscopically assisted continent catheterizable cutaneous appendicovesicostomy. J Endourol. 1993;7:517–20.
10. Strand WR, McDougall EM, Leach FS, Allen TD, Pearle MS. Laparoscopic creation of a catheterizable cutaneous ureter-ovesicostomy. Urology. 1997;49:272–5.
11. Pedraza R, Weiser A, Franco I. Laparoscopic appendicovesicostomy (Mitrofanoff procedure) in a child using the da Vinci robotic system. J Urol. 2004;171:1652–3.
12. Nguyen HT, Passerotti CC, Penna FJ, Retik AB, Peters CA. Robotic assisted laparoscopic Mitrofanoff appendicovesicostomy: preliminary experience in a pediatric population. J Urol. 2009;182:1528–34.
13. Famakinwa OJ, Rosen AM, Gundeti MS. Robot-assisted Laparoscopic Mitrofanoff appendicovesicostomy technique and outcomes of extravesical and intravesical approaches. Eur Urol. 2013;64(5):831–6.
14. Leslie B, Lorenzo AJ, Moore K, Farhat WA, Bägli DJ, Pippi Salle JL. Long-term followup and time to event outcome analysis of continent catheterizable channels. J Urol. 2011;185:2298–302.
15. El Ghoneimi A. Re: laparoscopic mitrofanoff procedure in children: critical analysis of difficulties and benefits. Blanc T, Muller C, Pons M, Pashootan P, Paye-Jaouen A, El Ghoneimi A. J Pediatr Urol 2015;11, 28.e1-8. J Pediatr Urol. 2015;11(5):303–4.

MIS Management of Posterior Urethral Valves (PUV)

61

Vincenzo Di Benedetto, Carmela Arena, and Maria Grazia Scuderi

61.1 Introduction

Posterior urethral valves (PUV) are the most common cause of bladder outlet obstruction in children. They occur in 1/5000–25,000 live births and constitute 10% of urinary obstruction diagnosed in utero [1–4]. PUV are associated with high fetal and neonatal mortality (30%) and considerable lifelong morbidity. The morbidity is related to the congenital obstruction of the urinary tract at the critical time in organogenesis which may have a profound and lifelong effect on kidney, ureter, and bladder function [4]. In severe cases, the disorder can lead to anhydramnios and pulmonary dysplasia during the canalicular phase of lung development. Mortality is related to ongoing renal damage in children.

61.2 Voiding Cystourethrography Imaging

The gold standard for postnatal diagnosis is voiding cystourethrography (VCUG), while prenatal diagnosis is dependent on routine screening ultrasonography. The diagnosis of PUV is sometimes difficult because of its wide spectrum in terms of severity and morphology. The most typical PUV is presented in neonates with history of prenatal bilateral hydronephrosis or in infants with acute pyelonephritis associated with massive vesicoureteral reflux (VUR). This group of PUV is easy to be diagnosed by typical findings in voiding cystourethrography (VCUG). More than half of the patients with PUV will have VUR at the time of diagnosis (Fig. 61.1) [2]. Secondary VUR may be difficult to detect in ordinary imaging studies because it does not present with conventional findings, such as dilatation of posterior urethra. Dilatation of posterior urethra is often transiently observed during the voiding phase of VCUG, or such dilatation may be totally absent, but segmental narrowing of the bulbomembranous urethra may be a single abnormality. Others abnormal urethral findings are transient urethral kink or angulation of the membranous urethra. It is crucial to take serial photographs during voiding to make an accurate diagnosis. Until recently there has been no references standard based on findings in VUCG and endoscopy [5].

61.3 Endoscopic Classification of PUV

Although Young's classification of PUV is well known, Douglas Stephens added a more precise explication for each type of Yong's classification

V. Di Benedetto · C. Arena (✉) · M. G. Scuderi
Pediatric Surgery Unit, University of Catania, Catania, Italy
e-mail: vdb@chirpedunict.it

C. Esposito et al. (eds.), *ESPES Manual of Pediatric Minimally Invasive Surgery*,
https://doi.org/10.1007/978-3-030-00964-9_61

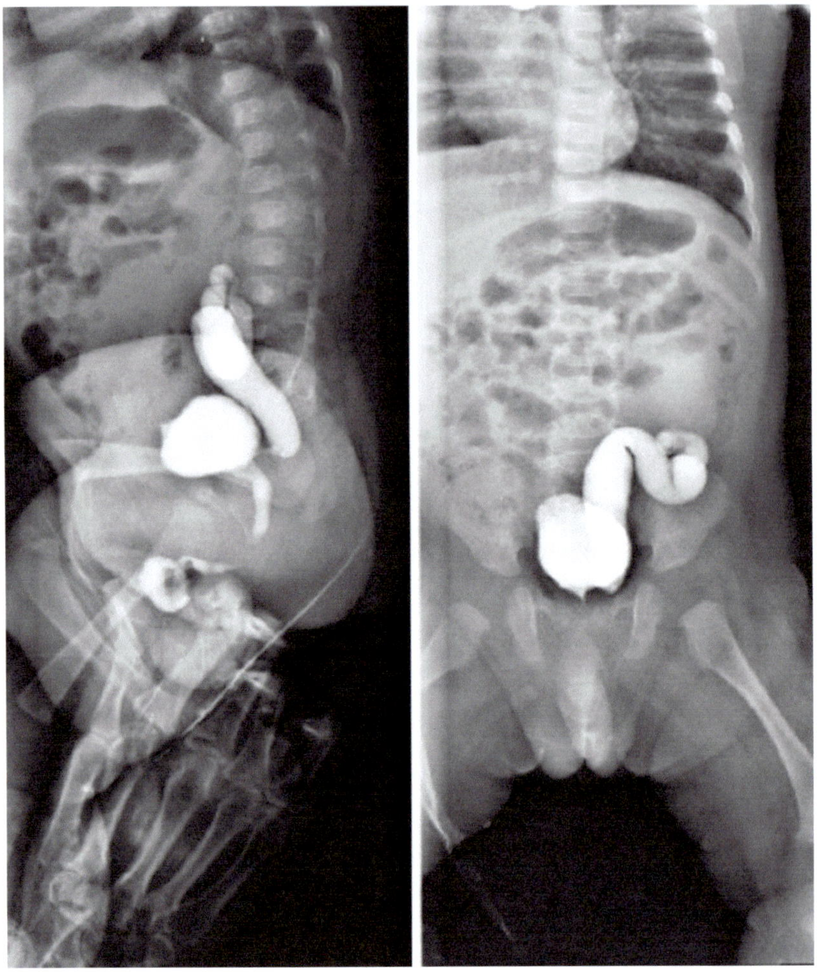

Fig. 61.1 Massive RVU in VCUG

Table 61.1 Douglas Stephens' description of PUV

Type	Embryology	Shape	Orientation to urethral axis	Continuity to verumontanum	Verumontanum	Inferior crest
1	Originate from abnormally located Wolffian duct orifices	Valvular	Oblique	Continuous	Big	Thick fin like
2	Overestimation or overclassification	–	–	–	–	–
3	Originate from persistent urogenital membrane	Membrane or diaphragm	Transverse	No	Small	Very fine
4	?	Deep infold of anterior and anterolateral walls	Transverse	No	–	–

in 1996. Stephens' detailed explanation is considered to be the most useful and easily understood in regard to structural characteristics based on embryology (Table 61.1). There are two main types of PUV: type 1 and type 3. Type 2 was originally defined by Young in 1919 but was later considered an overclassification. Type 4 is rare [5].

61.4 Management

The most common therapy for antenatal bladder outlet obstruction remains pregnancy termination [4]. Despite being introduced over 25 years ago, literature regarding antenatal intervention consists of case reports and small series. There was initial enthusiasm for fetoscopic ablation of VUP. However, therapeutic effectiveness of fetal cystoscopy compared with shunting has not been proven [4, 6]. Fetal valve ablation risks urethral and adjacent organ injury because laser energy can travel posteriorly [7].

In a full-term baby, the standard of care for PUV is cystoscopic valve incision. The current methods of incision include electrocautery incision, cold-knife incision, and laser fulguration [3, 4]. In infants with extremely low birth weight, the urethra might be too small to admit cystoscopy equipment safely. Long-term catheter drainage is inadvisable because of the risk of candidaemia. Rather than risking stricture with cystoscopic instrumentation, these babies should either undergo open vesicostomy or the rarely used Fogarty balloon valve ablation under fluoroscopic guidance [3]. Patients with severe disease often require multiple surgical intervention and may develop long-term complication, including urinary incontinence and loss of renal function [4].

61.5 Preoperative Preparation

All parents have to sign a specifically informed consent before procedure.

Anesthesia is general but it is possible to do valve resection in spinal anesthesia.

All patients receive antibiotic prophylaxis with i.v. ceftriaxone and gentamicin.

61.6 Positioning

The patient is placed in gynecological position. Surgeon's position is at the feet of the patient and the monitor is on the left of the surgeon.

61.7 Instrumentation

We use a 9.5 Fr pediatric cystoscope (Storz). We performed valve resection using a point electrocautery via a 3 Fr ureteric catheter with metal stylet passed through the cystoscope.

61.8 Technique

After filling the bladder with saline solution, we perform the urethro-cystoscopy using a 9.5 Fr cystoscope. After identifying the valves, a 3 Fr ureteric catheter is passed through the channel of the cystoscope, and electro-fulguration is performed. Fulguration is done mainly at 5, 7, and 12 o'clock position. For type 1 PUV, a major incision is made on the membranous lesion at the 12 o'clock position, and an additional incision was made if necessary on any valvular lesion in the 5 or 7 o'clock position (Fig. 61.2a, b). For type 3, an incision is made on the membranous lesion in the 12 o'clock position (Fig. 61.3). For both types, the incision on the membranous lesion in the 12 o'clock position is long and deep enough for complete excision.

The adequacy of the fulguration is confirmed intraoperatively by gentle pressure on the bladder with cystoscope positioned just distal to the verumontanum to look for the absence of valvular obstruction. Another method to check for adequacy of fulguration may be to observe the urinary stream by Crede maneuver with patient under anesthesia. The urethral catheter is placed after procedure.

61.9 Postoperative Care

The postoperative therapy included i.v. antibiotics (ceftriaxone and gentamicin) and paracetamol.

A small-size Foley urethral catheter is left in situ. Patients are discharged with an indwelling catheter the day after procedure, and they return 10 days after discharge to have a VCUG and remove the catheter.

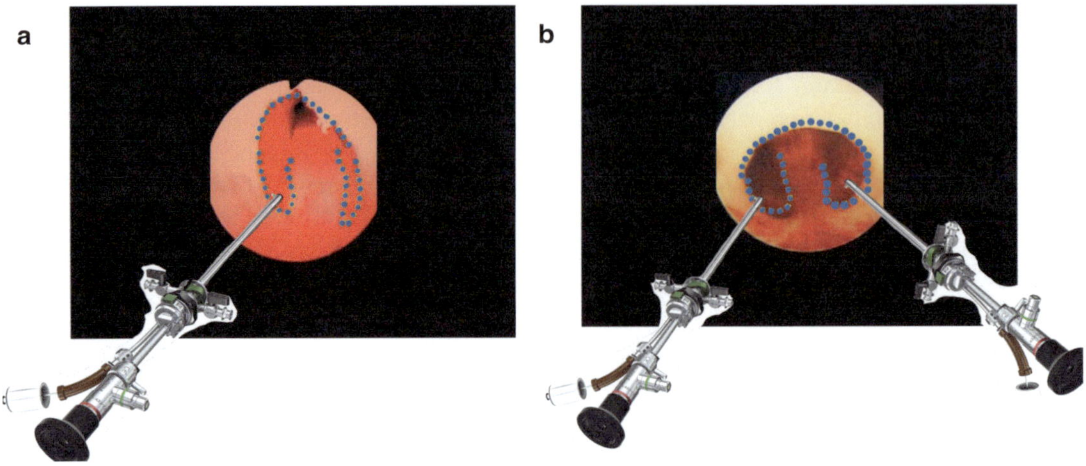

Fig. 61.2 (a) Incision at the 7 o'clock position for type 1 PUV. (b) Incision at the 5, 7, and 12 o'clock position for type 1 PUV

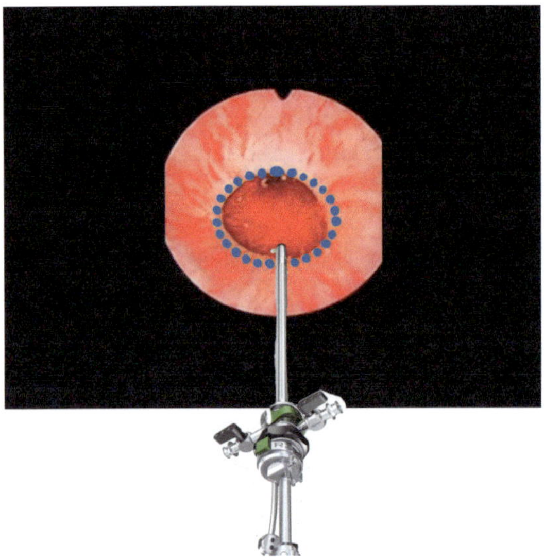

Fig. 61.3 Incision at the 7 o'clock position for type 3 PUV

61.10 Results

The timing of valve ablation varies according to age at presentation.

Successful voiding and improvement of stream are considered as the criteria of successful treatment.

Follow-up includes ultrasonography (US) to look for resolution of hydroureteronephrosis (HUN) at 2 weeks and 3 months after treatment, VCUG to look for the resolution of VUR and valve remnants at 3 and 6 months after treatment, and DTPA renal scan to evaluate renal function at 12 months. Urodynamic study is performed in selected patients.

Repeat cystourethroscopy is performed in patients who continue to have obstructive voiding at VCUG, persistence or deterioration of bilateral HUN, no decrease in posterior urethral dilatation, presence of valve remnants, non-resolution of bilateral VUR, and no improvement in renal function or new-onset renal insufficiency. Re-fulguration is performed in boys with valve remnants.

Complications after valve ablation reported in literature are in 5–25% of cases. Stricture formation occurs infrequently ranging from 0 to 25% and can be treated successfully with visual internal urethrotomy (VIU).

Up to 80% of VUR will resolve after valve ablation [3, 8]. Downgrading or resolving VUR and/or improvement in upper tract dilatation may be considered as indirect signs of urinary tract decompression. However, despite successful valve ablation, VUR and HUN may persist. Hence, VUR is expected to resolve after the release of urethral obstruction. Spontaneous resolution rates range between 27 and 79% at 2 weeks to more than 1 year following valve ablation. Some reflux can take as long as 3 years [2].

Those children with persistent upper tract dilation may have bladder emptying problems related to valve bladder syndrome or have a large urine output as a result of renal tubular damage, residual infravesical obstruction, or, rarely, ureterovesical junction obstruction [2].

Notwithstanding surgical relief of urethral obstruction, ongoing bladder dysfunction is a cause of morbidity and a potential threat to upper tract function. The prevalence of bladder dysfunction has been estimated to be 75–80% in boys studied urodynamically after PUV ablation [9]. A small, contracted bladder in infancy that progresses to a large capacity, poorly compliant bladder, often found in the presence of persistent upper tract dilatation and nephrogenic diabetes insipidus, has been termed valve bladder. This can create a self-injurious cycle, with persistent dilatation leading to a renal concentrating defect and creating more work for bladder at risk of muscular failure. Regular urodynamic monitoring is crucial in the management of these patients.

Abnormal renal development persists into childhood and adolescence: 30–42% of patients develop end-stage renal failure, making VUP the most common cause for pediatric renal transplantation [3].

61.11 Tips and Tricks

Early endoscopic resection of the valves has advantage, regarding bladder function, over long-term diversion. Small instruments are used to avoid urethral damage.

We try to minimize fulguration time and to avoid excessive deep fulguration for the risk of current injury to surrounding corpus spongiosum. We don't use loop resectoscope for risk of urethral strictures.

61.12 Discussion

The major goals in treatment of PUV are restoration of bladder voiding function, control of infections, preservation of renal function, maintenance of continence, and elimination of obstruction and VUR.

Several opinions for surgical management of infants with PUVs are available, and the mainstay of treatment is primary valve ablation [10–12].

Currently, surgeons have better instruments to treat valves endoscopically using different modalities under direct vision, with minimal incidence of complications [10, 13].

Various techniques of valve ablation were used: hot loop resectoscope, cold-knife urethrotome, hook diathermy electrode, Bugbee electrode, and Fogarty catheter.

Prevention of urethral stricture after valve ablation depends on many factors. These include gentle surgical technique, avoidance of oversized instrumentation in a small caliber urethra, minimizing fulguration time, avoiding excessive and deep fulguration, fulguration under direct vision, shortening the duration of preoperative catheterization, and use of nonreactive small-sized catheters. [10].

Bladder and renal function are often unstable and usually change during life, requiring lifelong monitoring.

It was found that neonatal valve ablation would protect the bladder functions and allow normal bladder cycling and healing. This underscores the importance of routine prenatal screening and early intervention for the valves. These findings suggest that the long-term prognosis of PUV might be improved by prenatal diagnosis [6, 14].

VUR and UTIs are not associated with worse renal outcomes, although these parameters remain vital in guiding treatment and may influence the number of surgeries a patient undergoes. Further investigation and longer follow-up are needed to identify patients at risk for late progression to CKD or end-stage renal disease (ESRD) [4].

Large retrospective studies of people with posterior urethral valves (PUV) have reported chronic renal insufficiency (CRI) in up to one third of the participants and end-stage renal failure in up to one quarter of them. Nadir creatinine (lowest creatinine during the first year following diagnosis) is the recognized prognostic indicator for renal outcome in PUV. Elevated nadir creatinine is the only independent risk factor for poor renal outcome as reported in literature [15].

The management of children with PUV is a continuous process that starts with the antenatal detection and early fulguration of the valves. The identification of the bladder dysfunction and its appropriate management will prevent the deleterious effects on the upper tracts and improves the long-term survival.

References

1. Oktar T, Acar O, Sancaktutar A, Sanli O, tefik T, Ziylan O. Endoscopic treatment of vesicoureteral reflux in children with posterior urethral valves. Int Urol Nephrol. 2012;44:1305–9.
2. Oktar T, Salabas E, Acar O, Atar A, Nane I, Ander H, Ziylan O. Residual valve and stricture after posterior urethral valve ablation: how to evaluate? J Pediatr Urol. 2013;9:184–7.
3. Diamond DA, Chan IHY, Holland AJA, Kurtz MP, Nelson C, Estrada CR Jr, Bauer S, Tam PKH. Advances in paediatric urology. Lancet. 2017;390:1061–71. www:thelancet.com.
4. Bilgutay AN, Roth D, Gonzales ET Jr, Janzen N, Zhang W, Koh CJ, Gargollo P, Seth A. Posterior urethral valves: risk factors for progression to renal failure. J Pediatr Urol. 2016;12:179.e1–7.
5. Nakai H, Hyga T, Kawai S, Kubo T, Nakamura S. Aggressive diagnosis and treatment for posterior urethral valves as an etiology for vesicoureteral reflux or urge incontinence in children. Investig Clin Urol. 2017;58(Suppl 1):46–53.
6. Kilby MD, Morris RK. Fetal therapy for the treatment of congenital bladder neck obstruction. Nat Rev Urol. 2014;11:412–9.
7. Sananes N, Favre R, Koh CJ, et al. Urological fistulas after fetal cystoscopic laser ablation of posterior urethral valves: surgical technical aspects. Ultrasound Obstet Gynecol. 2015;45:183–9.
8. Priti K, Rao KL, Menon P, et al. Posterior urethral valves: incidence and progress of vesicoureteral reflux after primary fulguration. Pediatr Surg Int. 2004;20:136–9.
9. Sarin YK, Sinha S. Efficacy of bladder neck incision on urodynamic abnormalities in patients with posterior urethral valves. Pediatr Surg Int. 2013;29:387–92.
10. Sarhan O, El-Ghoeneimi A, Hafez A, Dawaba M, Ghali A, Ibrahiem E. Surgical complications of posterior urethral valve ablation. 20 years of experience. J Pediatr Surg. 2010;45:2222–6.
11. Chertin B, Cozzi D, Puri P. Long-term results of primary avulsion of posterior urethral valves using a fogarty balloon catheter. J Urol. 2002;168:1841–3.
12. Farhat W, Mc Lorie G, Capolicchhio G, et al. Outcome of primary valve ablation versus urinary tract diversion in patients with posterior urethral valves. Urology. 2000;56:653–7.
13. Yohannes P, Hanna M. Current trends in the management of posterior urethral valves in the pediatric population. Urology. 2002;60:947–53.
14. Kousidis G, Thomas DF, Morgan H, Haider N, Subramaniam R, Feather S. The long-term outcome of prenatally detected posterior urethral valves: a 10 to 23-year follow-up study. BJU Int. 2008;102: 1020–4.
15. Coleman R, King T, Nicoara CD, Bader M, McCarthy L, Chandran H, Parashar K. Nadir creatinine in posterior urethral valves: how high is low enough? J Pediatr Urol. 2015;11(6):356.e1–5. https://doi.org/10.1016/j.jpurol.2015.06.008. Epub 30 Jul 2015.

Primary Obstructive Megaureter: Endourological Treatment

62

J. M. Angulo, A. Parente, B. Fernandez-Bautista, L. Burgos, and R. Ortiz

62.1 Introduction

Most patients with primary obstructive megaureter (POM) only need conservative management since functional obstruction resolves spontaneously during the first months of life without renal function impairment or appearance of symptoms [1]. Surgical treatment is then reserved for those cases that develop progressive hydro-ureteronephrosis with urinary tract infections (UTI) and/or renal loss of function. However, its management and surgical options remain controversial. Ureteral reimplantation with or without ureteral tapering has been considered the gold-standard procedure for these patients, but in small infants, reimplantation of a huge ureter is challenging and leads to potential complications [2].

Endoscopic balloon dilation (EBD) of the vesicoureteral junction (VUJ) was first described by Angulo et al. in 1998 as initial approach of complicated POM [3]. Since then several publications have shown that EBD is feasible, safe, and a less-invasive procedure in the initial management of POM even for very young patients [4–7]. In recent years the interest has been focused on the long-term effectiveness of this procedure, being reported good outcomes that maintain in time, suggesting EBD as a valid option for definitive treatment in POM [8–10].

In 2004 we established in our institution the EBD of the VUJ and temporary stenting as first surgical treatment in POM with surgical criteria. In this chapter we describe our experience with this technique, its results, its complications, and its outcomes after 100 treated cases.

62.2 Patients and Methods

One hundred of POM in 92 consecutive patients were treated by EBD between years 2004 and 2016. A total of 79 POM in 73 patients (6 patients had bilateral POM) with more than 18 months of follow-up after treatment were retrospectively analyzed.

Diagnosis and management of POM were done according to the European guidelines and consensus statement of this entity. Primary obstructive megaureter was considered in those that presented progressive hydro-ureteronephrosis with distal ureter diameter greater than 10 mm, obstructive pattern on MAG3 renogram scan, and absence of vesicoureteral reflux on cystography. Nevertheless, not all of these patients needed surgical repair (in our series only 13% of cases prenatally diagnosed). The indication for surgical

J. M. Angulo (✉) · A. Parente
B. Fernandez-Bautista · L. Burgos · R. Ortiz
Pediatric Urology Unit, Department of Pediatric Surgery, Hospital General Universitario Gregorio Marañón, Madrid, Spain
e-mail: josemaria.angulo@salud.madrid.org

C. Esposito et al. (eds.), *ESPES Manual of Pediatric Minimally Invasive Surgery*,
https://doi.org/10.1007/978-3-030-00964-9_62

intervention was established in those with one or more of the following conditions (Table 62.1):

- Breaking through febrile UTI in 30 cases (38%) despite antibiotic prophylaxis, with clinical scenario of pyonephrosis and sepsis in 6 patients at time of treatment
- Progressive worsening of hydro-ureteronephrosis with renal parenchyma thinning in 29 cases (36.7%)
- Impairment of renal function (differential renal function less than 40% at diagnosis or decreasing more than 10% during expectative surveillance) in 20 cases (25.3%)

Table 62.1 Indications for surgical treatment

	Number of cases
UHN worsening + UTI	30 (38%)
UHN worsening with renal parenchyma thinning	29 (36.7%)
UHN worsening + impairment of DRF	14 (17.7%)
UHN worsening + UTI + imapairment of DRF	6 (7.6%)
	79 POM

62.2.1 Technique

Under general anesthesia and with antibiotic prophylaxis, a cystoscopy with a 9.5 FG *Storz* cystoscope with 5F working channel is done. For some early cases of the series, we then performed retrograde pyelography before the dilation, using contrast through a 3 FG ureteral catheter.

A hydrophilic guidewire (0.014″ *Choice PT*™, *J-tip*, *Boston Scientific*) or (0.018″ *Radiofocus*® *Terumo)* is introduced through the VUJ, followed by the dilating balloon. The balloons used were semi-compliant dilation catheters with a size of 3.1 F and a nominal diameter from 5 to 7 mm and 2 cm length (*RX Muso*™, *Terumo*). Then, the balloons are filled with radiologic contrast with their nominal pressure (14 atm) with a pressure inflation device, under direct and fluoroscopic control until the complete release of the stenosis. Figure 62.1 illustrates the typical endoscopic and radiology sequence of dilation images.

When successful dilation is done, the cystoscope is introduced through the distal ureter to assess the UVJ, and a double-J stent is left in situ

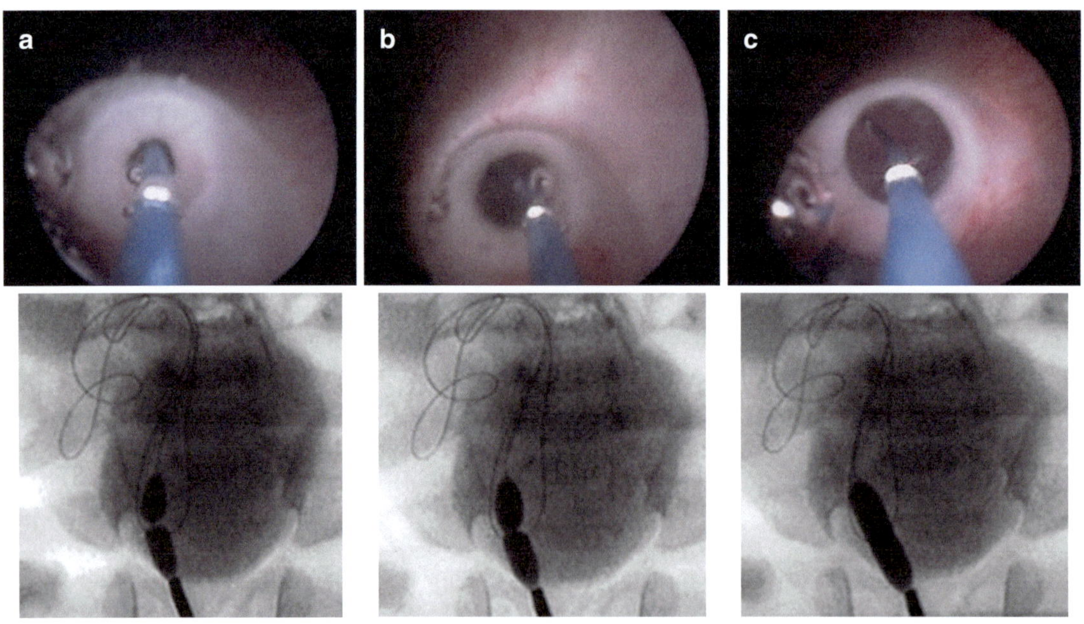

Fig. 62.1 Balloon inserted through right VUJ, endoscopic view and radiographic control. (**a**) Initial balloon inflation with the presence of stenotic ring; (**b**) progressive dilation; (**c**) complete expansion of the balloon and disappearance of the stenosis

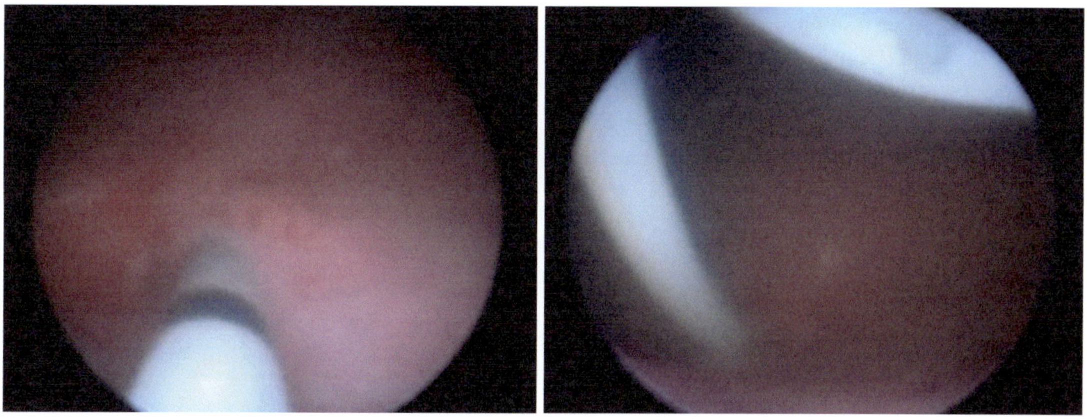

Fig. 62.2 Double-J stent placement after EBD of the VUJ

(3 Fr, 8–12 cm long, *Sof-Flex Multi-Length Ureteral Stent,* Cook Medical Europe™). After the procedure, a bladder catheter is placed during 24 h to prevent complications (Fig. 62.2).

Double-J stents are removed at 4–6 weeks at a second cystoscopy. At this time the VUJ is calibrated by distal ureteroscopy. When the cystoscope could be introduced through the VUJ, it is considered a satisfactory result. If not, a new balloon catheter is introduced and inflated to its nominal diameter to assess the VUJ diameter.

After several years performing this technique, we have done some modifications in order to achieve an easier and shorter procedure, avoiding unnecessary radiation in the majority of cases. Performing the retrograde ureteropyelography may be challenging due to the narrow ureteral meatus and may result in mucosal inflammation, edema, or bleeding. For these reasons in the last years, we are performing the balloon dilation without fluoroscopic control, only under cystoscopic vision. We then reserve retrograde pyelography and fluoroscopic guidance for those cases in which we want to check the upper urinary tract anatomy, when dilation is being difficult or when we have problems placing the double-J stent. In the same way, we actually don't try to reach the renal pelvis with the guidewire and the double-J catheter, which is left in the dilated ureter. Overcoming ureteral loops may be technically demanding and time-consuming and needs unnecessary radiation exposure for the baby.

62.2.2 Follow-Up

All children underwent a standard follow-up protocol after endoscopic treatment; this included a clinical review and US at 3, 6, 12, and 18 months and then annually and a MAG-3–furosemide renogram scan at 6 and 18 months. Voiding cystourethrography (VCUG) was performed only if patients presented UTI or persistent ureterohydronephrosis without obstruction at the renogram (Fig. 62.3).

62.3 Results

Median age at surgery was 4 months (0.5–44), with median operating time of 20 min (10–60) and median hospital stay of 1 day [1–7]. All patients had hospital admission of 24 h except three patients in whom the endoscopic approach was done at time of urinary sepsis with ureteropyonephrosis, requiring further medical assistance after the procedure.

There were no intraoperative complications in 75 cases (94.9%). In the remaining 4 patients (5.1%), EBD could not be performed because of failure of the guidewire to pass through the VUJ in two cases (requiring open ureteral reimplantation) and unsuccessful dilation with false path in the other two cases (requiring temporary nephrostomy and posterior ureteral reimplantation).

Early perioperative complications occurred in 6 cases (7.8%). Febrile UTI after endoscopic procedure or after double-J stent removement was reported in 5 (Clavien-Dindo 1). One patient presented ureteral double-J stent migration and developed early severe restenosis with pyonephrosis, requiring initial nephrostomy (Clavien-Dindo 3) and ureteral reimplantation weeks later.

Looking at US findings in patients who had successful initial endoscopic treatment (74/79), significant differences were observed in distal ureteral diameter before treatment, 15 mm range (10–23); at first postoperative US after endoscopic dilation, 10 mm (0–21); and in long term, 5 mm (0–22) ($p < 0.001$ Wilcoxon test).

All patients had significant improvement in hydro-ureteronephrosis ($p < 0.05$ T-test) except those who developed restenosis or high-grade secondary VUR during long-term follow-up. Initial renal function was preserved in all patients, with normalization of the renogram elimination curves.

Postoperative secondary VUR was found during long-term surveillance in 17 cases (23%), being diagnosed in 12 after UTI and 5 after VCUG control for contralateral reflux. Subureteral endoscopic injection of *Deflux*™ (*dextranomer copolymer in hyaluronic acid*) was successful in 13 patients (76.4%) and failed in 4 (23.6%) who finally needed ureteral reimplantation.

Long-term restenosis occurred in 9 cases (12.2%). A new EBD procedure was successfully done in 8 cases (88.9%) at a median postoperative period of 9.5 months (5–63). Only one patient developed recurrent restenosis and finally required ureteral reimplantation.

Endoscopic approach of POM including endoscopic balloon dilation of the VUJ and endoscopic management of 2° VUR had a long-term success rate of 87.3% (69/79) with a median follow-up of 5.6 years (1.5-13-5). Endoscopic management of POM failed in 10 cases (12.7%) that finally required ureteral reimplantation (see Figs. 62.4 and 62.5).

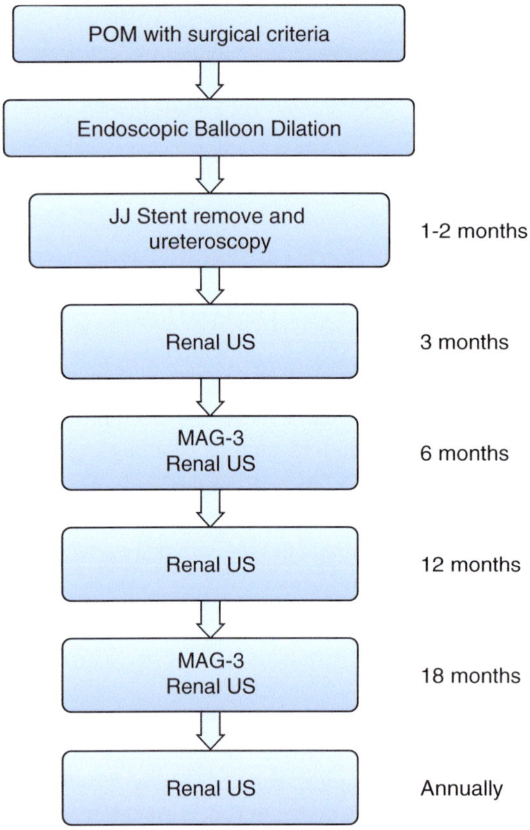

Fig. 62.3 Follow-up protocol

Fig. 62.4 Successful endoscopic management of POM

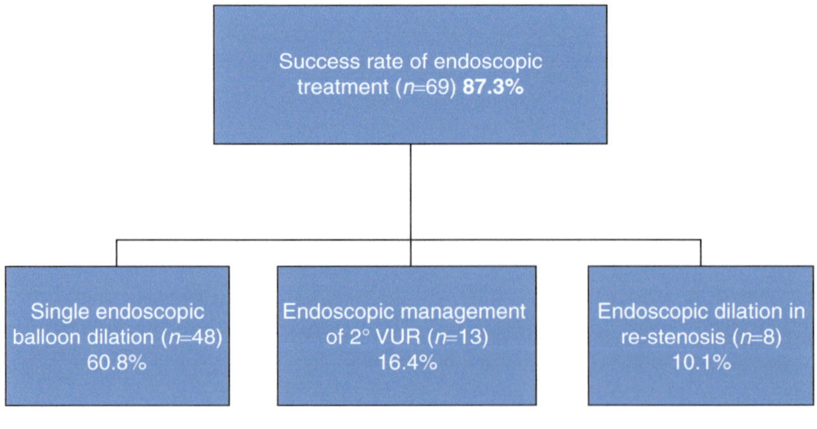

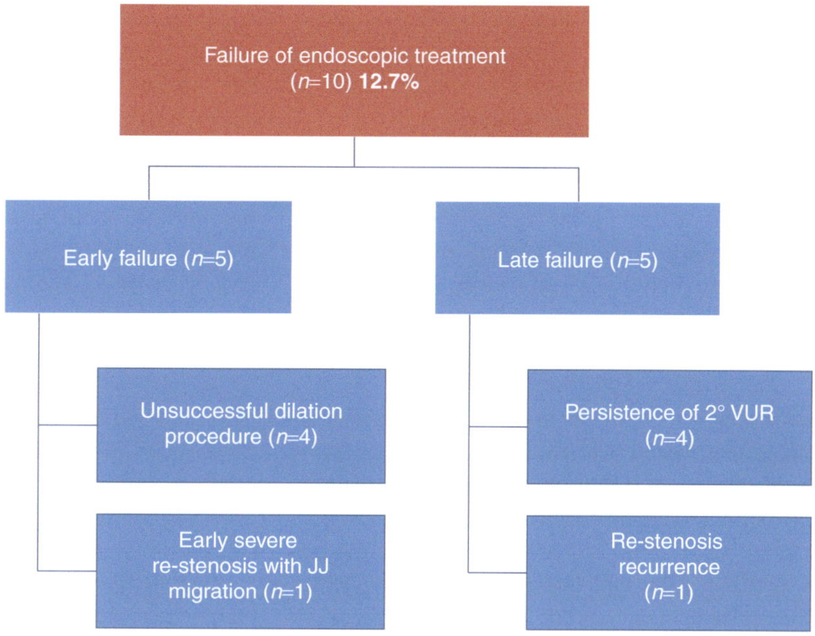

Fig. 62.5 Endoscopic failure in the management of POM

If we obviate secondary VUR and focus on the final result of EBD as treatment for ureteral obstruction, the long-term result for normalization of ureteral drainage and preserving renal function was 92.4% (73/79).

In 12 cases an ipsilateral paraureteral diverticulum coexisted with the POM. Ten of them were successfully treated by EBD showing good outcomes in long term; nevertheless, ureteral reimplantation was required in two cases (one persistent VUR and the case of recurrent restenosis).

62.4 Discussion

It is well known that POM resolves spontaneously in more than 70% of cases without impairment in renal function. However, there is a small group of patients who are going to present a progressive hydro-ureteronephrosis worsening with appearance of infectious complications and/or deterioration in renal function. These patients benefit from surgical treatment, which is usually indicated in the first months of life [1, 11].

Ureteral reimplantation with or without ureteral tapering is considered the gold-standard procedure for these patients, with a well-documented success rate between 90 and 95%. However, reimplantation of a grossly dilated ureter in a small infantile bladder could be challenging and leads to potential complications such as secondary obstruction, vesicoureteral reflux, and bladder dysfunction. For this reason temporary urinary diversions could be indicated during first months of life, but are not exempt of complications. External ureterostomies may present problems such as infections, skin irritations, and stenosis [12]. In addition parental tolerance is usually low, demanding early closure. Percutaneous nephrostomies could be done with external tubes but have limited durability in small infants. Internal urinary diversions have become popular as proposed by Lee and Kaefer [13] who perform a refluxing megaureter reimplantation through a small laparotomy during the first months of life. However, it remains a non-definitive open surgery and creates a high-grade secondary VUR.

The important development of minimally invasive techniques achieved in pediatric age in the last years has led to nonaggressive procedures for the surgical treatment of POM such as the laparoscopic, robotic, or endourological approach. Nevertheless, we cannot obviate that the main objective of any technique even minimally invasive must be to obtain similar outcomes to the gold standard or at least good results with less morbidity or complications.

Several authors have postulated the placement of double-J ureteral stent as a temporary internal derivation in the initial management of POM, with good outcomes in a group of patients that did not need any more procedure but controversial results and remarkable comorbidity in an important number of cases.

Since endoscopic balloon dilation was first described by Angulo et al. [3] as an initial treatment for children with complicated POM, several publications with few patients and short follow-up periods showed that EBD using the original technique or variations of the same principle was a feasible, safe, and less-invasive procedure for the initial management of POM with surgical criteria even for very young patients. In 2007 Angerri et al. [4] reported their initial experience with six patients in whom urinary obstruction disappeared without associated complications in a median follow-up of 31 months. Christman et al. [5] reported in 2012 their experience after the treatment of 17 children with a follow-up of 3.2 years. These authors added a laser incision in cases of ureteral stenosis greater than 2 cm and placed two double-J stents in the ureter simultaneously, reporting good long-term outcome with disappearance of hydro-ureteronephrosis in 71% of the series. García-Aparicio et al. [6] presented a series of 13 patients with a medium-term success rate of 84.6% (11 of 13), requiring ureteral reimplantation in 3 patients (2 persistence of UHN and 1 high-grade VUR).

Recent publications have focused on establishing long-term effectiveness of EBD as definitive treatment of POM, confirming good results with minimal associated morbidity. Romero et al. [8] reported in 2014 the experience of our institution in 29 patients treated until 2010, with a median age at treatment of 4 months and a median follow-up of 47 months. It was concluded that the patients who had a favorable evolution with disappearance of the UHN and adequate renal drainage confirmed by renogram remained asymptomatic and with stable situation during the subsequent follow-up. Five patients had secondary VUR and three of them were satisfactorily treated endoscopically. Finally, the endourological management of the POM including EBD of the VUJ and treatment of 2° VUR had a success rate of 86%. Bujons et al. [9] have reported excellent results in 19 patients, with a long-term success of 90% after the initial dilatation procedure and a follow-up of 6.9 years. One patient required a second dilatation due to restenosis and another one endoscopic treatment of 2° VUR, both with good outcome. Casal et al. [10] have just communicated good outcomes in a short series of 13 patients but with an important median follow-up of 10.3 years (4.7-12-2), asserting the value of balloon dilation as a definitive treatment for POM.

Technical variations to the initial procedure have been proposed with encouraging results. The group of Kajbafzadeh [14] reported in 2007 a long series of patients treated by endo-ureterotomy (ureterotomy and detrusorotomy at 6 h) leaving double-J stent for 1 week, without associated comorbidity and with a complete resolution of ureterohydronephrosis in 71% of cases. Capozza et al. [7] published the dilation of the VUJ with Cutting Balloon™ in three patients with persistence of the stenotic ring during the previous endoscopic high-pressure balloon dilation, obtaining a complete resolution of the stenosis and good postoperative course.

Even the advantages described of EBD, the endourological management of POM remains controversial. The aspects to be discussed focus on secondary VUR, the possibility of restenosis, and the use of radiation in young patients. Additionally, it is difficult to assess its value as a definitive treatment in POM attending to the short experience reported in the literature.

Regarding secondary VUR, García-Aparicio [15] analyzed it in his group of patients, reporting 27% (6 cases of 22 POM treated). Of these, two were treated endoscopically, and two were treated by ureteral reimplantation. The author concluded that the coexistence of ipsilateral paraureteral diverticulum is a risk factor for developing secondary VUR; however the number of cases was very low (two of four) to establish a reasonable conclusion. In the series published by Bujons et al. [10], only 1 case of 19 presented secondary VUR, and it was resolved endoscopically.

In our series secondary VUR was found during long-term surveillance in 17 cases (23%). Endoscopic treatment of it was successful in 13 patients (76.4%) and failed in 4 (23.6%) who required ureteral reimplantation. For these patients with 2° VUR, three had an ipsilateral para-meatal diverticulum and only one required reimplantation. In our experience, the presence of para-meatal diverticulum was not a bad prognosis factor for the endoscopic management of POM, since 10 of 12 cases of the series had an excellent outcome.

Long-term restenosis occurred in 9 cases of our series (12.2%). A new EBD was done with good long-term outcome in 8 cases (88.9%) till the date. Only one patient developed recurrent restenosis and finally required ureteral reimplantation. The role of Cutting Balloon™ dilation may be a useful option in these cases. We used it recently with excellent midterm outcome in three patients treated at other institutions who developed restenosis after initial EBD of the VUJ. Then, we actually reserve the Cutting Balloon™ dilation for future restenosis or in primary cases when the stenosis is not completely solved with the balloon catheter at time of initial EBD.

Attending to our experience and looking at the literature, we can consider EBD of the VUJ as a relatively simple technique, reproducible, and with a short learning curve compared to other procedures. However, its success lies in the use of adequate endoscopic material. Appropriate hydrophilic guidewires (0.014″–0.018″), balloon catheters with low profile (2.7CH), and double-J stents suitable for pediatric age are crucial both for the success of the technique and to avoid complications.

62.5 Conclusion

Endoscopic balloon dilation has shown to be a safe, feasible, and really less-invasive procedure in primary obstructive megaureter with surgical criteria even in small infants.

In our experience we can consider it an effective treatment with few postoperative complications and good outcomes that maintains at long-term follow-up. The main complication observed was secondary VUR; notwithstanding it did not result in significant morbidity for the patients and could also be treated endoscopically with a high success rate.

In comparison with the conventional surgery, EBD has the obvious advantages of being a minimally invasive procedure, with a shorter operating time, immediate recovery, and with no patient-age limitations. In our opinion, it may be considered first-line treatment in the management of POM in children, avoiding unnecessary bladder surgery in the vast majority of patients. Nevertheless, it doesn't invalidate ureteral reimplantation in case of failure.

References

1. Di Renzo D, Aguiar L, Cascini V, et al. Long-term followup of primary nonrefluxing megaureter. J Urol. 2013;190(3):1021–6.
2. Hendren WH. Complications of megaureter repair in children. J Urol. 1975;113(2):238–54.
3. Angulo JM, Arteaga R, Rodriguez Alarcon J, Calvo MJ. [Role of retrograde endoscopic dilatation with balloon and derivation using double pig-tail catheter as an initial treatment for vesico-ureteral junction stenosis in children]. Cir Pediatr. 1998;11(1): 15–8.
4. Angerri O, Caffaratti J, Garat JM, Villavicencio H. Primary obstructive megaureter: initial experience with endoscopic dilatation. J Endourol. 2007;21(9):999–1004.
5. Christman MS, Kasturi S, Lambert SM, Kovell RC, Casale P. Endoscopic management and the role of double stenting for primary obstructive megaureters. J Urol. 2012;187(3):1018–22.
6. Garcia-Aparicio L, Rodo J, Krauel L, Palazon P, Martin O, Ribo JM. High pressure balloon dilation of the ureterovesical junction—first line approach to treat primary obstructive megaureter? J Urol. 2012;187(5):1834–8.
7. Capozza N, Torino G, Nappo S, Collura G, Mele E. Primary obstructive megaureter in infants: our experience with endoscopic balloon dilation and cutting balloon ureterotomy. J Endourol. 2015;29(1):1–5.
8. Romero RM, Angulo JM, Parente A, Rivas S, Tardaguila AR. Primary obstructive megaureter: the role of high pressure balloon dilation. J Endourol. 2014;28(5):517–23.

9. Bujons A, Saldana L, Caffaratti J, Garat JM, Angerri O, Villavicencio H. Can endoscopic balloon dilation for primary obstructive megaureter be effective in a long-term follow-up? J Pediatr Urol. 2015;11(1):37 e1–6.
10. Casal Beloy I, Somoza Argibay I, García González M, García Novoa MA, Míguez Fortes LM, Dargallo Carbonell T. Endoscopic balloon dilatation in primary obstructive megaureter: long-term results. J Pediatr Urol. 2018;14(2):167.e1–5. pii: S1477-5131(17)30470-9.
11. Farrugia MK, Hitchcock R, Radford A, et al. British Association of Paediatric Urologists consensus statement on the management of the primary obstructive megaureter. J Pediatr Urol. 2014;10(1): 26–33.
12. Kitchens DM, DeFoor W, Minevich E, et al. End cutaneous ureterostomy for the management of severe hydronephrosis. J Urol. 2007;177(4):1501–4.
13. Kaefer M, Maizels M. Obstructed megaureter in the newborn—repair by temporary refluxing megaureter reimplantation. J Pediatr Urol. 2015;11(3):110–2.
14. Kajbafzadeh AM, Payabvash S, Salmasi AH, et al. Endoureterectomy for treatment of primary obstructive megaureter in children. J Endourol. 2007;21(7):743e9.
15. García-Aparicio L, Blázquez-Gómez E, de Haro I, et al. Postoperative vesicoureteral reflux after high-pressure balloon dilation of the ureterovesical junction in primary obstructive megaureter. Incidence, management and predisposing factors. World J Urol. 2015;33:2103–6.

63 Ureterocele: Minimally Invasive Endoscopic Treatment

P. Caione, M. Bada, S. Gerocarni Nappo, G. Collura, M. Innocenzi, L. Del Prete, G. Farullo, E. Mele, and N. Capozza

63.1 Definition and Epidemiology

Ureterocele is defined as cystic dilatation of the distal ureter ending that can be located within either the bladder or the bladder neck and urethra [1]. This enlargement usually interferes with the outlet of urine: the degree of obstruction varies based on the type of ureterocele and the amount of abnormal tissue development. It may be associated with a single or more frequently with a duplex system, and in duplex systems ureterocele is associated with the upper pole [2]. At autopsy, the incidence of ureteroceles has been reported as 1 in 500 alive newborns. Ureteroceles occur four to six times more frequently in females than in males and more commonly in Caucasians than in other races. Unilateral ureteroceles occur with similar frequency on the right and left, and in 10% of cases, bilateral involvement is present [3].

63.2 Pathogenesis

The underlying pathogenesis is unknown: several theories have been proposed. Embryologic mechanisms resulting in ureterocele development may include [4]:

- An incomplete breakdown of the ureteral membrane between the ureteral bud and the mesonephric duct, resulting in an obstruction that causes the development of a ureterocele. This theory explains the presence of the majority of obstruction in ureteroceles.
- Obstruction of the ureteral orifice by the bladder neck as a consequence of developmental delay in the timing of the ureteral bud insertion into the bladder.
- Abnormal induction of the bladder trigone development, resulting in the absence of trigonal musculature in the intravesical portion of ureteroceles.

63.3 Classification

Several classification systems have been proposed for ureteroceles, but the most useful divides ureteroceles based on their location. According to this point, ureteroceles are classified as intravesical or orthotopic (entirely within the bladder and above the bladder neck) and ectopic (some portion of ureterocele is situated permanently at the bladder neck or urethra). The last is the most common subtype [5]. Stephens published a descriptive subdivision of ureterocele types that include cecoureterocele. In cecoureterocele the

P. Caione (✉) · M. Bada · S. Gerocarni Nappo
G. Collura · M. Innocenzi · L. Del Prete · G. Farullo
E. Mele · N. Capozza
Division of Paediatric Urology, Department of Surgery, Bambino Gesù Children's Hospital, Rome, Italy
e-mail: paolo.caione@opbg.net

C. Esposito et al. (eds.), *ESPES Manual of Pediatric Minimally Invasive Surgery*,
https://doi.org/10.1007/978-3-030-00964-9_63

orifice is within the bladder, but the cavity extends beyond the bladder neck into the urethra. Ureteroceles also may be classified with either a single collecting system or a double collecting system. Approximately 80% of ureteroceles are associated with the upper pole of a duplex collecting system, 60% of these are ectopic [6]. They are more frequently observed in female patients.

63.4 Clinical Presentation

Ureterocele may be recognized before or after birth. Antenatal presentation is nowadays more frequent, as many ureteroceles are detected incidentally on antenatal ultrasonography. Approximately 2% of antenatal hydronephroses are caused by ureteroceles, which obstruct the distal end of the affected ureter. In postnatal presentation, the most common presentation is during an evaluation for urinary tract infection (UTI) in the first few months after birth [7]. Febrile UTI may occur frequently as a consequence of pyelonephritis with failure to recurrent abdominal or pelvic pain: haematuria is a rare presentation in elderly children. Some infants may present with a palpable abdominal mass due to the severe ureterocele obstruction of the dilated pyeloureteral system. In neonatal or infant females, a reddish vaginal mass may be observed as a consequence of a prolapsed ureterocele through the bladder neck. This situation causes usually severe bladder and bilateral upper tract dilatation with acute renal failure. A few patients, particularly older males with a single system intravesical ureterocele, may be diagnosed incidentally during imaging for other conditions [5, 7].

63.5 Diagnosis

The diagnosis is generally made by ultrasonography that shows a well-defined cystic intravesical mass in the trigonal portion of the bladder [8] (Fig. 63.1a–c). Dilatation of the upper tract is often observed, with kinked megaureter and pyelectasy of the related system. The dilatation may be present in both ureters of the ipsilateral side and sometimes in the contralateral system. Voiding cystourethrogram (VCUG) is used to detect vesicoureteral reflux (VUR). Reflux into the ipsilateral lower pole occurs in approximately 50% of patients and on the contralateral side in 25%. VCUG provides the most definitive evaluation of the bladder and distal ureters, as well as urethra. Nuclear medicine scan is used to evaluate the relative function of all renal segments [9] (Fig. 63.1d). In particular, in patients with duplex system, the pole associated with the affected ureter may contribute little or no function and may not be worth preserving when surgery is performed. In addition, a delay in the isotope washout demonstrates impaired urinary drainage, with a diagnosis of urinary flow obstruction [10].

63.6 Management

If ureterocele is asymptomatic without significant outflow obstruction, no treatment is needed, and follow-up is recommended. Observational management of ureteroceles in carefully selected patients is a reasonable option, with the potential for spontaneous decompression. Urinary tract infections are treated with antibiotics, if present [11]. If kidney function is good, the ureterocele can be treated using early endoscopic decompression. In case of poor kidney function, the kidney tissue may be removed surgically. The goals of therapy are preservation of renal function, elimination of UTI, releasing of outlet bladder and upper tract decompression with VUR resolution and maintenance of urinary continence [10].

63.7 Treatment Options

Ureteroceles are often complex anomalies, and a single approach for ureterocele's treatment is not possible. It seems reasonable to individualize the correct management according to specific endpoints oriented to:

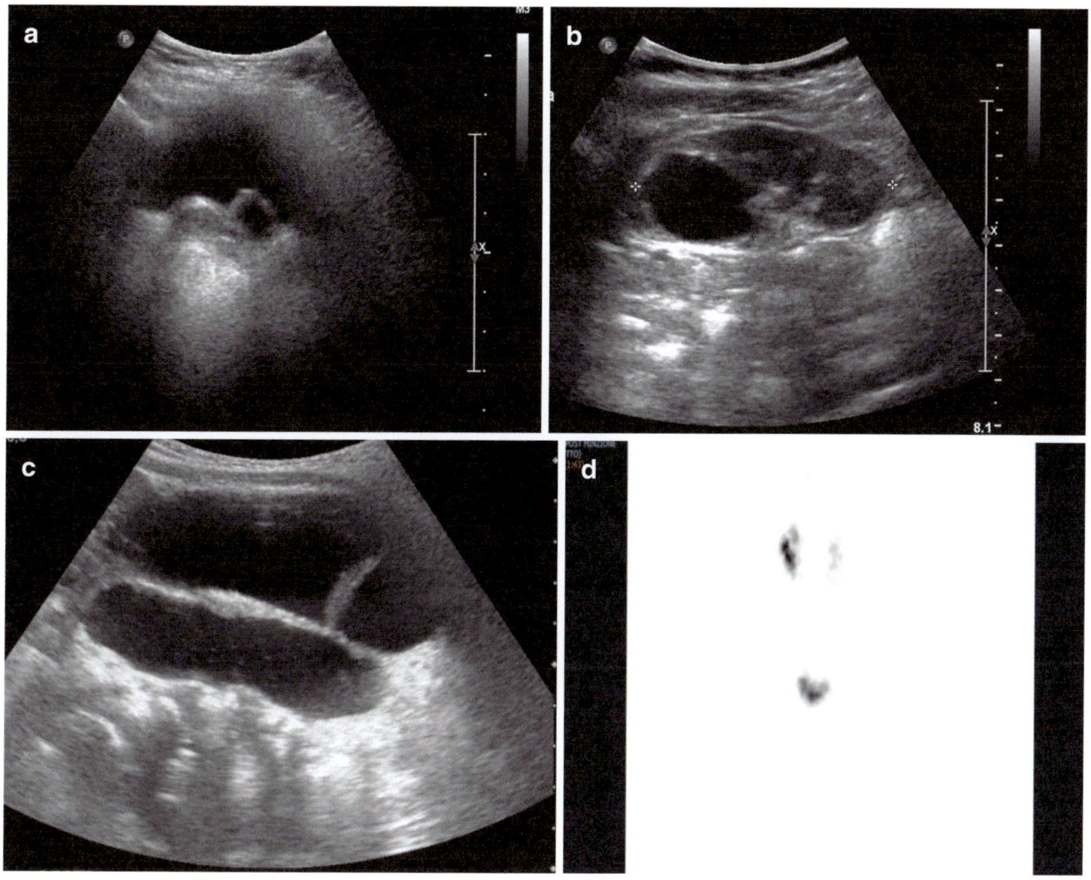

Fig. 63.1 (**a–d**) A 4-month-old female infant with prenatal diagnosis of hydronephrosis and ureteral dilatation. (**a**) Bladder ultrasound: ureterocele on bladder basis with dilated ureter ending. (**b**) Renal ultrasound: duplex collecting system with dilatation of the upper pole. (**c**) Abdominal ultrasound: upper pole megaureter. (**d**) DMSA nuclear renal scan: left upper pole reduced uptake in a duplex system

- Solve the outlet obstruction
- Prevent UTI
- Prevent/correct associated VUR
- Preserve the renal function

The management includes conservative approach, endoscopic decompression, partial nephroureterectomy or complete primary reconstruction [9, 10] (see Table 63.1).

Table 63.1 Management options of ureterocele

1. Conservative management
2. Minimally invasive procedures
(a) Transurethral incision (TUI)
(b) Laparoscopic upper pole heminephroureterectomy
– Transperitoneal access
– Retroperitoneal access
3. Open surgical procedures
(a) Upper pole heminephroureterectomy
(b) Ureteroureterostomy or ureteropyelostomy
(c) Ureterocele excision and ureteral reimplantation
(d) Complete one-stage primary reconstruction

63.8 Conservative Management

In highly selected cases, conservative management may be offered in asymptomatic patients, with absent hydronephrosis and reflux [11]. According to EAU guidelines 2017 [12], surgery may be avoided in patients with non-obstructing ureterocele. A careful follow-up is needed for long life.

Table 63.2 Urological indications to conservative treatment

– Asymptomatic patients
– Small, nonobstructive intravesical ureterocele
– Extravesical ureterocele or associated with multicystic dysplastic moieties in the absence of high-grade VUR or bladder outlet obstruction
– Absence of grade III or IV VUR
– Absence of bladder outlet obstruction
– Absence of obstruction in inferior renal moiety

The selection of the approach depends on:

- Clinical status of the patient (e.g. presence of urosepsis)
- Patient age
- Function of the upper pole renal parenchyma at scintigraphic scan
- Presence of reflux or obstruction of the ipsilateral or contralateral ureter
- Presence of bladder neck obstruction
- Position of the ureterocele intravesical or ectopic
- Parent's and surgeon's preference

Many authors have expressed a possible condition of overtreatment and unnecessary surgery in ideal candidates for a conservative approach to ureteroceles [8–10]. Several studies have shown that carefully selected, many asymptomatic children with ureteroceles can be safety managed initially without surgical approach. Han et al. reported no significant difference between the nonoperative and operative groups with regard to hydronephrosis grade, reflux grade or ureterocele size [8]. Direnna and colleagues also reported a watchful waiting for prenatally detected ureteroceles [9]. Current data suggest that urological indications to a conservative approach are summarized in Table 63.2.

In any patients managed conservatively, the development of complications should promptly consider for surgical repair [10].

63.9 Endoscopic Ureterocele Incision

Endoscopic ureterocele decompression is a minimally invasive procedure that can be performed under general or regional anaesthesia, to obtain a decreasing risk of UTI and decompressing the upper tract: in recent years, endoscopic puncture became a gold standard technique that supplanted the ureterocele wall incision [9, 10]. The incision offers more effective decompression with a potentially higher risk of de novo VUR. Endoscopic puncture represents the treatment of choice for patients with ureterocele resulting in systemic infection or high-grade obstruction. It's the first-line treatment in the case of the septic or acutely ill child with an obstructing ureterocele. Some authors have demonstrated the advantages of endoscopic puncture in the preservation of renal tissue, with rapid recovery of the related renal function reported in 85–100% of cases [11].

63.9.1 Technique of Endoscopic Puncture of Ureterocele

- Patient under general or regional anaesthesia.
- The most common technique consists of small 2–3 mm incisions or punctures made just above the distal junction of the ureterocele with the bladder, using a Bugbee electrode or a sharp electrode through a paediatric cystoscope. Paediatric resectoscope can be successful used with diathermy [12, 13]. The bladder should be poorly filled by not saline solution. The endoscopic punctures may be performed with high efficacy using laser energy, and holmium pulse laser and thallium continuous laser may be both used, with thin fibre (272 μm) and low energy (0.5 J). Multiple punctures of the ureterocele basis can be performed with high precision and no bleeding risk. Immediate decompression of the ureterocele is usually observed [14, 15] (Fig. 63.2a–c).
- A second endoscopic puncture should be considered in cases where a large ureterocele persists postoperatively.

According to Lewis [16] and Castagnetti [17], the indications to the endoscopic procedures are:

- Obstructing ureterocele with systemic infection

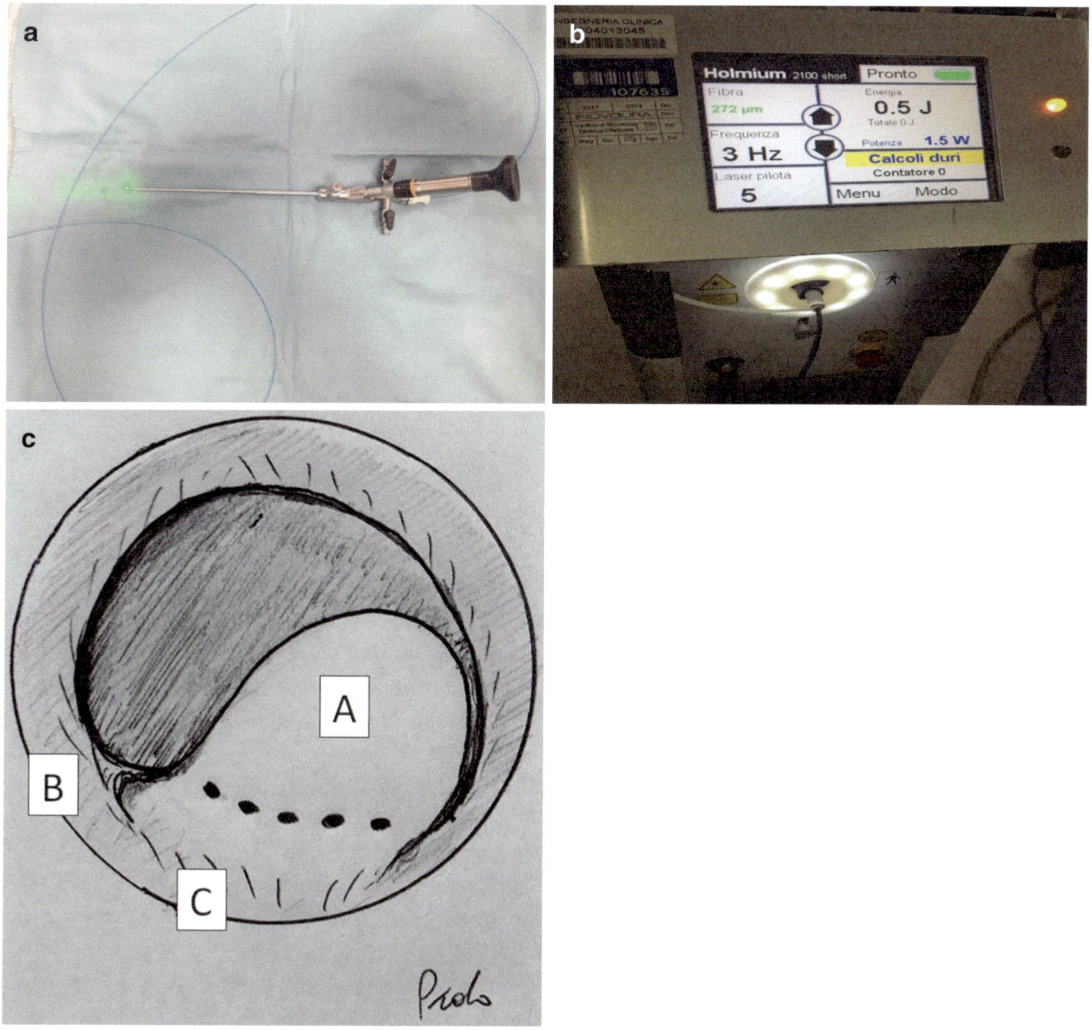

Fig. 63.2 Laser multiple endoscopic punctures technique. (**a**) Paediatric cystoscope with 272 μm fibre. (**b**) Holmium laser source. (**c**) Schematic picture of the multiple punctures site on the basis of ureterocele. (A) ureterocele. (B) Contralateral orifice. (C) bladder neck. Foley catheter is left into the bladder trigone for 24 h to increase the ureterocele wall collapse

- Obstructing ureterocele with severe non-refluxing hydroureteronephrosis
- Intravesical ureterocele within a single non-refluxing system

Successful decompression without reflux may be achieved in 70–80% of cases [14]. In ectopic and duplex system ureteroceles, the ectopic position is associated with higher reoperation rates after endoscopic incision. Husmann and colleagues found that in 28 patients with ectopic ureterocele undergoing endoscopic decompression, 18 (64%) required additional surgical treatment usually because of ipsilateral reflux [13]. In this setting, transurethral puncture represents an effective short-term correction of upper pole obstruction but may not represent definitive therapy in most cases. Many children require to repeat puncture to obtain adequate decompression or, more commonly, subsequent reconstructive surgery for persistent obstruction, recurrent infection and persistent or de novo reflux. Satisfactory postoperative urinary tract decompression has been reported in 85–100% of cases of endoscopic decompression, and recovery of renal function following endoscopic puncture or incision may be also achieved mostly in orthotopic ureteroceles. Surgeons in favour of the endoscopic puncture or incision as first-stage treatment in neonates with ureteroceles refer the following results [15, 16]:

- One third of these patients will be definitively cured by this technique.
- Early renal and ureteral decompression will allow improvement or stabilization of ipsilateral renal function, as well as a decreased risk of pyelonephritis.
- The endoscopic technique allows to delay the definitive surgical correction, when requested. Moreover a technically easier operation can be carried out after the neonatal period, due to decreased dilatation of the affected ureter.

Ureteroceles in duplex collecting systems may be more frequently complicated by VUR, obstruction or UTI, especially if ectopic.

63.10 Our Experience

From January 2012 to December 2017, a total of 64 endoscopic procedures for ureterocele have been performed at the Division of Paediatric Urology. The median age at the surgery was 19.7 months (from 1 month to 168 months). Ectopic ureteroceles were 41 and orthotopic 23. The other associated anomalies were duplex collecting system in 53 patients, renal agenesis in 5 infants and ipsilateral reflux in the lower kidney pole in 3 patients. We observed in nine cases contralateral reflux. Prenatal diagnosis of pyelocaliceal and ureteral dilatation was present in 38 cases. Ureterocele was recognized prenatally in 17 cases of them. Febrile UTI was the presenting symptom in 21 cases.

In the group of 64 patients, 12 required further surgery at 1–5 years from initial endoscopic puncture (18%): ureteral reimplantation in 7 cases and laparoscopic heminephroureterectomy in 5 cases (Table 63.3).

Table 63.3 Number of procedures per year, age at surgery and other associated anomalies in our series

Number procedures	64
2012	6
2013	9
2014	8
2015	12
2016	23
2017	6
Age at surgery (months)	
Median	19.7
Range	1–168
Other anomalies associated	
Duplex system	53
Ipsilateral reflux	4
Contralateral reflux	5
Renal agenesis	2

63.11 Open Surgical Options

The open surgical treatment is still a valid alternative to minimally invasive endoscopic procedures.

Four surgical approaches are available:

1. Heminephrectomy with total or partial ureterectomy, allowing the ureterocele to collapse spontaneously (upper tract approach)
2. Ureteroureterostomy (UU) to bypass the obstructed lower ureter and allow for adequate drainage of the upper pole
3. Excision or marsupialization of the ureterocele, reconstruction of the posterior bladder and reimplantation of the ureter (lower tract approach)
4. Combined upper and lower approach (complete primary approach)

63.12 Heminephroureterectomy (Upper Tract Approach)

The procedure of heminephroureterectomy can be performed in the traditional open technique, or by minimally invasive video surgical technique and laparoscopic- or robot-assisted technique. The laparoscopic partial (or polar) nephrectomy has good results reported but is widely considered to be one of the hardest laparoscopic procedures to perform [18]. The robotic approach removes many of the technical barriers to the laparoscopic approach. In both approaches upper pole ureter can then be identified: the upper pole ureter is dissected free from the surrounding tissue [19]. The lower pole ureter needs to be identified and dissected free, being careful to leave a sufficient amount of periureteral tissue in place to avoid devascularization. The dilated upper pole ureter is followed up towards the renal hilum. It is brought under the renal vessels, being careful not to injure them. The ureter can be followed to the upper pole segment, which can be dissected free from the healthy renal parenchyma. It is important to remove the entire pyelocalyceal structures of the upper renal pole and to carefully inspect the remaining kidney for the presence of any opened lower pole calyces, which need to be closed meticulously with absorbable sutures [16].

63.13 Ureteroureterostomy (UU) (Renal Parenchymal Conservative Upper Approach)

It's increasingly being used to repair duplex systems with reasonable function of the upper pole and relatively equal calibre of ureters, although it has been shown to be effective in systems with any degree of function and ureteral size [16]. The UU enjoys the advantage of avoiding to damage the renal vasculature of the lower pole of the kidney and eliminates the potential risk of injury to these structures [20].

63.14 Excision or Marsupialization of the Ureterocele, Reconstruction of the Trigonal Bladder Wall and Reimplantation of the Ureter (Lower Tract Approach)

The traditional open surgical approach involves the complete excision of the ureterocele with reconstruction of the bladder and bladder neck to create a functional bladder neck mechanism. This approach can involve injury in the bladder neck or creation of a vescicovaginal fistula. An alternative option involves the marsupialization of the ureterocele, which leaves the floor of the ureterocele intact and adhered to the bladder mucosa. One study has found no statistical difference between these two techniques [21]. Using a modified Pfannenstiel incision, the skin and anterior muscles are opened transversally. The filled bladder is incised longitudinally, taking care to avoid injury to the bladder neck. Several sponges are placed into the superior bladder. The ureterocele, the orifice of the lower renal pole ureter and the contralateral ureter are visualized. Each ureter is catheterized with an infant feeding tube or a ureteral catheter. Once the ureterocele is freed completely, the remaining intramural ureter is mobilized as with a standard intravesical ureteral reimplantation. Alternatively, the ureterocele can be marsupialized by excision at the anterior and lateral walls using cautery knife. At this stage, the ureters are reimplanted according to Cohen's technique. The bladder is then closed in a standard two-layer technique using resorbable sutures [22].

63.15 Combined Upper and Lower Approach (Complete Primary Approach)

Some authors [17, 18] proposed a combined upper and lower approach in a single surgical approach. This complete primary approach consists in a heminephroureterectomy of the dysplastic or hydronephrotic poorly functioning upper pole as first step. If the upper pole parenchyma is judged having a relatively good function at scintigraphy renal scan, ureteroureterostomy can be affered [20]. During the same surgery, ureterocelectomy with trigonal reconstruction and ureteral reimplantation of the lower pole is performed. Criticism to the complete upper and lower approach in a single step points out that this technique is very aggressive especially for young infants [23].

63.16 Conclusions

Ureterocele is a relatively uncommon urological malformation that involves all the urinary tract from renal parenchyma to bladder outlet.

Consequences may be severe with significant damage of kidneys, febrile UTIs and contralateral involvement in some cases. The female sex is more commonly involved. Nowadays, prenatal diagnosis may frequently demonstrate pyelocaliceal and ureteral dilated system and be confirmed by neonatal ultrasonographic scan. The presence of a cystic lesion on the bladder base is specific for diagnosis of ureterocele. Neonatal diagnosis allows early decompressive treatment with obstruction release, avoiding febrile UTIs and pyelonephritic episodes with further renal and urinary tract damages. Minimally invasive techniques are today progressively overwhelming the open surgical procedures, especially in young children and newborn. The endoscopic multiple puncture of the ureterocele basis allows immediate decompression of the related upper tract and often may avoid secondary reflux on the same reno-ureteral moiety in duplex system. Both diathermic cautery and laser energy may be used for the endoscopic technique, depending mostly from the surgeon preference. In our experience, in the last 5 years, we adopted laser energy for ureterocele multiple punctures, reducing the risk of intraoperative bleeding and decreasing significantly the need for further surgery to correct secondary VUR of persisting obstruction. The novel endoscopic procedures guarantee good results in the majority of ureteroceles in the first years of life with a very short hospitalization. It represents in our opinion a further significant step towards the use of minimally invasive video surgical techniques in children.

References

1. Godhio AB, Nunes C, et al. Ureterocele: antenatal diagnosis and management. Fetal Diagn Ther. 2013;34:188–91.
2. Zeng L, Huang G, et al. A new classification of duplex kidney based on kidney morphology and management. Chin Med J. 2013;126:615–9.
3. Dada SA, Rafiu MO, et al. Chronic renal failure in a patient with bilateral ureterocele. Saudi Med J. 2015;36:862–4.
4. Schultza K, Todab LY. Genetic basis of ureterocele. Curr Genomics. 2016;17:62–9.
5. Maizels M, Liu D, Gong, et al. Endoscopic ureterocelectomy-retrograde incision from orifice (RIO) of urethral segment of ureterocele and extending to bladder neck is a feasible and simple procedure. J Pediatr Urol. 2016;12:137–8.
6. Gander R, Asensio, et al. Evaluation of the initial treatment of ureteroceles. Urology. 2016;89:113–7.
7. Chowdhary SK, Kandpal DK, et al. Ureterocele in newborns, infants and children: ten year prospective study with primary endoscopic deroofing and double J (DJ) stenting. J Pediatr Surg. 2017;52:569–73.
8. Han MY, Gibbons MF, Belman AB, et al. Indications for nonoperative management of ureteroceles. J Urol. 2005;174:1652.
9. Direnna T, Leonard MP. Watchful waiting for prenatally detected ureteroceles. J Urol. 2006;175:1493.
10. Gutiérrez JM, Ortega, et al. Endoscopic incision of intravesical ureteroceles in patients with duplex system. Cir Pediatr. 2014;27:107–9.
11. Timberlake MD, Corbett ST. Minimally invasive techniques for management of the ureterocele and ectopic ureter: upper tract versus lower tract approach. Urol Clin North Am. 2015;42:61–76.
12. Adorisio O, et al. Effectiveness of primary endoscopic incision in treatment of ectopic ureterocele associated with duplex system. Urology. 2011;77:191.
13. Castagnetti M, et al. Management of duplex system ureteroceles in neonates and infants. Nat Rev Urol. 2009;6:307.
14. EAU guidelines 2017—ureterocele treatment.
15. Husmann D, Strand B, et al. Management of ectopic ureterocele associated with renal duplication: a comparison of partial nephrectomy and endoscopic decompression. J Urol. 1999;162:1406.
16. Lewis J, Cheng E, et al. Complete excision or marsupialisation of ureteroceles: does choice of surgical approach affect outcome? J Urol. 2008;180:1819.
17. Castagnetti M, Vidal E, et al. Duplex system ureterocele in infants: should we reconsider the indications for secondary surgery after endoscopic puncture or partial nephrectomy? J Pediatr Urol. 2013;9:11–6.
18. Hisamatsu E, Takagi S, et al. Nephrectomy and upper pole heminephrectomy for poorly functioning kidney: is total ureterectomy necessary? Indian J Urol. 2012;28:271–4.
19. Swana HS, Hakky TS, et al. Transurethral neoorifice (TUNO) a novel technique for management of upper pole obstruction in infancy. Int Braz J Urol. 2013;39:143.
20. Le HK, Chiang G. Long-term management of ureterocele in duplex collecting systems: reconstruction implications. Curr Urol Rep. 2018;19(2):14.
21. Kagantsov IM, Sizonov VV, et al. Laparoscopic heminephroureterectomy for duplex kidney in children. Urologia. 2017;(5):69–74.
22. Storm DW, et al. Laparoscopic ipsilateral ureteroureterostomy in the management of ureteral ectopia in infants and children. J Pediatr Urol. 2011;7:529.
23. Jesus LE, et al. Clinical evolution of vesicoureteral reflux following endoscopic puncture in children with duplex system ureteroceles. J Urol. 2011;186:1455.

Laparoscopic Adrenalectomy in Children

64

Andrzej Golebiewski, Marcin Losin, and Piotr Czauderna

64.1 Introduction

Laparoscopic approach to the adrenal gland was introduced in 1992; since then laparoscopic adrenalectomy (LA) becomes a gold standard in adult population, and many studies evaluating safety and results have been published [1–3]. In contradistinction to adult population, LA remains still challenging in children population despite the fact that it was first performed in a child over 20 years ago [4, 5].

Indications of LA remain unclear, but it is mainly used for neoplastic masses arising from adrenal glands like neuroblastomas (NB), ganglioneuroblastomas (GNB), and pheochromocytomas (PHE). Adrenal cortex tumors and congenital adrenal hyperplasia are very seldom to find in children, and NB remains the most common indication for LA [5, 6].

Transperitoneal laparoscopic approach remains the most commonly used among pediatric surgeons. Single-port surgery (SPS) and retroperitoneal approach are used only in a limited number of centers [7, 8].

A. Golebiewski · M. Losin · P. Czauderna (✉)
Department of Surgery and Urology for Children and Adolescents, Medical University of Gdansk, Gdansk, Poland
e-mail: pczaud@gumed.edu.pl

64.2 Preoperative Preparation

In all adrenal tumor (AT) cases, ultrasound (US) examination is obtained followed by computed tomography (CT) and/or magnetic resonance imaging (MRI).

Hormone levels are routinely examined, and adrenal MIBG scintigraphy is used in NB-suspected cases. In PHE patients hypertension has to be normalized prior to surgery; also proper antihypertensive premedication and intraoperative management are essential.

Before procedure blood tests are taken, IV central line is preferably established, and antibiotic prophylaxis is given. Twenty cubic centimeter per kilogram of packed red blood cells are prepared, and nasogastric tube and urinary catheter are inserted.

64.3 Positioning

The patient is placed supine with spread legs and small roll put under the back. The monitor is usually placed at the patients' head slightly moved laterally to the affected site. The surgeon stands between patients' legs with camera operator and scrub nurse standing on both sides of the table. In small babies it is convenient to position them transversely across the table.

In older children posterolateral positioning of the patient is used occasionally. In this case

C. Esposito et al. (eds.), *ESPES Manual of Pediatric Minimally Invasive Surgery*,
https://doi.org/10.1007/978-3-030-00964-9_64

surgeon and camera operator are standing on the same side of the operating table with scrub nurse facing them. We commonly use reversed Trendelenburg position as it helps to obtain a good insight to upper abdominal region.

64.4 Instrumentation

We never use a scope larger than 5 mm as HD tools provide great visualization. LigaSure Vessel Sealing System®, harmonic knife, or another vessel-sealing bipolar device is present at OR depending on surgeon's preferences. In order to close larger vessels, we often use HemoLock® instead of titanic clips. Specimen should be extracted in plastic endobag.

64.5 Technique

Procedure of laparoscopic adrenalectomy or biopsy taking is started with introducing the first trocar via umbilicus, usually by open approach as described by Hasson [9]. We often use 10 mm port as specimen will be extracted in most cases through the umbilicus. Pneumoperitoneum with CO_2 is created slowly to a pressure of 10–12 mmHg. Three additional 3 or 5 mm ports are placed depending on the patients' size. In majority of cases, we put two ports in midline, superior to umbilicus, and one port laterally on the level of umbilicus below the affected region. The procedure is started with lifting the right lobe of the liver or spleen by a self-locking grasper clipped on diaphragm. In order to get direct visualization of the right adrenal gland, lifting the liver is usually enough. On the left site, total colon splenic flexure mobilization is always performed by incising its lateral peritoneal and splenic attachments. Sometimes it is also necessary to mobilize the spleen and pancreatic tail medially. The retroperitoneal space is dissected (after opening renal fascia and fatty capsule of upper renal pole), and a tumor localized in adrenal gland is exposed (Fig. 64.1). Superior adrenal pole is mobilized first after dissecting connective tissue connected with diaphragmatic crura, and

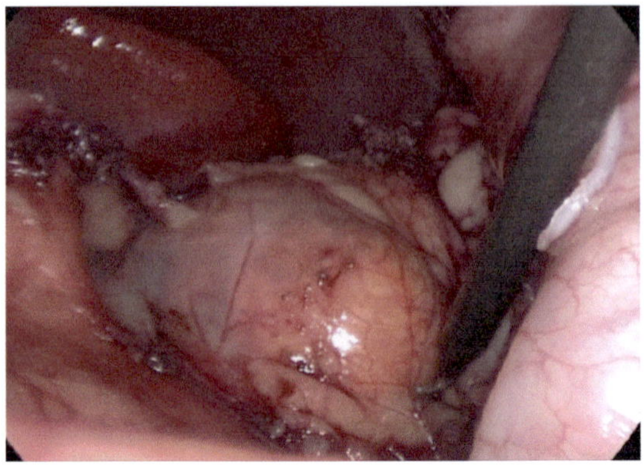

Fig. 64.1 Left adrenalectomy in neuroblastoma. Intraoperative view of affected site

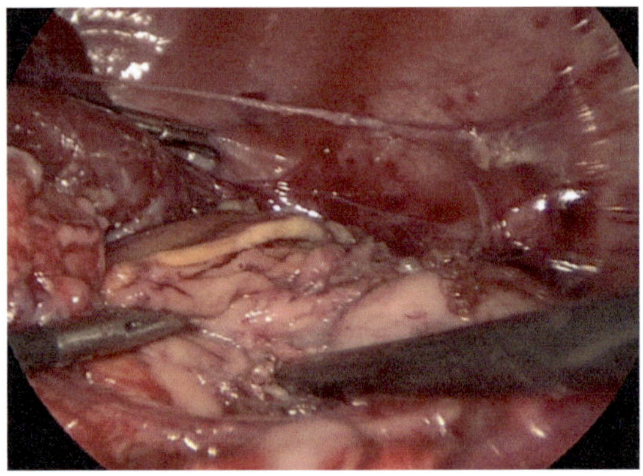

Fig. 64.2 Left adrenalectomy in neuroblastoma. Grasper clipped on diaphragm in order to elevate a spleen. Part of unaffected adrenal gland is visible at the center

then medial part of adrenal gland is approached (Fig. 64.2). Some surgeons prefer to start dissection medially, especially on the left side. In large adrenal or para-adrenal tumors, in order to have great anatomical view at the operative field, we dissect renal hilum and pull away renal vessels by placing rubber loops around them. After meticulous dissection of adrenal vessels (Fig. 64.3), they can be clipped separately with HemoLock® (Fig. 64.4); however in many children, especially younger ones, this part of the procedure is usually realized with vessel-sealing device. The rest of dissection is also performed with LigaSure® or harmonic knife and is usually safe as major vessels are taken down already. The specimen is extracted in a bag via slightly enlarged umbilical

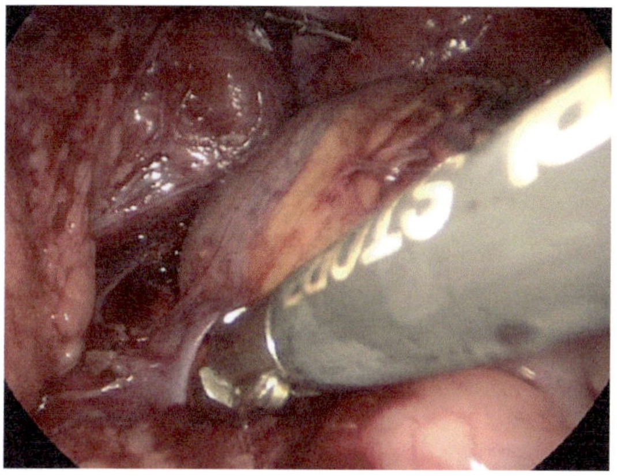

Fig. 64.3 Left adrenalectomy in neuroblastoma. Dissection of adrenal vessels

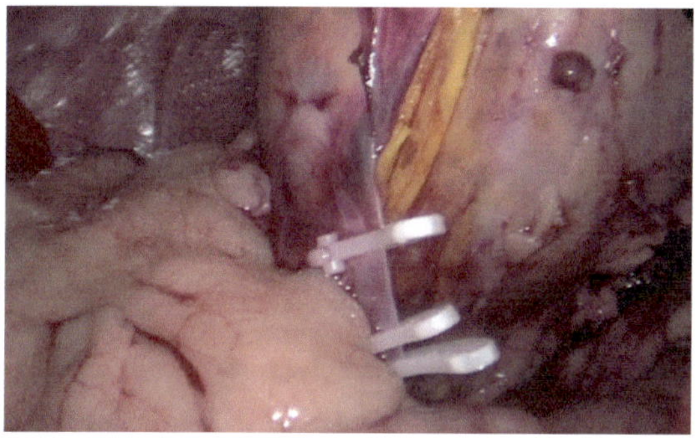

Fig. 64.4 Left adrenalectomy in neuroblastoma. Adrenal vessels closed with HemoLock

incision, and the abdomen is inspected for enlarged lymph nodes (LN) to perform eventual LN biopsy or more formal lymphadenectomy. Initial dissection is usually more difficult on the left side, since taking down the colon flexure is unnecessary on the right. On the contrary, closing of the right adrenal vein is more difficult, since it is a single and short one, as well as originates directly from internal vena cava (IVC) (Fig. 64.5). Be aware that larger adrenal tumors often reach behind the IVC, which makes dissection more hazardous due to small vessels connecting both structures and the risk of bleeding.

We have used single-port surgery in selected cases of adrenal tumors. We prefer to use the GelPort® (Applied Medical) which is introduced via 2.5 cm incision in umbilicus. The procedure is essentially done the same way as in typical

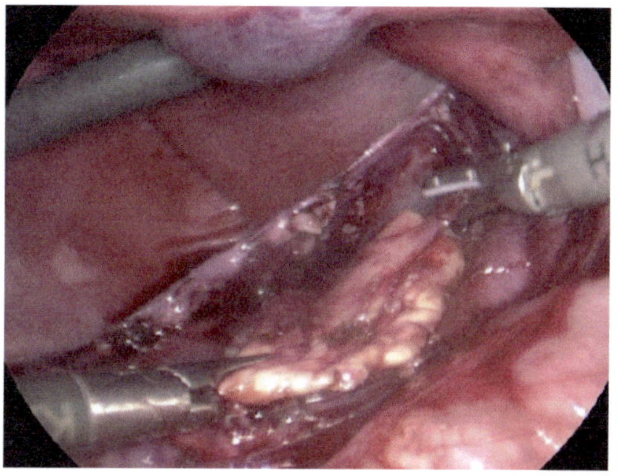

Fig. 64.5 Right adrenalectomy in neuroblastoma. Closing of adrenal vein close to ICV with harmonic knife. Grasper is clipped on diaphragm in order to elevate right liver lobe

laparoscopic surgery, but special articulated instruments (reusable or disposable ones) are helpful.

64.6 Postoperative Care

We usually remove nasogastric tube at the end of procedure. Child is transferred to postop ward with vital signs monitored overnight. Chest X-rays are performed to evaluate central line position and to exclude risk of pneumothorax. Opioids combined with paracetamol are administrated. Oral feeding is advanced when tolerated, IV fluids administrated in weight depend regime.

64.7 Results

Twenty-two patients have undergone laparoscopic adrenalectomy in two Polish centers including ours. Boys predominated and age at the time of operation varied from 2 months to 7 years. All but two lesions were unilateral, left-sided slightly predominant. In all cases standard transperitoneal laparoscopic approach has been selected with single-port technique used in three patients. In three cases laparoscopy required conversion to open approach because of tumor infiltration of inferior vena cava and diaphragm

[2] and lesion of renal vein with excessive hemorrhage [1]. Mean operation time was 2.5 h (1.5–3 h). We treated one port-site infection during postop course, and we found one renal atrophy in one patient as the result of renal artery persistent spasm.

Mean hospital stay was 4.5 days (1–14 days). Follow-up is 1–16 years.

64.8 Tips and Tricks

Right-sided adrenalectomy requires usually the use of four ports for liver retraction or percutaneous insertion of an additional self-locking grasper in a bayonet fashion.

64.8.1 Right Adrenalectomy

Closing adrenal vessels, especially the vein, may be more difficult as it originates directly from inferior vena cava. It is usually very short with no place for typical traction.

64.8.2 Left Adrenalectomy

The lienocolic ligament should be divided up to the level of the gastric fundus which improves exposure of the left adrenal gland by allowing the spleen to fall medially, pulling the tail of the pancreas with it.

Be aware of the proximity of the renal vessels due to medial location of the LT adrenal gland; hence use electrocautery with caution.

The inferior phrenic artery often runs along the upper edge of the adrenal glands and should be sought and ligated with clips and divided.

Manipulation and mobilization of the adrenal gland using graspers should be gentle, since it is very fragile and can be easily damaged causing bleeding and hemodynamic instability, which may occur in patients with pheochromocytoma. In cases of pheochromocytomas, it is especially important to close the vein first.

Large tumors require an abdominal incision to facilitate atraumatic extraction.

In the case of a thorough bleeding control, no additional abdominal drains are required.

64.9 Troubleshooting

64.9.1 Injury to the Vena Cava

- Small tear: press IVC with an endopeanut or a cotton tape inserted via the port for few minutes, and then place a hemostatic agent over the defect.
- If the bleeding persists: close the injury with forceps (preferably vascular clamp), insert another 5 mm port, and suture the defect.
- Large lesion: convert to open approach by making an incision between the two trocars, and fix lesion with standard technique.

Bleeding from small vessels: increase the intra-abdominal pressure, and use bipolar coagulation.

Pleural injuries: suture (check after the procedure with X-ray for pneumothorax), and consider the insertion of temporary chest tube.

Visceral injuries (spleen, liver): use argon plasma coagulator, bipolar coagulation, and topical hemostatic agents.

64.10 Discussion

The debate regarding optimal surgical management in the case of pathological adrenal masses in pediatric population is still open. In recent years, adrenal surgery has evolved considerably due to advances in diagnostic tools, the development of endocrine knowledge, and the emergence of minimally invasive techniques.

Since the first transperitoneal laparoscopic adrenalectomy, described by Gagner et al. [1] in 1992, minimal invasive surgery has revolutionized adrenal surgery and largely replaced the open approach. Therefore, laparoscopic adrenalectomy is presently considered the "gold standard" procedure for the surgery of benign and selected malignant adrenal masses in adult patients [2].

Many retrospective clinical studies have shown the benefits of laparoscopic adrenalectomy in adults. When compared to open surgery, minimally invasive adrenal surgery has resulted in shorter hospital stay, faster recovery, decreased requirements for analgesics, and better cosmetic results [3].

The first pediatric malignant case was performed on a small asymptomatic neuroblastoma identified by mass screening of children in Japan [4]. Laparoscopic adrenalectomy has progressively become an effective, feasible, reproducible, and safe procedure in children [5].

Nevertheless, in the pediatric population, the experience with laparoscopic adrenalectomy is limited. The reasons are the rarity of adrenal lesions in this population, a variable pathologic spectrum, and a higher incidence of malignancy in these patients (more than 90% of adrenal masses are neuroblastomas) [5, 6].

The most common childhood adrenal pathology, neuroblastoma, is in many instances not readily feasible to laparoscopic excision because it is not a well-encapsulated tumor but rather has an infiltrative and invasive nature and most often is not suitable for resection at diagnosis.

In addition, small children and especially infants, which is typical age for NB, present unique challenge related to small body size and inexperience with smaller laparoscopic instrumentation among surgeons.

Due to the rare occurrence of adrenal lesions in children which may be operated laparoscopically, the accumulation of information on pediatric LA is limited, and the experience in children consists of relatively small retrospective case series [6].

In these reports outcomes focused on operative parameters such as operative time, length of stay, and complications have shown that a laparoscopic adrenalectomy is feasible and safe in highly selected patients.

Thus, the use of minimally invasive adrenalectomy in children is superior to open surgery for the excision of benign tumors with low morbidity rates; its use for malignant tumors should be limited to selected cases [6].

Children with adrenal masses are either diagnosed coincidentally by imaging or by investigation of symptoms suggesting adrenal hormone excess. Adrenal masses can be palpated in smaller children. Once an adrenal mass is diagnosed, all patients should be studied with ultrasonography, computed tomography, or magnetic resonance imaging to assess the side, the size, the local extent, and the operability of the primary lesion. All patients should also undergo preoperative evaluations including endocrinologic investigation to determine secretory tumor activity [10].

Complete and thorough preoperative evaluation is essential for operative planning. Patients are suitable for laparoscopic resection if the preoperative imaging showed no vascular encasement and in a tumor with the greatest dimension ≤5 cm. Candidates for LA included low-risk adrenal tumors and tumors that were prenatally diagnosed and increased in size during follow-up. In children, an absolute limitation cannot be determined but should be evaluated individually, based on the size of mass relative to the size of child. Tumors that are radiologically unsuitable for laparoscopy have midline expansion/infiltration and major vessels invasion/encasement. Relatively large size tumors which have a predictable risk of macroscopically incomplete resection or tumor rupture should be rather managed by open surgery. Open access is still preferable for patients with suspicion of malignancy based on renal vein involvement or significant retroperitoneal lymphadenopathy, although there are some reports of using laparoscopic approach even in such cases [16]. The size of the tumor above 6 cm is a relative contraindication, depending on the age and size of the child [10–12].

To choose the correct approach, we follow the International Pediatric Endosurgery Group guidelines, which state that only lesions without vascular encasement and adjacent organ involvement and with the greatest dimension <6 cm on preoperative imaging are eligible for the laparoscopic approach [12].

For patients with pheochromocytoma, a preoperative preparation is required.

For most adrenal lesions requiring operation, minimally invasive adrenalectomy can be performed safely and effectively with either transperitoneal or the retroperitoneal approach.

Few studies have compared both procedures thoroughly, showing no superiority of either technique [13].

We preferred the transperitoneal approach for all of the adrenalectomies on both sides, and we found the lateral transperitoneal approach to be the procedure of choice.

The transperitoneal route demonstrated to have many advantages compared to retroperitoneal approach. Firstly, it offers a large working space with a clear view of the structures which allows the surgeon to see perfectly both adrenal glands and adjacent organs. Secondly, it has a shorter learning curve and shorter operative time and allows for resection of larger tumors and exploration and treatment of other intra-abdominal conditions.

Thus, the transperitoneal approach as technically easier is widely considered the most accepted procedure for laparoscopic surgery of the adrenal glands [7].

Single-site and robotic techniques have recently been widely used in adults, but experience in the pediatric population is very limited so far [8].

Walz et al. in their case–control study have demonstrated that single-site LA had a conversion rate of 14%, longer operative times, similar rate of complications, and a shorter hospital stay. They concluded that no age and size criteria applied to a well-trained surgical team [14].

Although the literature suggests that laparoscopy could potentially offer great short-term benefits in the pediatric population, few reports comment on tumor spillage, port-site disease recurrence, or overall survival in malignant tumors. However, Kelleher et al. state that laparoscopic resection of adrenal neuroblastoma is feasible and can be performed with equivalent recurrence and mortality rates in low-/intermediate-risk group patients and selected high-risk patients with neuroblastoma who were carefully selected to undergo laparoscopic adrenalectomy [10].

Leclair and colleagues reported a predicted disease-free survival of 84% at 5 years for 45 patients with abdominal neuroblastoma undergoing laparoscopic resection [15].

To reduce these risks, we found it important to gently manipulate the adrenal gland and to use an endosurgical bag to remove the specimen. In our patients, we did not observe neoplastic relapse.

Our experience indicates that laparoscopic adrenalectomy for neuroblastoma in patients who meet surgical selection criteria, i.e., tumor size smaller than 6 cm and absence of vascular encasement, is feasible and offers equivalent progression-free survival and overall survival regardless of other indicators of risk including age and stage.

These data suggest that laparoscopic resection of adrenal neuroblastoma should be considered in patients meeting the selection criteria, regardless of the risk group.

Although the patient group was limited, our experience proves the safety, feasibility, and advantages of a laparoscopic approach to the treatment of benign and malignant adrenal masses in children. All procedures were successfully performed with excellent intraoperative and postoperative results.

In addition, laparoscopic adrenalectomy showed good results in tumor resection >6 cm, suggesting that the dimensional limit of the tumors eligible for laparoscopy should be revised.

Peter et al. state that significantly bigger lesions >6 cm take greater operative times and the conversion rate is 10% higher with the larger lesions.

Our experience also suggests that laparoscopic adrenalectomy, if performed by a highly skilled laparoscopic surgeon, may be feasible and safe even for the treatment of larger, malignant adrenal lesions, without infiltration of surrounding structures, though.

64.11 Complications

Laparoscopic adrenalectomy carries the risk of typical laparoscopic injuries to abdominal structures and organs with trocar and instrument placement.

Based on literature, the main cause of conversion was adherence of the tumor to the surrounding organs and renal vein or vena cava thrombosis. In our own center series, we had no conversion, since we had no tumor ruptures or relevant bleeding, which are the most frequent reasons for conversion. We believe that this was due to our meticulous selection of patients.

In all our patients, the blood loss was negligible (<100 mL), without the need for a blood transfusion, which can be attributed to laparoscope magnification and gentle operative technique.

The only postoperative complication in our series was renal infarction after resection of a large left-sided neuroblastoma in an infant that required skeletonization of the renal vessels with resulting prolonged renal artery spasm.

Neuroblastoma should be excised to the extent that it is feasible without compromising surrounding organs. The International Pediatric Endoscopic Group published guidelines for the surgical treatment of adrenal masses in children, stating that although there were no absolute contraindications, cases should be carefully selected [12].

In conclusion, laparoscopic adrenalectomy offers a safe and effective surgical option for many pediatric adrenal lesions offering shortened hospital stay and minimal blood loss. Tumor vascular involvement (encasement) seems to be an obvious contraindication to MIS approach, while very large tumor size may be a relative contraindication on an individual case basis. Proper preoperative patient selection and planning seems to be a major criterion for success.

References

1. Gagner M, Lacroix A, Bolte E. Laparoscopic adrenalectomy in Cushing's syndrome and pheochromacytoma. N Engl J Med. 1992;327:1033.
2. Gil-Cardenas A, Cordon C, Gamino R, et al. Laparoscopic adrenalectomy: lessons learned from an initial series of 100 patients. Surg Endosc. 2008;22:991–4.
3. Guazzoni G, Montorsi F, Bocciardi A, et al. Transperitoneal laparoscopic versus open adrenalectomy for benign hyperfunctioning adrenal tumors: a comparative study. J Urol. 1995;153:1597–600.
4. Yamamoto H, Yoshida M, Sera Y. Laparoscopic surgery for neuroblastoma identified by mass screening. J Pediatr Surg. 1996;31:385–8.
5. Nerli RB, Reddy MN, Guntaka A, et al. Laparoscopic adrenalectomy for adrenal masses in children. J Pediatr Urol. 2011;7(2):182–6.
6. De Barros F, Romao RL, de Pinho-Apezzato ML, et al. Laparoscopic adrenalectomy in children for neuroblastoma: report of case series. Surg Laparosc Endosc Percutan Tech. 2012;22(1):79–81.
7. Fascetti-Leon F, Scotton G, Pio L, et al. Minimally invasive resection of adrenal masses in infants and children: results of European multi-center survey. Surg Endosc. 2017;31(11):4505–12.
8. Łosin M, Czauderna P, Gołębiewski A, et al. Single incision laparoscopic adrenalectomy—initial experience. Videosurg Other Miniinvasive Tech. 2010;3(3):104–6. https://doi.org/10.5114/wiitm.2010.16421.
9. Hasson HM. Open laparoscopy as method of access in laparoscopic surgery. Gynecol Endosc. 1999;8:353–62.
10. Kelleher CM, Smithson L, Nguyen LL, et al. Clinical outcomes in children with adrenal neuroblastoma undergoing open versus laparoscopic adrenalectomy. J Pediatr Surg. 2013;48(8):1727–32.
11. Brisse HJ, McCarville MB, Granata C, et al. Guidelines for imaging and staging of neuroblastic tumors: consensus report from the International Neuroblastoma Risk Group Project. Radiology. 2011;261(1):243–57. https://doi.org/10.1148/radiol.11101352
12. International Pediatric Endosurgery Group. IPEG guidelines for the surgical treatment of adrenal masses in children. J Laparoendosc Adv Surg Tech A. 2010;20(2):vii–x.
13. Berber E, Tellioglu G, Harvey A, Mitchell J, Milas M, Siperstein A. Comparison of laparoscopic transabdominal lateral versus posterior retroperitoneal adrenalectomy. Surgery. 2009;146:621–5.
14. Walz MK, Groeben H, Alesina PF. Single-access retroperitoneoscopic adrenalectomy (SARA) versus conventional retroperitoneoscopic adrenalectomy (CORA): a case–control study. World J Surg. 2010;34(6):1386–90.
15. Leclair M-D, de Lagausie P, Becmeur F, et al. Laparoscopic resection of abdominal neuroblastoma. Ann Surg Oncol. 2008;15(1):117–24.
16. Iwanaka T, Arai M, Ito M, et al. Challenges of laparoscopic resection of abdominal neuroblastoma with lymphadenectomy. Surg Endosc. 2001;15:489–92.

65 Endoscopic Management of Bladder Tumors in Children

Mohamed Abouheba and Sameh Shehata

65.1 Introduction

Urinary bladder tumors are not common in children and adolescents. They are either urothelial or non-urothelial (Fig. 65.1). The commonest is rhabdomyosarcoma (RMS) of the bladder or prostate/vagina followed by papillary urothelial tumors (Table 65.1) [1]. RMS, being the commonest childhood soft tissue sarcoma, ranks third commonest pediatric solid tumor (5–15%) [2, 3]. A recent analysis of 57 reports of pediatric urothelial bladder tumors which included 127 cases reported patients younger than 20 years old, of which only 21 patients (16.5%) were below 10 years old [4]. Both tumor categories exhibit a 3–9:1 male-to-female preponderance [5].

The histologic classification of RMS that was originally formulated in 1958 included four subtypes: embryonal, alveolar, pleomorphic, and undifferentiated [7]. Later, the pleomorphic type was considered an anaplastic variant of embryonal or alveolar RMS and hence culminated into only three histologic categories currently recognized: embryonal, alveolar, and undifferentiated [8].

Papillary urothelial tumors terminology has probably generated the greatest debate in oncology literature until recently in 2004 when the World Health Organization (WHO)–International Society of Urologic Pathology (ISUP) has formulated a widely accepted classification of urothelial neoplasms of the urinary bladder. The former transitional cell carcinoma of the urinary bladder (TCCB) [9] is now split into a papillary urothelial neoplasm of low malignant potential (PUNLMP) and a low-grade carcinoma of the urinary bladder (LGCB), depending on the amount of atypia [10]. The current classification is built on histopathologic criteria and correlates to the clinical outcome and prognosis of different bladder papillary tumor subtypes (Table 65.2) [5].

While RMS usually presents by obstructive uropathy [12], papillary tumors usually present with painless hematuria followed by dysuria and rarely pyelonephritis [13]. Diagnosis is usually delayed probably due to underestimation of hematuria in children [14]. Although about 75% of tumors are unifocal in the trigone that usually turn out to be non- or minimally invasive [15], yet still invasive TCCB is seen in older children and adolescents [12].

Transurethral resection of bladder tumors (TURBT) is done as the definitive surgery for the common PUNLMP as well as to provide specimens for pathologic staging and grading the less common TCC.

M. Abouheba · S. Shehata (✉)
Pediatric Surgery Division, Children's Hospital, Alexandria University, Alexandria, Egypt
e-mail: sameh_shehata@alexmed.edu.eg

C. Esposito et al. (eds.), *ESPES Manual of Pediatric Minimally Invasive Surgery*,
https://doi.org/10.1007/978-3-030-00964-9_65

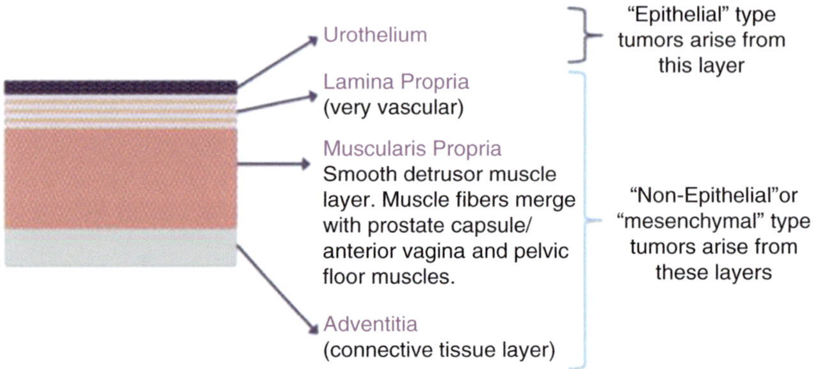

Fig. 65.1 Urinary bladder wall histological layers and their respective tumors [6]

Table 65.1 Most common bladder tumors in children [1]

Tumor	Age- and sex-related features
Urothelial tumors	
Infiltrative urothelial carcinoma (high grade)	Infiltrative urothelial carcinoma and noninvasive urothelial carcinoma are more common in adolescents; they occur in individuals younger than 10 years in only one-third of cases
Noninvasive urothelial carcinoma (low grade)	(PUNLMP) Age range of affected individuals is variable in childhood
Urothelial papilloma	Age range of affected individuals is variable in childhood
Fibroepithelial polyp	Manifests in individuals with a mean age of 9 years; more common in males
Mesenchymal tumors	
Rhabdomyosarcoma	Manifests in individuals in a bimodal age distribution (within first 2 years of life and during adolescence); certain genetic syndromes, such as Li-Fraumeni cancer syndrome and neurofibromatosis type 1, are associated with increased risk
Leiomyoma	Rare in children, with only two case reports to date; more common in women aged 30–60 years
Neurofibroma	Majority of tumors are first detected in individuals younger than 18 years; manifests
IMT	Manifests in individuals with a mean age of 7 years
Leiomyosarcoma	Exceedingly rare in children; the youngest affected person reported in the literature was aged 10 years
Angiosarcoma	Extremely rare; more common in males; manifests in individuals with an average age of 2 years
Hemangioma	Rare; usually occurs in individuals younger than 5 years
Neuroendocrine tumors	
Paraganglioma	Exceedingly rare in children; more common in individuals aged 30–60 years; the youngest affected patient reported was aged 10 years

65.2 Preoperative Preparation

Since urological ultrasound is the first tool to assess dysuria or gross/microscopic hematuria, it usually raises the suspicion of RMS by finding "frank invasive bladder tumor" [11] or TCCB by finding "papillary urothelial ingrowths" [13]. For suspected RMS, definitive CT or MRI imaging is needed to detect tissue of origin, LN status, and proper staging. For suspected TCCB, the next step better be the noninvasive urine cytology rather than insensitive VCUG owing to dye density often masking (and missing) papillary ingrowths [5].

Urinary cytology is obtained as a baseline and to establish the likelihood of high-grade TCCB. Dysplasia dictates careful bladder examination during cystoscopy. Cystoscopic transurethral resection of bladder tumor (TURBT) under

Table 65.2 Classification of bladder tumors in children [11]

Parameter	TCCB	PUNLMP	LGCB
Classification reference	WHO (1973)	WHO (2004)	WHO (2004)
Cellular features			
Cell density	Increased	Increased	Less increased
Size of cells	Irregularity	Minimal variations	Variations
Cellular polarity	Disturbances	Preserved	Variations
Differentiation	Failure from the base to the surface	Basal layers show palisading, minimal to absent cytologic atypia	Orderly overall appearance of urothelium, typical cytologic atypia
Mitotic figures	Displaced or abnormal	Rare, basal location	Infrequent and may occur at any level but are more frequent basally
Typical cells	Giant cells	Umbrella cell layer preserved	
Nuclear features	Crowding	Impression of predominant order with absent to minimal variation	Variations
Nuclear shape	Variations	Minimal variations	Mild differences
Nuclear size	Enlarged	Slightly enlarged	Uniformly enlarged
Nucleoli	Present	Absent	Present but inconspicuous
Chromatin pattern	Variations	Fine	Mild differences
Expression of cytokeratin 20, CD44, p53, and p63	+ to ++	+	++

TCCB Transitional cell carcinoma of the bladder, *PUNLMP* Papillary urothelial neoplasm of low malignant potential

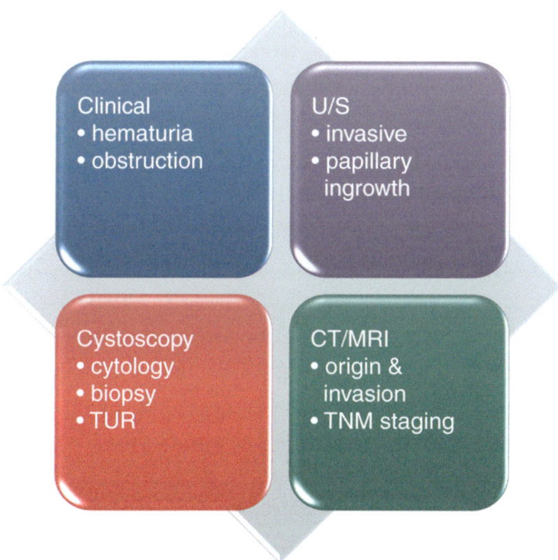

Fig. 65.2 Diagnostic workup

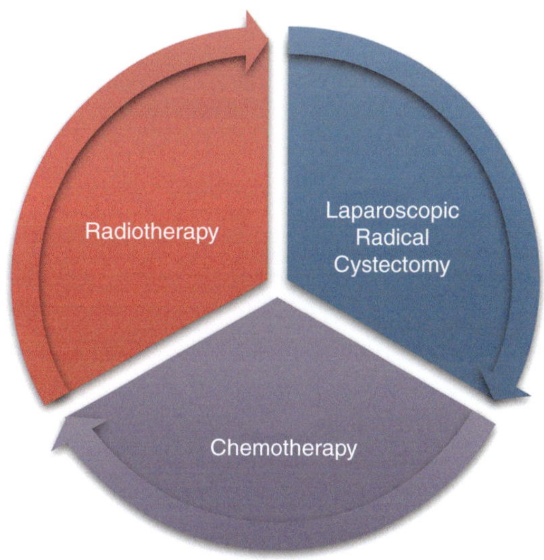

Fig. 65.3 Multimodal approach to RMS treatment

general anesthesia by loop electrode facilitates excision of visible tumors and provides specimens for histologic confirmation of tumor grade and stage (Fig. 65.2). Tumor invasion into ureteric orifices or involvement of prostatic urethra guides further surgery.

Verified RMS patients proceed to risk-stratification treatment regimen of the multimodal approach devised by Children Oncology Group (COG) (Fig. 65.3) with the aim of preserving functional organ and minimizing radiation while achieving comparable outcome. Papillary tumors, on the other hand, are usually low-grade and noninvasive, and hence cystoscopic TUR is usually sufficient with regular surveillance [5].

65.3 Positioning

- General anesthesia
- Lithotomy
- IV broad-spectrum antibiotic prophylaxis

65.4 Instrumentation

65.4.1 Equipment

- Rigid cystoscope set
- 9.5-,11-, or 14-Fr pediatric scope
- 70° lens optics (for visualization) or 12 or 30° lens optics (for resection)
- Resectoscope, cup biopsy forceps, and loop electrode
- Endoscopic camera and stack
- Light source
- Irrigation channel
- Irrigation fluid—water if monopolar diathermy is used, saline if bipolar electrocautery

65.5 Technique

65.5.1 Diagnostic Visualization

Male	Female
• Hold the penis in vertical position	• Separate the labia to view the urethra
• Holding the cystoscope vertically, gently insert the tip into the urethra	
• Slowly advance the scope with slow irrigation to keep the lumen in view until the bulbar urethra and external sphincter are identified	• Cystoscope advances to the bladder easily
• Once the external sphincter is identified, the scope must be dropped down below the horizontal and advanced upward into the posterior urethra. The verumontanum and bladder neck are inspected, and the scope may need to be dropped further to clear a prominent bladder neck	
• Inspect the bladder in a stepwise fashion: trigone, ureteric orifices, and four quadrants of the bladder. Locate any papillary growths	
• Empty the bladder	

65.5.2 Resection Biopsy

An examination of the bladder may be helpful in adolescents under general anesthesia before preparation and draping and throughout the procedure may reveal a RMS mass but often misses small papillary tumors. Mass mobility or fixation should be assessed before and after resection [10].

Small tumors are often easily scooped en masse, but pedicled tumors are resected piecemeal, using stalk for countertraction until the end. Friable, low-grade papillary tumors can often be resected with a cold loop to lower risk of bladder perforation and "frying" specimens, whereas solid high-grade tumors usually require powered loop for hemostatic control of tumor bed.

After "complete" resection of all "visible" tumor, an extra chip is scooped with the loop electrode, or a cold-cup biopsy is punched out and sent separately for histopathology to exclude muscle invasion that invariably impacts diagnosis. Vigorous irrigation to ensure proper hemostasis at tumor bed concludes resection.

Introduction of bipolar electroresection is reported to allow TUR in saline and to minimize the risk of the obturator reflex, which can predispose to bladder perforation [1].

Although diverticular tumors are rare in children, yet owing to their muscle invasiveness involving perivesical fat, their complete resection often transgresses the bladder wall which theoretically may spread malignancy [1, 13]. Therefore, conservative resection is preserved for low-grade diverticular tumors followed by fulguration of their base. This could be repeated if final histology confirms high-grade. On the other hand, high-grade diverticular tumors must be sampled at the base (including perivesical fat), despite risking bladder perforation. Partial or radical cystectomy is the definitive surgery for such tumors, however.

Manual compression of the lower abdominal wall may bring anterior bladder wall or dome tumors closer to resectoscope to facilitate resection of such inaccessible lesions. Periureteric tumors represent a technical challenge. Resection of the orifice itself or even the intramural ureter can be done if indicated yet risks refluxing malignant cells [14].

The Bugbee electrode ensures good hemostasis if placed on the biopsy crater with the bladder underfilled, by firing energy to crumble mucosa around the electrode. Light irrigation clears all clots and bubbles to visualize the coagulum painting biopsy crater.

If a tumor appears frankly muscle-invasive, multiple biopsies of the tumor edge and base to confirm invasion could be done instead of complete resection to avoid bladder perforation, since cystectomy will likely follow. On the other hand, low-grade tumors have low risk of muscle invasion obviating the need of transmural biopsy to avoid bladder perforation [15].

65.6 Postoperative Care

Transient hematuria, dysuria, and urgency are common complaints in the immediate postoperative period. However, massive hematuria and pelvic pain raise the suspicion of a missed bladder perforation that may complicate less than 5% of TURs.

A postoperative urinary catheter is usually not needed unless there is a risk of perforation. However, if intraoperative bladder perforation is detected, an indwelling urinary catheter for urinary diversion usually permits healing in few days.

Perioperative antibiotic prophylaxis is preferable, but extended broad-spectrum antibiotic coverage is needed for suspected or confirmed bladder perforation.

65.7 Results

Most bladder perforations are extraperitoneal, but intraperitoneal rupture has been reported after TUR of dome tumors (Fig. 65.4) [1]. Risk of malignant seeding is negligible [11] yet theoretically exits [13]. Extraperitoneal perforations usually resolve on prolonged indwelling urethral catheter drainage. Intraperitoneal perforations, however, usually require open or laparoscopic surgical repair. Extended antibiotic prophylaxis is required in both.

Ureteral obstruction rarely complicates ureteral orifice resection due to scarring. Using pure cutting current minimizes this risk. Confirmation is done by cystoscopic visualization of efflux of IV indigo carmine or methylene blue to exclude obstruction. Strictures usually yield to balloon

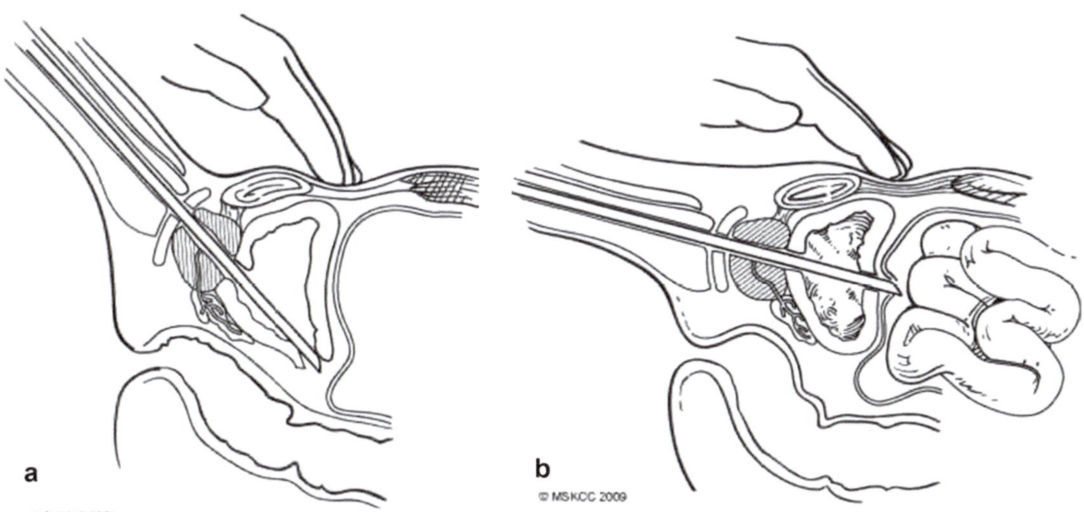

Fig. 65.4 Bladder perforations. (**a**) Extraperitoneal bladder rupture during transurethral resection (TUR) of a bladder tumor. (**b**) Intraperitoneal bladder rupture during TUR of a bladder tumor with subsequent intraperitoneal leakage of irrigant and urine. (**a** and **b**, ©2009 Memorial Sloan Kettering Cancer Center)

dilation of the ureteric orifice or at times may need endoscopic laser incision. Rarely, failures may require formal reimplantation [1].

65.8 Tips and Tricks

- Video TUR allows magnification, facilitates resident teaching, allows documentation of findings, and reduces the risk of body fluid exposure to the surgeon.
- Lifting the tumor edge away from detrusor lessens the chance of perforation.
- Repeated slow fulguration may complicate the ability of the pathologist to determine grade or invasion status.
- Bladder perforations could be avoided by few tricks:
  - Continuous open irrigation avoids bladder overdistension and detrusor thinning.
  - Minimizing energy usage, preferably using bipolar rather than unipolar electrocautery.
  - Using anesthetic paralysis for lateral wall lesions to abolish obturator reflex.
  - Staging rather than complete resections of large muscle-invasive tumors.
- Biopsy cup forceps causes a smaller perforation, if any, than does the cutting loop.
- An increase in abdominal girth or fullness after resection suggests intraperitoneal perforation.
- Using pure cutting electrode for periurethral lesions and avoiding fulguration are advisable to minimize risk of scarring obstruction.

65.9 Discussion

Transitional cell carcinoma (TCC) of the bladder is an uncommon lesion in children and adolescents. In contrast to adult disease that is associated with smoking and other environmental toxins, postulated risk factors in children include cyclophosphamide and dantrolene treatments [1].

Ultrasonography is the standard diagnostic tool with 100% sensitivity and is the preferred surveillance tool [13, 14]. On the contrary, VCUG is far less sensitive as dye density may obscure small lesions [5]. Definitive diagnosis by cystoscopy provides biopsy for histopathological grading and staging, and in many papillary tumors, TUR is enough treatment [15].

Most lesions are superficial, low-grade tumors, seldom invasive fatal disease [1]. Pediatric TCC is best treated with transurethral resection, while intravesical therapy has no defined role. Bacille Calmette-Guérin (BCG) is of questionable benefit in arresting TCC progression in children yet is generally beneficial for high-grade papillary tumors and CIS in older children and adolescents [15].

Staged tumor resection whether planned beforehand (due to bulky tumor mass, surgically inaccessible, perforation risk, or anesthetic event) or dictated by imaging during follow-up is beneficial for high-grade tumors since residual tumor is identified at the initial resection site in 26–83% of patients and corrected clinical staging errors in half of those patients [1, 6].

Repeat resection within 1–6 weeks is usually indicated in patients with high-grade disease, especially if no muscle was present in the initial TURBT. All suspicious lesions should be sampled, but random biopsies are not required. Repeat TURBT can detect worse prognostic factors in 25% of T1 tumors especially if no muscle is identified on initial pathology. Survival was 63% in patients who underwent a second TURBT versus 40% for those who did not, and recurrences appear to be lower after repeat TUR [1, 9].

Typically, pediatric bladder TCC does not involve the upper tracts; hence no current guidelines for routine upper tract surveillance exist [13]. Recurrence appears to be rare, even with high-grade disease [5]. Periodic surveillance with ultrasonography is therefore recommended owing to its sensitivity, obviating the need for serial invasive cystoscopy.

References

1. Berrettini A, Castagnetti M, Salerno A, Nappo SG, Manzoni G, Rigamonti W, Caione P. Bladder urothelial neoplasms in pediatric age: experience at three tertiary centers. J Pediatr Urol. 2015;11(1):26.

2. Lerena J, Krauel L, Garcia-Aparicio L, et al. Transitional cell carcinoma of the bladder in children and adolescents: six-case series and review of the literature. J Pediatr Urol. 2010;21:75–8.
3. Shelmerdine SC, Lorenzo AJ, Gupta AA, Chavhan GB. Pearls and pitfalls in diagnosing pediatric urinary bladder masses. Radiographics. 2017;37:1872–91.
4. Umlauf VN, Coerdt W, Leuschner I, et al. How to name papillary tumors of the bladder in children: transitional cell carcinoma or papillary urothelial neoplasm of low malignant potential? Urology. 2015;86:379–83.
5. Rodeberg DA, Anderson JR, Arndt CA, et al. Comparison of outcomes based on treatment algorithms for rhabdomyosarcoma of the bladder/prostate: combined results from the Children's Oncology Group, German Cooperative Soft Tissue Sarcoma Study, Italian Cooperative Group, and International Society of Pediatric Oncology Malignant Mesenchymal Tumors Committee. Int J Cancer. 2011;128:1232–9.
6. Williamson SR, Lopez-Beltran A, MacLennan GT, Montironi R, Cheng L. Unique clinicopathologic and molecular characteristics of urinary bladder tumors in children and young adults. Urol Oncol. 2013;31(4):414–26.
7. Spiegelberg C, Giedl J, Gaisa NT, Rogler A, Riener MO, Filbeck T, Burger M, Ruemmele P, Hartmann A, Stoehr R. Frequency of activating mutations in FGFR2 exon 7 in bladder tumors from patients with early-onset and regular-onset disease. Int J Clin Exp Pathol. 2014;7(4):1708–13.
8. Kojima S, Yagi M, Asagiri K, Fukahori S, Tanaka Y, Ishii S, Saikusa N, Koga Y, Yoshida M, Masui D, Komatsuzaki N, Nakagawa S, Ozono S, Tanikawa K. Infantile neuroblastoma of the urinary bladder detected by hematuria. Pediatr Surg Int. 2013;29(7):753–7.
9. Huppmann AR, Pawel BR. Polyps and masses of the pediatric urinary bladder: a 21-year pathology review. Pediatr Dev Pathol. 2011;14(6):438–44.
10. Ray B, Grabstald H, Exelby PR, Whitmore WF Jr. Bladder tumors in children. Urology. 1973;2(4):426–35.
11. Klochko PI, Kononenko NG. Diagnosis of bladder tumors in children. Urol Nefrol (Mosk). 1987;(5):58–60.
12. Hartman C, Williamson AK, Friedman AA, Palmer LS, Fine RG. Bladder ganglioneuroma in a 5-year-old girl presenting with a urinary tract infection and hematuria: case report and review of the literature. Urology. 2015;85(2):467–9.
13. Stein R, Frees S, Schröder A, Russo A, Gutjahr P, Faber J, Thüroff JW. Radical surgery and different types of urinary diversion in patients with rhabdomyosarcoma of bladder or prostate—a single institution experience. J Pediatr Urol. 2013;9(6 Pt A):932–9.
14. Chen H, Niu ZB, Yang Y. Bladder leiomyoma in a 6-year-old boy. Urology. 2012;79(2):434–6.
15. Yan C, Kim YW, Ha YS, Kim IY, Kim YJ, Yun SJ, Moon SK, Bae SC, Kim WJ. RUNX3 methylation as a predictor for disease progression in patients with non-muscle-invasive bladder cancer. J Surg Oncol. 2012;105(4):425–30.

Part V

Gynaecology

Laparoscopic Management of Ovarian Cysts

66

Juan Carlos de Agustín-Asensio
and David Peláez-Mata

66.1 Introduction

Ovarian cysts can be diagnosed in the fetal period, most of them in the third trimester of pregnancy. The incidence of presentation is of 1:2500 at referral centers. Three to five percent of children have small incidental ovarian cysts detected on ultrasound (US) [1]. It can be detected from the fetal period until adolescence. It is considered a pathological cyst when it has a diameter greater than 2 cm. However, it does not have the same meaning at one age or another. In neonates the pathological diagnoses usually are follicular cysts, intrauterine torsions, and, exceptionally, teratomas. In older girls, they are usually follicular cysts whose transcendence depends on the acquired size. When the cyst is accompanied by a solid component, we should suspect malignancy (teratomas or stromal tumors). In prepubertal girls with an ovarian mass or cyst, they should be operated if they are symptomatic or have poorly defined radiological signs. In adolescents, ovarian cysts must be related to the clinical history of menstruation and their sexual relations (Fig. 66.1).

The indication for laparoscopy will be made for patients with symptoms of abdominal pain, when there is a presence of a cyst greater than 5 cm in diameter, or when a tumor is suspected.

J. C. de Agustín-Asensio · D. Peláez-Mata (✉)
Department of Pediatric Surgery, Hospital General Universitario Gregorio Marañón, Madrid, Spain

In neonates, laparoscopy is performed if the cyst does not regress or is complicated (it is not a simple follicular cyst). Conservative surgery of the ovary should be performed whenever possible, except in cases of malignancy. Even with the suspicion of ovarian torsion, surgery must be conservative with detorsion and not with excision, and the cyst can be removed.

In this chapter we describe the laparoscopic treatment of ovarian conservative surgery, either by fenestration or by enucleation of the cyst (cystectomy).

66.2 Preoperative Preparation

Parents of patients and older girls should be informed of the effects of laparoscopy and intervention. They must sign the written informed consent. In all patients a non-cuffed bladder catheter should be placed just after being anesthetized to properly observe the minor pelvis. Antibiotic prophylaxis is not used unless there is suspicion of infection or ovarian torsion. A blood sample will be taken for tumor markers when we suspect malignancy (alpha-fetoprotein, human chorionic gonadotropin).

66.2.1 Positioning

The patient is placed in the supine position. In the case of neonates and infants, the patient is placed

C. Esposito et al. (eds.), *ESPES Manual of Pediatric Minimally Invasive Surgery*,
https://doi.org/10.1007/978-3-030-00964-9_66

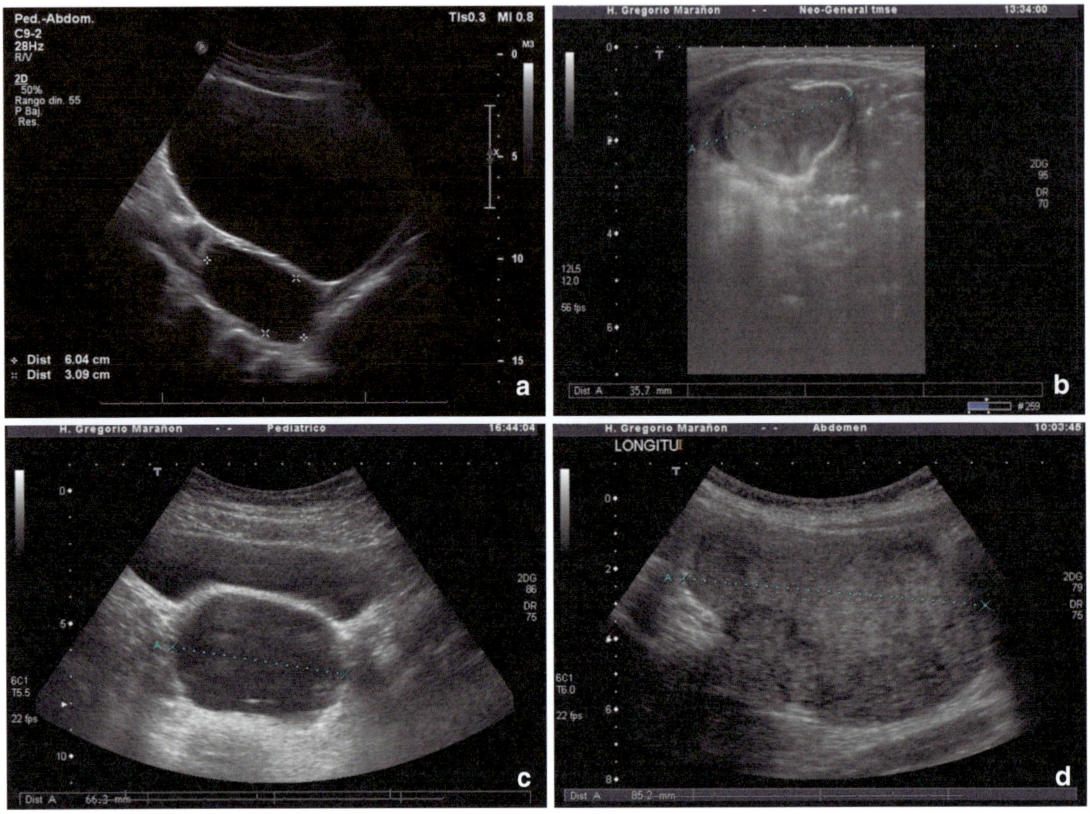

Fig. 66.1 Ultrasonographic images of ovarian cystic and solid lesions. (**a**) Simple cyst. (**b**) Complicated cyst. (**c**) Cystic teratoma. (**d**) Solid tumor

crosswise to the operating table and the surgeon at the head of it. In older girls and adolescents, the surgeon will be placed to the left of the patient and the assistant to the right. The monitor should be placed at the patient's feet. The operation will begin with the introduction of the optic by the navel with a trans- or infraumbilical incision with an open technique. The working ports will be placed on both sides of this trocar and in the same plane just to the sides of the lateral edge of the rectus abdominis muscles. In neonates the first trocar can be placed at the epigastrium or at the upper quadrant opposite to the cyst, in order to gain more intra-abdominal working space (Fig. 66.2). One or more trocars are then positioned as needed.

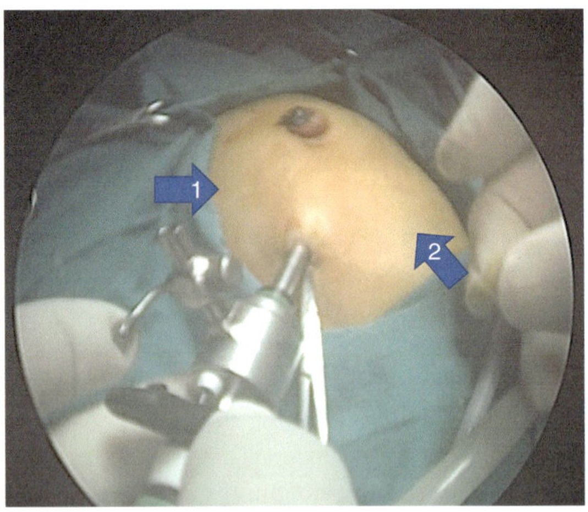

Fig. 66.2 Position of trocars

66.2.2 Instrumentation

It is necessary to have two grasping forceps, a dissector, a monopolar electrode (hook), a scissors, two needle holders, suction cannula, and extraction bag. If possible, an electronic vascular sealing device greatly facilitates hemostasis. The ideal lens should be 30° and a diameter of 5 mm.

A 3 mm lens can be used in neonates. The length of the instruments will vary depending on the size of the patient.

66.2.3 Technique

Controlled pneumoperitoneum is achieved using 2–3 liters per minute of CO_2 flow to reach a mean intra-abdominal pressure of 8–10 mmHg.

66.2.3.1 Fenestration

In cases of simple (follicular) cysts, the cyst can be partially emptied by aspiration puncture from outside and then opening thereof by cutting with scissors or a bipolar tissue sealing device. Hemostasis will be done by applying the energy of the monopolar scalpel to the scissors electrode. It will be left open to prevent re-accumulation of liquid inside (Fig. 66.3a, b).

66.2.3.2 Cystectomy

Cystectomy is performed by incising the ovary on its antimesenteric border. The hook can be used for initial incision delimitation. Blunt dissection separates the cyst wall from the ovarian capsule using gentle traction by two graspers, and the cyst will be removed in one piece. Suture of the capsule could be used to control hemostasis, but in absence of bleeding, it could be left open. With this technique the ovarian tissue contained in the capsule is preserved (Fig. 66.4a, b).

Benign cystic teratoma can be also managed by enucleating the mass leaving the normal ovarian parenchyma in the capsule.

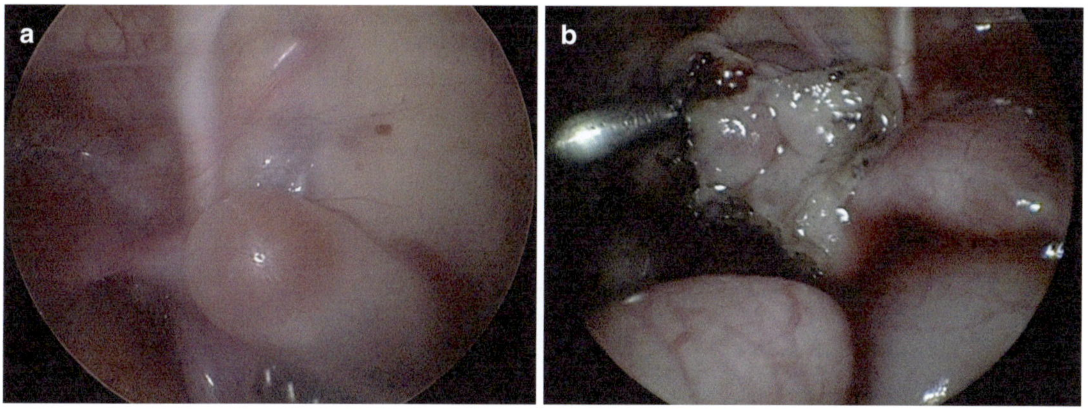

Fig. 66.3 (**a**) Simple ovarian cyst. (**b**) Ovarian cyst opened (fenestration)

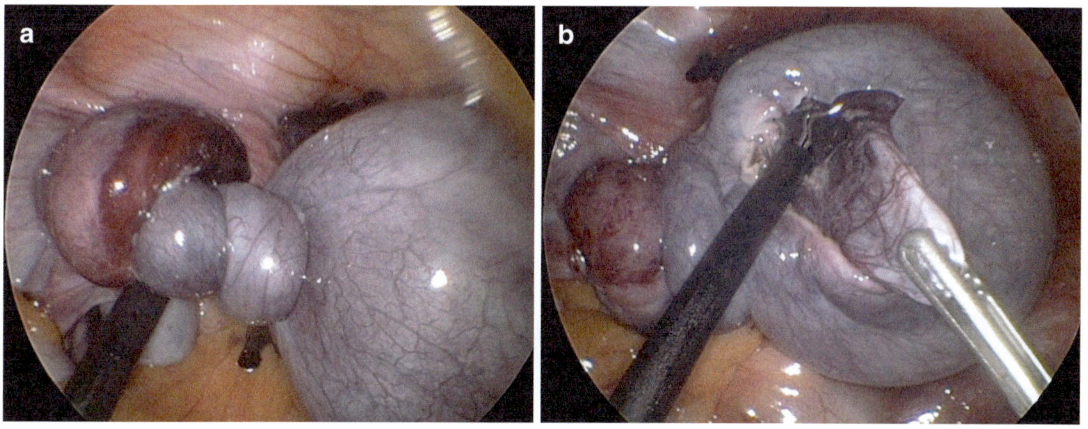

Fig. 66.4 (**a**) Torsion of ovarian cyst. (**b**) Opening ovarian capsule after detorsion and cyst wall traction and removal (striping)

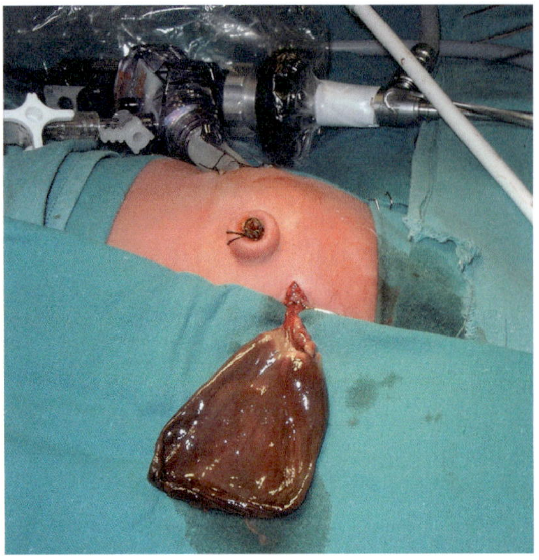

Fig. 66.5 Ovarian necrotic torsion in neonate

66.2.3.3 Oophorectomy

When malignancy is suspected, oophorectomy and tissue lymphatic sampling are performed. Many surgeons suggest to convert to open operation for proper periaortic lymphatic sampling technique. In this case sub-umbilical midline incision is recommended. Oophorectomy is also done in neonatal completely necrotic ovarian torsion (Fig. 66.5).

66.3 Postoperative Care

Postoperative pain can be reduced using low intra-abdominal pressure and local anesthetic infiltration of ports. Nonsteroidal anti-inflammatory drugs (paracetamol, metamizol) can be administered every 6 h for the first 24–48 h. Oral feeding can be initiated after the patient is fully awakened and advanced it accordingly. Shower can be allowed after 48 h after surgery, and wound dressing is changed after it. Patient can be discharged on the first or second postoperative day if asymptomatic.

66.4 Results

Ultrasonographic follow-up studies have shown ovarian anatomy recovery and preservation of follicular tissue after fenestration or cystectomy.

66.5 Discussion

In a multicenter retrospective study, Tyraskis et al. showed that prenatally diagnosed simple cysts resolved in 32% of cases, while 38% resolved postnatally. Fourteen percent underwent surgery postnatally, and 16% had torsion of the ovary. The torsion rate increased with size from 0% in cysts <20 mm to 33% in cysts >50 mm. In between 0 and 40 mm, there is a higher rate of spontaneous resolution, and the median time to postnatal resolution was 10 (5–27) weeks in those treated conservatively [2]. Other publications suggest a similar pattern of spontaneous resolution [3]. So, it is recommended a conservative approach and postnatal ultrasound monitoring. Those cysts which exceed 5 cm and do not shrink postnatally may require surgical treatment [4].

Complex ovarian cysts lead to problems even after regression in the postnatal period and require operative intervention sooner or later. In a series of 38 patients, Karakuş et al. found that three out of seven complex ovarian cysts that initially regressed presented with intestinal obstruction, and oophorectomy plus adhesiolysis had to be performed. In another series, surgical treatment was required in 7 out of 11 (64%) complex ovarian cysts [5].

In prepubertal girls, visualization of ovarian follicles is perfectly physiological, as the diameter does not exceed 10 mm. Ovarian cysts are well defined for fluid images of >20 mm. If asymptomatic they are usually discovered incidentally by ultrasound. The natural history of functional cysts is eventually regression; persistence is suggestive of malignancy. The onset of pain is a sign of complication, and abrupt pain with vomiting is a sign of torsion [6].

Bolli et al. explore a predictive score of torsion complication. They found that the presence of vomiting, short duration of abdominal pain, and elevated C-reactive protein level have a predictive value for the diagnosis of ovarian torsion in girls between 2 and 12 years old [7].

If operative intervention is necessary, ovary-preserving techniques should be utilized as describe in this chapter. Precocious pseudopuberty in girls is associated to an autonomous ovarian cyst or in patients with McCune-Albright syndrome and occurs as a result of estrogen production. These patients have suppressed LHRH testing and have simple ovarian cysts producing estradiol. Current management involves surgery (cystectomy) and endocrinological therapy (pharmacological suppression) [8].

Papic's group found, by histopathology, viable ovarian tissue in all three oophorectomies performed. Also, postnatal torsion occurred in 1/25 observation patients (4%) or in 1/8 (13%) with cysts ≥50 mm [9]. So, stripping of benign ovarian cysts has been reported to be preferable to cyst wall ablation. It is shown that no ovarian tissue is removed together with the cyst if the cyst is non-endometriotic [10].

Finally, in a big series of adolescents and young adults, there were only 4 malignant cysts (1.4%). Cystectomy was performed in 205 cases (72.7%), fenestration of cyst wall was performed in 53 cases (18.8%), and aspiration was applied in 22 cases (7.8%). The types of operation were not significantly different among adolescents and young adults ($P > 0.05$) [11].

In summary, prenatally simple cysts can be managed expectantly, as complicated cysts have to be operated. In older girls, cyst greater than 5 mm in diameter has a great chance of torsion, and laparoscopy is indicated. Conservative surgery can be done in majority of cases, by fenestration, cystectomy of even simple aspiration.

References

1. Millar DM, Blake JM, Stringer DA, et al. Prepubertal ovarian cyst formation: 5 years' experience. Obstet Gynecol. 1993;81:434–7.
2. Tyraskis A, Bakalis S, Scala C, Syngelaki A, Giuliani S, Davenport M, David AL, Nicolaides K, Eaton S, De Coppi P. A retrospective multicenter study of the natural history of fetal ovarian cysts. J Pediatr Surg. 2018;53(10):2019–22. pii: S0022-3468(18)30103-9. https://doi.org/10.1016/j.jpedsurg.2018.02.049.
3. González N, Ruiz de Temiño M, Riazuelo G, Elías J, Esteban JA. Prenatal ultrasound in the diagnose of ovarian cysts. Cir Pediatr. 1999;12:22–5.
4. Moreno R, Savirón R, Corona C, LermA D, Corbacho T. Diagnóstico prenatal de 10 quistes de ovario fetal: manejo postnatal. Rev Chil Obstet Ginecol. 2013;78(1):19–25.
5. Karakuş OZ, Ateş O, Hakgüder G, Olguner M, Akgür FM. Complex fetal ovarian cysts cause problems even after regression. Eur J Pediatr Surg. 2014;24(4):337–40.
6. Pienkowski C, Cartault A, Carfagna L, Ernoult P, Vial J, Lemasson F, Le Mandat A, Galinier P, Tauber M. Ovarian cysts in prepubertal girls. Endocr Dev. 2012;22:101–11.
7. Bolli P, Schädelin S, Holland-Cunz S, Zimmermann P. Ovarian torsion in children: development of a predictive score. Medicine (Baltimore). 2017;96(43):e8299.
8. Papanikolaou A, Michala L. Autonomous ovarian cysts in prepubertal girls. How aggressive should we be? A review of the literature. J Pediatr Adolesc Gynecol. 2015;28(5):292–6.
9. Papic JC, Billmire DF, Rescorla FJ, Finnell SM, Leys CM. Management of neonatal ovarian cysts and its effect on ovarian preservation. J Pediatr Surg. 2014;49(6):990–3; discussion 993–4.
10. Palmara V, Sturlese E, Romeo C, Arena F, De Dominici R, Villari D, Impellizzeri P, Santoro G. Morphological study of the residual ovarian tissue removed by laparoscopy or laparotomy in adolescents with benign ovarian cysts. J Pediatr Surg. 2012;47(3):577–80.
11. Seckin B, Ozdener T, Tapisiz OL, Batioğlu S. Laparoscopic treatment of ovarian cysts in adolescents and young adults. J Pediatr Adolesc Gynecol. 2011;24(5):300–3.

Laparoscopy for Ovarian Tumors

67

Henri Steyaert and G. Rodesch

67.1 Introduction

Management of ovarian tumors depends on the age, the radiologic (sonographic) appearance, but also the type of symptoms (acute or not).

In order to describe more accurately the technical options, this chapter will be divided into three parts:

1. Laparoscopy in functional ovarian cysts in neonates
2. Laparoscopic ovary-sparing surgery in symptomatic children and adolescents
3. Laparoscopy in solid tumors of the ovary

67.2 Laparoscopy in Functional Ovarian Cysts in Neonates

67.2.1 Introduction

There is still a controversy in the management of prenatal and postnatal functional ovarian cysts depending on their ultrasound pattern, the diameter of the cyst, and expertise of gynecologist, radiologist, and surgeon [1].

H. Steyaert (✉) · G. Rodesch
Department of Pediatric Surgery, Université Libre de Bruxelles (ULB), HUDERF Children's Hospital, Brussels, Belgium
e-mail: henri.steyaert@huderf.be

Prenatal management varies from simple oversight to evacuating puncture that has sometime to be repeated [2]. In our institution gynecologists prefer an evacuating puncture just before birth the risk of torsion seeming increased close to birth.

After birth there are two scenarios [3]: first is the presence of a complex cyst at ultrasound. The ovary is lost, and surgery will be delayed for several weeks; second is a simple cyst of more than 5 cm. In this case a US-guided transcutaneous evacuating puncture may be tried, or patient is put on the operating table for a punction under laparoscopic control very soon after birth in order to avoid torsion and loss of the ovary [4, 5].

67.2.2 Preoperative Preparation

No special preparation is needed. A nasogastric tube is not necessary. Urinary catheter may be helpful but is not mandatory. No antibiotics are needed.

67.2.2.1 Positioning

The patient is placed in a supine position transversally across the operating table. This allows surgical and anesthetic teams to be close to the baby. Depending on surgeon's habit, he can stay on the legs or on the head of the patient. With the surgeon on the head, the trocars are inserted

C. Esposito et al. (eds.), *ESPES Manual of Pediatric Minimally Invasive Surgery*,
https://doi.org/10.1007/978-3-030-00964-9_67

into the umbilicus and laterally on each side of the umbilicus. If the surgeon stays on the legs, the operating trocars are moved to the right and left iliac fossa. The first position is probably easier for handling; the second one is cosmetically better certainly in case 5 mm trocars are used. Our preferred trocars are 3 mm ones at that age.

67.2.2.2 Instrumentation

No special equipment is required.

67.2.2.3 Technique

A three-trocar technique (5 mm scope at 30° and two 3 mm operating trocars) is used. Open access for introduction of the first trocar is the rule in pediatric surgery whatever the age. This is certainly the case in newborns. A "smile" umbilicoplasty in the inferior fold of the umbilicus or a vertical transumbilical opening may be preferred. Access to the peritoneum takes mostly few seconds due to a frequent patent umbilical process.

US-guided transcutaneous puncture is preferred in case of very large cyst. Evacuation is controlled by the scope. After puncture, insufflation is maintained between 4 and 8 mmHg.

If an auto-amputed ovary is discovered, the ovary has to be searched everywhere in the abdominal cavity but may be missing. By experience we notice that the ovary is frequently situated in the hepatic region. Extraction through the umbilical incision is mostly easy even if some adhesions have to be cut using a monopolar hook or scissors. In case of necrotic ovary still attached to the fallopian tube, the easiest way is to aspirate the content and attract the ovary through the umbilicus. Oophorectomy is done outside the abdominal cavity before reintroducing the tube into the peritoneum. Intraperitoneal oophorectomy is, notwithstanding, perfectly possible. Addition of a retracting forceps in the suprapubic region may help to stabilize the ovary for this purpose (2 mm single-use trocarless instrument). A cystectomy is possible in case of uncomplicated cyst, but mostly an evacuating puncture is enough because the neonatal cysts have less tendency to recur.

67.2.3 Postoperative Care

Feeding is usually started within the first 6 postoperative hours, and patient leaves the hospital at day 1 or 2 post-op.

67.2.4 Tips and Tricks

- Before surgery, future porthole sites may be infiltrated with bupivacaine 0.2% up to a total dosage of 1.5 mg/kg.
- A sleeve around the trocars may help to fix them to the abdominal wall and ensure a good position of the end of the trocar just into the peritoneum in order to increase the available space.
- Use of 20 cm short instrument set is recommended in neonates.

67.2.5 Discussion

Actually most of the ovarian cysts are seen prenatally. Diagnosis is often made during the third trimester of pregnancy. Differential diagnosis includes mesenteric cysts and duplications. Postnatally, cysts are mostly asymptomatic. Rarely adhesions between the tube and an amputated cyst may cause bowel obstruction.

There is still no consensus about the best approach of those cysts after birth. Several teams decide just to follow them because resolution is frequent with time. Others decide, as in our department, to operate in order to be sure not to have an eventual torsion. The question of the size (diameter) needing surgery is also not known. Mostly the cutoff is around 5 cm in diameter.

It is possible to preserve the neonatal ovary in non-complicated cysts. That's why we are in favor of an early surgical treatment (punction under laparoscopic control) soon after birth in those cases. In case of torsion, experience shows that the fallopian tube is frequently twisted at the junction of the proximal 2/3 and terminal 1/3. In those cases gynecologists suggest a complete resection of the ipsilateral tube in order to avoid problems later (implantation difficulties or extra uterine pregnancy). This is also controversial [6].

67.3 Laparoscopic Ovary-Sparing Surgery in Symptomatic Children and Adolescents

67.3.1 Introduction

As a result of hormones, stimulation of the ovary occurs during puberty and adult fertile life. Follicular cysts may sometimes increase in size and become real "functional ovarian" cysts. Once the diameter reaches 5 cm, the majority of authors estimates that the risk for torsion is high and surgical management mandatory. Indication is obvious in case of accompanying symptoms (pain, severe dysmenorrhea), mostly in emergency, but waiting may be discussed (4–8 weeks) in asymptomatic patients.

In some cases, symptoms are acute, and ultrasound examination diagnoses a mass containing solid or semisolid content (blood) eventually accompanied with a torsion. Torsion is not always easy to diagnose with a transabdominal ultrasound. Torsion of the vessels has to be searched for.

67.3.2 Preoperative Preparation

A nasogastric tube is placed in case of emergency surgery. Broad-spectrum antibiotics are started in case a complicated cyst is suspected. A urine catheter is useful in order to free the pelvic cavity.

67.3.2.1 Positioning

Patient is placed in a supine Trendelenburg position. Surgeon stays on the opposite side of the affected ovary. The video screen is located at the foot of the patient on the side of the affected ovary and must be in line with surgeon's eyes. Accessory screens may help scrub nurse and/or anesthesiologist to follow the operation.

67.3.2.2 Instrumentation

Bipolar electrocautery should be available. Mini-laparoscopic transcutaneous instruments are interesting to have in order to grasp the tissue for presentation. Mostly a four-trocar technique is used. Either a suprapubic and a contralateral lower quadrant port or both lower quadrant ports can be used + an accessory trocar of percutaneous instrument in the suprapubic region. The scope is as usual a 5 mm 30° one. A suction/irrigation device is needed. An endobag device is also helpful.

67.3.2.3 Technique

In children, laparoscopic technique is always open. The first blunt trocar is inserted after vertical transumbilical or infraumbilical "smile" incision.

Once the scope is in place, insufflation may start. After a quick overview of the abdomen, the two accessory trocars are inserted under visual control and eventually a fourth trocar (of instrument) just suprapubic for retraction.

In girls ovarian surgery should always be preceded by careful inspection of the pelvic peritoneum, contralateral ovary, and abdominal content.

In case of non-complicated cyst, a line is drawn with the monopolar hook on the ovarian capsule (in the long axis of the ovary) that is gently opened using scissors just following the line. The suprapubic instrument may help to stabilize the ovary during operation. Bluntly a plane is created between the cystic wall and the ovarian cortex spreading progressively the two lips of the cortex. Once widely separated from the ovary, the content of the cyst is aspirated with a fine needle. At that moment, the cyst may be opened and inspected with the help of the scope. Once the cyst is empty, it can be grasped with a large forceps and detached using the "spaghetti" maneuver. The last attachments of the cyst are mostly the most solid and may bleed. Sometime a bipolar cautery may be helpful. Once the cyst freed, extraction can be done. Best is to use an endobag except if surgeon is 100% sure that it's a functional cyst. The ovary doesn't need to be closed except in case of difficult hemostasis. Thorough irrigation of the pelvis is performed at the end of surgery.

In case of twisted ovary, the first thing to do is a detorsion. The additional suprapubic instrument is particularly helpful for this purpose. Once untwisted the ovary is to be let in place whatever the aspect (even if the ovary is black or green) (Figs. 67.1 and 67.2). Recovery is surprisingly good for ovaries, and a second look few

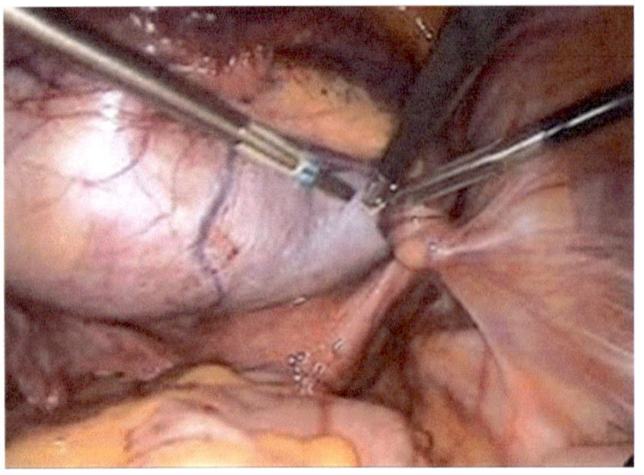

Fig. 67.1 Untwisting ovary with the help of a suprapubic instrument

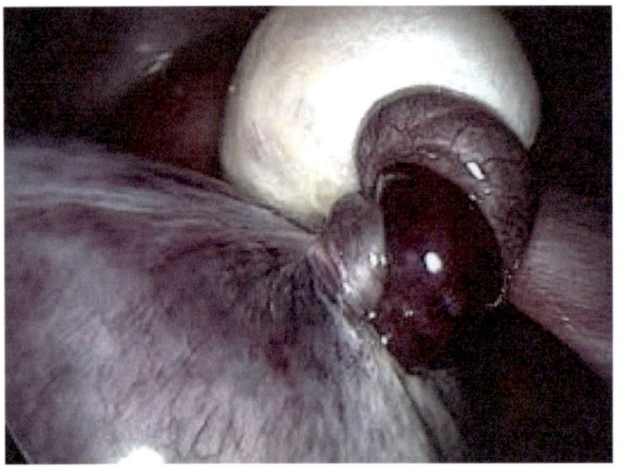

Fig. 67.2 Blue/black ovary and tube. Oophorectomy is quite never done at first operation

weeks after detorsion (or US with Doppler study) is the best option in case of doubt.

An untwisted ovary is never opened for cyst removal even if the risk for malignancy in a twisted ovarian mass is small (less than 3%). Postoperative workup may conclude that a tumor may have been responsible for the torsion and proper management scheduled in much better conditions.

67.3.3 Discussion

Functional cyst is the most encountered ovarian pathology in prepubertal and pubertal girls [7]. Most are diagnosed incidentally or during nonspecific abdominal symptoms. Risk of torsion depends on the size, but there is no real consensus about that size [8]. Most authors write that over 5 cm of size cyst management will be needed. Laparoscopy is an excellent tool in order to deal with functional cysts. Large cysts, however, may bleed and finally rupture or twist with loss of the ovary. Some of those cysts are paraovarian from mesothelial, paramesonephric, or mesonephric origin. They can sometimes reach impressive diameters. They can also twist. Laparoscopy may be difficult in large cysts due to the lack of space [9].

Laparoscopy increases the risk of cyst rupture, in particular in large cysts. Surgeons must be certain of the benignity of the tumor before any minimal invasive manipulation. In case of any doubt about eventual presence of a tumor, conversion is probably the safest option. In case of torsion, the ovary has to be let in place whatever the aspect of the tissue after detorsion [10]. The success of laparoscopy not only depends on the skill of the surgeon but also and even more importantly on the proper preoperative evaluation and patient selection [7].

67.4 Laparoscopy in Solid Tumors of the Ovary

67.4.1 Introduction

The risk of malignancy for ovarian tumors in girls, including both solid and cystic lesions, is around 10–25%. Laparoscopic surgery seems to be a safe option in most of the cases encountered in children [11].

The most common solid ovarian tumors are mature teratomas [12]. Those tumors are mostly benign and tumor markers (alpha-fetoprotein) normal. Adult series of laparoscopic enucleation are published. In children there are only case reports. Cystadenoma is another benign tumor that may be bilateral in more than 10% of the cases. Laparoscopic enucleation is also described.

67.4.2 Preoperative Preparation

Same as for cyst removal. Tumor markers such as alpha-fetoprotein, CEA 125, and beta-hCG are determined.

67.4.2.1 Positioning
Same as above.

67.4.2.2 Instrumentation
Same as above. A thermofusion instrument may be helpful in case of large tumor.

67.4.2.3 Technique
Technique of enucleation is the same as for a cyst. Spillage of cyst contents must be avoided but is not always easy to confirm, in particular in tumors containing solid and cystic parts. All specimen have to be extracted with the help of an endobag. In case of a large tumor, we prefer to enlarge one of the lower abdomen portholes in order to control completely the extraction.

67.4.3 Tips and Tricks

- Hydrodissection is a good tool in order to help separation between ovarian cortex and cyst wall.
- The size of the bag must be chosen regarding the size of the tumor at preoperative ultrasound (from 5 to 15 mm).
- Some gynecologists advocate to let around 100 mL liquid in the pelvis at the end of the operation because it seems to avoid adhesion formation and decreases pain.
- A drain is mostly pushed into the pelvis for 24–48 h.

67.4.4 Discussion

When there are no clear tumor characteristics that define malignancy and as the risk of malignancy is significant, these doubtful pediatric ovarian lesions should always be managed and completely staged in the assumption that they are malignant [13]. This assumption would say that, in such cases, the ovary may not be opened (for any reason) and that a complete oophorectomy has to be conducted avoiding any damage even to the capsule. For that reason authors advocate a laparoscopic staging (abdominal and omental exploration, contralateral ovary exploration, intraperitoneal fluid sampling) continued by a conversion to a Pfannenstiel incision for proper excision of the tumor. In that case, even an enucleation may be sufficient and safe because eventual spilling will take place outside the abdomen. Recently some communications were made about peritoneal carcinomatosis after enucleation of mature teratomas (with a little part of immature cells not seen even at pathologic examination). Authors found also a publication with one case of immature teratoma in a series of supposed mature teratomas [14]. All those arguments convinced the authors to go back to a more conservative attitude using laparoscopy only for excision of functional cysts, untwisting ovaries, and staging.

Mostly a malignant tumor will be recognized at exploration [15, 16]. Surface of the tumor is irregular, eventual cyst wall is thick, there are adhesions with the adjacent organs and peritoneal implants, and there is presence of ascites. In those cases, sampling by laparoscopy and conversion to a Pfannenstiel incision is the most secure way to go. Each case has to be discussed with oncologists and radiologists because chemotherapy is actually of great efficiency in treating malignant ovarian tumors.

But the main question is always: in case of proper surgery (without opening of the capsula, etc.), is chemotherapy necessary? If not, surgery must be absolutely perfect if a minimal invasive surgery is chosen. At the end of the operation the tumor (of the ovary) has to be extracted by at least an enlargement of one of the lower trocar holes. For all those reasons, authors are actually convinced that laparoscopy is a perfect tool for exploration and sampling but that conversion is the best option for the tumor resection.

References

1. Bailez MM. Laparoscopy in functional ovarian cysts in neonates. In: Endoscopic surgery in infants and children. New York: Springer; 2008. p. 771–6.
2. Noia G, Riccardi M, Visconti D, Pellegrino M, Quattrocchi T, Tintoni M, Manzoni C, Pintus C, Masini L, Caruso A. Invasive fetal therapies: approach and results in treating fetal ovarian cysts. J Matern Fetal Neonatal Med. 2012;25(3):299–303.
3. Papic JC, Billmire DF, Rescorla FJ, Finnell SM, Leys CM. Management of neonatal ovarian cysts and its effect on ovarian preservation. J Pediatr Surg. 2014;49(6):990–3; discussion 993–4.

4. Cho MJ, Kim DY, Kim SC. Ovarian cyst aspiration in the neonate: minimally invasive surgery. J Pediatr Adolesc Gynecol. 2015;28(5):348–53.
5. Schenkman L, Weiner TM, Phillips JD. Evolution of the surgical management of neonatal ovarian cysts: laparoscopic-assisted transumbilical extracorporeal ovarian cystectomy (LATEC). J Laparoendosc Adv Surg Tech A. 2008;18(4):635–40.
6. Boukaidi SA, Delotte J, Steyaert H, Valla JS, Sattonet C, Bouaziz J, Bongain A. Thirteen cases of isolated tubal torsions associated with hydrosalpinx in children and adolescents, proposal for conservative management: retrospective review and literature survey. J Pediatr Surg. 2011;46(7):1425–31.
7. Bailez MM. Laparoscopy of functional ovarian cysts and mesosalpinx cysts in peripuberal girls. In: Endoscopic surgery in infants and children. New York: Springer; 2008. p. 777–81.
8. Steyaert H, Meynol F, Valla JS. Torsion of the adnexa in children: the value of laparoscopy. Pediatr Surg Int. 1998;13(5–6):384–7.
9. Lim S, Lee KB, Chon SJ, Park CY. Is tumor size the limiting factor in a laparoscopic management for large ovarian cysts? Arch Gynecol Obstet. 2012;286(5):1227–32.
10. Nur Azurah AG, Zainol ZW, Zainuddin AA, Lim PS, Sulaiman AS, Ng BK. Update on the management of ovarian torsion in children and adolescents. World J Pediatr. 2015;11(1):35–40.
11. Bailez MM. Laparoscopic ovary-sparing surgery in benign ovarian neoplasms. In: Endoscopic surgery in infants and children. New York: Springer; 2008. p. 782–5.
12. Zhang M, Jiang W, Li G, Xu C. Ovarian masses in children and adolescents—an analysis of 521 clinical cases. J Pediatr Adolesc Gynecol. 2014;27(3):e73–7.
13. Ure B, Valla JS. Laparoscopy in (doubtful) malignant adnexal pathology, ovarian torsion beyond the neonatal period, endometriosis, and pelvic inflammatory disease. In: Endoscopic surgery in infants and children. New York: Springer; 2008. p. 786–90.
14. Amies Oelschlager AM, Sawin R. Teratomas and ovarian lesions in children. Surg Clin North Am. 2012;92(3):599–613.
15. Özcan R, Kuruoğlu S, Dervişoğlu S, Eliçevik M, Emir H, Büyükünal C. Ovary-sparing surgery for teratomas in children. Pediatr Surg Int. 2013;29(3):233–7.
16. Papic JC, Finnell SM, Slaven JE, Billmire DF, Rescorla FJ, Leys CM. Predictors of ovarian malignancy in children: overcoming clinical barriers of ovarian preservation. J Pediatr Surg. 2014;49(1):144–7; discussion 147–8.

68 Laparoscopic Approach to Paratubal and Paraovarian Cysts

Maria Escolino, Giorgia Esposito, and Ciro Esposito

68.1 Introduction

Paratubal and paraovarian cysts represent approximately 10% of all adnexal masses [1, 2]. The peak incidence occurs during the third and fourth decades of life with only 4% occurring in adolescents [3]. The lifetime prevalence is thought to be 5–15% [4]. Paratubal and paraovarian cysts are benign and commonly found as incidental findings during other surgical procedures (Fig. 68.1) [5].

Paratubal cysts (PTCs) are seen in women of all ages and are simple cystic structures filled with serous fluid that are located along the ampulla of the fallopian tube, usually arising from the broad ligament or mesosalpinx. They originate from mesothelium or are thought to be remnants of paramesonephric (Mullerian) and mesonephric (Wolffian) ducts. These Wolffian remnants are destined to become male reproductive structures in the presence of androgen secretion during embryonic development. It has been postulated that these Wolffian remnants found in females, in the form of PTCs, might also have androgen sensitivity [6]. Paramesonephric duct remnants tend to occur more commonly within the broad ligament rather than at the fimbriated ends of the fallopian tube. The size of the PTCs seen in the broad ligament might range from 1 to 8 cm in diameter; however, cysts up to 10 cm have been documented in case studies, and under the influence of hormonal factors, they can reach huge sizes [7–9]. Stimulating hormonal factors have been postulated for PTC development, but no direct association has been determined. Although malignancy has been described, it is extremely rare, with an incidence of 2–3% among those diagnosed with paratubal or paraovarian cysts [10, 11]. Characteristics of PTCs are highly variable because some may be septated and have an ovoid appearance or they may be sonolucent and have a tubular appearance [12]. PTCs usually consist of either unciliated epithelium, ciliated

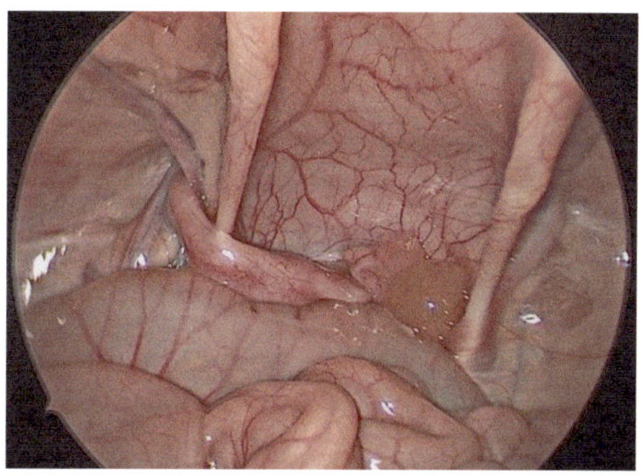

Fig. 68.1 A right paraovarian cyst incidentally found during laparoscopy performed for left ovarian inguinal hernia

M. Escolino (✉) · G. Esposito · C. Esposito
Pediatric Surgery Unit, Department of Translational Medical Sciences (DISMET), University of Naples "Federico II", Naples, Italy
e-mail: maria.escolino@unina.it; ciroespo@unina.it

C. Esposito et al. (eds.), *ESPES Manual of Pediatric Minimally Invasive Surgery*,
https://doi.org/10.1007/978-3-030-00964-9_68

cuboidal epithelium, or ciliated columnar epithelium [1]. A paratubal cyst is a closed, fluid-filled sac that grows beside or near the ovary and fallopian tube but is never attached to them. It is located at the ligament between the uterus and the ovary, and usually it is unilateral and benign. When a PTC is pedunculated and located near the fimbria of the fallopian tube, it is referred to as a hydatid cyst of Morgagni, which is usually smaller than 2 cm. Hydatids of Morgagni are among the most common benign, noninflammatory conditions of the fallopian tubes. These Wolffian duct remnants are simple cysts filled with serous fluid that occur near the fimbriated ends of the fallopian tube. Hydatid cysts of Morgagni are classified as PTCs but differ in that they tend to be smaller and are typically attached to the fimbria of the fallopian tube. Because of their small size of less than 2 cm, they were previously hard to distinguish from ovarian cysts during transabdominal ultrasound [1, 13].

Paraovarian cyst arises in the part of the broad ligament between the fallopian tube and ovary. Gartner's duct cyst, unilocular serous cystadenomas, and ovarian cysts, such as follicle cyst or corpus luteum cyst, may have a similar appearance, and the accurate preoperative diagnosis of paraovarian cyst is difficult. In the literature, it was reported that paraovarian cysts are probably more common in women between 30 and 40 years of age, while they are very uncommon in children, and most paraovarian cysts are incidentally discovered during pelvic surgery [1].

68.2 Clinical Presentation

Although paratubal and paraovarian cysts are not uncommon, they rarely cause symptoms and are usually incidentally found [1]. A certain diagnosis of these cysts is not usually possible preoperatively. Therefore, they are usually found incidentally during operative procedures for other indications [5, 14]. A preoperative misdiagnosis as true ovarian cysts is very common and creates a major problem [15]. The symptoms occur when they grow excessively or in case of hemorrhage, rupture, or torsion. Their enlargement presents more frequently in the early menarchal female due to secretory activity of the tubal epithelium, which is subject to hormonal influence after the postpubertal years. The associated physical examination findings are vague with deep pain in the pelvis and/or abdomen on palpation and a concomitant large cyst on ultrasound. Most hydatids of Morgagni achieve the size of about 1 cm, and they can rarely undergo torsion with infarction by strangulation of their mesentery. After torsion they may become symptomatic causing intermittent chronic pelvic pain or acute abdominal pain.

Torsion of paratubal and paraovarian cysts is rare due to their location; however, if torsion does occur, the infundibulopelvic ligament and ipsilateral ovary are frequently involved [16, 17]. The right adnexa undergo torsion more commonly than the left with a ratio of 3:2 [18]. This is due to the support of the left adnexa by the fixed sigmoid colon in the left lower quadrant. The diagnosis of tubal torsion is often difficult because symptoms are nonspecific [19, 20]. The only consistent presenting symptom is intermittent abdominal pain. Nausea and vomiting are less common. Physical findings include abdominal tenderness with or without peritoneal signs and adnexal tenderness on pelvic examination. A specific mass is not always palpable. Laboratory values are usually nonspecific; occasionally there may be an elevated white blood cell count. Ultrasound is the best imaging modality [11]. Characteristic features include an elongated, cystic mass with variable septations and scattered internal echoes, which often tapers near the uterine cornua. While these features are not always seen, if such a mass and normal ovarian parenchyma on that side are observed on ultrasound, diagnosis is fairly certain. If the ovary is twisted as well, diffuse swelling of the ovarian parenchyma and follicular enlargement in the cortical zone may be seen on the sonogram. Color Doppler may be helpful in such cases [11, 12].

Symptomatic paratubal cysts complicated by acute tubo-ovarian torsion share a common clinical presentation with other more common conditions, and the differential diagnosis in an adolescent female includes acute appendicitis, kidney stones, incarcerated hernia, pelvic inflammatory disease, gastroenteritis, and ectopic pregnancy [19]. Adnexal torsion should therefore be kept in mind in the differential diagnosis of all pediatric patients including those of prepubertal age who present with acute abdominal pain [13].

68.3 Diagnosis

Diagnosis of paratubal and paraovarian cysts has proven difficult. The best imaging modality available is ultrasonography (US); however, in many studies, only 30–44% of paratubal cysts were correctly identified prior to surgery [14]. Typically, uncomplicated paraovarian cysts are solitary, thin-walled, and unilocular, separate from the ovary with no septa or folds, and are sonographically anechoic or hypoechoic [12]. The dissociation of the cyst from the ovary when pushing the probe is a useful sign, called as "split sign," for discriminating paraovarian masses (Fig. 68.2) [15, 19]. Multilocular paraovarian cysts have rarely been described.

Paratubal cysts appear as round cysts attached to the fimbriated end of the fallopian tube by a pedicle [12, 14]. Other imaging techniques like computerized tomography (CT) and magnetic resonance imaging (MRI) can also be used in differential diagnosis. MRI features of paraovarian cysts were described as homogeneous cystic masses near the ipsilateral round ligament and the uterus. Especially demonstration of a normal ovary separate from the cyst is an important MRI finding [15].

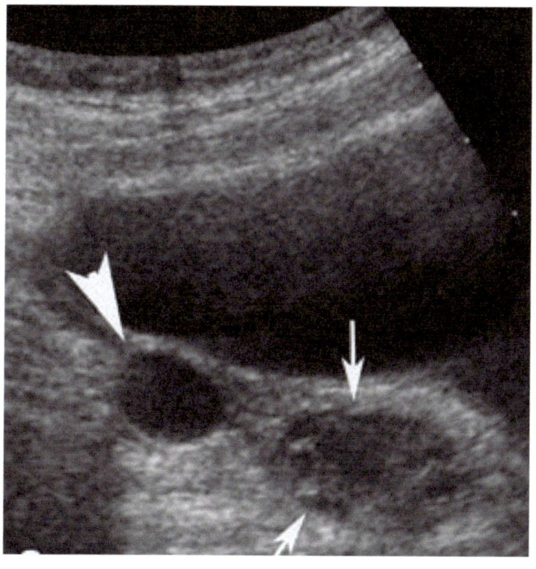

Fig. 68.2 Asymptomatic paraovarian cyst, separated from the ovary

There is no specific finding on CT other than unilocular cystic masses near the adjacent ovary showing fluid attenuation or signal.

In cases of secondary adnexal torsion, the sonographic features of the tubal component include the visualization of the twisted vascular pedicle and a dilated tubular structure with thickened echogenic walls and internal debris or hemorrhage, situated between the uterus and the ovary. Color and spectral Doppler sonography of the intraovarian vascularity has been found to be of limited value in the exclusion of torsion [16]. While the absence of blood flow does usually indicate torsion, blood flow can still be demonstrated in torsed ovaries in up to 64% of cases [17]. Diagnostic features of ultrasound color Doppler may show a high impedance waveform with reversal of diastolic flow in the affected tube (Fig. 68.3) [11].

A CT scan may be useful to rule out other causes of lower abdominal pain such as acute appendicitis. CT features of tubal torsion are a thickened fallopian tube and smooth eccentric cyst wall thickening, and CT is suggested as an alternative for overweight patients where US may be of limited value [13]. In case of diagnostic doubts, the MRI is preferable to clarify the diagnosis, avoiding radiation damage on the ovary, especially in young girls [18].

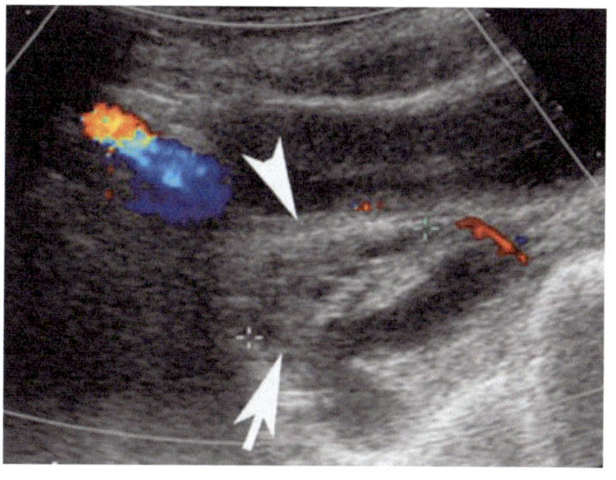

Fig. 68.3 US appearance of a torsed tube: US images show a complex structure next to the right ovary, with no flow apparent on the Doppler image

68.4 Laparoscopic Treatment

Since paratubal and paraovarian cysts are generally asymptomatic, they can be incidentally discovered during a laparoscopy performed for another indication [9, 14]. In this latest occurrence, their resection is indicated considering the risk that they could later enlarge and/or be subjected to torsion. In addition, in several cases, these lesions are discovered during laparoscopies performed for right lower quadrant pain since torsion of right adnexal lesions produces symptoms similar to acute appendicitis [14].

Traditional midline laparotomy has been the conventional surgical approach for the removal of symptomatic giant paraovarian and paratubal cysts [9, 19]. Oophorectomy or tubal excision is sometimes required. Because of the well-recognized advantages of the laparoscopic procedures, recently paraovarian and paratubal cysts have been managed by the mini-invasive approach [9, 10]. Different minimally invasive approaches have been described until now.

68.4.1 Single-Incision Single-Instrument (SISI) Approach

This approach uses a 12-mm standard laparoscopy trocar introduced transumbilically, after placement of an indwelling bladder catheter. Then an operating endoscope, which combines a 10-mm, 0° lens with an offset eyepiece and a 5-mm port through which a long instrument, such as a grasper or suction, can be introduced, is adopted. Ovarian torsions can almost always be reduced with this instrument. For large simple cystic lesions, aspiration of the cyst fluid is performed with a spinal needle introduced through the anterior abdominal wall under direct vision while stabilizing the lesion with the grasper or by cauterizing a hole in the cyst with the long suction and then inserting it inside the cyst. Such decompression affords increased mobility of the adnexa. If the cystic lesion is so large that it extends out of the pelvis and can be directly visualized through the umbilical incision, it is grasped with an atraumatic clamp. Once the adnexa are mobile, they are extruded through the umbilical incision, using a fascial extension if needed. Ovarian-sparing procedures are attempted when possible, with the cystic lesions being dissected off the normal ovarian parenchyma, which is dropped back into the abdomen after achieving hemostasis.

Conversion to standard laparoscopy is dependent upon the experience and comfort of the surgeon with each individual case [12, 13].

68.4.2 Single-Incision Laparoscopic Surgery (SILS) Approach

After urinary decompression via Foley catheter performed prior to the procedure, entry into the abdomen is accomplished through a 2-cm longitudinal incision in the umbilicus. The underlying midline fascia is opened over a length of 1.5–2.5 cm to enter the peritoneal cavity. Two different devices may be used, (1) TriPort or (2) a homemade port, using a plastic ring rolled up onto the wrist portion of a surgical glove and then inserted through the umbilical incision site. A 5-mm endoscope is introduced into the port, and the patient is placed in moderate Trendelenburg position to get maximum exposure of the lower abdomen. With reusable 5-mm standard straight laparoscopic instruments, the adnexa are mobilized, and a straight electrocautery instrument is used for unroofing the cyst. More complex adnexal dissection and/or resection can be carried out with the use of the Harmonic scalpel, an endoloop, or an endostapler [14, 15].

68.4.3 Three-Trocar Laparoscopic Approach

A carbon dioxide pneumoperitoneum is created using the open laparoscopy technique under vision through an umbilical incision. A three-trocar laparoscopy is performed. The primary 10-mm port is inserted through the umbilicus for the 10-mm 0° optic, and 2 secondary 3- or 5-mm working ports are inserted for laparoscopic instruments (Fig. 68.4).

Laparoscopic inspection of the pelvis is carried out to inspect the pelvic organs and to identify the cystic lesions. In case of a voluminous fluid-filled cyst, aspiration of the cyst fluid is performed with a spinal needle introduced through the anterior abdominal wall under direct vision while stabilizing the lesion with a grasper. Then the cyst is excised using monopolar scissors or sealing devices (Fig. 68.5). At the end of the procedure, the specimen is extracted through the central umbilical 10-mm port without the need to use an endobag [16–18].

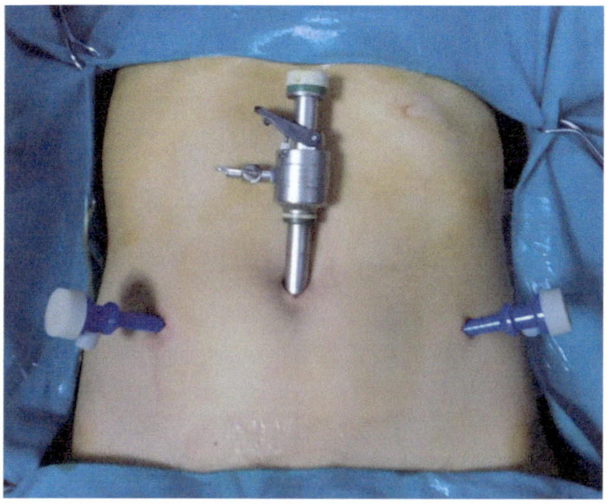

Fig. 68.4 Trocars' position

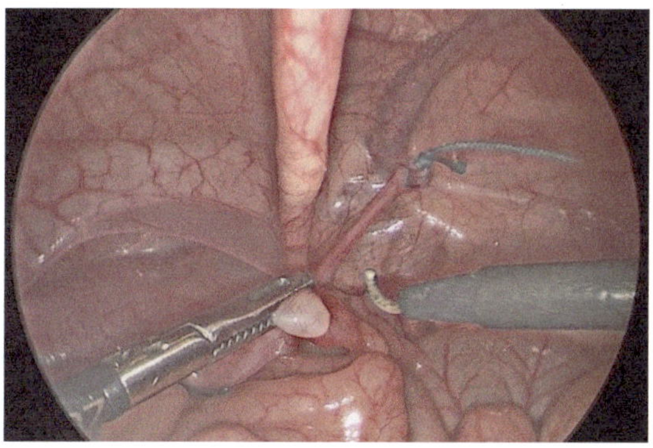

Fig. 68.5 A paratubal cyst, incidentally discovered during a laparoscopic inguinal hernia repair, was excised using a monopolar hook

68.4.4 Laparoscopic Treatment of Adnexal Torsion

Early diagnosis and immediate intervention are necessary in cases of ovarian and/or tubal torsion in order to preserve long-term ovarian function and fertility. The gold standard of diagnosis and treatment is operative laparoscopy. With isolated tubal torsion, the tube can be untwisted unless there is evidence of necrosis and/or rupture. The current surgical approach is laparoscopic detorsion without removal of the fallopian tube/ovary accompanied by removal of any tubal and/or ovarian mass that may have precipitated the torsion. Fixation of the torted isolated tube or accompanied ovary (if present) is controversial. If the torsion is due to an adnexal mass, excision of the mass with detorsion should be curative. If the torsion is due to a spontaneous event, fixation to the peritoneum of the sidewall or cul-de-sac with permanent suture may be an option [19]. However, if, after detorsion maneuver, the tube and ovary appear clearly necrotic, the sole therapeutic option is to perform an oophorosalpingectomy (Fig. 68.6).

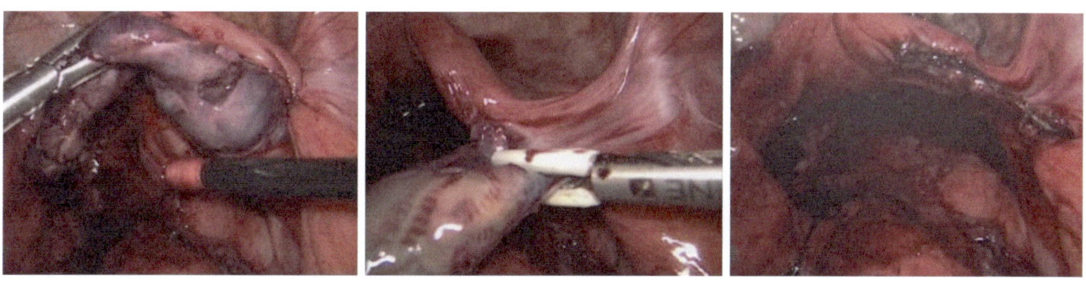

Fig. 68.6 After laparoscopic detorsion, the tube and ovary appeared clearly necrotic, and an oophorosalpingectomy was performed using a sealing device

68.5 Discussion

Laparoscopic surgery is considered the gold-standard treatment for the management of adnexal lesions in the pediatric and adolescents population. One reason is that postoperative adhesions are usually rare after laparoscopic surgery and this increases chances for future fertility in this age group [13]. Also, the cosmetic advantages of laparoscopic surgery are more profound in pediatric and adolescent patients (Fig. 68.7) [20]. For adults, previous reports have documented similar rates of major postoperative complications between laparoscopy and laparotomy for the management of benign gynecologic lesions. However, minor postoperative complications like fever and postoperative wound and urinary tract infections are less commonly seen in patients who undergo laparoscopic surgery [11].

Because of the benign nature of these cysts and the lack of spontaneously resolution based on its Wolffian origin, it is reasonable to consider definitive surgical management in cases of persistent or enlarging cysts noted on serial ultrasounds in order to decrease the risk of cyst recurrence and ovarian torsion in the future [20]. Because these cases may present with adnexal torsion, all efforts should be made to salvage the adnexa whenever possible, and, in the absence of tissue necrosis, definitive treatment involves excision of the cyst alone [16]. Paraovarian cysts larger than 5 cm in diameter are the most symptomatic, necessitating surgical intervention [14]. Although rare, paraovarian cysts containing neoplasm have been reported [10, 11]. Neoplasms constituted 2.9% of the reported cases, and most neoplasms were carcinoma, such as cystadenocarcinoma and papillary carcinoma. Most neoplasms occurred in adults, but it should be noted that paraovarian carcinoma can also occur in young patients [14]. Also female hydatids of Morgagni, although rare in premenarchal patients, may become symptomatic due to torsion [15]. The mechanisms of torsion are the following: (a) torsion of the hydatids of Morgagni on its pedicle with intact adnexa, (b) torsion involving the adnexa, and (c) torsion and entanglement of the hydatids of Morgagni's pedicle around the distal fallopian tube [1]. In theory, cystic dilatation of these Wolffian duct remnants is thought to be more frequent in adult women owing to secretory activity of the tubal-type epithelium under the hormonal influence after the postpubertal years and in pregnancy. However, it has been reported that the torsion of hydatids of Morgagni may be encountered in acute onset lower quadrant pain in premenarchal adolescent girls in the presence of normal inflammatory markers and ultrasound results of the pelvic region. In cases of a normal-appearing appendix on laparoscopy in adolescent girls, it is important for the pediatric surgeon to be aware of this condition and inspect the adnexal region thoroughly [15].

In addition, since these formations are often incidental findings during laparoscopies performed for other indications, most frequently being laparoscopic exploration for right lower quadrant (RLQ) acute or chronic pain, it seems that a thorough search of the adnexa for the presence of paratubal or paraovarian cysts during laparoscopic exploration for RLQ pain is a useful procedure [17]. The intraoperative diagnosis

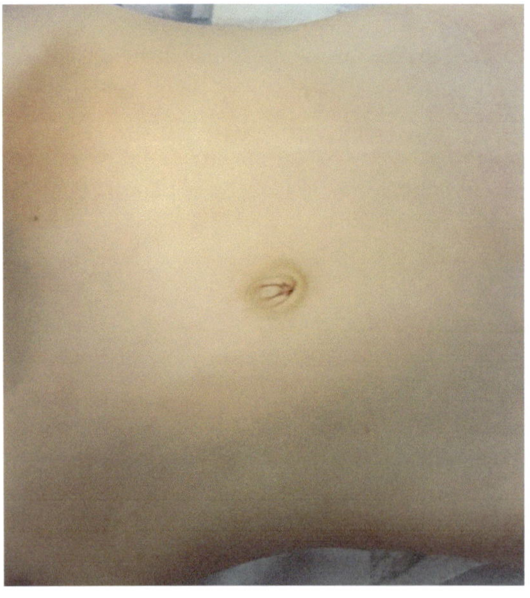

Fig. 68.7 Cosmetic outcome of laparoscopic procedure

during the thorough inspection of the adnexal region in the setting of a normal-looking ovary seems to be easier during laparoscopy compared with an open operation. This may not only lead to resection of a cyst that could later enlarge and/or be subjected to torsion but would also allow detection of other pathological lesions of the right adnexa that often produce symptoms similar to acute appendicitis. This procedure could also prove beneficial in cases of future infertility, considering that excision of a paratubal cyst may result in pregnancy in a substantial number of infertile women [20]. The significant effect of paratubal cystectomy on tubal patency supports the concept of routine removal of any paratubal or paraovarian cyst discovered at laparoscopy. An additional value of removal of these cysts detected at laparoscopy is the exclusion of the rare possibility of malignancy (2–3%) and obtaining sufficient tissues for histopathologic evaluation. Lastly, its extraction is relatively easy and less time-consuming. In general, it is not necessary to use an endobag for specimen extraction, but the specimen is exteriorized through the umbilical port, unless there is a suspicion of malignancy of the adnexal mass.

The classic advantages of laparoscopy include low morbidity, excellent cosmetic results, short hospital stay, and rapid return to normal activities. In addition, laparoscopy gives an excellent view of the pelvic structures, including the genital organs. Because of magnification of the image in laparoscopy, this feature may allow a better chance to preserve ovary and ovarian tube, especially in cysts located closely to these structures, which otherwise cannot be achieved. Preservation of the pelvic organs, while performing the laparoscopic paraovarian or paratubal cystectomy, is needed in young nulliparous patients, in order to preserve their fertility.

References

1. Perlman S, Hertweck P, Fallat ME. Paratubal and tubal abnormalities. Semin Pediatr Surg. 2005;14(2):124–34. Review.
2. Kiseli M, Caglar GS, Cengiz SD, Karadag D, Yilmaz MB. Clinical diagnosis and complications of paratubal cysts: review of the literature and report of uncommon presentations. Arch Gynecol Obstet. 2012;285(6):1563–9.
3. Muolokwu E, Sanchez J, Bercaw JL, Sangi-Haghpeykar H, Banszek T, Brandt ML, Dietrich JE. The incidence and surgical management of paratubal cysts in a pediatric and adolescent population. J Pediatr Surg. 2011;46(11):2161–3.
4. Vlahakis-Miliaras E, Miliaras D, Koutsoumis G, Miliaras S, Spyridakis I, Papadopoulos MS. Paratubal cysts in young females as an incidental finding in laparotomies performed for right lower quadrant abdominal pain. Pediatr Surg Int. 1998;13:141–2.
5. Muolokwu E, Sanchez J, Bercaw JL, Sangi-Haghpeykar H, Banszek T, Brandt ML, Dietrich JE. Paratubal cysts, obesity, and hyperandrogenism. J Pediatr Surg. 2011;46(11):2164–7.
6. Letourneur B, Grandjean S, Richard P, Parant O. Management of a giant paraovarian cyst. Gynecol Obstet Fertil. 2006;34:239–41.
7. Terek MC, Sahin C, Yeniel AO, Ergenoglu M, Zekioglu O. Paratubal borderline tumor diagnosed in the adolescent period: a case report and review of the literature. Pediatr Adolesc Gynecol. 2011;24(5):e115–6.
8. Athey PA, Cooper NB. Sonographic features of paraovarian cysts. AJR. 1985;144:83–6.
9. Thakore SS, Chun MJ, Fitzpatrick K. Recurrent ovarian torsion due to paratubal cysts in an adolescent female. J Pediatr Adolesc Gynecol. 2012;25(4):e85–7.
10. Kiseli M, Caglar GS, Cengiz SD, Karadag D, Yılmaz MB. Clinical diagnosis and complications of paratubal cysts: review of the literature and report of uncommon presentations. Arch Gynecol Obstet. 2012;285(6):1563–9.
11. Low SC, Ong CL, Lam SL, Beh ST. Paratubal cyst complicated by tubo-ovarian torsion: computed tomography features. Australas Radiol. 2005;49(2):136–9.
12. Barloon TJ, Brown BP, Abu-Yousef MM, et al. Paraovarian and paratubal cysts: preoperative diagnosis using transabdominal and transvaginal sonography. J Clin Ultrasound. 1996;24:117–22.
13. Kishimoto K, Ito K, Awaya H, et al. Paraovarian cyst: MR imaging features. Abdom Imaging. 2002;27:685–9.
14. Darwish AM, Amin AF, Mohammad SA. Laparoscopic management of paratubal and paraovarian cysts. JSLS. 2003;7(2):101–6.
15. Dural O, Yasa C, Bastu E, Ugurlucan FG, Yilmaz G, Yuksel B, Akhan SE, Buyru F. Laparoscopic outcomes of adnexal surgery in older children and adolescents. J Pediatr Adolesc Gynecol. 2017;30(1):128–31.
16. Loux T, Falk GA, Gaffley M, Ortega S, Ramos C, Malvezzi L, Knight CG, Burnweit C. Single-incision

single-instrument adnexal surgery in pediatric patients. Minim Invasive Surg. 2015;2015:246950.

17. Macarthu M, Mahomed AA. Laparoscopy in the diagnosis and management of a complicated paraovarian cyst. Surg Endosc. 2003;17(10):1676–7.
18. Okada T, Yoshida H, Matsunaga T, Kouchi K, Ohtsuka Y, Takano H, Horie H, Ohnuma N. Paraovarian cyst with torsion in children. J Pediatr Surg. 2002;37(6):937–40.
19. Muthucumaru M, Yahya Z, Ferguson P, Cheng W. Torsion of hydatids of Morgagni in premenarchal adolescent girls—a case report and review of literature. J Pediatr Surg. 2011;46(9):e13–5.
20. Pansky M, Smorgick N, Lotan G, et al. Adnexal torsion involving hydatids of Morgagni: a rare cause of acute abdominal pain in adolescents. Obstet Gynecol. 2006;108:100–2.

Laparoscopic-Assisted Vaginoplasty

69

Maria Marcela Bailez

69.1 Introduction

Providing its excellent visualization, access to pelvic structures, and less postoperative adhesion, laparoscopy has been an important tool for the treatment of uterovaginal anomalies. We have used it to define the anomaly, monitor endometriosis or a hysteroscopic procedure, replace an absent vagina, and resect abnormal Müllerian structures.

We have reported technical details and results of the use of operative laparoscopy for the treatment of uterovaginal anomalies in children and adolescents and described a simple classification according to the procedure required for the multiple varieties [1].

There are a variety of conditions with total or partial absence of vagina in which a neovagina has to be created. In group 1 we included those patients with complete absence of vagina and uterus treated with a laparoscopic sigmoid vaginal replacement. Patients with Müllerian dysgenesis (Mayer-Rokitansky syndrome) and selected DSD patients are included in this group.

If a vaginal orifice is present, the treatment of choice is passive or active elongation [2].

M. M. Bailez (✉)
Pediatric Surgery Unit, Surgical Department
Garrahan Childrens Hospital, Buenos Aires, Argentina

When this technique fails either because of lack of motivation or in cases of a flat perineum, a surgical correction should be attempted.

Surgical approach varies according to clinical and emotional condition of the affected adolescent and surgeon's experience.

Techniques that have been used more frequently are the McIndoe operation and its modifications and vaginoplasty. These techniques are successful in 75–85% of the cases [3, 4]. Other techniques described include Williams' operation (which uses vulvar skin), Johnson's operation (using skin from the back), Vecchietti's operation (laparoscopic elongation), use of buccal mucosa, or Pratt operation which uses the sigmoid colon [5–7].

Even though the use of the sigmoid colon is not frequently quoted in the gynecological literature, the good results obtained with this technique repairing complex malformations or those associated with absence of vagina such as a cloaca or anorectal malformations with rectovulvar or rectovestibular fistula, which should be repaired in a single operation, encouraged us to optimize this technique for isolated vaginal replacement [8–11]. The use of sigmoid for vaginal replacement is a well- quoted operation in the pediatric surgical literature [12]. With this technique a tubular vagina is created. Two major advantages of this procedure are as follows: there is no need for dilatation or use of some kind of a mold in the vagina, and the neovagina has natural

C. Esposito et al. (eds.), *ESPES Manual of Pediatric Minimally Invasive Surgery*,
https://doi.org/10.1007/978-3-030-00964-9_69

lubrication [13]. One of its major disadvantages was the need for a laparotomy, implicating pain and discomfort. We started doing it laparoscopically in 1998.

This aim of this presentation is to analyze this technique.

69.2 Preoperative Preparation

All patients and their parents have to sign a specifically formulated informed consent before the procedure. Patients participate actively in the selection of the technique for the vaginal replacement. When dealing with patients with Müllerian dysgenesis or DSD, we only indicate this technique in patients mature enough to discuss and select from different options. In other occasions we had the opportunity to do it earlier: selected patients with cloacas or combined anorectal malformations and vaginal agenesis, peripubertal patients with a functional Müllerian structure and a complete absent vagina, or an infant with an uterovaginal rhabdomyosarcoma requiring total vaginectomy who underwent a simultaneous laparoscopic vaginal replacement.

We always rule out familial history of colonic polyposis or colonic cancer before using the colon.

We indicate ambulatory bowel preparation preoperatively.

We use antibiotic prophylaxis with i.v. ampicillin sulbactam.

69.2.1 Positioning

The patient is placed in lithotomy position, supine with the legs elevated, abducted, and supported in stirrups (Fig. 69.1). If only one monitor is available, it should be placed at the left side down. The surgeon is positioned on the right side of the patient with a nurse on his side, and the cameraman is also on tistanthe right cephalic to the surgeon. The assistant stands on the left side (Fig.69.2).

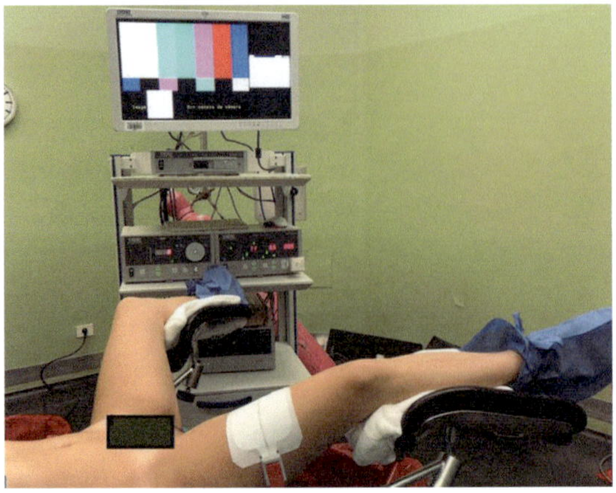

Fig. 69.1 The patient has to be positioned on the operative table in lithotomy position

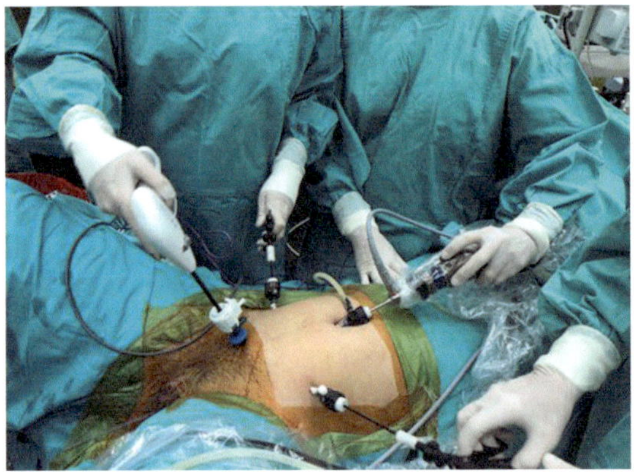

Fig. 69.2 Team position. The surgeon and cameraman on the right. The assistant on the left. The surgeon is using the suprapubic port for the right hand (bipolar sealer) and the right lower quadrant port for the left hand. The assistant is using the left lower quadrant port for contratraction

69.2.2 Technique and Instrumentation

69.2.2.1 Evolution of Surgical Technique

In the 2000 we reported the first patient who underwent a laparoscopic sigmoid vaginal replacement and the results of its use later [14]. Our experience with the next 14 patients was published in 2004 and 2008 [15, 16].

The initial operative technique is available in WebSurg (www.websurg.com). At that time, we used four ports: a 10 mm (umbilical), a 12 mm (right lower quadrant), and two 5 mm (left lower quadrant and hypogastric). The lens was initially introduced through the umbilical port but later on was moved to the right lower quadrant one in order to achieve better visualization of the vascularization of the sigmoid colon.

A segment of 15 cm of the sigmoid colon was isolated using bipolar HFE, or the bipolar sealer (LigasureTM), and two linear endostaplers. The sigmoid may be transilluminated with a 5 mm lens inserted through the port in the left lower quadrant to facilitate vessel visualization. This maneuver was abandoned with increased experience.

Colocolonic continuity was reestablished using a circular mechanical suturing device. The proximal end of the colon was exteriorized through the umbilicus, the proximal part of the circular stapling device inserted, and the colon returned to the abdominal cavity.

The remaining part of the stapling device was inserted through the rectum. Both parts of the stapling device were assembled intra-abdominally under laparoscopic control, and the stapling device was fired.

Then a space was created between the urethra and rectum by perineal dissection but under laparoscopic verification.

The peritoneum near the Douglas' space was incised in order to allow the passage of a forceps from the perineum, which enabled the descent of the isolated bowel segment The vaginoplasty was completed from the perineal side using 5/0 absorbable sutures avoiding a circular ending and rather opening the bowel ending widely to avoid stenosis (Fig. 69.3).

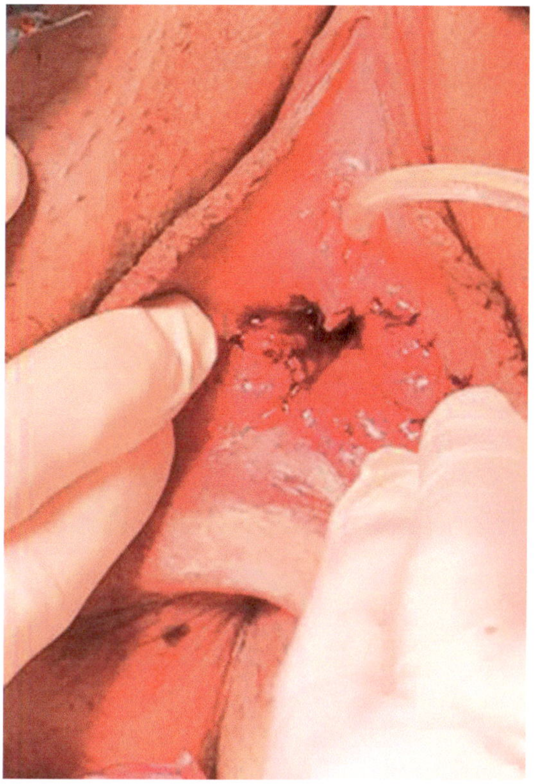

Fig. 69.3 Aspect of vaginoplasty

69.2.2.2 Last Technical Modifications

We modified the original technique in 2010: (1) reduce the port size, (2) use a different hemostatic device, and (3) use the NOTES (Natural Orifice Transendoscopic Surgery) concept.

1. We reduced the port sizes using a 4 mm 30-degree lens in the umbilicus, two 3 mm operative ports in each lower quadrant, and one 5 mm suprapubic port, avoiding a 12 mm port in the abdomen (Fig. 69.4).

   With the advent of HD cameras, it is possible to have an excellent view of the pelvis with low diameter lens in a nearly adult pelvis. We still need a 5 mm port for the use of the hemostatic device, and we choose the suprapubic port for cosmetic and ergonomic reasons. The surgeon uses the 3 mm right lower quadrant port for his left hand and the suprapubic 5 mm port for his right hand.

   The assistant retracts the colon using traction and contratraction maneuvers using the left 3 mm port.
2. We started using a 5 mm bipolar sealer with a monopolar cautery tip, all hand activated, avoiding changing instruments as much as possible.
3. After isolating vessels and creating the mesenteric windows of the selected piece of sigmoid as previously described (Fig. 69.5), we

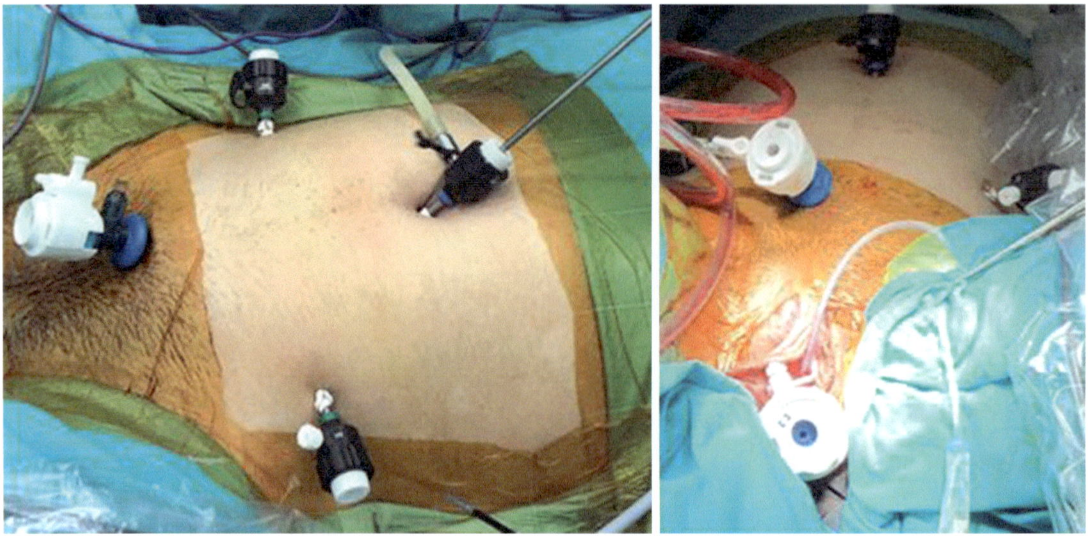

Fig. 69.4 Port setting. Four millimeters port in the umbilicus for the lens. Two 3 mm in each lower quadrant and one 5 mm suprapubic for the sealer and scissors or suction. In the last modification, the 12 mm port to introduce the linear stapler is initiated through the space dissected between the rectum and urethra in the perineum

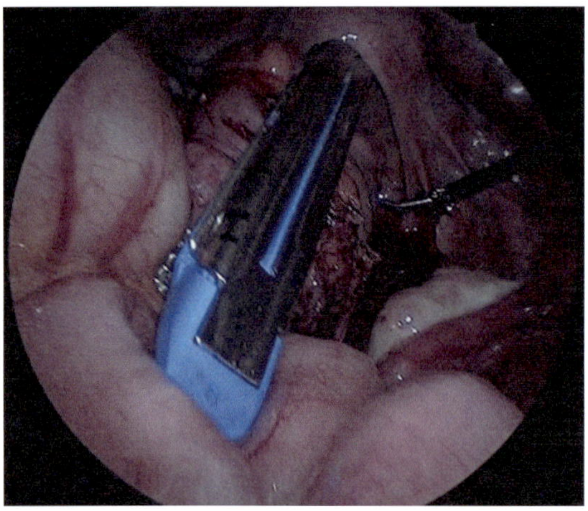

Fig. 69.5 Isolated sigmoid segment. Both mesenteric windows created with the bipolar sealer

proceed to dissect the space between the urethra and rectum, a 12 mm port and the linear stapler sutures inserted through it (Figs. 69.4 and 69.6).

The proximal transected colon is also exteriorized through this space to introduce the anvil of the circular stapler and reintroduced into the abdomen afterward.

In this way we use the space created for the neovagina as a natural orifice to introduce a 12 mm port and stapler (NOTES concept), achieving better cosmetic results.

The colocolonic anastomosis is assembled under laparoscopic vision (Fig. 69.6).

An important detail is keeping the isolated sigmoid to the right of the anastomosis for an easier descent.

69.3 Postoperative Care

A urinary catheter is left for 24 h.

The patients can restart full oral feeding usually after 24 h after surgery. The analgesic requirement is generally limited to 72 postoperative hours. Most patients are discharged on the third postoperative day.

Parents are instructed on how to treat the perineal suture (introitoplasty) by maintaining it clean and dry for about 1 week after surgery.

Between 7 and 15 postoperative days, a digital exam of the introitus is done. We advise to start using tampons with estrogen cream during the night for the first 2 or 3 weeks on a daily schedule

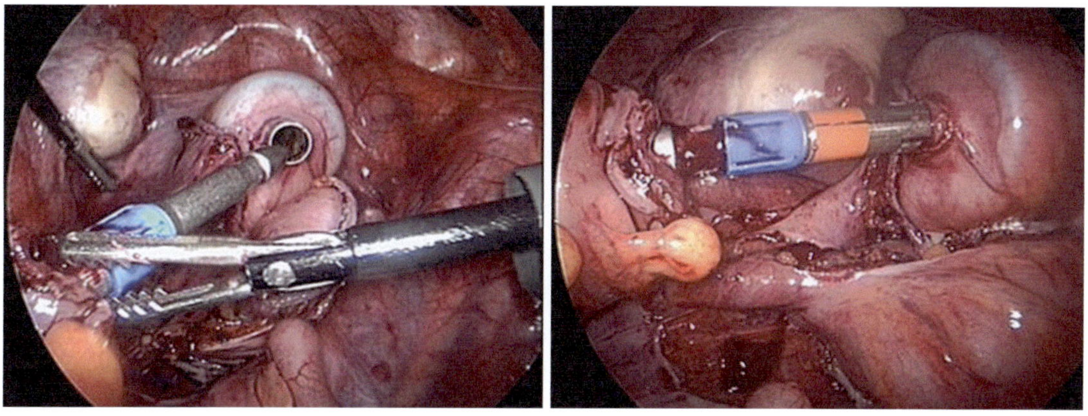

Fig. 69.6 Colocolonic anastomosis under laparoscopic vision

to become familiar with the neovagina. We don't use routine dilatation or molds.

A follow-up is carried out by clinical examinations at 1 week, 2 weeks, and then at 1, 6, and 12 months after surgery. We follow them in a once-a-year basis after the first year.

69.4 Results

The average length of surgery is 120 min (range from 90 to 300 min).

One hundred and thirty patients were operated using a laparoscopic sigmoid vaginoplasty. Mean age was 16.5 years (range 15–41 years). One hundred and twenty-five had a Mayer-Rokitansky syndrome and six were 46XY DSD patients, of which three had complete androgen insensitivity and had previously underwent a laparoscopic bilateral orchidectomy. Six patients had a single pelvic kidney. Four patients had an ARM previously operated through a sagittal-posterior approach with a colostomy. Two underwent a simultaneous resection of a Müllerian functional remnant. Three patients had a previously failed skin or muscular vaginoplasties.

In this report, we are excluding patients with partial vaginal agenesis and a single medial functional uterus requiring uterine communication to a neovagina or vaginal agenesis with a medial uterus with cervix atresia or hypoplasia for considering them a different population with more demanding an expert care.

There was one accidental opening of the bladder that was sutured laparoscopically. The urine catheter was left for 3 days.

Care needs to be taken with the technical changes to avoid descending the colocolonic anastomosis instead of the isolated bowel. Explanation may be that the proximal end of the colon exteriorized through the perineum has a sort of memory to go down again so it is advisable to double check every segment before opening the distal exteriorized end to create the neovagina. This event occurred once.

Two patients presented transient rectal bleeding.

All patients were able to tolerate food 24 h after the procedure, and 125 patients were discharged 48 h after the operation. The average time to return to full daily activities was 7 days.

Viability and patency of neovagina are excellent in 124 patients after a mean follow-up of 68 months (range 6–220 m), and 80 patients are sexually active.

Two patients developed mucosal prolapse and four needed introital revisions. Excessive mucous secretion was not observed, except in one patient; it may be explained by the length of bowel used.

69.5 Tips and Tricks

69.5.1 Right Pedicle

Selecting the right pedicle is crucial. This is a team maneuver. It is important to use the 30 degrees of the lens accurately and expose with traction and contratraction maneuvers to have a frontal view of the sigmoid pedicles, always preserving the superior rectal vessels.

A right pelvic kidney made the procedure more difficult and required more "camera work." In contrast, a left pelvic kidney exposed the sigmoidal vessels very well, which made the isolation of a sigmoid colon segment easier.

69.5.2 Urethrorectal Space Dissection

A complete dissection of the vesicorectal space is required before trying to open it from above to prevent accidental opening of the bladder and a blunt dissection from below using both fingers until they can be seen under laparoscopic vision (can maneuver) [15]. Only at this point, the 12 mm port is inserted in this space.

69.5.3 Colocolic Anastomosis

If you are planning to use the NOTES concept, the proximal end of the colon has to be well dissected to exteriorize in the perineum to insert the anvil. If it cannot be achieved, the suprapubic port incision might be widened and the maneuver made through it.

Choosing the right diameter of the circular suture prevents postoperative bleeding.

We use the suprapubic 5 mm instrument to assembly the 2 ends of the circular stapler.

69.5.4 Descending the Isolated Bowel

As we previously described, avoid losing the pneumoperitoneum and vision while grabbing the neovagina from the perineum and double check. A regular bowel conventional graper is our preference for this maneuver.

69.6 Discussion

The Mayer-Rokitansky syndrome is characterized by the absence of the vagina with or without uterine remnants. Most of the patients in this group are adolescents presenting with primary amenorrhea. Associated renal and skeletal malformations are frequent like renal agenesis, horseshoe kidney, and cervical scoliosis, and diagnosis can be made earlier if a routine genital exam is indicated in these high-risk group of patients. There are many options to treat vaginal absence as we have described.

Laparoscopic-assisted sigmoid vaginal replacement is one of them.

Nowadays many young females ask for it because they prefer to undergo a 2- or 3-h-long surgical procedure under general anesthesia to have their corporal squema [scheme] complete without any need of repeated and somehow painful elongations. Decreasing the size of ports, as well as improving cosmesis and outcome, is our goal.

We have also indicated it in selected 46XY DSD patients with very little space between the urethra and rectum.

With the widespread culturing of vaginal epithelium, it is likely that an ideal vaginoplasty material will become available.

References

1. Bailez M. Advanced endoscopic surgery in children. Semin Pediatr Surg. 2007;16(4):278–87.
2. Ingram JM. The bicycle seat stool in the treatment of vaginal agenesis and stenosis: a preliminary report. Am J Obstet Gynecol. 1981;140:867–9.
3. Tjaden BL, Rock J. Uterovaginal anomalies. In: Carpenter SE, Rock J, editors. Pediatric and adolescent gynecology, vol. 20. New York: Raven Press; 1992. p. 313–30.
4. Strickland JL, Cameron WJ, Krantz KE, et al. Long-term satisfaction of adults undergoing McIndoe vaginoplasty as adolescents. Adolesc Pediatr Gynecol. 1993;6:135–7.

5. Muran D, Frederick R, Shell D. Modified Williams vulvovaginoplasty: the role of tissue expanders. Adolesc Pediatr Gynecol. 1992;5:81–3.
6. Samuelson M, Baker L. Autologous buccal mucosa vulvovaginoplasty for high urogenital sinus. J Pediatr Urol. 2006;2(5):486–8.
7. Pratt JH. Vaginal atresia corrected by use of small and large bowel. Clin Obstet Gynecol. 1972;15:639–49.
8. Bailez M, Heinen F, Solana J. Absent vagina in patients with anorectal anomalies. BJU. 1998;81:76.
9. Giovanni B, Zaffaroni G, Milena D, et al. Proctoperineovaginohysterstomy and sigmoid colon pull-through for vaginal agenesis, hematocervicometra and vestibular anus. Adolesc Pediatr Gynecol. 1993;6:95–8.
10. Hendren H. Management of cloacal malformations. Semin Pediatr Surg. 1997;6:217–27.
11. Peña A. Atlas of surgical management of anorectal malformations. New York: Springer Verlag; 1990. p. 19.
12. Rock JA, Sclaff WD. The obstetrical consequences of uterovaginal anomalies. Fertil Steril. 1985;43:681–92.
13. Novak F, Kos L, Plesko F. The advantages of the artificial vagina derived from sigmoid colon. Acta Obstet Gynecol Scand. 1978;57:95–7.
14. Bailez MM, Scherl H, Dibenedetto V, et al. Laparoscopic vaginal replacement with sigmoid colon. Pediatr Endosurg Innov Tech. 2000;4:90.
15. Bailez MM, Dibenedetto V, Elmo G, Korman L. Laparoscopic sigmoid vaginal replacement. What we learned? Pediatr Endosurg Innov Tech. 2004;8(4):295–301.
16. Bailez MM. Laparoscopy in uterovaginal anomalies. In: Bax K, Georgeson K, Rothenberg S, Valla JS, Yeung CK, editors. Endoscopic surgery in infants and children. Berlin: Springer; 2008. p. 791–803.
17. McIndoe A. The treatment of congenital absence and obliterate conditions of the vagina. Br J Plast Surg. 1950;2(4):254–7.
18. Rock JA. The double uterus associated with an obstructed hemivagina and ipsilateral renal agenesis. Am J Obstet Gynecol. 1980;138:339.

70 Ovarian Cryopreservation

Mario Lima and Michela Maffi

70.1 Introduction

Ovarian tissue collection for cryopreservation is a technique for fertility preservation. Gonadal tissue is collected laparoscopically and then is processed and cryopreserved, and it can be reimplanted to restore endocrine and reproductive function.

Patients eligible for this procedure are all those females, especially prepubertal, who are exposed to a risk of premature ovarian failure. Premature ovarian failure is associated with exposure to chemotherapy and radiation [1, 2] (Table 70.1).

Ovarian tissue cryopreservation was firstly described in 1996 by Hovatta et al. [3] Even if this technique is still to be considered experimental, it is currently the only option applicable in prepubertal girls. The following are the three mainly feasible techniques for tissue collection:

- Ovarian cortical tissue biopsy: it consists of obtaining several specimens of cortical tissue away from the hilum using a laparoscopic biopter.
- Partial oophorectomy: it consists of partial excision of ovarian cortical tissue. Different authors report from 1/4 to 2/3 of ovarian tissue to be removed leaving the hilar part intact.
- Unilateral ovariectomy: it consists of the collection of the whole ovary including vascular pedicle that will be used during the reimplantation.

The collected tissue is then harvested and prepared for cryopreservation. The most used method is slow freezing, which represents the standard of care, but also vitrification is an available method [4]. Vitrification differs from slow freezing for concentration of cryoprotectant (higher in vitrification) and rate of cooling (faster in vitrification) [5]. The tissue can be cryopreserved for about 7 years [5].

Table 70.1 Conditions associated with the risk of premature ovarian failure

Malignant diseases	Nonmalignant conditions
Pelvic diseases	Autoimmune diseases
Pelvic rhabdomyosarcoma	Systemic lupus erythematosus
Sarcoblastoma	Nephritic syndromes
Sacral tumors	Bone marrow transplantation
Extrapelvic diseases	Sickle cell anemia
Ewing osteosarcoma	Thalassemia major
Wilms' tumor	Endocrine/genetic diseases
Hepatoblastoma	Turner's syndrome
Neuroblastoma	Galactosemia
Systemic diseases	Family history of premature ovarian failure
Hodgkin's/non-Hodgkin's lymphomas	
Leukemias	

M. Lima (✉) · M. Maffi
Pediatric Surgery Unit, S. Orsola Hospital, University of Bologna, Bologna, Italy
e-mail: mario.lima@unibo.it; michela.maffi@libero.it

C. Esposito et al. (eds.), *ESPES Manual of Pediatric Minimally Invasive Surgery*,
https://doi.org/10.1007/978-3-030-00964-9_70

When the fertility has to be restored, after the end of therapies, the harvested tissue can be reimplanted in an orthotopic or heterotopic position. The rest of the native ovary or a peritoneal fold near the fimbriae are considered orthotopic positions as they allow spontaneous pregnancies. The forearm or abdominal wall are the most used heterotopic sites. The reactivation of the tissue appears 4–9 months after the reimplantation [5].

70.2 Preoperative Preparation

All patients undergo a preoperative assessment which consists of the following investigation and laboratory tests:

- Pelvic US to explore dimensions and structure of ovaries
- Follicle-stimulating hormone (FSH), luteinizing hormone (LH), progesterone, estradiol, prolactin, testosterone, 17-hydroxyprogesterone, thyroid hormones, D4-androstenedione, inflammatory cytokines, dehydroepiandrosterone (DHEA), inhibin B, anti-Müllerian hormone, HIV 1–2 Ab and p24 Ag, HBV HbsAg, core Ab IgG and IgM, HCV IgG Ab, *T. pallidum* Ab

All patients and their parents have to sign a specifically formulated informed consent before the procedure. Patients receive general anesthesia.

70.2.1 Positioning

The patient is placed in a slight tilt supine position. Two monitors are placed at the feet of the patient, one for the surgeon and the other for the assistant. The surgeon's position is opposite to the ovary to be treated, with a nurse on his side, and the cameraman is in front of the surgeon. A first 10 mm Hasson trocar is placed in the umbilicus, and two operative 5 mm trocars are placed in the right and left flank, respectively.

70.2.2 Instrumentation

A 10 or 5 mm 0° camera can be used. Other useful instruments are atraumatic grasper; cold scissors; instruments for hemostasis such as monopolar hook, bipolar electrocautery, or argon gas device; and instruments for suction and irrigation.

70.2.3 Technique

The camera is inserted through the umbilical trocar. Atraumatic grasper is used to hold the ovary (Fig. 70.1), and most of the gonadal tissue is cut with cold scissor (Fig. 70.2). The collected tissue is then exteriorized through the umbilical wound paying attention not to grasp it strictly to avoid damage to follicles. The tissue is entrusted to the cryopreservation managers who immediately start the processing.

Hemostasis is achieved with monopolar hook, or bipolar forceps, or argon gas device if available (Fig. 70.3). It is important to leave a little layer of ovarian tissue and vascular pedicle to promote the engraftment of the tissue in case of reimplantation. At the end of the procedure, if there are doubts on hemostasis achievement, an abdominal drainage is left in the pelvis to monitor risk of hemorrhagic complication in postoperative period.

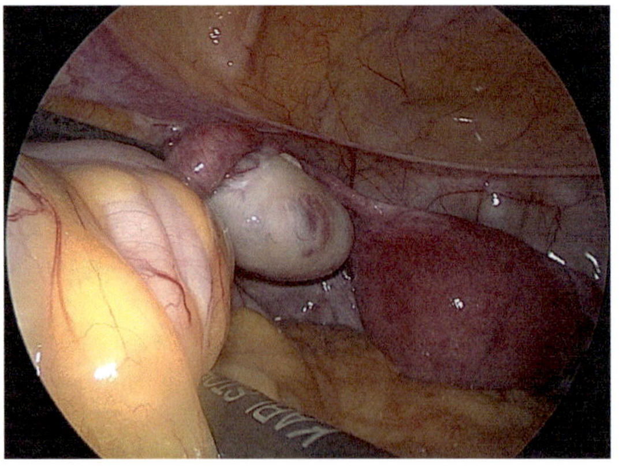

Fig. 70.1 The ovary is exposed and stabilized with atraumatic grasper

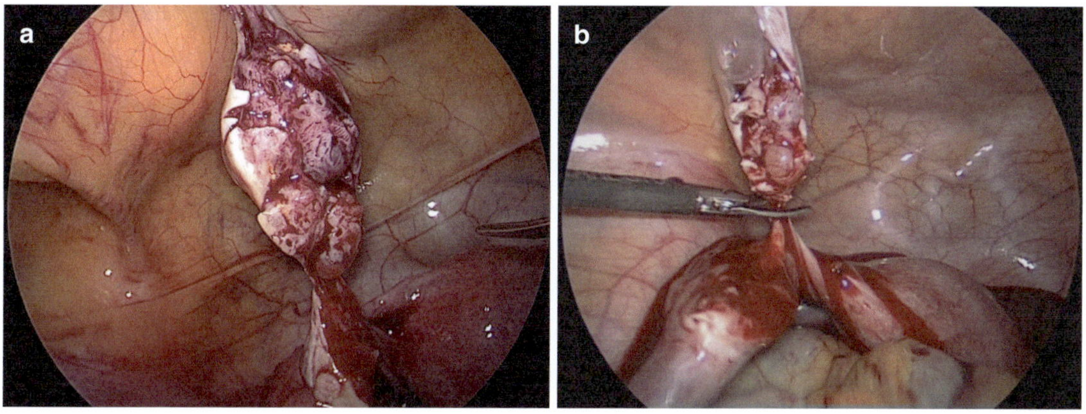

Fig. 70.2 The ovarian cortex is cut with cold scissors preserving the visible follicles (**a**, **b**)

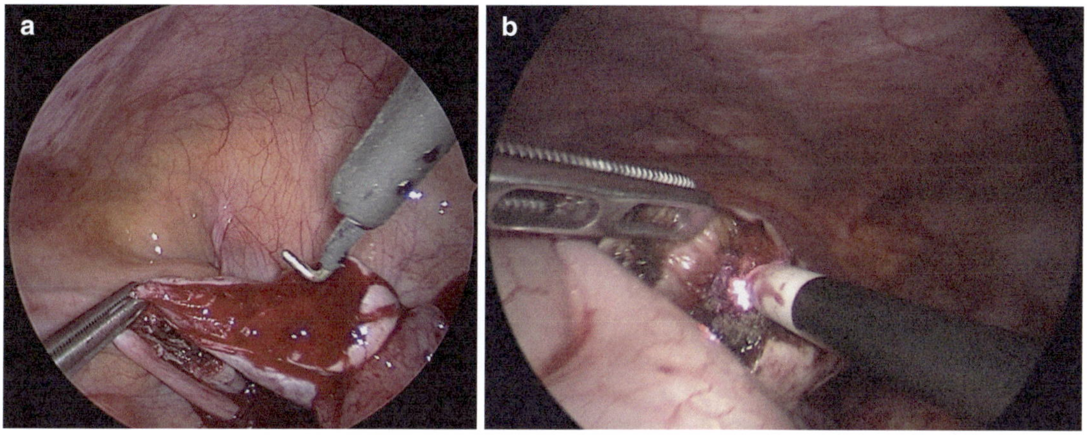

Fig. 70.3 The hemostasis can be achieved with monopolar hook (**a**), bipolar electrocautery, or argon gas device if available (**b**)

70.3 Postoperative Care

Fluid and oral feeding can be restarted after a few hours. The day after surgery, we usually test hemoglobin and platelets levels, and we remove the drainage. Pain control is usually obtained with paracetamol 15 mg/kg every 6 h for the first 48 h after surgery. The patient is usually discharged in postoperative day 1 or 2.

70.4 Results

We started our experience with laparoscopic collection of ovarian tissue in 2002, and till now 162 patients have been treated. The median age is 13.38±3.71. About 41.8% of patients had solid tumors, 41.2% systemic diseases, 10.6% genetic diseases, 2.2% autoimmune diseases, and 4.2% other diseases. Till 2016 we used to collect about 2/3 of both ovaries; by 2017, according to the indications of our biologists, we started to collect most of the parenchyma of only one ovary leaving the pedicle for the future reimplantation. The mean operative time has been 40 ± 15 min. We used to leave a drainage that has been removed in p.o. day 1. The patients have been discharged in p.o. day 2. In one case we had an intraoperative bleeding requiring red blood cell transfusion. Till now we haven't received requests for reimplantation. At follow-up there have been a mortality of 10% of patients due to oncologic disease [6, 7].

70.5 Tips and Tricks

The technique is quite simple even if it can hide some difficulties. First of all, stabilization of the ovary can require some time especially if the patient has a peripubertal age. Usually an atraumatic grasper that holds the ovary near the pedicle is sufficient to enable the surgeon to perform a precise cut. In case of excessive difficulties, a further instrument can be added in the suprapubic region to help stabilization. The collection should be made with cold instruments and with a cut as linear as possible to avoid both thermal and mechanical damages to the follicles. The specimen should be held with a gentle grip in one edge for the same reason and extracted from the umbilical wound avoiding squeezing while passing through the abdominal wall. A mild pressure to the vascular pedicle can help the hemostasis that can usually be achieved with monopolar hook or bipolar electrocautery.

70.6 Discussion

The survival rate of children affected by oncologic diseases has been increased in the last decades from about 60 to 80% [8]. For this reason, all efforts leading to the restoration of a normal quality of life including fertility have to be attempted.

Loss of reproductive potential depends mainly on the type, dose, of chemo- and radiotherapy, and age of the patient. Alkylating agents and pelvic radiotherapy are the most toxic therapies for gonadal tissue [9]. Several studies estimated the risk of premature ovarian failure on the basis of administrated therapies and age of patients [9]. If the risk is estimated to be high, the patient should be offered an option for fertility preservation. Ovarian tissue collection doesn't require hormonal stimulation so it can be used in prepubertal girls or in young adult patients who cannot delay chemo- or radiotherapy. A recent report [10] made an account of the children born following transplantation of freeze-thawed ovarian tissue: they are approximately 130 according to the last published data. The data are encouraging and reassuring, and even if experimental, ovarian tissue cryopreservation is becoming an established fertility preservation method.

Nevertheless several concerns are still debated. First of all it can be difficult to demonstrate if the reported pregnancies have resulted from ovulation of the transplanted tissue or the residual one [5]. The reported delivery rate per transplant or per woman amounts to 23% and 32%, respectively, according to recent reports [11, 12], while the first pregnancy in a woman undergoing ovarian tissue preservation in pediatric age was reported only in 2015 [13].

Another active problem is the risk of oncologic contamination of the collected tissue with the risk of reintroduction with autotransplantation [5]. This risk is obviously higher in patients with blood-borne malignancies or cancers that metastasize to the ovary or in patients with a predisposition to ovarian cancer. So in these cases, it is not recommended. Stating this risk, several efforts have been made to identify markers of tissue contamination or techniques to "wash" immature follicles avoiding reintroduction of malignancies with transplantation [14, 15].

As this procedure requires a general anesthesia, it should be coordinated with other needed procedure such as central venous line placement, lumbar puncture, bone marrow biopsy, or imaging investigations requiring anesthesia.

It has to be mentioned that alternatives to ovarian tissue cryopreservation and autotransplantation exist but have currently some limitations. Among alternative option there is ovarian transposition that can be used in case of pelvic radiotherapy. It consists of moving the ovaries as far as possible from the site to be irradiated. Another option is in vitro maturation. This option requires collection of the native ovarian tissue but aims at maturation of immature follicle to avoid autotransplantation with the connected risk of reintroduction of malignancy. Unfortunately this technique is still not well established and has led to live birth only in animal models [5].

In conclusion, the efforts to restore fertility potential in pediatric oncologic girls are mandatory. Currently, ovarian tissue cryopreservation, even if experimental, is the only option applicable to prepubertal patients that has led to pregnancies and live births. Nevertheless several concerns have to be discussed.

References

1. Jensen AK, Rechnitzer C, Macklon KT, Ifversen MR, Birkebæk N, Clausen N, Sørensen K, Fedder J, Ernst E, Andersen CY. Cryopreservation of ovarian tissue for fertility preservation in a large cohort of young girls: focus on pubertal development. Hum Reprod. 2017;32(1):154–64.
2. Wallace WH, Kelsey TW, Anderson RA. Fertility preservation in pre-pubertal girls with cancer: the role of ovarian tissue cryopreservation. Fertil Steril. 2016;105(1):6–12. https://doi.org/10.1016/j.fertnstert.2015.11.041.
3. Hovatta O, Silye R, Krausz T, Abir R, Margara R, Trew G, Lass A, Winston RM. Cryopreservation of human ovarian tissue using dimethylsulphoxide and propanediol-sucrose as cryoprotectants. Hum Reprod. 1996;11(6):1268–72.
4. Corkum KS, Laronda MM, Rowell EE. A review of reported surgical techniques in fertility preservation for prepubertal and adolescent females facing a fertility threatening diagnosis or treatment. Am J Surg. 2017;214(4):695–700. https://doi.org/10.1016/j.amjsurg.2017.06.013.
5. Practice Committee of American Society for Reproductive Medicine. Ovarian tissue cryopreservation: a committee opinion. Fertil Steril. 2014;101(5):1237–43. https://doi.org/10.1016/j.fertnstert.2014.02.052.
6. Lima M, Gargano T, Fabbri R, Maffi M, Destro F. Ovarian tissue collection for cryopreservation in pediatric age: laparoscopic technical tips. J Pediatr Adolesc Gynecol. 2014;27(2):95–7. https://doi.org/10.1016/j.jpag.2013.11.002.
7. Fabbri R, Vicenti R, Macciocca M, Pasquinelli G, Lima M, Parazza I, Magnani V, Venturoli S. Cryopreservation of ovarian tissue in pediatric patients. Obstet Gynecol Int. 2012;2012:910698. https://doi.org/10.1155/2012/910698.
8. El Issaoui M, Giorgione V, Mamsen LS, Rechnitzer C, Birkebæk N, Clausen N, Kelsey TW, Andersen CY. Effect of first line cancer treatment on the ovarian reserve and follicular density in girls under the age of 18 years. Fertil Steril. 2016;106(7):1757–1762.e1. https://doi.org/10.1016/j.fertnstert.2016.09.001.
9. Salama M, Isachenko V, Isachenko E, Rahimi G, Mallmann P. Updates in preserving reproductive potential of prepubertal girls with cancer: systematic review. Crit Rev Oncol Hematol. 2016;103:10–21. https://doi.org/10.1016/j.critrevonc.2016.04.002.
10. Jensen AK, Macklon KT, Fedder J, Ernst E, Humaidan P, Andersen CY. 86 successful births and 9 ongoing pregnancies worldwide in women transplanted with frozen-thawed ovarian tissue: focus on birth and perinatal outcome in 40 of these children. J Assist Reprod Genet. 2017;34(3):325–36. https://doi.org/10.1007/s10815-016-0843-9.
11. Van der Ven H, Liebenthron J, Beckmann M, Toth B, Korell M, Krüssel J, Frambach T, Kupka M, Hohl MK, Winkler-Crepaz K, Seitz S, Dogan A, Griesinger G, Häberlin F, Henes M, Schwab R, Sütterlin M, von Wolff M, Dittrich R, FertiPROTEKT Network. Ninety-five orthotopic transplantations in 74 women of ovarian tissue after cytotoxic treatment in a fertility preservation network: tissue activity, pregnancy and delivery rates. Hum Reprod. 2016;31(9):2031–41. https://doi.org/10.1093/humrep/dew165.
12. Jensen AK, Kristensen SG, Macklon KT, Jeppesen JV, Fedder J, Ernst E, Andersen CY. Outcomes of transplantations of cryopreserved ovarian tissue to 41 women in Denmark. Hum Reprod. 2015;30(12):2838–45. https://doi.org/10.1093/humrep/dev230.
13. Demeestere I, Simon P, Dedeken L, Moffa F, Tsépélidis S, Brachet C, Delbaere A, Devreker F, Ferster A. Live birth after autograft of ovarian tissue cryopreserved during childhood. Hum Reprod. 2015;30(9):2107–9. https://doi.org/10.1093/humrep/dev128.
14. Soares M, Saussoy P, Maskens M, Reul H, Amorim CA, Donnez J, Dolmans MM. Eliminating malignant cells from cryopreserved ovarian tissue is possible in leukaemia patients. Br J Haematol. 2017;178(2):231–9. https://doi.org/10.1111/bjh.14657.
15. Grèze V, Brugnon F, Chambon F, Halle P, Canis M, Amiot C, Grémeau AS, Pereira B, Yáñez Peralta Y, Tchirkov A, Kanold J. Highly sensitive assessment of neuroblastoma minimal residual disease in ovarian tissue using RT-qPCR-A strategy for improving the safety of fertility restoration. Pediatr Blood Cancer. 2017;64(5). https://doi.org/10.1002/pbc.26287.

Part VI

Miscellanea

71 Laparoscopic Inguinal Hernia Repair

Ciro Esposito, Maria Escolino, Alessandra Farina, Marta Iannazzone, Giuseppe Cortese, Fulvia Del Conte, Mario Mendoza-Sagaon, and Philippe Montupet

71.1 Introduction

A surgical intervention for inguinal hernia (IH) is one of the most common types of surgery performed in children. The advent of minimal access techniques has changed completely conventional management for the treatment of inguinal hernia [1].

The proposed advantages of the laparoscopic technique are visualization of contralateral defects, diminished postoperative pain, improved cosmetic results, and more rapid return to normal function [2, 3]. Regarding the technical point of view, there are many techniques now described for laparoscopic hernia (LH) repair [4, 5]. The different repair options can be categorized as either intracorporeal or extracorporeal/percutaneous [6–9]. In regard to intracorporeal repairs, it consists in a purse-string suture performed on the periorificial peritoneum at the level of the internal ring [2, 9, 10]. In 1998, Schier introduced his technique, consisting in an "N"-shaped suture on the periorificial peritoneum [8, 9]. The extracorporeal techniques all involve the placement of a suture circumferentially around the internal ring and tying the knot using percutaneous techniques [7, 10, 11]. Loads of variations of this approach have been described. The laparoscopic approach can be performed either transperitoneally or through a preperitoneal approach (using special needles) with transperitoneal visualization [8, 9, 11, 12].

The laparoscopic classic approach is the transperitoneal approach using three ports.

In this chapter we describe mainly the classic laparoscopic three-port approach.

71.2 Preoperative Preparation

All patients and their parents have to sign a specifically formulated informed consent before the procedure. No specific preparation is needed in patient older than 1 year of age. In neonates and in infants, we perform an intestinal preparation using simethicone a couple of days before surgery to reduce the intestinal loop distension diminishing the gas into the intestinal loops with the aim to have a larger operative chamber.

C. Esposito (✉) · M. Escolino · A. Farina
M. Iannazzone · G. Cortese · F. Del Conte
Pediatric Surgery Unit, Department of Translational Medical Sciences (DISMET), University of Naples "Federico II", Naples, Italy
e-mail: ciroespo@unina.it

M. Mendoza-Sagaon
Pediatric Surgery Unit, Bellinzona Children Hospital, Bellinzona, Switzerland

P. Montupet
Pediatric Surgery Unit, CHU Bicetre, Paris, France

C. Esposito et al. (eds.), *ESPES Manual of Pediatric Minimally Invasive Surgery*,
https://doi.org/10.1007/978-3-030-00964-9_71

Before surgery the bladder is emptied with a Nelaton catheter; in this way we have a clear view of the pelvic area to identify rare hernias as femoral or crural hernias.

71.2.1 Positioning

As for the patient's position on the operative table, in case of laparoscopic hernia repair, the patient is positioned always in supine position with a 15–20° Trendelenburg position to keep low the intra-abdominal pressure (IAP). The video column is positioned at the feet of the patient, the surgeon positioned at the head of the patient, and the cameraman contralateral to the pathology to treat.

71.2.2 Instrumentation

A 0° telescope of 5–10 mm through an umbilical port is used, allowing direct visualization of the deep inguinal rings, followed by the use of two 3-mm trocars in triangulation to keep a good ergonomics (Fig. 71.1). As for the optic, the use of a 5- or 10-mm optic gives the same invisible scar in the navel; for this reason the use of a 5- or 10-mm optic depends on the instruments available. As for the operative 3-mm trocars, the majority of authors prefer to adopt screw trocars. The advantage of using screw trocars is fundamental above all in infants under 10 kg; in fact in these categories of patients, the tissues and the skin are very thin, and the smooth trocars exit all the time creating a subcutaneous emphysema. Screw trocars are more stable, and in addition you can change instruments rapidly, without dislodgement of the trocars and without gas leaks. In case you have only smooth trocars, you can put a piece of Nelaton catheter around the cannula and then fix the piece of Nelaton catheter to the skin to stabilize the trocar (Fig. 71.2a, b). Some surgeons prefer to use instruments without the assistance of trocars (stub incision) also if

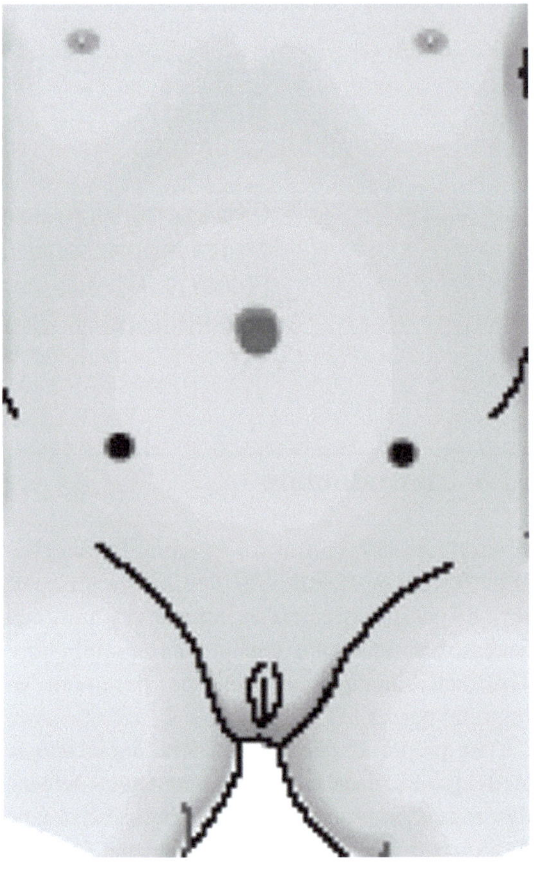

Fig. 71.1 Trocar's position

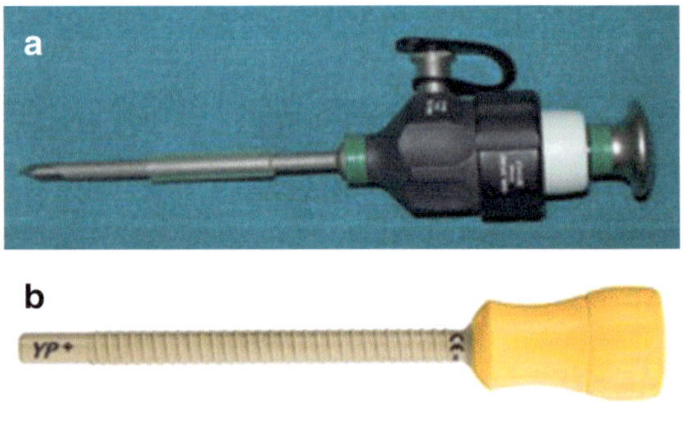

Fig. 71.2 We use two 3-mm working ports. If you use trocars with smooth cannulas (**a**), you have to position a peace of Nelaton catheter around the cannula to fix the trocar to the skin with a stitch. In our experience we prefer to use screw trocars (**b**) that are more stable on the skin

using this technique can be difficult to change instruments. As for the instruments, all of 3 mm, we need a needle holder, a contralateral grasping forceps, and scissors.

71.2.3 Technique

As for the technical point of view, the needle has to be introduced in the abdominal cavity transparietally and then removed transparietally or preferably transumbilically (Fig. 71.3). The preferred needle to use is 3/8 of circle with a 20–22-mm needle. To perform a unilateral closure, the length of suture has to be 13–15 cm; for a bilateral repair, it has to be 15–20 cm, according to the surgeon's preference. The laparoscopic technique affords confirmation of the diagnosis, as well as inspection of the contralateral side for the presence of a hernia or a contralateral patent processus vaginalis (CPPV) (Fig. 71.4). The deep ring is then closed, after sectioning the periorificial peritoneum (Fig. 71.5), with a non-resorbable suture either as purse-string suture as described by Montupet or similar type an N suture as described by Schier (Figs. 71.6 and 71.7). Analyzing the literature, these two techniques seem to give similar results with a long-term outcome. In the preperitoneal approach (needlescopic approach), a small hook, loaded with a suture, is passed around the deep ring after mak-

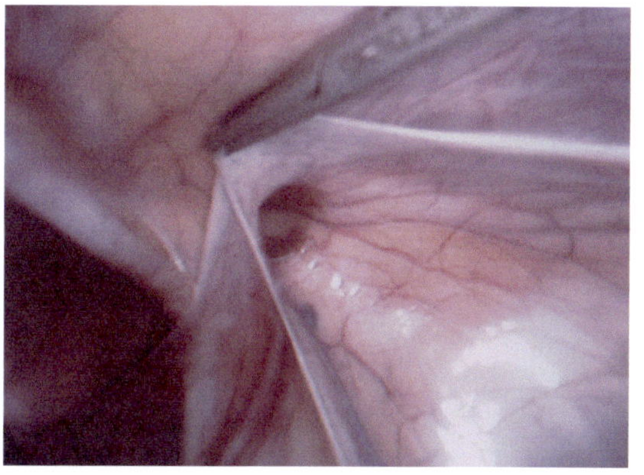

Fig. 71.4 It is extremely easy to identify the patency of peritoneo-vaginal duct responsible of the inguinal hernia

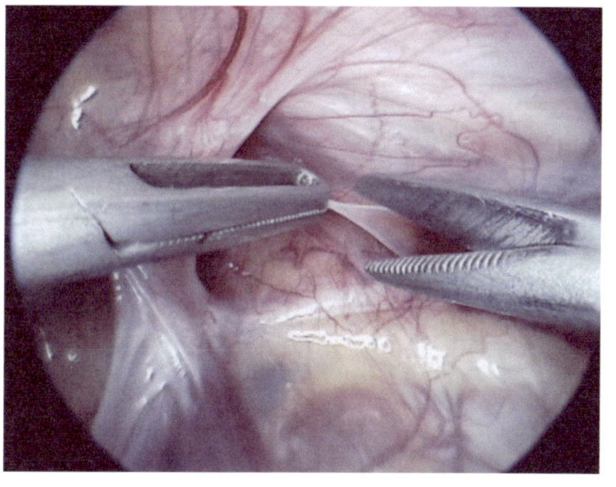

Fig. 71.5 The first step of the procedure is to section the periorificial peritoneum circumferentially to permit the distal part of the hernia sac to collapse

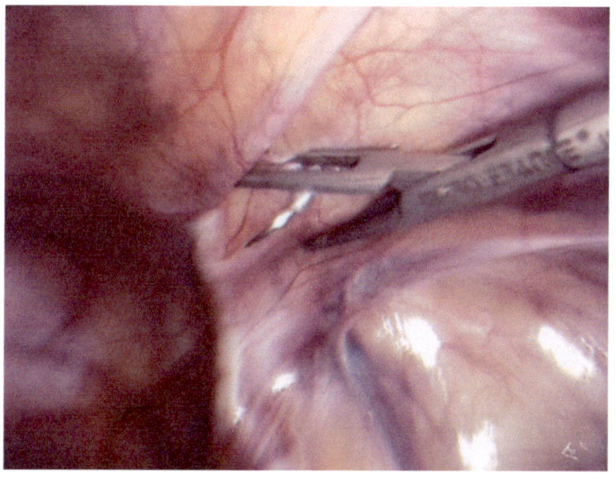

Fig. 71.3 Considering that we use 3-mm trocars, the needle has to be introduced into the abdominal cavity transparietally

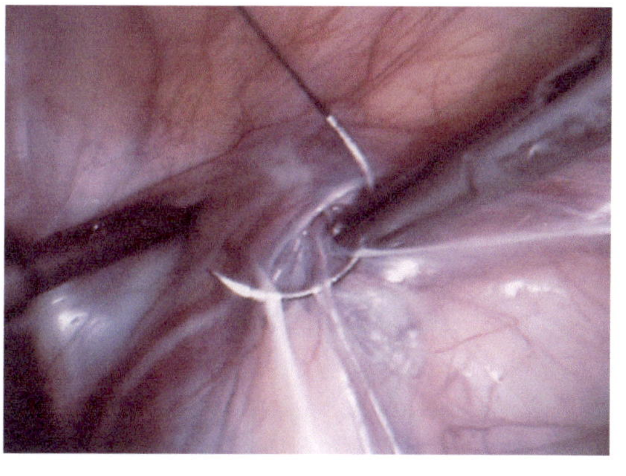

Fig. 71.6 To perform the hernia repair, we prefer to perform a purse-string suture around the periorificial peritoneum

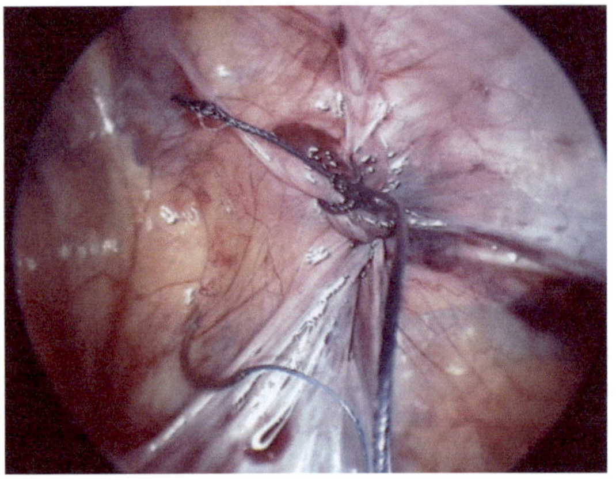

Fig. 71.7 The final aspect of the procedure

ing a small inguinal skin incision. The passage of the suture is observed via an endoscope at the umbilicus. The ligature is then brought extracorporeally and tied, thus closing the hernial orifice. In case of direct hernia, a key point of the technique is to remove the lipoma always present in this pathology and to close the defect using a purse-string suture or separated stitches. In case of huge hole, to reinforce the closure, a lateral bladder ligament can be adopted.

71.3 Postoperative Care

No particular postoperative care is necessary. Patients start feeding 2–3 h after surgery, and they are discharged from the hospital the same day or the day after surgery.

As for postoperative pain, no treatment is needed except paracetamol treatment only once in the evening. The timing of postoperative control is only two clinical controls a POD 7 and POD 31.

71.4 Results

The average operative time for the repair of unilateral inguinal hernia was about 30 min via the open approach (OH) and about 23 min via laparoscopy (LH), with no significant difference between the two techniques. For the repair of bilateral disease, it was significantly longer for the open inguinal hernia repair (46 min) compared to laparoscopy (30 min).

A conversion rate was reported in 10 studies and ranged between 0 and 1.7%, but in the majority of these studies, there was a 0% conversion rate.

Recurrence rate after LH repair is less than 1%.

As for other complications, such as wound infection, hydrocele, iatrogenic cryptorchidism, and testicular atrophy, the rate of these complications was significantly higher for OH (2.7%) compared to LH (0.9%) ($P = 0.001$).

As for the incidence of rare hernias, all of them are identified in the LH studies, with an incidence ranging from 0.3 to 7.2%. Several studies reported the coexistence of a unilateral inguinal hernia with a contralateral patent processus vaginalis (CPPV), for an incidence of contralateral patency between 19.9 and 66%.

71.5 Tips and Tricks

The key points of the success of LH repair are the standardization of the technique.

Here are reported some tips and tricks to remember to have a successful procedure. First of all is the simethicone preparation in infants to enlarge working chamber and to reduce IAP. It's preferable to use screw trocars or to fix the trocars to the skin. A 3-mm set instrumentation is essential to perform the procedure. The needle is introduced transparietally. In order to obtain a low to zero recurrence rate, you have to use non-resorbable suture to close the inguinal orifice, and always you have to cut the periorificial peritoneum before closing the ring to reduce the tension on the closure. In case of direct hernia, it's important to cut and to remove the lipoma before closing the defect. At the end of the procedure, it's easier to remove the needle through the umbilical orifice.

71.6 Discussion

Laparoscopic inguinal hernia repair in children was firstly described 25 years ago by Montupet in 1993 [2, 10, 11].

Since then, several retrospective studies but few prospective studies, meta-analysis, or systematic reviews have been published on the subject, and there is ongoing discussion about the best management of an inguinal hernia in children [12].

An interesting finding, analyzing the international literature on inguinal hernia in children, is that the majority of the studies published in the last 20 years are focused on the laparoscopic approach [7, 13].

On the other hand, literature focused on open inguinal hernia repair is scanty, and we think that the real incidence of complications of inguinal hernia repair is probably underestimated.

Analyzing the international literature, it seems that LH repair is easier, in particular in infants, and with fewer complications compared to inguinal hernia repair [5, 8, 13]. In two studies, similar time to full feeds and length of hospital stay were reported in the LH and OH groups [4, 7, 14].

From a technical point of view, the laparoscopic approach is easier but technically more demanding for the surgeon because he or she has to be able to suture intracorporeally and to work in a very small space above all in infants [2, 15].

We analyzed the international literature, searching articles comparing OH and LH, to give to the readers of this chapter a general idea on the results of both techniques.

Our review examined different aspects of both procedures. The results of this review of more than 50 studies with regard to operative time suggested that there was no significant difference between the two approaches for unilateral inguinal hernia repair [8, 9, 14]. On the contrary, in the patient with bilateral disease, there was a significant reduction in the operative time for LH compared to OH [9]. However, the operative time showed wide variations depending on the technique and experience of the surgical team [7, 9].

As for recurrence rate, no significant difference was observed between the two techniques, while the rate of other complications such as wound infections, hydrocele, iatrogenic cryptorchidism, and testicular atrophy was significantly higher for OH compared to LH [2, 5, 9]. In addition, it seems that recurrence rate and wound infections in infants were always higher after OH than after LH. However, the length of follow-up in reviewed series was less for the laparoscopic approach compared to the open operation [9, 14, 15].

In our opinion, the higher wound infection rate following OH may be due to the fact that the laparoscopic scars are located higher on the abdominal wall compared to inguinal scars that are inside the diaper area; for this reason they are subject to urine or fecal contamination which may lead to a higher infection rate [6, 8]. In fact, LH reported fewer wound infections compared to the infants of similar age operated through the inguinal approach [3, 9].

As for other complications, complications after OH (vas deferens injuries, iatrogenic cryptorchidism, testicular atrophy) have been rarely reported in the last 15–20 years. For this reason, we have had to analyze older published series to gain adequate data for comparison purposes.

We found five studies that reported an incidence of postoperative cryptorchidism and testicular atrophy that was higher after OH compared to LH [2, 5, 9]. Accurate comparisons between the two approaches for these other complications suffer from the use of historical controls. Also, there was a shorter follow-up in the LH series compared to the OH ones.

The advantages of LH are believed to include better visualization of vital cord structures, which makes dissection of these structures safer [3, 9]. The dissection field of LH is limited to the peritoneal layer, with the vas deferens and cord left untouched. Therefore, injury to the vas is not thought to occur very often.

This review also reinforces the usefulness of the laparoscopic approach for the diagnosis of contralateral patency, which may avoid the need for a second surgery and anesthesia in patients with a metachronous contralateral hernia. It is our feeling that repair of a CPPV should be offered to all families as most desire to have the CPPV repaired at the same operative setting.

In conclusion in case of inguinal hernia in children, laparoscopy seems to be a very good alternative to open surgery.

It is mandatory to remember that to have a successful laparoscopic hernia repair in children, you have to follow the details of technique that was described 25 years ago and nowadays is well standardized as we reported in the technical part of this chapter. Analyzing the international literature, in summary, LH appears faster for bilateral hernia repair when compared to the inguinal crease approach. Recurrence rates appear similar, but the follow-up is less in the LH studies. Wound infection appears more likely after OH, but the incidence is low. Time to resume normal activity is similar with both approaches.

However there is no evidence in the literature about which technique (laparoscopy or inguinal approach) is preferable to repair an inguinal hernia. Probably a surgeon has to offer to the patient both techniques, and above all, considering the importance of the parental role in the decision-making process, the parents have to know that, to repair an inguinal hernia, two different approaches exist and the advantages and disadvantages of both procedures.

References

1. Esposito C, Escolino M, Cerulo M, et al. Two decade of history of laparoscopic pediatric inguinal hernia repair. J Laparoendosc Adv Surg Tech A. 2014;24(9):669–70.
2. Gorsler CM, Schier F. Laparoscopic herniorrhaphy in children. Surg Endosc. 2003;17:571–3.
3. Miltenburg DM, Nuchtern JG, Jaksic T, et al. Laparoscopic evaluation of the pediatric inguinal hernia: a meta-analysis. J Pediatr Surg. 1998;33(6):874–9.
4. Parelkar SV, Oak S, Gupta R, et al. Laparoscopic inguinal hernia repair in the pediatric age group—experience with 437 children. J Pediatr Surg. 2010;45:789–92.
5. Holcomb GW 3rd, Brock JW 3rd, Morgan WM 3rd. Laparoscopic evaluation for a contralateral patent processus vaginalis. J Pediatr Surg. 1994;29(8):970–3; discussion 974.
6. Esposito C, Montinaro L, Alicchio F, et al. Technical standardization of laparoscopic herniorrhaphy in pediatric patients. World J Surg. 2009;33:1846–50.
7. Schier F. Laparoscopic inguinal hernia repair: a prospective personal series of 542 children. J Pediatr Surg. 2006;41(6):1081–4.
8. Schier F. Laparoscopic herniorrhaphy in girls. J Pediatr Surg. 1998;33:1495–7.
9. Esposito C, St Peter SD, Escolino M, et al. Laparoscopic versus open inguinal hernia repair in pediatric patients: a systematic review. J Laparoendosc Adv Surg Tech A. 2014;24(11):811–8.
10. Ostlie DJ, Ponsky TA. Technical options of the laparoscopic pediatric inguinal hernia repair. J Laparoendosc Adv Surg Tech A. 2014;24:194–8.
11. Montupet M, Esposito C. Laparoscopic treatment of congenital inguinal hernia in children. J Pediatr Surg. 1999;34:420–3.
12. Esposito C, Escolino M, Settimi A. Laparoscopic pediatric inguinal hernia repair using purse-string suture: technical recommendations after 20 years experience. J Laparoendosc Adv Surg Tech A. 2016;26(9):748–9.
13. Esposito C, Turial S, Escolino M, et al. Laparoscopic inguinal hernia repair in premature babies weighing 3 kg or less. Pediatr Surg Int. 2012;28:989–92.
14. Esposito C, Montinaro L, Alicchio F, et al. Laparoscopic treatment of inguinal hernia in the first year of life. J Laparoendosc Adv Surg Tech A. 2010;20(5):473–6.
15. Schier F, Montupet P, Esposito C. Laparoscopic inguinal herniorrhaphy in children: a three center experience with 933 repairs. J Pediatr Surg. 2002;37:395–7.

Laparoscopic Management of Pediatric Varicocele

72

Mario Mendoza-Sagaon, Philippe Montupet, and Ciro Esposito

72.1 Introduction

Varicocele is defined as the abnormal dilatation or enlargement of the veins of the pampiniform plexus. Mostly affects the left side but can also compromise the right side or be bilateral. The pediatric population has an incidence of 15% [1]. It is associated with the risk of harming the testicular development and the risk of infertility [2, 3]. Many controversies still exist regarding the etiology and the physiopathology of this entity mostly related to anatomical aspects, the increase in the testicular blood flow, the increase in testicular temperature, the roll of reflux of renal and adrenal metabolites into the dilated spermatic veins, the low oxygen concentration into the dilated veins with consequent local tissue hypoxia and the paracrine imbalances [4]. The diagnosis is based on the clinical exam and the degree of severity according to the classification of Dubin and Amelar [5].

M. Mendoza-Sagaon (✉)
Department of Pediatric Surgery, Regional Hospital of Bellinzona–EOC, Bellinzona, Switzerland
e-mail: mario.mendozasagaon@eoc.ch

P. Montupet
Department of Pediatric Surgery, University Hospital of Bicêtre, Paris, France

C. Esposito
Pediatric Surgery Unit, Department of Translational Medical Sciences (DISMET), University of Naples "Federico II", Naples, Italy

In the pediatric population, the decision regarding the best treatment is still challenging and controversial, first of all because the real benefits between the conservative non-surgical follow-up or the preventive surgical treatment are still not clear [6]. Secondarily, when the surgical treatment has been chosen, the next question is which could be the best technique and approach in order to avoid recurrences and decrease the risk of complications.

The main indications for surgical treatment in the pediatric population are: (1) testicular asymmetry (involved testicle with a lower volume difference of more than 20% in comparison with the contralateral testicle), (2) grade III according to Dubin and Amelar classification, (3) bilateral varicocele in end-stage testicular development, (4) psychological or physical discomfort, and (5) pain [7].

Several surgical techniques have been described for the varicocelectomy and the surgical approach [8], but this chapter is intended to focus only on the laparoscopic approach for the treatment of varicocele in children and adolescents.

Regarding the laparoscopic approach, we can divide them into two main groups: (1) Multi-trocar conventional laparoscopic approach and (2) Laparoendoscopic single-site (LESS) approach. Another mini-invasive approach that could also be considered is the retroperitoneoscopic approach [9].

C. Esposito et al. (eds.), *ESPES Manual of Pediatric Minimally Invasive Surgery*, https://doi.org/10.1007/978-3-030-00964-9_72

72.2 Preoperative Setup

The parents or the parental authority of the patients must sign the surgical/anesthesia consensus information form and a pre-assessment visit with the anesthesiologist is performed previous to any surgical procedure.

Generally, no particular medical therapy or special preparation is required.

72.3 Patient Positioning and Trocar Placement

Under general anesthesia, for a *transperitoneal laparoscopic approach* the patient is positioned in a supine position. The anesthesia team is positioned at the head of the patient. In case of a left varicocelectomy, the surgeon and the assistant are placed at the right side of the patient. The laparoscopic tower is at the lower left side of the patient. In case of a right varicocele, the positions are inverted. For a transperitoneal laparoscopic multi-trocar approach, a 5 or 10 mm trocar is placed at the umbilicus according to the Hasson's technique for the telescope and two other trocars of 3 or 5 mm for instrumentation are placed, one in the left flank and the second in the hypogastrium (Fig. 72.1).

For a transperitoneal LESS approach, a transumbilical incision is created. The length of the incision will depend on the device that will be used. Two 5 mm trocars (one for a 5 mm 30° telescope and the other for 5 mm bending special instruments) and one 3 mm trocar for instrumentation are generally required (Figs. 72.2 and 72.3).

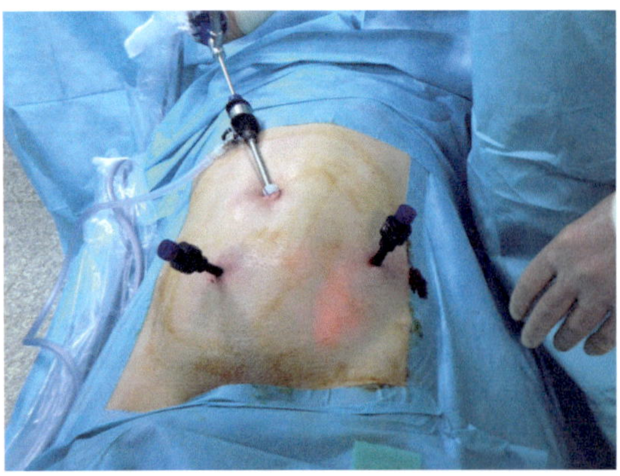

Fig. 72.1 Transperitoneal multi-trocar position

Once the trocars are placed, the table is positioned in slightly Trendelenburg and lateralized to the right in order to expose the retroperitoneal spermatic vessels and decrease the blood flow in the pampiniform plexus.

In case of a *retroperitoneoscopic approach* for a left varicocelectomy, the patient is positioned in right lateral decubitus or supine position with moderate lateralization to the right side. The table is slightly bending at the lumbar level. The surgeon and the assistant are placed at the back of the patient and the laparoscopic tower in the front side of the patient. The first trocar is positioned at the middle of the distance between the tip of the 12th rib and the iliac crest. A muscular splitting dissection is performed in order to create the retroperitoneal space for working and then introduce two other 5 or 3 mm trocars for instrumentation.

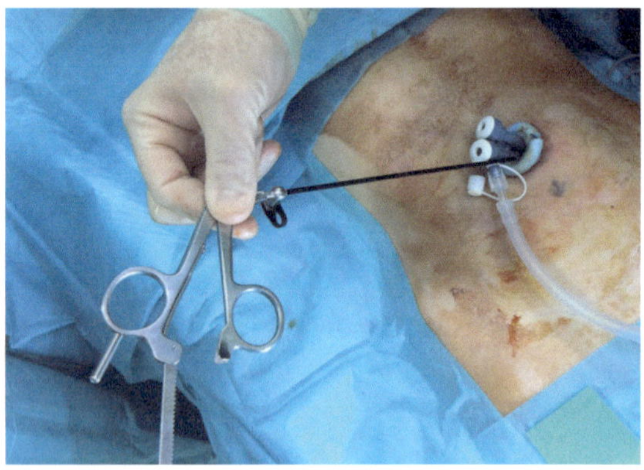

Fig. 72.2 LESS approach

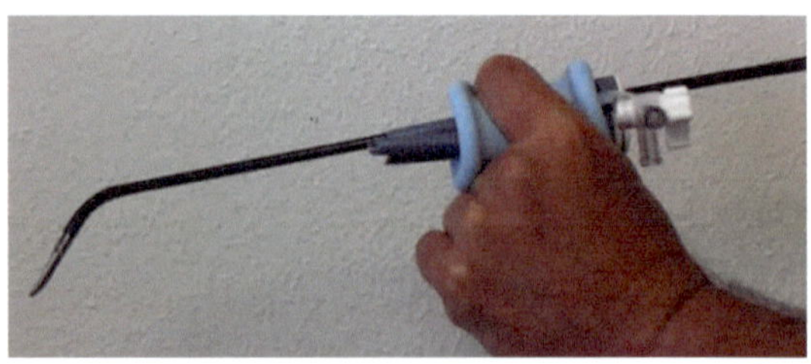

Fig. 72.3 LESS 5-mm bending instruments

72.4 Surgical Technique

For most transperitoneal and retroperitoneal procedures, the CO_2 pneumoperitoneum is established around 10–12 mmHg. The retroperitoneal spermatic vessels and the internal inguinal ring are identified (Fig. 72.4). Using monopolar/laparoscopic scissors and atraumatic graspers, the retroperitoneum is open and the spermatic vessels are dissected as high as possible, with a minimum distance distally of 2 cm above the internal inguinal ring (Fig. 72.5). A ligature or a silicon band could be used to retract the vessels in order to simplify their proximal and distal dissection (Fig. 72.6).

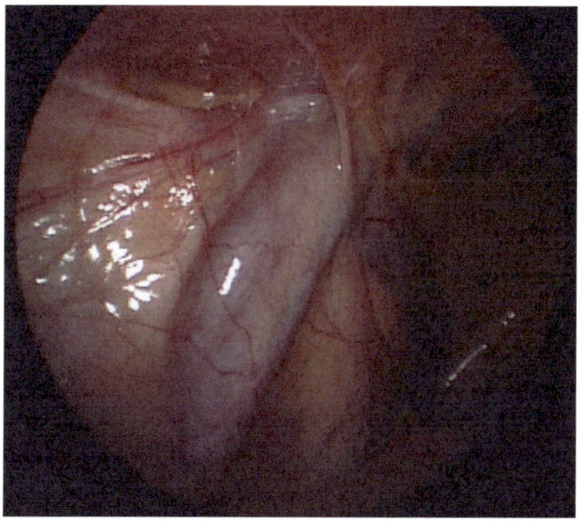

Fig. 72.4 Identification of the internal inguinal ring and the spermatic vessels

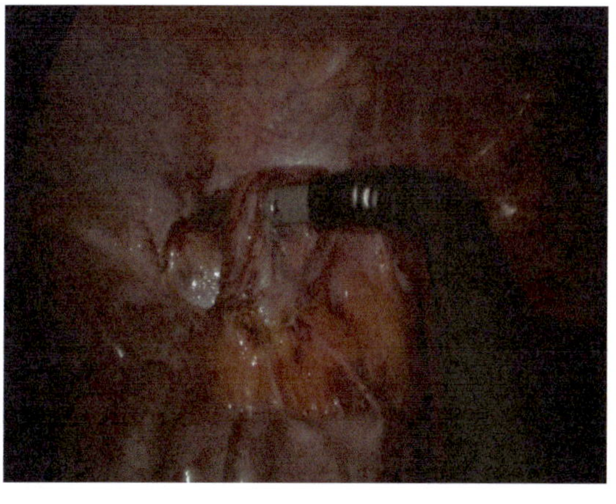

Fig. 72.5 Dissection of the spermatic vessels

The two main techniques performed are:

1. Palomo's technique which includes dissection and section of the spermatic artery and the spermatic veins.
2. Modify Palomo's technique which includes only dissection and section of the spermatic veins with sparing of the spermatic artery.

The occlusion of the spermatic vessels could be performed with absorbable, non-absorbable ligatures or clips (Figs. 72.6 and 72.7).

In recent years, the lymphatic sparing technique is gaining popularity. This technique consists in the intra-dartos or intratesticular injection of blue dyes such as Isosulfan blue few minutes before surgery in order to evidence the lymphatic spermatic vessels avoiding their dissection thus

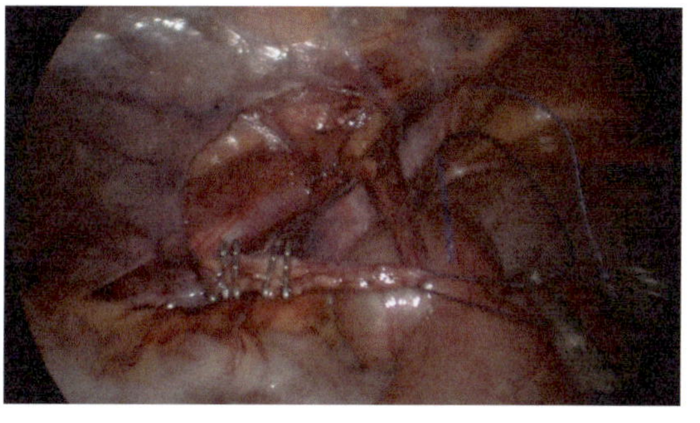

Fig. 72.6 Palomo's technique using clips

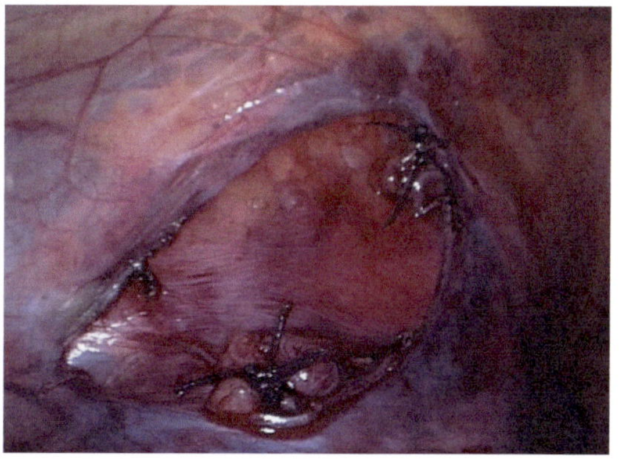

Fig. 72.7 Palomo's technique using ligatures

decreasing the risk of postoperative hydrocele [10, 11].

In the transperitoneal approach, at the end of the procedure, it is not necessary to close the retroperitoneum. The trocars are removed and the abdominal wall orifices are closed with absorbable sutures.

These patients could be treated in the majority of the cases in an ambulatory (day hospital) setting.

72.5 Postoperative Care

Besides 10 days of no sportive activity, no other particular postoperative therapy is necessary. Long-term follow-up to control testicular development and complications such as hydrocele, recurrence, and testicular atrophy (rare) is advocated. When possible, follow-up to adulthood could be useful to assess fertility and paternity.

72.6 Results and Complications

Laparoscopic varicocelectomy offers good results. Besides the less operative pain, better cosmesis and faster return to normal life, one of the main advantages of the minimally invasive approach is the possibility to perform a high dissection and ligation of the spermatic veins near their drainage. This decreases the necessity to dissect less tributary spermatic veins and harm collateral vessels and to identify collateral spermatic veins, lowering the risk of recurrence and bleeding. Moreover, at this level the spermatic artery is sometimes easier to identify and this is particularly helpful when performing a modified Palomo's technique. Operative time varies from 20 to 60 min depending of the surgeon's experience, skills, and technique [12].

The general overall rate of complications is around 8–12%, and these include bleeding, subcutaneous emphysema, genitofemoral nerve injury, hydrocele, recurrence, testicular atrophy, and intestinal injury [10, 13, 14]. Hydrocele is secondary to accidental ligation of the lymphatic vessels and is the most common postoperative complication encountered with a rate of 7–15% [13, 15]. Recent reports advocate the use of the lymphatic sparing technique with blue dyes that allows to distinguish and preserve the lymphatic vessels decreasing the rate of postoperative hydrocele to 0–3% [11, 16]. Recurrence is reported in 6–15% and has been correlated to the presence of collateral/aberrant spermatic veins, incomplete ligation of the spermatic veins while performing the sparing of the spermatic artery in the modified Palomo's technique and dilatation of other preexisting collateral gonadal veins [17]. Testicular atrophy following laparoscopic varicocelectomy, even with the Palomo's technique, is very rare and is reported in 0–2%. This complication is mainly correlated with the open inguinal or sub-inguinal approach [17, 18].

72.7 Discussion

Varicocele is present in 15% of the pediatric population. Prevalence begins predominantly in children over 12 years old and increases during testicular development in adolescence. The main challenges in pediatric varicocele are: (1) to establish the degree of severity and the potential risks for the testicular development and fertility and (2) to establish when and which could be the best treatment to perform. Establishing the degree of severity and the potential risks is not easy because until now the general classification used to evaluate severity is merely clinical based on the testicular volume and the Dubin and Amelar classification [5]. These data do not consider the size of the varicocele independently of the Amelar classification as well as the intensity and consequences of the venous blood flow reflux into the testicular parenchyma. Iosa and Lazzarini proposed a new classification based on a scrotal Doppler sonography that evaluates the type and degree of venous reflux, offering a better assessment of the severity and the hemodynamic repercussion of the venous reflux [19]. To elucidate if this new hemodynamic classification, associated to the clinical evaluation, could offer a better estimation of the degree of severity of the varicocele and its risk for the testicular development and the fertility in the pediatric population, more studies are necessary.

Regarding the second challenge, choosing when and which therapy should be performed in the pediatric population is still controversial. The main indications for varicocelectomy in children and adolescents are: (1) testicular asymmetry (involved testicle with a lower volume difference of more than 20% in comparison with the contralateral testicle), (2) grade III according to Dubin and Amelar classification, (3) bilateral varicocele in end-stage testicular development, (4) psychological or physical discomfort, and (5) pain [7]. However, these indications are still controversial because in children and adolescents varicocelectomy seems to be mainly prophylactic than therapeutic especially because the real impact of the varicocele itself or a varicocelectomy during the adolescence in the adulthood fertility and paternity is not clear [2, 6]. The parameter of testicular catch-up growth after varicocelectomy in children is controversial due to the influence of the testicular development and the normal asymmetric speed of growing [6]. Moreover, the recommendations for varicocelectomy in adults published in the latest European Guidelines for male infertility are: (1) Varicocele treatment is recommended for adolescents with progressive failure of testicular development documented by serial clinical examination. (2) No evidence indicates benefit from varicocele treatment in infertile men who have normal semen analysis or in men with subclinical varicocele. In this situation, varicocele treatment cannot be recommended. (3) Varicocele repair should be considered in case of a clinical varicocele associated to oligospermia, infertility duration of $\geq$2 years, and otherwise unexplained infertility in the couple [20]. In contrast, in adults with varicocele that have fulfilled the indications for varicocelectomy, an improvement in semen quality and reverse of the DNA fragmentation after surgery have been reported [21].

Laparoscopic varicocelectomy has been reported to be safe, feasible, and an excellent indication to treat varicocele in the pediatric population. When compared to the open approach, laparoscopy showed no statistical differences regarding rate of success and complications but superiority in better cosmesis, faster return to normal activities, less postoperative pain, treating bilateral cases, and allowing to perform concomitantly procedures through the same laparoscopic approach such as inguinal hernia repair, orchidopexy, appendectomy, and removal of peritoneal adhesions [17]. The disadvantages of the procedure include the high cost (depending on the technique and instrumentation), the necessity of general anesthesia, and in some cases hospital stay over 1 day.

The two main techniques performed are: (1) Palomo's technique which includes dissection and section of the spermatic artery and the spermatic veins and (2) modification of Palomo's technique which includes only dissection and section of the spermatic veins with sparing of the spermatic artery. When comparing these two techniques, Palomo's technique seems to offer better results such as less intraoperative time, less intraoperative bleeding, lower risk for recurrence, the same very low risk of testicular atrophy (0–2%) but a slightly higher risk of hydrocele [10, 15]. Moreover, the risk of hydrocele could be decreased from 15% to 0–3% when performing a lymphatic sparing technique with blue dyes [11, 16].

In conclusion, varicocele in the pediatric population represents a challenge to establish the degree of severity and the consequent risk of impairing the testicular development and function and to establish the best timing for surgical therapy. The real impact in future adulthood fertility and paternity in pediatric patients with varicocele or in those operated of varicocelectomy is not clear and more studies are necessary to elucidate this concern. When a surgical treatment is indicated, the laparoscopic varicocelectomy in children offers excellent results with a low risk of complications. Moreover, the association of a lymphatic sparing technique reduces significantly the risk of postoperative hydrocele.

References

1. Locke JA, Noparast M, Afshar K. Treatment of varicocele in children and adolescents: a systematic review and meta-analysis of randomized controlled trials. J Pediatr Urol. 2017;13(5):437–45.
2. Jacobson DL, Johnson EK. Varicoceles in the pediatric and adolescent population: threat to future fertility? Fertil Steril. 2017;108(3):370–7.
3. Damsgaard J, Joensen UN, Carlsen E, Erenpreiss J, Blomberg Jensen M, Matulevicius V, Zilaitiene B, Olesen IA, Perheentupa A, Punab M, Salzbrunn A, Toppari J, Virtanen HE, Juul A, Skakkebæk NE, Jørgensen N. Varicocele is associated with impaired semen quality and reproductive hormone levels: a study of 7035 healthy young men from six European countries. Eur Urol. 2016;70(6):1019–29.
4. Eisenberg ML, Lipshultz L. Varicocele-induced infertility: newer insights into its pathophysiology. Indian J Urol. 2011;27(1):58–64.
5. Dubin L, Amelar RD. Varicecele size and results of varicocelectomy in selected subfertile men with varicocele. Fertil Steril. 1970;21:606–9.
6. Moursy EE, ElDahshoury MZ, Hussein MM, Mourad MZ, Badawy AA. Dilemma of adolescent varicocele: long-term outcome in patients managed surgically and in patients managed expectantly. J Pediatr Urol. 2013;9(6 Pt B):1018–22.
7. Zampieri N, Corroppolo M, Zuin V, Cervellione RM, Ottolenghi A, Camoglio FS. Longitudinal study of semen quality in adolescents with varicocele: to treat or not? Urology. 2007;70(5):989–93.
8. Chan P. Management options of varicoceles. Indian J Urol. 2011;27(1):65–73.
9. Mancini S, Bulotta AL, Molinaro F, Ferrara F, Tommasino G, Messina M. Surgical retroperitoneoscopic and transperitoneoscopic access in varicocelectomy: duplex scan results in pediatric population. J Pediatr Urol. 2014;10(6):1037–42.
10. Esposito C, Escolino M, Castagnetti M, Cerulo M, Settimi A, Cortese G, Turrà F, Iannazzone M, Izzo S, Servillo G. Two decades of experience with laparoscopic varicocele repair in children: standardizing the technique. J Pediatr Urol. 2018;14(1):10.e1–7. pii: S1477-5131(17)30287-5.
11. Esposito C, Iaquinto M, Escolino M, Cortese G, De Pascale T, Chiarenza F, Cerulo M, Settimi A. Technical standardization of laparoscopic lymphatic sparing varicocelectomy in children using isosulfan blue. J Pediatr Surg. 2014;49(4):660–3.
12. Li M, Wang Z, Li H. Laparoendoscopic single-site surgery varicocelectomy versus conventional laparoscopic varicocele ligation: a meta-analysis. J Int Med Res. 2016;44(5):985–93.
13. Esposito C, Monguzzi GL, Gonzalez-Sabin MA, Rubino R, Montinaro L, Papparella A, Amici G. Laparoscopic treatment of pediatric varicocele: a multicenter study of the italian society of video surgery in infancy. J Urol. 2000;163(6):1944–6.
14. Muensterer OJ. Genitofemoral nerve injury after laparoscopic varicocelectomy in adolescents. J Urol. 2008;180(5):2155–7.
15. Pini Prato A, MacKinlay GA. Is the laparoscopic Palomo procedure for pediatric varicocele safe and effective? Nine years of unicentric experience. Surg Endosc. 2006;20(4):660–4.
16. Parrilli A, Roberti A, Escolino M, Esposito C. Surgical approaches for varicocele in pediatric patient. Transl Pediatr. 2016;5(4):227–32.
17. Borruto FA, Impellizzeri P, Antonuccio P, Finocchiaro A, Scalfari G, Arena F, Esposito C, Romeo C. Laparoscopic vs open varicocelectomy in children and adolescents: review of the recent literature and meta-analysis. J Pediatr Surg. 2010;45(12):2464–9.
18. de Los Reyes T, Locke J, Afshar K Varicoceles in the pediatric population: diagnosis, treatment, and outcomes. Can Urol Assoc J. 2017;11(1–2 Suppl 1):S34–9.
19. Iosa G, Lazzarini D. Hemodynamic classification of varicoceles in men: our experience. J Ultrasound. 2013;16(2):57–63.
20. Jungwirth A, Diemer T, Dohle GR, Giwercman A, Kopa Z, Krausz C, et al. Guidelines on male infertility. European Association of Urology. March 2014. http://uroweb.org/wp-content/uploads/17-Male-Infertility_LR1.pdf. Accessed 1 Dec 2015.
21. Smit M, Romijn JC, Wildhagen MF, Veldhoven JL, Weber RF, Dohle GR. Decreased sperm DNA fragmentation after surgical varicocelectomy is associated with increased pregnancy rate. J Urol. 2013;189(1 Suppl):S146–50.

MIS Management of Pilonidal Sinus Disease

73

Ciro Esposito, Maria Escolino, Marco Severino, Fulvia Del Conte, Giuseppe Cortese, Marta Iannazzone, F. Turrà, and Giovanni Esposito

73.1 Introduction

Pilonidal sinus disease (PSD) is a chronic and inflammatory disease that often occurs at the sacrococcygeal region [1]. PSD affects an estimated 26 per 100,000 persons, occurring primarily in young adults with a 3:1 male predilection [2]. PSD is more common in men and in hirsute people.

It usually occurs after puberty. In addition, there is a high recurrence rate of PSD after a traditional surgical excision. Although many techniques for surgical treatment of pilonidal sinus have been described until now, there is no consensus about the gold standard treatment [3]. The traditional open excision is extremely invasive, with a long and painful postoperative course, and patients are generally doubted whether to submit themselves to this procedure [4].

We describe in this chapter the pediatric endoscopic pilonidal sinus treatment (PEPSiT), a mini-invasive approach to PSD that gives excellent results in our hands.

C. Esposito (✉) · M. Escolino · M. Severino
F. Del Conte · G. Cortese · M. Iannazzone
F. Turrà · G. Esposito
Pediatric Surgery Unit, Department of Translational Medical Sciences (DISMET), University of Naples "Federico II", Naples, Italy
e-mail: ciroespo@unina.it

73.2 Preoperative Preparation

All patients and their parents have to sign a specifically formulated informed consent before the procedure. Patients received a specific type of subarachnoid anesthesia and antibiotic prophylaxis with IV ceftriaxone.

73.2.1 Positioning

The patient is placed in prone position with buttocks separated by two big plasters (Fig. 73.1). There are two monitors, the first one at the feet of the patient and the second one at the head of the patient, because you have to check the fistula's traject up and down. The surgeon's position is on the right side of the patient with a nurse on his side; the cameraman is in front of the surgeon (Fig. 73.2). To have a better ergonomy for the shoulders, the surgeon sometimes stands on a stool. No trocar is needed to perform this procedure, and the fistuloscope is inserted directly through the fistula's hole(s) (Fig. 73.3).

73.2.2 Instrumentation

From the technical point of view, also if we used a cystoscope to perform the procedure at the beginning of our experience, in the last 2 years, we always adopted a fistuloscope, with a dedicated

C. Esposito et al. (eds.), *ESPES Manual of Pediatric Minimally Invasive Surgery*,
https://doi.org/10.1007/978-3-030-00964-9_73

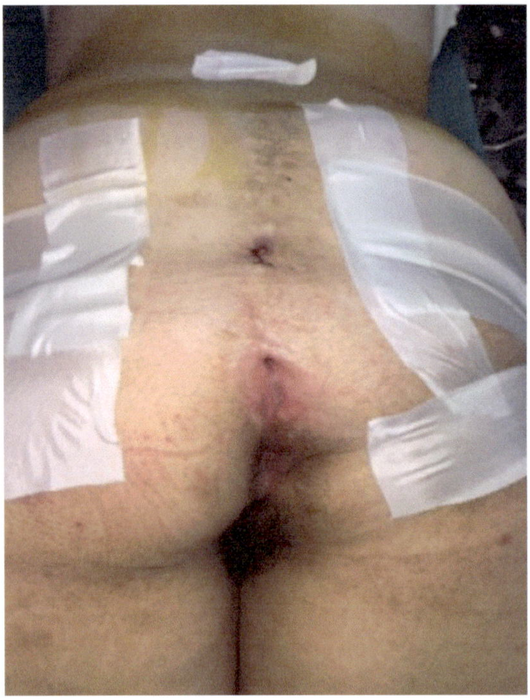

Fig. 73.1 The patient is placed in a prone position with buttocks separated by two big plasters

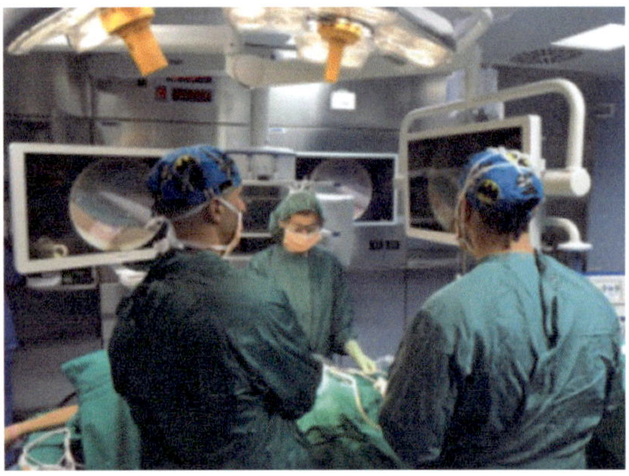

Fig. 73.2 Team position

set of instruments as a monopolar electrode, an endoscopic grasping forceps, and an endoscopic brush. The fistuloscope has an 8° angled eyepiece and is equipped with an optical channel and a working and irrigation channel. Its diameter is 3.2 × 4.8 mm, and its operative length is 18 cm.

A removable handle allows easier maneuvering and better ergonomy for the surgeon (Fig. 73.4). In addition you need a standard set of

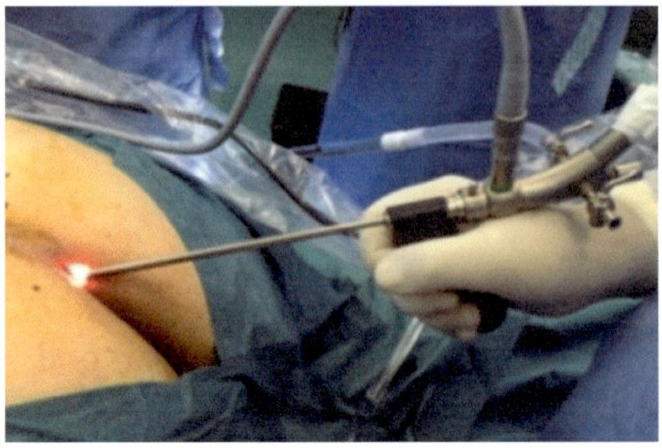

Fig. 73.3 Fistuloscope introduction into fistula hole

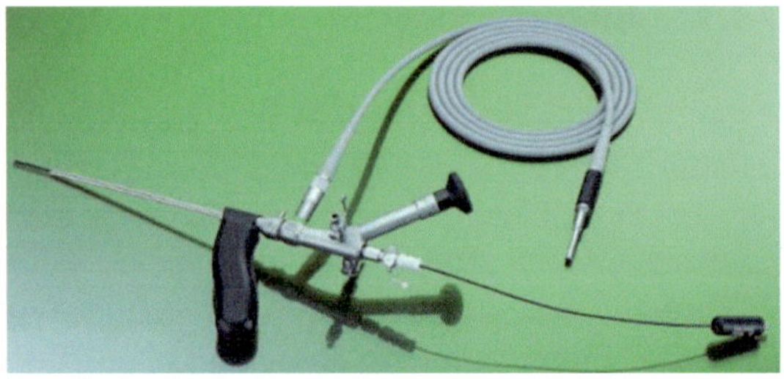

Fig. 73.4 The fistuloscope gives an excellent ergonomy to the surgeon

instruments for traditional open surgery and a monopolar electric cautery. To have a good view of the operative field, we use saline solution to irrigate (as in cystoscopy) the operative field during the entire procedure.

73.2.3 Technique

The technique is divided in two phases, the diagnostic phase and the therapeutic phase. In the diagnostic phase, we identify the anatomy of pilonidal sinus and any secondary tracts and/or abscess cavities. We introduce the fistuloscope through a fistula hole, and a clear view is possible, thanks to a continuous infusion of saline solution. In the operative phase, the endoscopic forceps is inserted through the operative channel of the fistuloscope to remove all the hairs and bulbs under vision (Fig. 73.5). Once this step is completed, the brush is then inserted to well scarify the fistula tract in order to facilitate

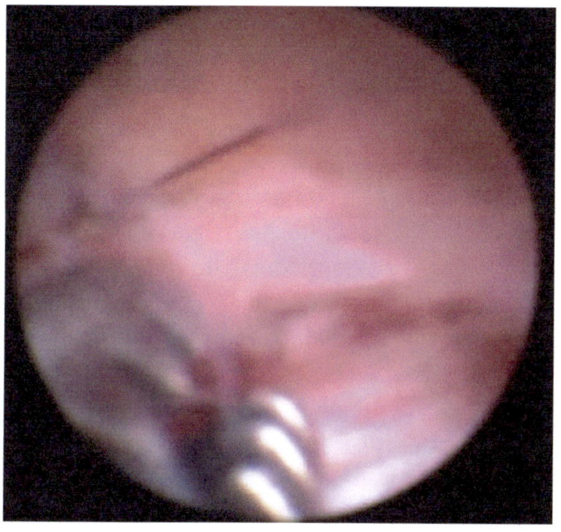

Fig. 73.5 During the procedure it easy to identify and to remove hair thanks to the grasper

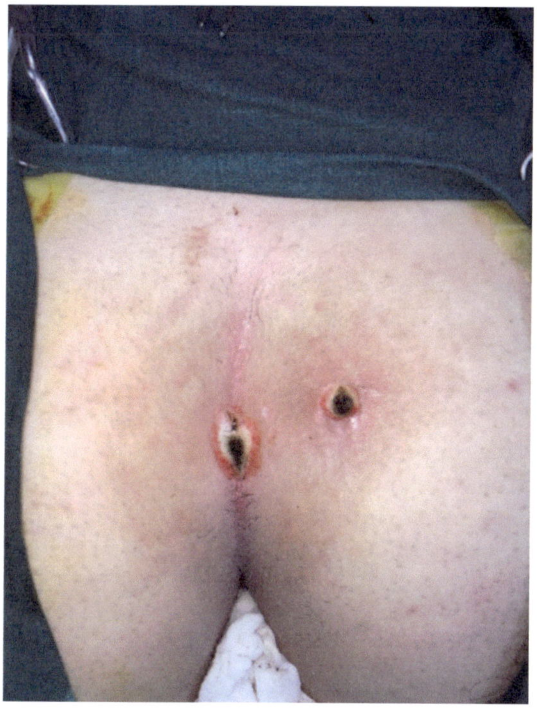

Fig. 73.6 At the end of the procedure, there are only two holes in a patient with a fistula with a double tract

its healing in the postoperative period. Finally, the monopolar electrode is connected to an electrosurgical knife power unit for cautery ablation of the sinus granulation tissue, starting in the main tract and where appropriate traversing secondary tracts and abscess cavities. The granulation tissue is then removed using the grasping forceps.

Particular attention should be paid to the hemostasis during the procedure to avoid bleeding in the postoperative period. External openings are not closed but only coagulated using a standard monopolar cautery (Fig. 73.6). At the end of the procedure, a dressing is applied on the incision(s).

73.3 Postoperative Care

In the postoperative period, the patients can keep a normal decubitus.

They can restart full oral feeding few hours after surgery. The analgesic requirement (paracetamol every 6 h) is generally limited to the first 24 postoperative hours. All patients are discharged on the first or maximum on the second postoperative day. No shower is admitted for 1 week after surgery.

Parents are instructed on how to treat the wound daily by applying topically an antiseptic solution of eosin 2% and a silver sulfadiazine spray for about 3 weeks after surgery.

73.4 Results

The average length of surgery is about 30 min. We did not report intraoperative neither postoperative complications in our series of a 4-year period.

Follow-up is carried out by clinical examinations at 1 week, 2 weeks, and then at 1, 3, 6, 12, and 18 months after surgery.

In general, at 1 month postoperatively, the external openings are closed in all patients.

In our recent series of more than 50 patients, no recurrence was recorded at a median follow-up of 18 months (range 1–48 months).

The average time to return to full daily activities was 2.5 days (range 1–4), and all patients were highly satisfied of the postoperative outcome and cosmetic results.

73.5 Tips and Tricks

Also if the original technique described by the adult surgeon reported the use of mannitol solution for irrigation, in our experience, we always used saline solution without any problem.

If the fistula's hole is too small to introduce the optic, please retract the hole with a small grasper forceps before introducing the fistuloscope.

As for the technical point of view and also if at the beginning of our experience we adopted a cystoscope to perform the procedure, we think that it is preferable to use the fistuloscope to perform PEPSiT, because thanks to the fistuloscope handle you have an excellent ergonomy, without work-related problems for surgeon's shoulders and wrists. In addition, it is very important to completely remove all the hairs and bulbs, to scarify the fistula tract with the brush and to coagulate very well the fistula's walls after removing the granulation tissue. You should check all fistulas' tracts up and down. At the end of surgery, it is important to remember to coagulate the borders of external hole(s) with a monopolar cautery.

73.6 Discussion

There is an ongoing debate regarding the optimal surgical management for pilonidal sinus disease in the pediatric population [5, 6]. The treatment is virtually the same as reported for adults. Various primary or secondary flap methods in open surgery, accompanied by one of the local curettages, phenol application, electrocauterization, and total sinus excision methods, have been described for the treatment of pilonidal sinus [7]. The main problem after a traditional open repair of PSD is the very bad and long postoperative period, and the healing process is very long and painful in several cases.

In addition, following the pilonidal sinus surgery, patients may encounter problems such as esthetical problems, infection, hematoma, dehiscence, and recurrence [8]. Despite various surgical techniques that have been described, reported recurrence rates are as high as 30%, with prolonged recovery times, increased use of resources, repeat surgeries, and patient's frustration [9].

Analyzing literature reports there are interesting data. A retrospective review about an over 35-year pediatric surgeon's experience at a Canadian children's hospital concluded that the excision and packing open produced a longer morbidity but had the same results in terms of recurrences, when compared with both marsupialization or excision and primary closure without drainage [3, 5, 10].

Minimally invasive surgical techniques are becoming widespread in recent years due to the increased experience and development of new instruments. New minimally invasive techniques derive from the concept of operating endoscopically and removing all the infected area by way of small circular incisions. One of these options is endoscopic pilonidal sinus treatment (EPSiT) that was inspired by video-assisted anal fistula treatment (VAAFT) described by Meinero in 2006 [8, 9, 11–14].

We renamed EPSiT procedure applied to pediatric patients PEPSiT.

PEPSiT includes two phases: a diagnostic phase and an operative phase. In the diagnostic phase, the aim is to identify the anatomy of the pilonidal sinus and any secondary tracts and/or abscess cavities [3, 7, 15]. The spontaneously draining opening which is normally situated on the midline cleft must be removed by enlarging the opening with a grasper. The same manoeuver is made also for the holes of secondary fistula tracts or abscesses. The operative phase consists in cautery ablation of the sinus granulation tissue, starting in the main tract and where appropriate traversing secondary tracts and abscess cavities and scarification of fistula walls with the brush. Necrotic material is removed with a grasping forceps passed through the fistuloscope. Where two holes have been used because the infected area is extensive, the brush, designed with bristles in the middle part of a flexible metallic thread, is passed through the incision site.

We have applied PEPSiT in the pediatric population with some modifications of the original EPSiT described for adult patients, and we obtained excellent results. In contrast to the technique described by Meinero, we adopt a continuous jet of saline solution instead of glycine-mannitol to ensure during the procedure a clear visual field but optimizing the economic impact of the procedure [4, 7, 11].

The PEPSiT procedure demonstrated to have many advantages compared to traditional open techniques. First of all, the direct vision allows the surgeon to see perfectly not only the pilonidal sinus but also any possible fistula tracts or abscess cavities. The fistula's tract treatment can be modulated, and there is the certainty of the complete removal of the infected area. Moreover, the hemostasis is done thoroughly under direct vision. This direct vision also allows the complete removal of the hairs and their follicles, often located not only in the pilonidal sinus but also in the surrounding tissue.

The aesthetic result is excellent so as the patient's quality of life and satisfaction. There is no need for painful dressings as reported for open surgery, and healing occurs within 3–4 weeks, as reported in our series.

In addition, the spinal saddle anesthesia with the savings of general anesthesia and its related risks, the low dose of local anesthetic, and the concomitant light sedation provided all components of balanced anesthesia, performing the same with minimum cardiorespiratory disturbances, early ambulation, and high level of satisfaction of patient, of surgical team, and of patient's caregivers. Furthermore, the anesthesiologic technique used allowed a good postoperative pain control without the need of pharmacological overtreatment.

In our experience PEPSiT represents the technique of choice for surgical treatment of pilonidal sinus disease in children. Until a few months ago, many patients refused surgery for important postoperative pain, prolonged hospital stay, and long time for healing. In the last months, we have seen an increased number of patients who choose to undergo this procedure. In fact, it is technically easy and quick to perform, with a short and painless hospital stay, and it allows to the operated patients an early return to full daily activities without restrictions as happened for the classic treatment technique.

References

1. Bascom J. Pilonidal disease: long-term results of follicle removal. Dis Colon Rectum. 1983;26(12):800–7.
2. Ali H, Oner M, Selim K, et al. Sacrococcygeal pilonidal disease: analysis of previously proposed risk factors. Clinics (Sao Paulo). 2010;65(2):125–31.
3. Chintapatla S, Safarani N, Kumar S, et al. Sacrococcygeal pilonidal sinus: historical review, pathological insight and surgical options. Tech Coloproctol. 2003;7:3–8.
4. Meinero P, Mori L, Gasloli G. Endoscopic pilonidal sinus treatment (E.P.Si.T.). Tech Coloproctol. 2014;18(4):389–92.
5. Amit K, John LR. Pilonidal disease. Clin Colon Rectal Surg. 2011;24(1):46–53.
6. Burhan HK, Selim S. Disease that should be remembered: sacrococcygeal pilonidal sinus disease and short history. World J Clin Cases. 2015;3(10):876–9.
7. Esposito C, Izzo S, Turrà F, Cerulo M, Severino G, Settimi A, Iannazzone M, Masieri L, Cortese G, Escolino M. Pediatric endoscopic pilonidal sinus treatment, a revolutionary technique to adopt in children with pilonidal sinus fistulas: our preliminary experience. J Laparoendosc Adv Surg Tech A. 2018;28(3):359–63.
8. Bütter A, Hanson M, VanHouwelingen L, et al. Hair epilation versus surgical excision as primary management of pilonidal disease in the pediatric population. Can J Surg. 2015;58(3):209–11.
9. Dahmann S, Lebo PB, Meyer-Marcotty MV. Comparison of treatments for an infected pilonidal sinus: differences in scar quality and outcome between secondary wound healing and Limberg flap in a prospective study. Handchir Mikrochir Plast Chir. 2016;48(2):111–9.
10. Küçükkartallar T, Tekin A, Vatansev C, et al. The comparison of the results of different operation techniques for pilonidal sinus disease. Genel Tıp Derg. 2007;17:95–7.
11. Williams RK, Adams DC, Aladjem EV, et al. The safety and efficacy of spinal anesthesia for surgery in infants: the Vermont Infant Spinal Registry. Anesth Analg. 2006;102:67–71.
12. Pini Prato A, Mazzola C, Mattioli G, Escolino M, Esposito C, D'Alessio A, Abati LC, Leonelli L, Carlini C, Rotundi F, Meinero PC. Preliminary report on endoscopic pilonidal sinus treatment in children: results of a multicentric series. Pediatr Surg Int. 2018;34(6):687–92.
13. Zagory JA, Golden J, Holoyda K, et al. Excision and primary closure may be the better option in the surgical management of pilonidal disease in the pediatric population. Am Surg. 2016;82(10):964–7.
14. Meinero P, Mori L. Video-assisted anal fistula treatment (VAAFT): a novel sphincter-saving procedure for treating complex anal fistulas. Tech Coloproctol. 2011;15(4):417–22.
15. Nasr A, Ein SH. A pediatric surgeon's 35-year experience with pilonidal disease in a Canadian children's hospital. Can J Surg. 2011;54(1):39–42.

74 Laparoscopic Approach to Nonpalpable Testis

Baran Tokar

74.1 Introduction

Undescended testis has a prevalence of 1% in infants at 1 year of age, of these testes approximately 20% are nonpalpable [1].

While operative approach is well defined and straightforward in palpable undescended testis, evaluation and management of nonpalpable testes (NPT) still have some controversial points.

Decision-making process is challenging in the management of NPT. Physical examination is the first and most important determinant for the diagnosis. After confirmation of the diagnosis, a management plan is made according to whether NPT is unilateral or bilateral. Since the first report of diagnostic laparoscopy for NPT in 1976, laparoscopy has been the main determining factor in the diagnosis and treatment process [2].

The aim of this review is to give tips and tricks on laparoscopic approach for NPT while addressing the importance of preoperative assessment, laparoscopic exploration, and interpretation of exploration findings.

B. Tokar (✉)
Division of Pediatric Urology, Department of Pediatric Surgery, School of Medicine, Eskisehir Osmangazi University, Eskisehir, Turkey
e-mail: btokar@ogu.edu.tr

74.2 Preoperative Assessment

Before definitive diagnosis of NPT, it is necessary to make a double check to confirm whether it is a real NPT or the testicle is in inguinoscrotal region but could not be palpated due to size and consistency of the testis or patient's condition. It is difficult to palpate testis in obese patients and severe orthopedic deformities. Testis may also be at ectopic location or in an abdominoinguinal retractile form within a hernia sac. For preoperative evaluation and diagnosis of unilateral NPT, physical examination is all needed, and no laboratory investigation is necessary. In unilateral NPT, compensatory hypertrophy of the contralateral testis may suggest testicular absence or atrophy. Monorchidism was observed in 95% of patients with a contralateral testis 2 cc or larger in the series of Belman and Rushton [3], but this sign is not specific and does not preclude surgical exploration.

In cases of bilateral NPT or unilateral NPT accompanied by anomalies of genital region such as severe hypospadias or scrotal hyperpigmentation, disorders of sex development (DSD) should be considered in differential diagnosis, and further genetic and endocrinological evaluations are needed [4].

Preoperative radiological evaluation was not recommended in the guidelines on NPT [4, 5]. Computerized tomography and magnetic resonance have no significant contribution to the

C. Esposito et al. (eds.), *ESPES Manual of Pediatric Minimally Invasive Surgery*,
https://doi.org/10.1007/978-3-030-00964-9_74

diagnosis. Ultrasonography (USG) is the most frequently requested radiological examination, and some physicians need USG to confirm physical examination findings. USG is an easy to perform noninvasive tool with no risk of anesthesia and radiation; but it has low efficacy at diagnosis to detect the presence of the testis or the absence of an intra-abdominal testis and is dependent on who performs. However, USG may be helpful in obese children, in cases of suspected DSD, to identify Mullerian structures and for determination of the exact size of pathologic and contralateral testes [6].

The testes that remain nonpalpable by 6 months are unlikely to descend spontaneously. Surgery should be started to plan at the age of 6 months and should be finished by 18 months at the latest [4, 5]. Adult studies on spermatogenesis, hormone production, and risk of tumor development also suggest the early timing of surgery [7]. Laparoscopic exploration as early as 6 months also decreases parental anxiety.

The parents should clearly understand the aim of the surgery which is to determine whether a testis is present or not, and if it is found, it could be removed or brought down to the scrotum with a single or two stage surgery. Informed consent should describe all these possibilities.

There are three options for initial surgical approach in NPT. Depending on the findings, the surgeon may prefer scrotal, inguinal, or laparoscopic approach. Laparoscopy as an initial procedure is the most accurate way to identify the condition of spermatic vessels, vas deferens, and if present the intra-abdominal testis [2, 4]. The next step could be easily planned following a complete laparoscopic exploration.

The current laparoscopic approach with tips and tricks, including some ongoing controversies, will be presented in the following section.

74.3 Surgical Technique

Reexamination and confirmation of NPT under general anesthesia is the first step in surgery. Testis could be palpated, and subsequently the surgical approach might be switched to standard inguinal orchidopexy [4, 5, 8]. This is especially important for obese patients.

For laparoscopic exploration, the patient is placed on the table in a supine position. The monitor is placed close to the patient's feet (Fig. 74.1). The surgeon, the camera, the target, and the monitor should be on the same line. First, the camera port is inserted at the level of the umbilicus using Hasson technique. A 4 mm port and a 4 mm 30° optic are used in infants and small children. A 5 mm optic might be preferred for older ages. Following the camera insertion, the table is brought to Trendelenburg position, allowing for better exploration of the inguinal and intrapelvic region. For unilateral NPT, exploration is initiated from the contralateral side. Entrance of spermatic vessels and vas deferens into internal ring without any associated pathology is confirmed. The camera then focuses on the side where the testis cannot be palpated. The spermatic vessels, vas deferens, and, if present, the condition of the intra-abdominal testis are evaluated. A full urinary bladder or dilated intestinal segments might cause difficulty in exposure of surgical anatomy. Exploration should not be questionable, and it has to be completed with a clear exposure of the

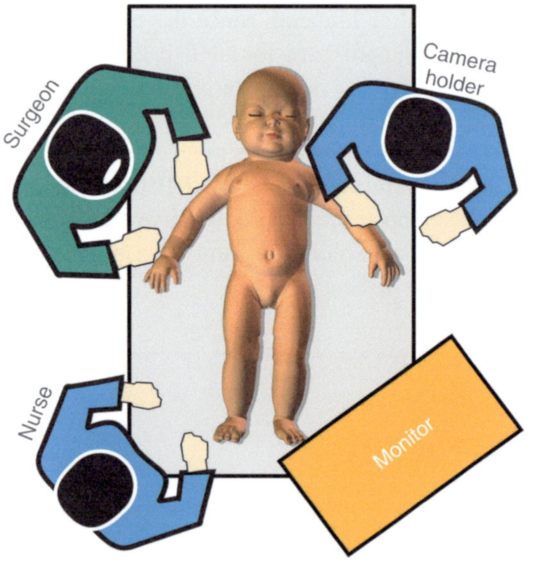

Fig. 74.1 Surgeon, patient, and monitor positions for laparoscopic exploration of nonpalpable testis at the left side

region of surgical interest. If needed, muscle relaxation might be asked to the anesthesiologist, and Trendelenburg angle could be increased. Emptying the full bladder and decompression of the colon may provide a better vision.

At this point of exploration, two possibilities exist: Either a testis is found, or signs of testicular agenesis and inguinal or vanishing testis are observed. In the case of spermatic vessels entering inguinal ring, laparoscopy is terminated, and inguinal exploration is performed. Atrophic or a healthy testis might be found on inguinal exploration. Atrophic one should be removed; standard orchidopexy is performed for healthy testis. If exploration shows peeping testis which is located right on the internal ring, it can be brought down in the scrotum laparoscopically or via an inguinal incision.

If blind-ending spermatic vessels are observed (Fig. 74.2), the European Association of Urology/European Society for Paediatric Urology and AUA Guidelines suggest not going further and terminating the surgery [4, 5]. Inguinoscrotal nubbin is not removed according to those guidelines. However, residual germ cells in an extra-abdominal testicular nubbin theoretically have the potential for malignant transformation, so that the decision regarding whether not doing an inguinal exploration or exploring the scrotum or inguinal canal to excise the testicular nubbin remains controversial [8]. Guidelines support the belief on nubbin removal being unnecessary and risk being negligible. The author of this manuscript prefers to make exploration of the scrotum and inguinal canal to excise the testicular remnant.

Testis, spermatic vessels, and vas deferens may not be found in laparoscopic exploration of the inguinal region. Intrapelvic or retrocolic testis might be present in such cases. If the bladder is full, first it is emptied, and if necessary Trendelenburg angle is increased to expose an intrapelvic testis hidden behind the bladder. If the testis is not found in rectovesical pouch, the retroperitoneum from the internal inguinal ring up to the lower pole of the kidney should be examined because the testis might be found anywhere along that tract.

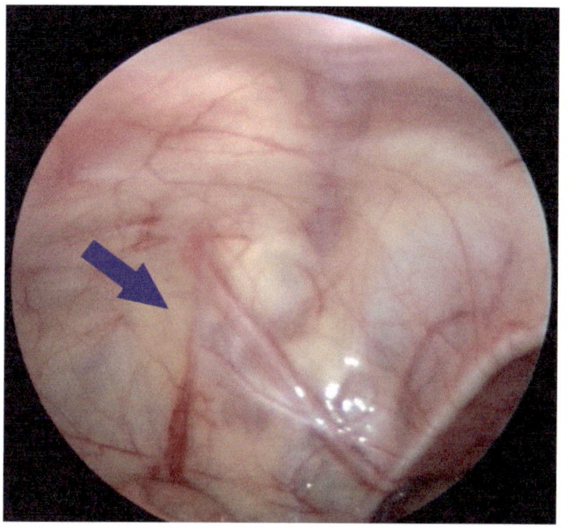

Fig. 74.2 Blind-ending left spermatic vessels

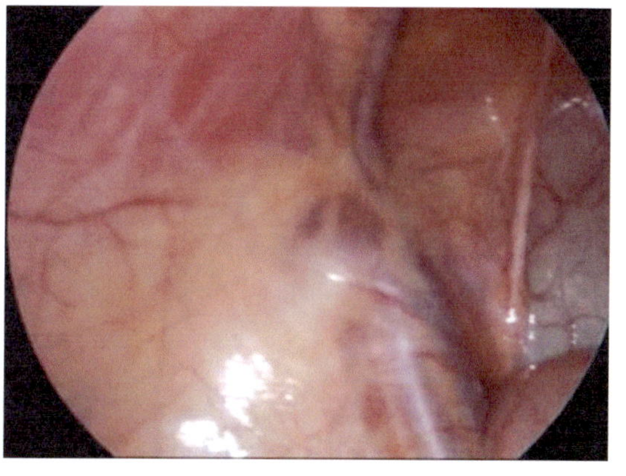

Fig. 74.3 Absence of left spermatic vessels with the diagnosis of testicular agenesis

Failure of testicular development also called as testicular agenesis can occur in early or late developmental phase (Fig. 74.3). Early-onset testicular agenesis results in the absence of the testis, spermatic vessels, and Wolffian structures. In later failure, testosterone is produced locally and induces development of Wolffian structures, so that the vas is observed in a late-onset testicular agenesis. Once the diagnosis is testicular agenesis, no further treatment is necessary. Congenital agenesis of the vas deferens is a rare pathology but could be observed during inguinal exploration. If testis and spermatic vessels are present, laparoscopic or inguinal orchidopexy is

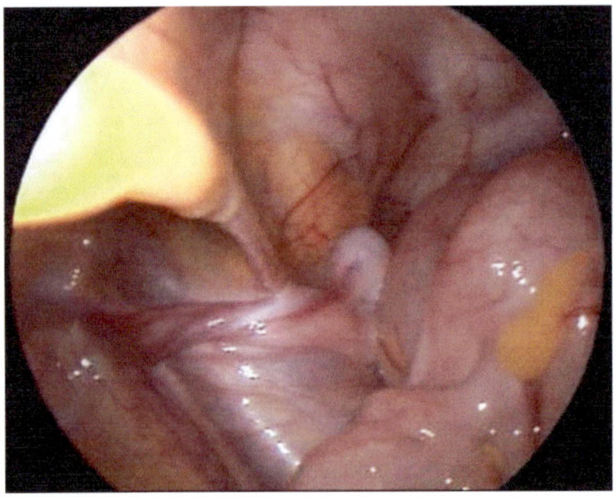

Fig. 74.4 Intra-abdominal left testis that can be brought down to scrotum by primary orchidopexy

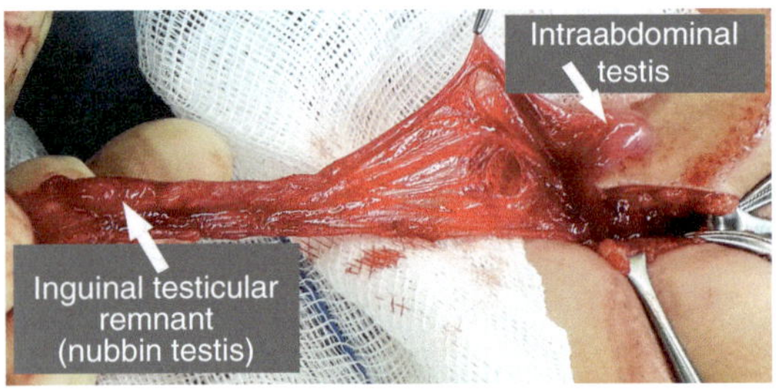

Fig. 74.5 Polyorchidism: intra-abdominal testis sharing the vas with an inguinal rudimentary testis

performed to save the viable testis. Associated congenital genitourinary malformations like renal agenesis might be observed and should be investigated. The parents should be informed on the late consequences of single or bilateral absence of the vas deferens.

Testis is absent in 20% of NPT and atrophic or rudimentary in 30% [4]. The rest are intra-abdominal, canalicular, or peeping on the internal inguinal ring. If intra-abdominal testis is found (Fig. 74.4) and if the testis can reach the dependent scrotum without tension after careful dissection, primary orchidopexy without vessel division is performed. As a general rule, if the abdominal testis is able to reach the contralateral inguinal ring, a primary orchidopexy can be performed. A testis within 2 cm of the internal ring can be brought down without vessel division. Laparoscopy orchidopexy could be performed with vessel sparing. Depending on the surgeon preference, the gubernaculum might be spared or dissected and cut. After complete mobilization, the surgeon may use neohiatus lateral to the urinary bladder and medial to the inferior epigastric vessels or may prefer to bring testis down to the scrotum via the internal inguinal ring and inguinal canal. A dartos pouch was made and a 10-mm port was inserted from the scrotum into the abdominal cavity. Testis is brought down in the scrotum and placed in dartos pouch. An alternative approach in such cases is to make an inguinal incision and perform laparoscopy-assisted standard inguinal orchidopexy. The author prefers that method. Inguinal exploration and orchidopexy via inguinal canal have several advantages. Following laparoscopic complete mobilization of the testis, inguinal exploration might provide a better exposure for inguinal hernia repair together with additional retroperitoneal dissection of spermatic vessels and vas. If needed, inguinal Prentiss maneuver could also be performed. There is also possibility of polyorchidism associated with intra-abdominal testis. An inguinal rudimentary testis sharing the vas with intra-abdominal testis could be found (Fig. 74.5). The author observed polyorchidism in 4.5% of the patients who had laparoscopic exploration for NPT [9]. Combined laparoscopic and inguinal explorations might be suggested for intra-abdominal testis with the aim of not missing an associated inguinal polyorchidic rudimentary testis and making inguinal orchidopexy [10].

Testis lying high beyond 4 cm of the internal ring may not reach the scrotum without division of the testicular vessels (Fig. 74.6); the distance between 2 and 4 cm is a gray area [11]. While some surgeons accept the distance more than 2 cm as high position and perform vessel division [4, 12], some others perform primary orchidopexy for the testis in gray area, and if the testis cannot reach down into the scrotum, the testis is left in high scrotal position at this stage, and later the second look is done.

If vessel division is needed, a single- or two-stage Fowler-Stephens (FS) orchidopexy could be performed. The main point in FS procedure is to divide the spermatic vessels with conservation of the collateral vascular supply.

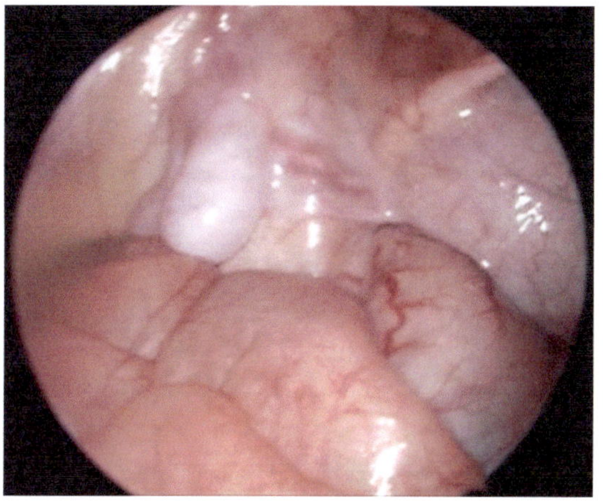

Fig. 74.6 Testis lying high and needs two-stage Fowler-Stephens orchidopexy

To perform FS procedure, the table is kept in Trendelenburg position and inclined 15° ipsilateral. Ports and instruments are 3 mm in infants; 5 mm might be preferred in older patients. At first, the peritoneum alongside of the spermatic vessels is cut, and then high dissection and ligation of vessels by sutures or clips are performed. If the surgery is planned as a single stage, laparoscopic orchidopexy is completed with preservation of deferential vessels.

If division of spermatic vessels is needed, the author prefers two-stage FS technique. Two-stage FS orchidopexy allows development of collateral blood supply and provides greater testicular mobility. Time interval between the first and second procedures is around 6 months. Sparing gubernaculum with less dissection may also decrease the chance of testicular atrophy. Preserving the gubernacular collaterals together with deferential vessels increases the chance of testicular survival [13].

At the second stage of FS, adequacy of the testis and collateral blood supply along the vas are confirmed. Spermatic vessels are divided between the proximal and distal ligation. The testis and the vas with a wide strip of peritoneal covering are mobilized. Meticulous dissection is needed to protect collateral vessels. One must also pay attention to avoid injury to ureter and iliac vessels. During dissection, the testis is moved toward the contralateral side to check the adequacy of mobilization. Dissection of peritoneum continues until enough length is gained. During dissection, it is better to use bipolar diathermy with the aim of not causing any harm to the collateral blood supply. Following a complete mobilization, the testis is brought down to the scrotum by either laparoscopic orchidopexy or laparoscopy-assisted standard inguinal orchidopexy described above. The gubernaculum has to be dissected and cut if laparoscopic orchidopexy is preferred. If the neohiatus lateral to the urinary bladder and medial to the inferior epigastric vessels is going to be made, the urinary bladder is emptied by catheterization prior to the insertion of scrotal port into the abdominal cavity via the neohiatus. After the laparoscopic mobilization, if the procedure is completed by an inguinal incision and standard inguinal orchidopexy, the gubernaculum and associated collateral vessels could be spared.

If the patient has bilateral intra-abdominal testis, concurrent bilateral orchidopexy could be performed. When ipsilateral testicular viability is questionable, a staged approach should be considered for the contralateral testis [14].

Surgical procedures for NPT do not involve an overnight stay in hospital. Postoperatively, follow-up of the patient is scheduled at the first week, the first month, and the third month of the operation and subsequently decreased on a yearly basis. The size, position, and condition of the testes are checked by both physical examination and Doppler USG.

74.4 Discussion

Physical examination followed by laparoscopic exploration answers most of the questions that might be asked in NPT. Laparoscopy has been widely accepted as the main determining factor in the diagnosis and treatment. Reexamination and confirmation of NPT under general anesthesia should be done routinely to avoid unnecessary laparoscopic exploration. Radiological investigations to find the testis or concentration on the changes of contralateral testis such as compensatory hypertrophy does not contribute significantly to decision-making process [4, 5]. Laparoscopy provides a perfect exposure of the inguinal region. The surgeon may easily figure out what the pathology is and what to do in the next step.

Ideal age for the surgery is starting from 6 months up to 18 months, but a child in an older age with NPT also needs laparoscopic exploration to delineate the pathology [15]. The management is planned accordingly.

Surgeons who prefer scrotal or inguinal approach as an initial procedure should consider the possibility of missing an intra-abdominal testis. Inguinal exploration might be subsequently combined to the laparoscopy, but initial procedure should be the laparoscopy to decide on whether to go further or not.

Depending on the experience, the surgeon may have difficulty in exposure and interpretation of intra-abdominal findings. In such cases, positions of the patient and the surgical team should be reevaluated. The patient should be in Trendelenburg position. Emptying the bladder, decompression of the colon, or muscle relaxation might be needed to create an intra-abdominal working space.

At the end of the laparoscopic exploration, either a testis is found intra-abdominally, or signs of testicular agenesis and inguinal or vanishing testis are observed. Laparoscopy is terminated with observation of spermatic vessels entering inguinal ring or findings of testicular agenesis. Before the final diagnosis of testicular agenesis, the rectovesical pouch and the retroperitoneum from the internal inguinal ring up to the lower pole of the kidney should be carefully explored to find an intra-abdominal testis. Guidelines also suggest to terminate surgical procedure in the case of blind-ending spermatic vessels [4, 5]. Although the risk is accepted as negligible, residual germ cells in testicular remnant left in inguinoscrotal region theoretically have the potential for malignant transformation. Since any intra-abdominal atrophic testis found at laparoscopic exploration should always be excised due to the high incidence of residual germ cells, we need prospective studies to show whether the risk is really negligible for extra-abdominal testicular nubbin or not.

When intra-abdominal testis is present, primary orchidopexy should be the primary goal. If it is not possible and if we need vascular division, then the goal becomes to preserve maximum vascular collateral. Two-stage FS orchidopexy allows development of collateral blood supply. Gubernaculum-sparing two-stage FS procedure done with attentive mobilization of a wide strip of peritoneum between the testis and the vas protects collateral vessels.

Postoperative follow-up with regular interval is highly important in NPT. Relative or complete testicular atrophy and testicular ascent may occur [8]. Parents should be informed on operative findings and the possible future scenarios.

References

1. Levitt SB, Kogan SJ, Engel RM, et al. The impalpable testes: a rational approach to management. J Urol. 1978;120:515–20.
2. Cortesi N, Ferrari P, Zambarda E, et al. Diagnosis of bilateral abdominal cryptorchidism by laparoscopy. Endoscopy. 1976;8:33–4.
3. Belman AB, Rushton HG. Is an empty left hemiscrotum and hypertrophied right descended testis predictive of perinatal torsion? J Urol. 2003;170:1674.
4. Radmayr C, Dogan HS, Hoebeke P, et al. Management of undescended testes: European Association of Urology/European Society for Paediatric Urology Guidelines. J Pediatr Urol. 2016;12(6):335–43.
5. Kolon TF, Herndon CD, Baker LA, Baskin LS, et al. American Urological Association. Evaluation and treatment of cryptorchidism: AUA guideline. J Urol. 2014;192(2):337–45.
6. Tasian GE, Copp HL, Baskin LS. Diagnostic imaging in cryptorchidism: utility, indications, and effectiveness. J Pediatr Surg. 2011;46(12):2406–13.
7. Engeler DS, Hösli PO, John H, et al. Early orchiopexy: prepubertal intratubular germ cell neoplasia and fertility outcome. Urology. 2000;56(1):144–8.
8. Shepard CL, Kraft KH. The nonpalpable testis: a narrative review. J Urol. 2017;198(6):1410–7.
9. Tokar B, Çiftçi M, Şimşek E, et al. Polyorchidism may not be as rare as thought: how valuable is a combined laparoscopic and inguinal exploration in a nonpalpable testis? In: 3rd Annual Scientific Meeting of ESPES, P020, Marseille, France, 2013, p. 93.
10. Tokar B. Do we need laparoscopic abdominal exploration for a testicular nubbin palpated in the inguinal region? A case with type IV polyorchidism. Eur J Pediatr Surg. 2010;20(3):203–4.

11. Francis XS, Mark FB. Abnormalities of the testes and scrotum and their surgical management. In: Alan JW, editor. Campbell-Walsh urology. 9th ed. Philadelphia: Elsevier Saunders; 2007. p. 3761–98.
12. Kirsch AJ, Escala J, Duckett JW, et al. Surgical management of the nonpalpable testis: the Children's Hospital of Philadelphia experience. J Urol. 1998;159(4):1340–3.
13. Mahomed A, Adams S, Islam S. Initial success with gubernacular-sparing laparoscopic-assisted Fowler-Stephens orchidopexy for intra-abdominal testes. J Laparoendosc Adv Surg Tech A. 2012;22(2):192–4.
14. Kaye JD, Palmer LS. Single setting bilateral laparoscopic orchiopexy for bilateral intra-abdominal testicles. J Urol. 2008;180(4 Suppl):1795–9.
15. Bracho-Blanchet E, Unda-Haro S, Ordorica-Flores R, et al. Laparoscopic treatment of nonpalpable testicle. Factors predictive for diminished size. J Pediatr Surg. 2016;51(7):1201–6.

Complications in Pediatric MIS 75

Holger Till, Jürgen Schleef, and Ahmed El Haddad

75.1 Introduction

Prevention and management of complications represent essential responsibilities of every pediatric surgeon. "Things just don't happen," but complications can be anticipated (by awareness, education), can be avoided (by training, experience), and must be managed well (on a mastery level). Especially in pediatric minimally invasive surgery (MIS), the spectrum of techniques ranges from neonatal to adolescent and from thoracic, abdominal, urological, to oncological procedures (and many others). All of these techniques imply a specific learning curve and a variety of complications. The following article shall deal with general complications of pediatric MIS, while procedure-specific challenges are dealt with in the corresponding chapters.

75.2 Complications of Access Techniques

The basic principles of access techniques to the body's cavities have already been elucidated in Part I of this book.

H. Till (✉) · J. Schleef · A. El Haddad
Department of Paediatric and Adolescent Surgery, Medical University of Graz, Graz, Austria
e-mail: holger.till@medunigraz.at

In general access techniques can be divided into open and closed methods. Usually the umbilicus serves as the primary entry site. Specifically in newborns and small infants, the umbilicus may cover persistent embryological structures like omphaloenteric duct, urachus, or patent umbilical vein. Direct insufflations of CO_2 into the patent umbilical vein and cardiac arrest have been described [1]. Consequently in such small children, the primary incision at the umbilicus should rather be made on the left side to avoid false entry. Furthermore blind puncture with the Veress needle for installation of the pneumoperitoneum and the open introduction (Hassan technique) imply a certain risk of intraabdominal organ damage including bowel or major vessels [2]. "The smaller the child, the greater the risk" may serve as a general guideline for the initial access.

75.3 Interaction Between the Pneumoperitoneum and Anesthesia

Pneumoperitoneum and pneumothorax represent unphysiological conditions with many possible side effects especially due to absorption of the gas and pressure within the compartment. Many elaborate studies about consequences for anesthesia, respiratory function, and hemodynamic parameters are available [3] and will be discussed elsewhere. Complications as such occur when

C. Esposito et al. (eds.), *ESPES Manual of Pediatric Minimally Invasive Surgery*,
https://doi.org/10.1007/978-3-030-00964-9_75

these side effects exaggerate or remain undetected. High-risk patients like newborns or children with cardiopulmonary insufficiency (like CDH) or elevated cranial pressure are exceptional vulnerable. Anyhow pressure and flow of CO_2 should be limited and adjusted according to the operative space and the size, age, and status of the patient [4].

75.4 Ports and Port Site Complications

Following the installation of the optical port and CO_2 insufflation, several working ports must be introduced "under optical control." There is a tremendous variety of ports and trocars available today. For pediatric MIS, the size and the length matter most, i.e., ergonomically they should fit to the size of the child. For example, thoracoscopic CDH repair should not be attempted with 5 mm and long ports; instead 3 or 3.5 mm seems adequate. All of these principles are dealt with in Part I "Basics" but seem worth mentioning again, because inadequate instrumentation will inevitably translate into inadequate performance or complications.

Complications from the introduction of the working ports do not differ much from those of the first port, especially perforation and bleeding. Port placement for laparoscopy should avoid the epigastric vessels and penetration of the abdominal muscle. Instead the lateral border of the rectus sheath or the aponeuroses of the lateral abdominal muscles should be preferred. For thoracoscopy the ports should avoid cutting the intercostal vessels and rather spread the intercostal muscles.

Final removal of ports should be guided with the scope. In case of port dislocation during the procedure, it must be reintroduced with a blunt trocar and again under optical control, preferably through the same defect. But remember that the leakage of gas may "blow" parts of the omentum up and into the defect, which later may cause herniation [5] and adhesions [6]. So during the final closure, one should inspect such complications carefully. In any case all port sites should be sutured!

75.5 Complications by Instruments and Sizes

The technical development of instruments suitable for pediatric MIS has been enormous in the last two decades. In fact some procedures have become much safer and easier since the introduction of special devices like a 3 mm sealer or 5 mm stapler, which seem just right for infant lung resections. The knowledge on how to use such devices correctly has increased in parallel. Basic straight instruments for pediatric surgery may be as small as 2 mm and 15 cm short. However, small instruments do not translate automatically into atraumatic handling. Instead grasping tissue with a small jaw of a 3 mm may inflict more pressure or damage than by a 5 mm instrument. Especially in newborns, gentle tissue handling with small instruments seems essential to avoid tissue damage, tissue perforation, tears, or leaks.

75.6 Complications During Retraction of Tissues and Organs

In many pediatric procedures, adequate exposure can only be facilitated with sufficient retraction of adjacent structures. Many different devices are available to retract the bowel, stomach, liver, and many other organs. They may cause bleeding, bowel perforation, or even partial organ damage like it has been described for the Nathan retractor causing partial liver necrosis during laparoscopic gastric surgery in an adult [7]. All tissue and organs, which have been retracted or grasped, should be controlled at the end of the procedure to avoid an unrecognized damage.

75.7 Complications by Cutting and Sealing with Energy Sources

Complications with cutting and sealing devices have been reported since the beginning of the development of MIS and must always be kept in mind.

Hook cautery with monopolar energy should be discussed first. Many experts are very fond of this instrument because it allows for delicate dissection. To avoid major burns, the entire non-insulated hock should be watched during activation. Furthermore it remains the surgeon's responsibility to check the "dispersive electrode" to avoid malfunction. Tissue damage, which occurred accidentally, must be repaired immediately. Severe thermal damage to the bowel, which remained unrecognized, could lead to necrosis, perforations, and systemic sepsis and peritonitis.

Several alternatives to monopolar coagulation exist carrying their distinct potential for complications, such as bipolar currency, Ultracision™, LigaSure™, laser, and JustRight™ 3 mm vessel sealing system. Of course surgeons should be familiar with the technical finesse before using them. Nevertheless when sealing a major vessel of, e.g., 5 mm in diameter, some companies claim that the sealer closes the vessel and allows cutting at the same time. Experts in the field however have experienced disastrous malfunction [8] and would rather prefer to (a) create enough length on the vessel, (b) make two independent seals, and (c) partially cut in between to check the complete occlusion before cutting completely. Such surgical details may avoid major complications.

75.8 Complications with Clip Applier and Stapler

Clips and staplers have eliminated tedious suture tying and knotting, especially in small spaces.

Clip appliers come in various sizes and mechanisms and are commonly used to occlude smaller blood vessels or luminal structures such as the cystic duct. As far as their complications are concerned, it seems important to use adequate sizes to occlude the entire width of that structure. Note that especially straight titanium clips may fall off, when the stability of the clip does not match the rigidity of the structure, especially when a major bronchus is clipped. Furthermore they may be pulled off during a procedure by repetitive manipulation. Postoperative clip failure represents another major complication. One reason could be the intraoperative combination of cautery and clips when sealing a vessel. This must absolutely be avoided, because heat causes collateral necrosis and the tissue within the clip will not scar but may fall off.

Staplers come in different sizes (12–5 mm by JustRight™), with different functions (roticulating Y/N) and in different lengths of the cartridge. The most common type is a linear stapler. Most models fire three rows of staples on each side and cut in between (linear cutter). Different staple heights must be selected depending on tissue thickness. The color of the cartridge codes for the height of the staples and thus for the tissue to be used on (e.g., white for vessel or blue for parenchyma). This point seems trivial to many experts, but stapler failure like bleeding or leaks is often based on this detail. Latest generation staplers combine various heights of staples in one cartridge to cope with different functions "all in one." Special care must be taken when stapling edematous intestine (e.g., the appendix [9] or thin tissue like dilated bowel), where the staples cannot hold the tissue. Finally most minimally invasive surgeons have experienced laparoscopic linear stapler malfunction causing adverse events which require mastery complication management to cope with [10]. One should be prepared.

75.9 Devices for Specimen Removal

Specimens have to be removed during many different procedures like splenectomy, cholecystectomy, colonic resection for Hirschsprung disease, and tumor biopsies or resection. Many harvesting devices and specimen bags in 5, 10, or 15 mm sizes (splenomegaly) are available. Possible complications include spillage of contaminated debride, loss of stones, or tissue fragments and malfunction. Finally especially in splenectomy for hematological disorders, when the spleen is being morcellated within the bag still, which is partially still in the abdomen, tears and cuts of the bag may cause spillage and autotransplantation of splenic tissues. So specimen bags should be checked carefully for small holes to avoid these very unpleasant complications.

75.10 Discussion

The field of endosurgery in children is constantly expanding and growing. Many reports in the literature can be found about new procedures, new techniques, and modified approaches. Mastering delicate procedures requires delicate complication management or even better the prevention. Unfortunately academic information about the true incidence of complications related to technical mistakes or instrument malfunction is rather limited. Thus recommendations for the management of minor and major technical complications lack a higher level of evidence. Nevertheless such complications occur, and most advanced centers for pediatric MIS have implemented their quality and risk management systems including a standardized surveillance of surgical complications. More specifically the classification by Esposito [2] supports detailed tracking of MIS complications (a) related to the time at which they occur (preoperative, intraoperative, postoperative); (b) the phase of the laparoscopic procedure (creation of pneumoperitoneum, positioning of trocar, dissection, coagulation, extraction, closure of trocar orifice); (c) complications related to the specific procedure performed; (d) failure or malfunction of the device or equipment used; and (e) other causes (non-trained surgeon, wrong indication for the patient, anesthesia). From these data each unit should develop its specific strategy on how to improve future care. Moreover individual training and teaching remain essential [11] conveying that complications must be anticipated (by awareness, education), can be avoided (by training, experience), and must be managed well (on a mastery level).

References

1. Kudsi OY, Jones SA, Brenn BR. Carbon dioxide embolism in a 3-week-old neonate during laparoscopic pyloromyotomy: a case report. J Pediatr Surg. 2009;44(4):842–5.
2. Esposito C, Mattioli G, Monguzzi GL, Montinaro L, Riccipetiotoni G, Aceti R, Messina M, Pintus C, Settimi A, Esposito G, Jasonni V. Complications and conversions of pediatric videosurgery: the Italian multicentric experience on 1689 procedures. Surg Endosc. 2002;16(5):795–8.
3. Ure BM, Suempelmann R, Metzelder MM, Kuebler J. Physiological responses to endoscopic surgery in children. Semin Pediatr Surg. 2007;16(4):217–23.
4. Kuebler JF, Schukfeh N, Vieten G, Osthaus WA, Huber D, Dennhard N, Suempelmann R, Ure BM, Metzelder ML. Arterioportal shunting, splanchnic capillary perfusion, and the effects of colloids during capnoperitoneum in neonatal and adolescent pigs. Surg Endosc. 2018;32(6):2923–31.
5. Nakajima K, Wasa M, Kawahara H, Hasegawa T, Soh H, Taniguchi E, Ohashi S, Okada A. Revision laparoscopy for incarcerated hernia at a 5-mm trocar site following pediatric laparoscopic surgery. Surg Laparosc Endosc Percutan Tech. 1999;9(4):294–5.
6. Bunting DM. Port-site hernia following laparoscopic cholecystectomy. JSLS. 2010;14(4):490–7.
7. Tamhankar AP, Kelty CJ, Jacob G. Retraction-related liver lobe necrosis after laparoscopic gastric surgery. JSLS. 2011;15(1):117–21.
8. Igai H, Kamiyoshihara M, Ibe T, Kawatani N, Osawa F, Yoshikawa R. Troubleshooting for bleeding in thoracoscopic anatomic pulmonary resection. Asian Cardiovasc Thorac Ann. 2017;25(1):35–40.
9. Escolino M, Becmeur F, Saxena A, Till H, Holcomb GW 3rd, Esposito C. Endoloop versus endostapler: what is the best option for appendiceal stump closure in children with complicated appendicitis? Results of a multicentric international survey. Surg Endosc. 2018;32(8):3570–5. https://doi.org/10.1007/s00464-018-6081-8.
10. Kwazneski D, Six C, Stahlfeld K. The unacknowledged incidence of laparoscopic stapler malfunction. Surg Endosc. 2013;27(1):86–9.
11. Esposito C, Escolino M, Draghici I, Cerulo M, Farina A, De Pascale T, Cozzolino S, Settimi A. Training models in pediatric minimally invasive surgery: rabbit model versus porcine model: a comparative study. J Laparoendosc Adv Surg Tech A. 2016;26(1):79–84.

76 Fetoscopy: The Minimally Invasive Fetal Surgery

Jose L. Peiro and Federico Scorletti

76.1 Introduction

Fetal surgery aims to correct congenital malformations in utero to prevent progressive deterioration and severe consequences on fetal development. Nowadays, prenatal diagnosis allows high rate of fetal anomaly detection since early in gestation. Open fetal surgery provides direct access to fetal anatomy but carries significant risk for the pregnant mother due to large laparotomy and hysterotomy and for the fetus, mainly preterm delivery. Improvement in pathophysiological knowledge of major fetal anomalies and the development of therapeutic tools allow fetoscopic procedures in some specific cases [1].

Selective fetoscopic laser photocoagulation (SFLP) is the goal standard for treatment of twin-to-twin transfusion syndrome (TTTS) in monochorionic twin gestations to fulgurate and block the placental vascular anastomosis [2]. The evidence for fetal intervention in congenital diaphragmatic hernia (CDH) by fetoscopic placement of an endoluminal detachable balloon for fetal tracheal occlusion provides promising benefits in outcomes and currently is still under formal investigation [3]. Selection of patients for prenatal intervention is becoming more precise and accurate. In other less common diseases, such as amniotic constrictive bands, obstructive uropathy, intrathoracic cyst lesions, or pleural effusion, indications for prenatal intervention should be evaluated case by case. Prenatal repair of myelomeningocele (MMC) has proved effective in reducing neurologic sequelae of this condition, improving limb function, and reducing the need for ventricular shunt [4]. So far, the gold standard for prenatal MMC repair is open procedure, through a controlled hysterotomy. Ongoing research studies aim to improve the minimally invasive approach also for this congenital malformation. Some groups are using percutaneous access with two or three inserted trocars to achieve the neurosurgical repair in utero [5]. In our institution, we externalize the uterus through a maternal laparotomy and proceed with the strict fetoscopy. This technique allows a better control of the fetus that can be manipulated and put in correct position, optimal insertion of the trocars, less pressure of CO_2 for the amniodistention, and closure of the amniotic orifices at the end of the procedure.

In this chapter, we describe the basic principles of minimally invasive fetal surgery by fetoscopy with both externalized uterus and percutaneous approaches.

J. L. Peiro (✉) · F. Scorletti
Pediatric General and Thoracic Surgery Division, Cincinnati Fetal Center, Cincinnati Children's Hospital Medical Center (CCHMC), Cincinnati, OH, USA
e-mail: jose.peiro@cchmc.org

C. Esposito et al. (eds.), *ESPES Manual of Pediatric Minimally Invasive Surgery*,
https://doi.org/10.1007/978-3-030-00964-9_76

76.2 Preoperative Preparation

Before any fetal intervention, every pregnancy should undergo a detailed diagnostic imaging (including high-resolution prenatal ultrasounds, Doppler, fetal echocardiography, and fetal MRI) to describe the anatomy of the fetus and the uterus (localization of placenta, insertion of umbilical cord, etc.) and an amniocentesis to exclude other major anomalies and genetic disease.

A full well-being evaluation of the mother is also paramount. Some maternal diseases, such hypertension, diabetes, or obesity, could be a contraindication for surgery.

Specific informed consent must be signed before the procedure. If the surgery is performed after 23 weeks of gestation, when newborn is potentially viable, the discussion should include the course of action to take in case of unforeseen fetal instability and delivery of the baby in the OR.

Fetal anesthesia is provided primarily through the transplacental passage of the volatile anesthetics. However, this takes about an hour to reach 70% of the maternal levels. If any intervention is expected directly on the fetus, we administer an anesthetic cocktail comprising 10–20 mg/kg fentanyl, 20 mg/kg atropine, and 0.2 mg/kg vecuronium intramuscularly to the fetus.

Tocolytic agents are administered the day before, in the OR, and, based on the type of procedure, continued in the postoperative period. IV antibiotic is administered to the mother before the incision, and, also, it is recommended to administer another dose into the amniotic fluid at the end of the procedure.

76.3 Positioning

Fetoscopic procedures can be performed with local, epidural, or general endotracheal anesthesia. The patient is placed on the OR table supine or in lateral position, based on the type of procedure and placenta position. In addition to endoscopic video, a monitor with intraoperative US imaging should be visible to all surgeons during for the entire procedure. Screens are usually positioned at the head of the patient. In our institution, the surgical team includes at least one pediatric surgeon and one maternal-fetal medicine specialist, one at each side of the table. Some specific fetal surgeries also require the contribution of pediatric sub-specialties such as cardiology, neurosurgery, ENT, or urologists.

76.4 Instrumentation

Ultrasound must be on the sterile field for the whole surgical procedure to guide surgery and constantly monitor the well-being of the fetus. Before the procedure, it also identifies the position of the fetus or fetuses and the placenta and reviews the specific anatomic anomalies (spinal defect, amniotic band, bladder, etc.). Several purpose-designed fetoscopic instruments were developed (Fig. 76.1). Currently, we use a 10 Fr

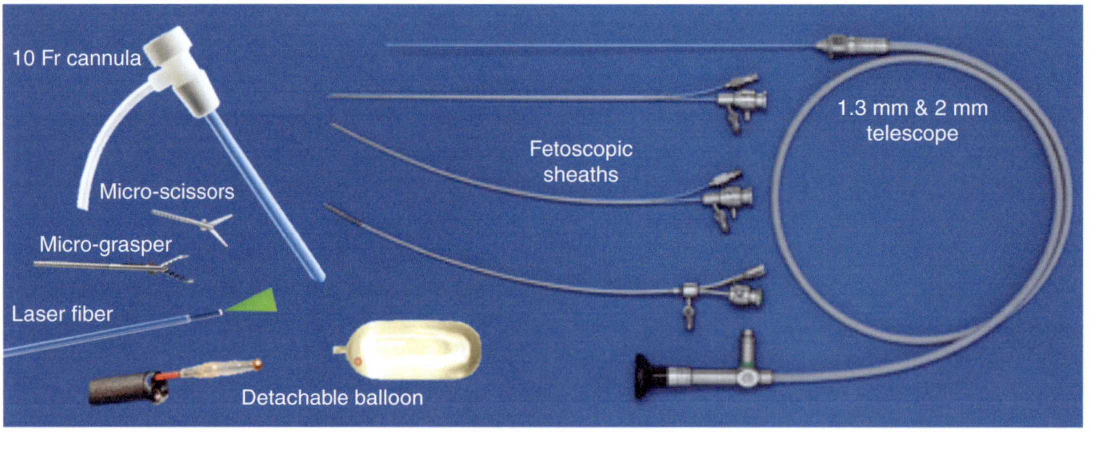

Fig. 76.1 Basic instruments and accessories for fetoscopic procedures

or 12 Fr valved cannulas inserted by Seldinger technique and semiflexible telescopes of 1.3 and 2 mm that fit inside a 2.7 mm rigid metallic sheath. The last can be curve, semi-curve, or straight, with working channels for amnioinfusion and instrumentation. Depending on the procedure, the instrumentation includes long needles, laser fiber, double-J urinary catheter, micro-graspers, micro-scissors, or a catheter connected to a detachable balloon.

Infusion apparatus of warm Ringer's lactate is also essential to clear our endoscopic visualization and replace the amniotic fluid lost.

76.5 Technique

Fetoscopic technique strictly defines the minimally invasive procedure on the uterus. Depending on the procedure and specific case, the uterus can be accessed percutaneously or be exteriorized through maternal laparotomy, for example, in the case of anterior placenta, fetal cystoscopy for urethral valves ablation, or fetoscopic spina bifida repair.

If oligohydramnios is present, amnioinfusion with warm Ringer's lactate may be performed to facilitate the fetoscopic surgery. Trocars' placement can't rely on external landmarks and depends completely on intraoperative ultrasound to assess the fetus, placental position, and desired target. In the case of percutaneous approach, after local anesthesia, a stab incision is made on the skin, and trocars are placed with Seldinger technique. Under continuous ultrasound guidance, the uterus is accessed with the needle, and a round-tipped guide wire is advanced; the trocar is then passed over the guide wire into the cavity. This procedure is repeated for all the needed access. A sharp tip on the sheath can be also used to introduce the fetoscope in the amniotic sac without cannula. By this technique we are not able to remove and enter repeatedly the fetoscope, which should stay intra-amniotic during the whole procedure to avoid multiple amniotic orifices.

In the case of externalized uterus, a maternal laparotomy is performed and the uterus exposed before accessing it. The needle is introduced without stub incision. In these cases, we advise to secure the trocars to the abdominal or uterine wall with a stitch to avoid dislodgement.

Once the fetoscope is introduced, the first step of all procedures is the direct visualization of the fetus, including limbs and umbilical cord. Surgeon must be always aware of these elements during his navigation in the amniotic cavity and during the actual procedure. Then he proceeds with the examination of the target and its accessibility.

In SFLP, a single trocar or sheath is placed in the sac of the recipient twin. Once inserted the fetoscope, a complete mapping of the vessels on the placental surface must be performed before any intervention. Umbilical cord placental insertions must be interrogated, and then, we list all vascular anastomosis between donor and recipient twins to recognize the vascular equator. These connections can be AA, VV, VA, and AV anastomosis. The inter-twin membrane serves as guidance to see vessels crossing, but we need to explore all 360° around to rule out any atypical vascular trajectory and peripheral anastomosis. Diode or Nd:YAG Laser photocoagulation (usually at 30–45 W of power) should be as selective as possible, directed only on connecting vessels without compromising the vascular support to the umbilical cords and the fetuses (Fig. 76.2).

In this condition, under some circumstances, an umbilical cord occlusion could be required. Laser energy can be used only early in gestation. Using a 10 Fr cannula, we can interrogate the umbilical cord anatomy and position and then introduce a 3 mm bipolar forceps to occlude the cord by diathermia (Fig. 76.2). There are optical forceps with the telescope integrated for direct visualization; otherwise, ultrasound guidance is required. This technique is used mostly in the twin reversed arterial perfusion (TRAP) sequence where an acardiac/acephalic monochorionic twin receives all of its blood from the normal or "pump" twin, and, as a result, the heart of the pump twin does extra work to sustain both fetuses and is at risk for heart failure and death.

Alternatively, radio-frequency ablation (RFA) is often used to stop the blood flow to the abnormal twin by percutaneous insertion of a

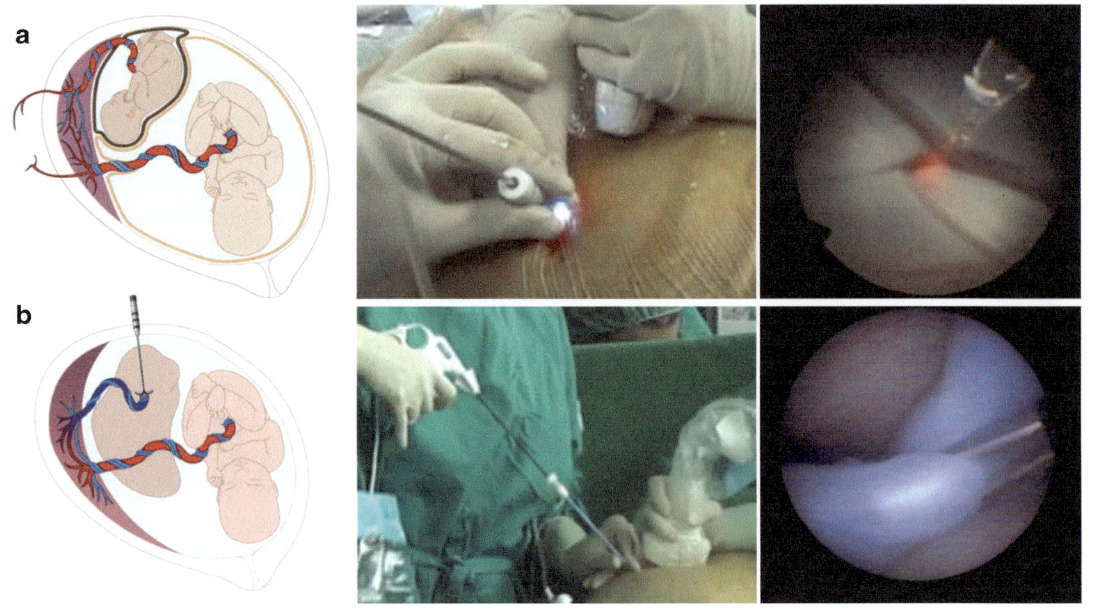

Fig. 76.2 (**a**) Monochorionic diamniotic twin pregnancy with TTTS. Percutaneous selective fetoscopic laser photocoagulation (SFLP) access and intrauterine vision. (**b**) Monochorionic twin pregnancy with TRAP. Percutaneous fetoscopic cord coagulation with bipolar diathermy

thick needle in the abdominal insertion of the cord of the acardiac twin under ultrasound guidance.

Fetoscopic endoluminal tracheal occlusion (FETO) performed for fetal endotracheal balloon placement for severe CDH prenatal therapy requires only one percutaneous trocar (Fig. 76.3). The fetoscope is guided into the fetal larynx and vocal cords to access fetal trachea with a combination of ultrasound guidance and direct visualization. Tracheal rings confirm the correct position and lead to the carina. The specific detachable balloon is then inserted pushing the catheter through the fetoscopic sheath and placed halfway between the carina and the vocal cord; the balloon is inflated with sterile saline and detached. The balloon can be removed fetoscopically in the same fashion or punctured under ultrasound guidance if necessary, around 34 weeks of gestation.

This same technique and approach can be used in congenital high airway obstruction syndrome (CHAOS) for re-permeabilization of bronchial, tracheal, or laryngeal web/atresia by means of laser fiber in contact with the obstructive tissue. Ultrasound guidance is crucial for an appropriate alienation of the fetoscope, laser fiber, and distended trachea before applying energy to make an orifice.

Constrictive amniotic bands can be approached with one or more trocars. Bands must be defined in all their lengths, courses, and connections with the fetus to determine the area of intervention. The surgeon can also visually confirm distal edema of the limb or possible amputations of fingers or toes. The bands can be released with graspers, if visible and accessible, or laser (usually at 40–50 W of power) to cut the point of constriction perpendicularly (Fig. 76.4). Umbilical cord appears involved in half of the cases (in 11 of 20 cases we did), so an accurate release of these bands is mandatory to avoid fetal demise by cord strangulation in the short term.

Fetal cystoscopy is used to diagnose and treat fetal low urinary tract obstructions (LUTO) or also called bladder outlet obstruction (BOO). Vesicoamniotic shunt (VAS) placement was the first procedure described to treat BBO, and it is still the most common procedure. VAS placement is currently performed as a percutaneous

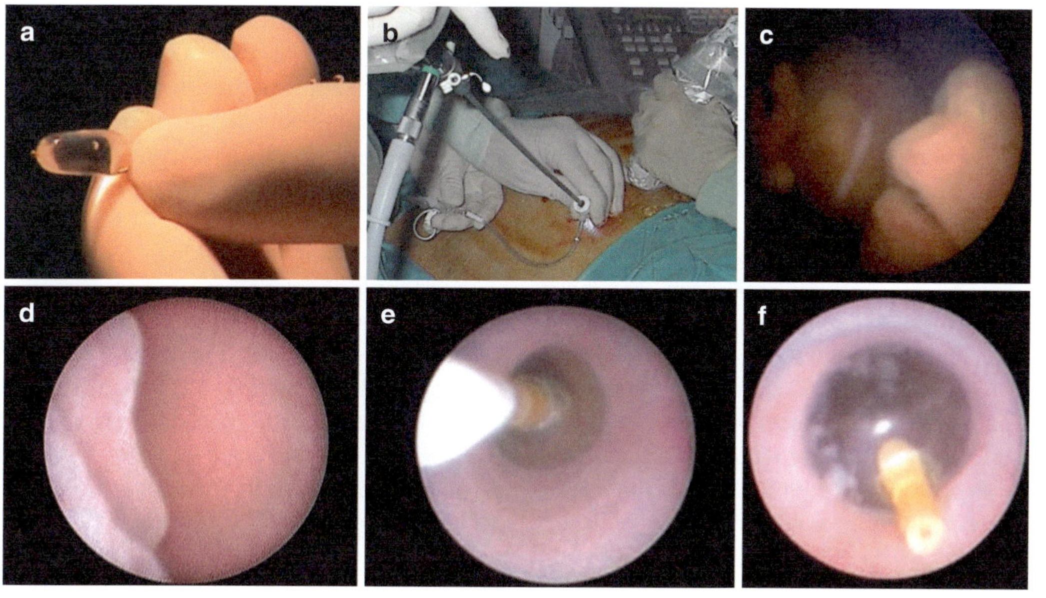

Fig. 76.3 FETO. (**a**) Detachable balloon inflated. (**b**) Percutaneous fetoscopy through intrauterine 10 Fr cannula. (**c**) Intrauterine view of fetal face and mouth. (**d**) Fetal epiglottis as an important landmark. (**e**) Inflation of the endotracheal balloon. (**f**) Detached inflated balloon for fetal tracheal occlusion

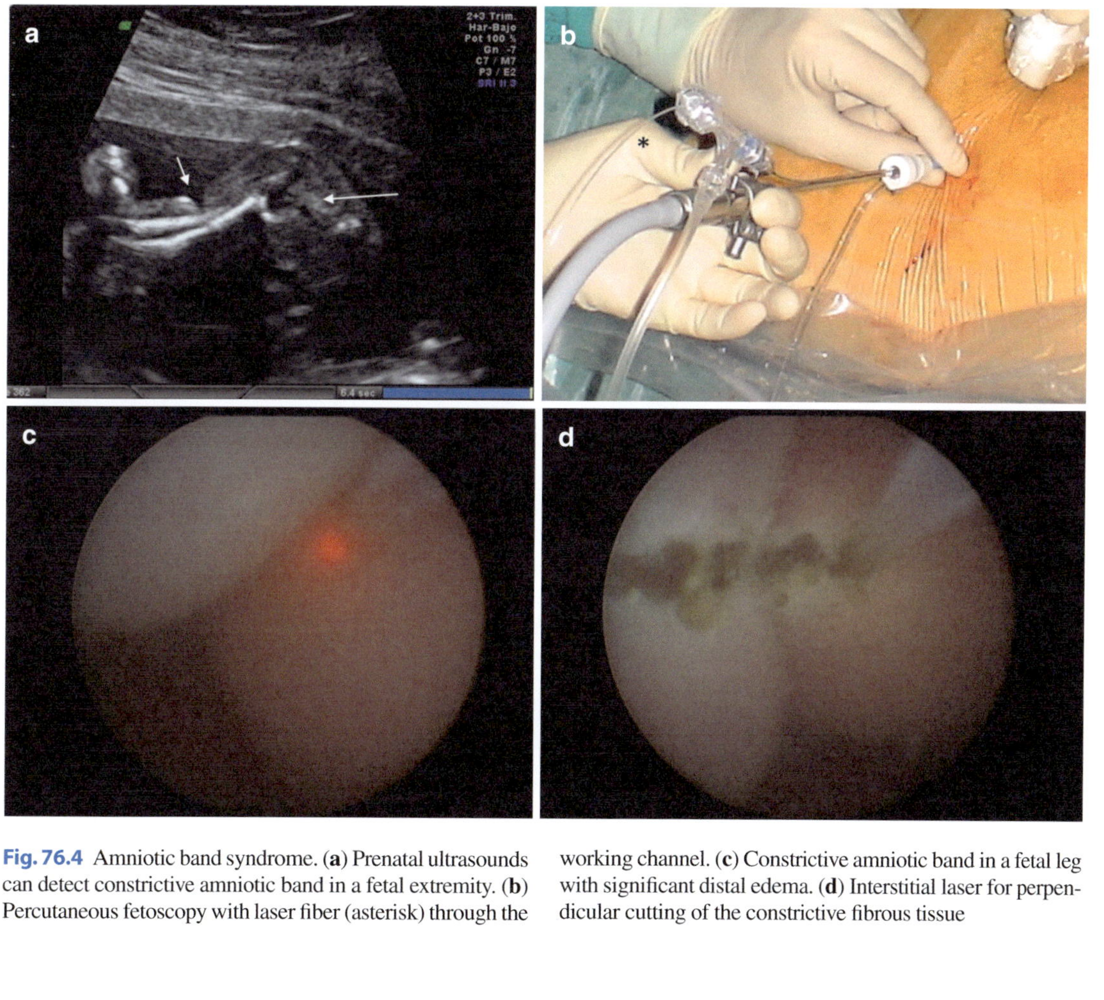

Fig. 76.4 Amniotic band syndrome. (**a**) Prenatal ultrasounds can detect constrictive amniotic band in a fetal extremity. (**b**) Percutaneous fetoscopy with laser fiber (asterisk) through the working channel. (**c**) Constrictive amniotic band in a fetal leg with significant distal edema. (**d**) Interstitial laser for perpendicular cutting of the constrictive fibrous tissue

procedure under ultrasound guidance. Fetal bladder can be easily identified, and one end of the double-pigtailed shunt can be pushed into the bladder to allow urine egression into the amniotic space. However, fetal cystoscopy is emerging as a useful technique to define the altered anatomy and introduce new treatment by a small fetoscope inserted percutaneously in the uterus with the previously described Seldinger technique. However, in this case, the sheath traverses both the maternal and fetal abdominal walls into the fetal bladder. The scope is then used to inspect the bladder neck and fetal posterior urethra. If posterior urethral valve (PUV) is visualized, these can be ablated with laser, and Doppler US can confirm the urine flow through the penile urethra (Fig. 76.5). Alternatively a transurethral catheter can be left for bladder decompression to the amniotic cavity.

As mention above, we use the fetoscopy with exposed uterus technique also in selected *fetal MMC* cases for neurosurgical repair of the spinal defect. A chamber of warm CO_2 is used to have better visualization of the neural placode that should be completely released and untethered before being covered by a protective dural substitute patch and a watertight suture of the skin in the midline (Fig. 76.6).

After maternal laparotomy, the uterus is exposed, and ultrasound is used to confirm the position of the fetus and the location of the defect. We find it useful to also mark the edges of the placenta. With gentle manipulation, the fetus can be positioned with the defect facing anteriorly and position of the trocars is decided. After the positioning of the trocars (in number of 3, to form a triangulation directed to the target) with the previously described Seldinger technique, we remove a part of the amniotic fluid (300–500 cc), and the uterine cavity is distended with warm carbon dioxide. The fetus can be fixed and kept in position with a transuterine stitch anchored on

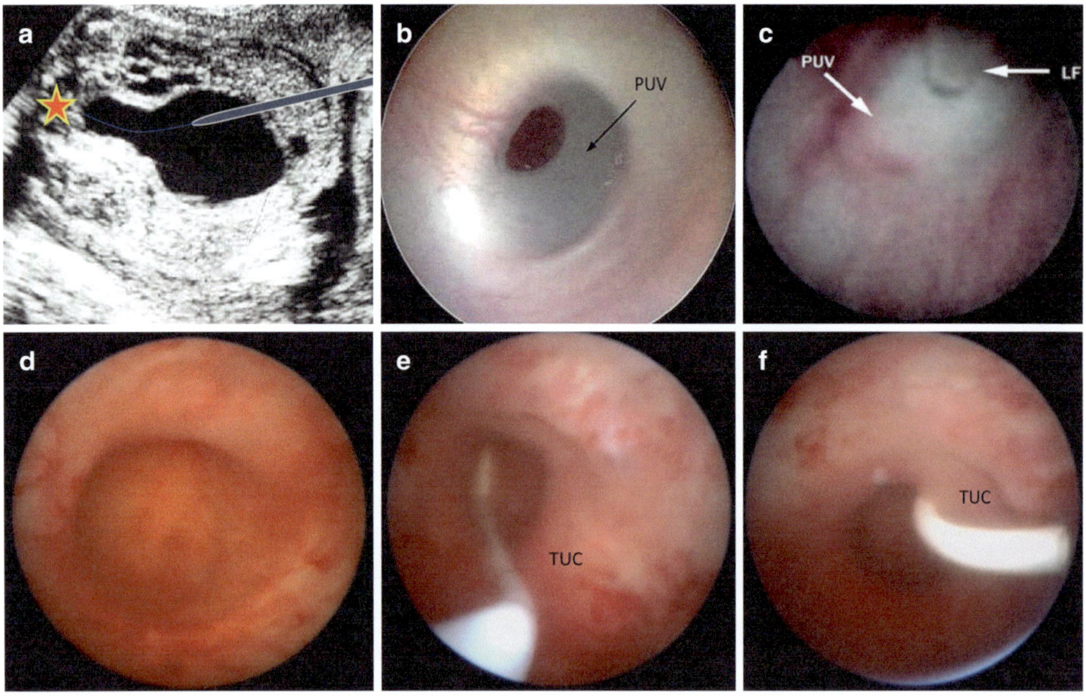

Fig. 76.5 Bladder outlet obstruction. (**a**) Prenatal ultrasounds detect oligohydramnios, distended bladder, and dilated posterior urethra (keyhole sign). (**b**) Intravesical image of posterior urethral valves (PUV). (**c**) Laser fiber (LF) fulgurating urethral valves. (**d**) Dilated fetal posterior urethra with difficult visualization of valves. (**e**) Introduction of a probe catheter through the urethral valves. (**f**) Double-J transurethral catheter (TUC) in place to decompress fetal urinary tract

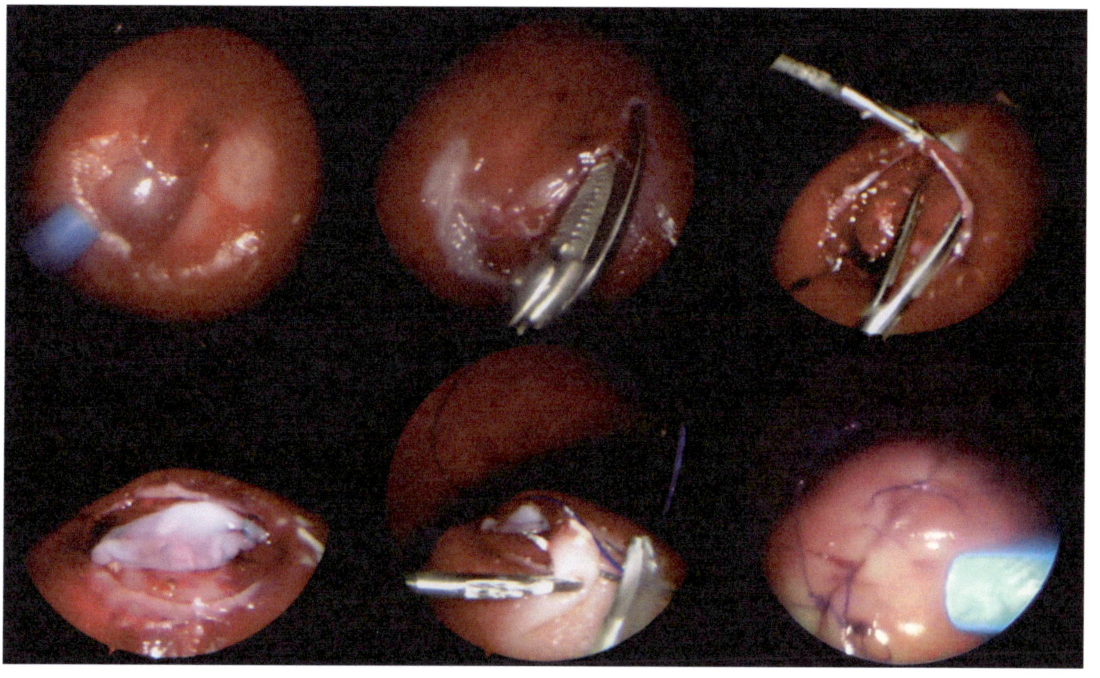

Fig. 76.6 Sequence of images in fetoscopic spina bifida prenatal repair. Release of the neural placode, removal of MMC sac, subcutaneous pocket for skin flaps, placement of a dural substitute patch, and skin closure with a barbed suture

the back. At this point, the repair of the spinal defect follows the usual steps: the sac is opened and resected, the placode is released from the surrounding tissue until it falls nicely in the spinal canal, and the defect is closed with a dural patch and skin flap or cutaneous substitute patch. At the end of the procedure, the trocars are removed, and transuterine U-shaped sutures are tied to close the port sites. The uterus is then repositioned into the peritoneal cavity, and the laparotomy is closed in the usual fashion.

In all procedures, intra-amniotic antibiotic is administered through the fetoscope before it is withdrawn entirety under ultrasound guidance. A loading dose of magnesium sulfate or other tocolytic agent is administered to the mother at the end of the procedure to avoid uterine contractions.

76.6 Postoperative Care

All patients must stay bed rest for at least 24 h. Tocolysis is one of the most important aspects in the postoperative care of fetal surgery; common medications are magnesium sulfate, nifedipine, terbutaline, nitroglycerin, and indomethacin. In Europe, atosiban, an inhibitor of oxytocin, is also widely used for tocolysis.

Another key aspect is the follow-up of fetus conditions and the impact of the surgery on the congenital malformation. Serial ultrasounds are scheduled usually once or twice a week. For CDH fetus and intrathoracic lesions, we schedule also a repeated MRI around 34 weeks' gestation to categorize the severity of the pulmonary hypoplasia and define a plan for delivery.

C-section is not mandatory after fetoscopic surgery, like what happens in open fetal surgery, so delivery can be vaginal unless there are other specific or obstetric contraindications.

76.7 Results

Fetoscopy still carries some risks when rupture of membranes and early delivery are the most common complications, but still significantly less than the open approach. One of the biggest ongoing trials using a fetoscopic procedure is the international TOTAL trial for fetoscopic tracheal occlusion in severe and moderate CDH [3]. In these studies, preliminary data reported premature rupture of membrane in 16.7% of pregnancies within 3 weeks from the procedure. Overall mean delivery was at 35.3 weeks of gestation, but 1/3 occurred before 34 weeks. The comparison with the historical registry for CDH shows an increased survival in severe left CDH from 24.1 to 49.1% [6]. Other randomized studies using FETO [7] showed similar results in survival, improving it up to 55% with tracheal occlusion from the 5% without fetal intervention, in severe CDH patients. Fetal pulmonary response after FETO is the most important factor associated with survival, independently from the gestational age at delivery [8].

As mentioned, the fetoscopic approach for MMC varies in different centers, and an analysis on the real results of these techniques compared to the standard open approach is difficult. Nevertheless, fetoscopic approach to repair neural tube defect does not appear to increase the risk for maternal-fetal complication when compared to repair by hysterotomy and allows vaginal delivery [9]. Moreover, experimental studies are ongoing to further reduce the number of the trocars. On an animal model, we were able to repair a surgically created fetal MMC with single-access fetal endoscopy (SAFE). With this technique, patch and glue can successfully repair the defect and restore gross neurologic function in the lamb [10], but seems not to be the same in human where a more permanent glue is required to warrant the watertightness during whole gestation.

Now, techniques using two or three mini-ports are developed and under study in clinical trials.

The benefit of SFLP for perinatal survival and quality of life has been reported in literature, and clinical trials have proved their superiority compared with amnioreduction only [11]. A European randomized trial showed improvement in survival of at least one of the twins with SFLP (76% vs. 56% with amnioreduction only) as well as in gestational age at delivery (pregnancy lasted 4 weeks more) and neurological outcomes of the survivors. Many groups add a Solomon technique using laser to fulgurate the line in between the selective coagulations to avoid missing any tiny vascular connection on the vascular equator [12]. In our series, after more than 1000 cases of SFLP performed for TTTS indication, the overall survival is 84%, being survival of both twins in 75% and achieving at least one twin alive in 92% of the operated cases.

In a systematic review, Tan et al. [13] show that acardiac twin ablation is technically easy and safe, with low preterm delivery or PROM before 32 weeks (7 out of 31) with a high survival of the pumping twin of 26 out of 31 in his experience for the treatment of TRAP sequence. Bipolar coagulation of the acardiac cord is very effective. Anyway, we usually use percutaneous radiofrequency ablation (RFA) needle to block the blood flow in the abdominal insertion of the acardiac mass, with excellent results.

In a large cohort of 111 fetuses with lower urinary tract obstruction (LUTO), Ruano et al. reported a significantly higher probability of survival with fetal cystoscopy and vesicoamniotic shunt compared to no intervention (adjusted relative risk (ARR), 1.86 (95% CI, 1.01–3.42; $P = 0.048$), and ARR, 1.73 (95% CI, 1.01–3.08; $P = 0.04$), respectively). They reported also a trend for normal renal function in the group treated with fetal cystoscopy (ARR, 1.16 (95% CI, 0.86–1.55; $P = 0.33$)) that was not observed in the vesicoamniotic shunt group [14].

With the advent of less-invasive fetal surgery techniques, nonlethal disorders are considered amenable to intrauterine treatment when they result in severe disabilities in the postnatal life such as amputating constrictive amniotic bands. This condition can cause an intrauterine amputation as a result of a mechanical effect with progressive strangulation of a limb or umbilical cord. In this last case, the cord involvement can potentially be lethal. These consequences can be avoided by fetoscopic amniotic band release using laser or micro-instruments after prenatal detection [15]. We have performed 20 cases of fetoscopic constrictive band release between 17 and 31 weeks of gestation (average 23 weeks), affecting mostly left leg and significantly involving umbilical cord in half of cases. Survival of 90% and good functional recovery of the operated extremities reflect the efficacy of this prenatal therapy.

76.8 Tips and Tricks

76.8.1 SFLP for TTTS

Selection of percutaneous site for amniotic access is crucial to have a good visualization of the vascular equator, and complete mapping can be possible. Obviously, anterior placenta makes this more difficult, since we need to look for a window free of placenta (transplacental access is not an option because the size of the fetoscope will produce significant bleeding). Fetal MR imaging and accurate ultrasounds/color Doppler guidance will facilitate to determine the optimal lateral window to introduce the curved fetoscope as much posterior and far away from the placental margin as possible. We recommend to put the patient in a lateral position and break the operating table to open the space between iliac crest and ribs.

Once inside the amniotic sac, we can have blur vision for the characteristics of amniotic fluid in gestations after 24 weeks or because of some bleeding of the insertion site. If this impaired vision affects our ability to do an appropriate mapping, then amnio-exchange will be useful by suctioning fluid and replacing it with clear warm Ringer's lactate.

Identify both umbilical cord insertions in placenta, and use intertwin membrane as a guide to see vessels crossing is essential. A 360-degree exploration around the intertwin membrane is recommended to not miss any atypical peripheral anastomosis outside placental surface. Complete mapping and remapping before starting laser also is crucial. With that, we can reduce significantly the time of lasering. Never contact the vessels to avoid bleeding, and in the case of a large-size vessel, laser first both sides to narrow its caliber, and then fulgurate the center. Always complete amnioreduction and administer intra-amniotic antibiotic.

76.8.2 FETO for Severe CDH

In this percutaneous fetoscopic procedure, appropriate fetal position is crucial. So, fetal external eversion is recommended until achievement of an optimal fetal position and then ultrasound-guided intramuscular injection of the fetal anesthetic cocktail for immobilization. Starting this procedure on a sub-optimal position can be a nightmare. It's always better to cancel the case and reschedule it 1 or 2 days later to try again for a better fetal position and head orientation. Once the scope is in the amniotic sac, use ultrasounds to orientate the tip of the fetoscope looking for the tip of the nose. Then use direct visualization, to navigate on the fetal face surface until you can identify the upper lip and gum. Introduce the scope over the tongue flushing warm Ringer's solution, and try to identify mucosal creases of the palate.

I recommend advance slowly and stay some time in this oral position until fetus helps deflecting the neck and head. Then we can go forward flushing fluid and opening structures.

Polyhydramnios can make this progression difficult when the fetus is floating in a distended amniotic cavity, so it could be helpful to limit the use of amnioinfusion or drain some amniotic fluid.

An important landmark is fetal epiglottis. If you don't identify it easily, a useful maneuver is to enter into the esophagus and then go back slowly until arytenoid folds or epiglottis is identified.

Once in the fetal trachea, where you can see cartilage rings and floppy posterior membrane, watch out! Identifying the actual carina can be difficult when you have a shifted mediastinum, characteristic of CDH. The main bronchus can be alienated with the direction of trachea, and carina can be unnoticed laterally. Inflation of the balloon in a main bronchus will produce severe damage in the fetal airway with ruptured bronchus and hydrothorax. So, don't go too deep; use guidance of ultrasounds, and be careful to identify the carina properly.

At the time of second fetoscopy for unplugging the fetal trachea, sometimes it is tough to pop the balloon with a needle. Laser fiber active in contact with balloon surface is an easy way to create a pore and deflate it.

76.8.3 Amniotic Band Release

Once the amniotic sac is accessed with the fetoscope, try to use the working channel to introduce laser fiber or micro-instruments like scissors or forceps. When the angle of those tools isn't optimal, use a second trocar if necessary to achieve the perpendicular projection to the constrictive band.

If the band is deep because of significant distal edema, use laser energy by tissue contact to cut perpendicularly the constrictive line, but always do it over the lateral external side of the extremity, avoiding injuries to the vascular or nerve elements of the limb.

Always double-check if the umbilical cord is not involved, and review all four extremities for other potential non-constrictive amniotic bands at that point.

76.8.4 Fetal Cystoscopy for BOO

Some authors use percutaneous access to the bladder, but sometimes the angle with the distended posterior urethra is so high and doesn't allow good visualization of the posterior urethral valves. We prefer to expose the uterus through a mini-laparotomy to insert our needle in a better angle entering the dome of the dilated fetal bladder. We use two T-fasteners before we insert the cannula and fetoscope in between for traction of the fetal bladder wall to the fetal abdominal wall during procedure to avoid fetal ascites and bladder leak. We use a probe urologic catheter to identify the valves in the posterior urethra under direct visualization. If the angle still doesn't allow perfect access to the valves for a safe laser ablation, we insert a double-J transurethral catheter for fetal bladder decompression. In case the diagnosis is urethral atresia on the fetal cystoscopy, a vesicoamniotic shunt (Harrison or Rodeck) is inserted through the same access and cannula.

76.8.5 Fetoscopic MMC Prenatal Repair

This is a technique still on evolution and under study. It should be limited to fetal centers with large experience in fetoscopy and prenatal treatment of spina bifida. Recently we created an international consortium for registry and study group. Still time and publications of these studies are required before globally recommending this minimally invasive approach for the prenatal repair of MMC.

Exposed uterus has been useful in our experience for allowing optimal intrauterine amniodistention and space with minimal CO_2 pressure, for better repositioning and orientation of the fetus, for better location access for trocar insertion, and for allowing the possibility to close the amniotic holes at the end of the procedure.

We recommend the use of warm and humidified CO_2 to maintain the appropriate fetal body temperature and avoid instability or acidosis. Humidification can play an important role in preserving the integrity of the amnion to avoid postoperative rupture of membranes and preterm delivery. When the fetus requires better position and stabilization, to apply a transuterine traction stitch in the fetal back becomes really useful. Use of lateral relaxing skin incisions or skin substitute patches allows close the skin in the midline to watertight cover the defect in almost all cases.

76.9 Discussion

Severe congenital anomalies can lead to the demise of the fetus during pregnancy or shortly after birth, as in the case of TTTS or CDH. Some other conditions, such as MMC or amniotic bands, although nonlethal, can cause severe disability and limb amputation. Unfortunately, at the moment, only few fetal malformations can be addressed or improved with prenatal intervention. Moreover, the decision to perform fetal intervention is complex. With progression in this field, survival outcomes have also improved over the last decades. Ongoing prospective trials aim to characterize fetuses that can benefit from surgery. Indeed, every prenatal intervention must balance the risk not only for the fetus but also for the mother. For this reason, fetal therapy is undoubtedly moving toward minimally invasive approach to minimize the hazard of the procedures.

Some fetoscopic procedures are simply adaptations of open technique. MOMS study, published in 2011, showed that prenatal surgery increases the possibility of ambulation, can revert hindbrain herniation, decreases the need for ventriculo-peritoneal shunt, and improves neurological development. On the other hand, open technique resulted in maternal morbidity and preterm delivery (13% of babies were born before 30 weeks). As in the open procedure, fetoscopy for MMC aims to watertight close the spinal defect, but the approach varies in different centers, with three ports placed percutaneously or accessing the uterus with two or three ports though maternal laparotomy [4].

Other procedures were specifically developed for prenatal treatment, as, for example, in the case of CDH, where the purpose of the procedure is to stimulate growth and development of the lung rather than correct the primary defect.

A crucial factor contributing the success of fetal therapy is the multidisciplinary approach, joining the skills of various specialists. Beside the pediatric surgeon, the core group must include neonatologists, anesthesiologist, radiologists, and maternal-fetal-medicine specialists among many others. Certain cases require specific specialists, such as neurosurgeons or urologists.

Currently, fetoscopy is effective for treating many fetal conditions. Nonetheless, rupture of membranes still remains the main disadvantage of these procedures, and research should focus on this fact to find solutions. Refinement of the techniques and technologic advances will allow future use of minimally invasive interventions for other fetal anomalies that will broaden the frontiers of fetoscopic surgery.

References

1. Peiró JL, Carreras E, Guillén G, Arévalo S, Sánchez-Durán MA, Higueras T, Castillo F, Marhuenda C, Lloret J, Martínez-Ibáñez V. Therapeutic indications of fetoscopy: a 5-year institutional experience. J Laparoendosc Adv Surg Tech A. 2009;19(2):229–36.
2. Khalek N, Johnson MP, Bebbington MW. Fetoscopic laser therapy for twin-to-twin transfusion syndrome. Semin Pediatr Surg. 2013;22(1):18–23.
3. Deprest J, Brady P, Nicolaides K, Benachi A, Berg C, Vermeesch J, Gardener G, Gratacos E. Prenatal management of the fetus with isolated congenital diaphragmatic hernia in the era of the TOTAL trial. Semin Fetal Neonatal Med. 2014;19(6):338–48.
4. Adzick NS, Thom EA, Spong CY, Brock JW 3rd, Burrows PK, Johnson MP, Howell LJ, Farrell JA, Dabrowiak ME, Sutton LN, Gupta N, Tulipan NB, D'Alton ME, Farmer DL, MOMS Investigators. A randomized trial of prenatal versus postnatal repair of myelomeningocele. N Engl J Med. 2011;364(11):993–1004.
5. Kohl T, Hering R, Heep A, Schaller C, Meyer B, Greive C, Bizjak G, Buller T, van de Vondel P, Gogarten W, Bartmann P, Knöpfle G, Gembruch U. Percutaneous fetoscopic patch coverage of spina bifida aperta in the human—early clinical experience and potential. Fetal Diagn Ther. 2006;21:185–93.
6. Jani J, Nicolaides KH, Keller RL, Benachi A, Peralta CF, Favre R, Moreno O, Tibboel D, Lipitz S, Eggink A, Vaast P, Allegaert K, Harrison M, Deprest J, Antenatal-CDH-Registry Group. Observed to expected lung area to head circumference ratio in the prediction of survival in fetuses with isolated diaphragmatic hernia. Ultrasound Obstet Gynecol. 2007;30(1):67–71.
7. Ruano R, Yoshisaki CT, da Silva MM, Ceccon ME, Grasi MS, Tannuri U, Zugaib M. A randomized controlled trial of fetal endoscopic tracheal occlusion versus postnatal management of severe isolated congenital diaphragmatic hernia. Ultrasound Obstet Gynecol. 2012;39(1):20–7.
8. Sananes N, Rodo C, Peiro JL, Britto IS, Sangi-Haghpeykar H, Favre R, Joal A, Gaudineau A, Silva MM, Tannuri U, Zugaib M, Carreras E, Ruano R. Prematurity and fetal lung response after tracheal occlusion in fetuses with severe congenital diaphragmatic hernia. J Matern Fetal Neonatal Med. 2016;29(18):3030–4.
9. Belfort MA, Whitehead WE, Shamshirsaz AA, Bateni ZH, Olutoye OO, Olutoye OA, Mann DG, Espinoza J, Williams E, Lee TC, Keswani SG, Ayres N, Cassady CI, Mehollin-Ray AR, Sanz Cortes M, Carreras E, Peiro JL, Ruano R, Cass DL. Fetoscopic open neural tube defect repair: development and refinement of a two-port, carbon dioxide insufflation technique. Obstet Gynecol. 2017;129(4):734–43.
10. Peiro JL, Fontecha CG, Ruano R, Esteves M, Fonseca C, Marotta M, Haeri S, Belfort MA. Single-access

fetal endoscopy (SAFE) for myelomeningocele in sheep model I: amniotic carbon dioxide gas approach. Surg Endosc. 2013;27(10):3835–40.
11. Senat MV, Deprest J, Boulvain M, Paupe A, Winer N, Ville Y. Endoscopic laser surgery versus serial amnioreduction for severe twin-to-twin transfusion syndrome. N Engl J Med. 2004;351:136–44.
12. Ruano R, Rodo C, Peiro JL, Shamshirsaz AA, Haeri S, Nomura ML, Salustiano EM, de Andrade KK, Sangi-Haghpeykar H, Carreras E, Belfort MA. Fetoscopic laser ablation of placental anastomoses in twin-twin transfusion syndrome using 'Solomon technique'. Ultrasound Obstet Gynecol. 2013;42(4):434–9.
13. Tan TY, Sepulveda W. Acardiac twin: a systematic review of minimally invasive treatment modalities. Ultrasound Obstet Gynecol. 2003;22(4):409–19.
14. Ruano R, Sananes N, Sangi-Haghpeykar H, Hernandez-Ruano S, Moog R, Becmeur F, Zaloszyc A, Giron AM, Morin B, Favre R. Fetal intervention for severe lower urinary tract obstruction: a multicenter case-control study comparing fetal cystoscopy with vesicoamniotic shunting. Ultrasound Obstet Gynecol. 2015;45(4):452–8.
15. Peiró JL, Carreras E, Soldado F, Sanchez-Duran MA, Aguirre M, Barber I, Martinez-Ibañez V. Fetoscopic release of umbilical cord amniotic band in a human fetus. Ultrasound Obstet Gynecol. 2009;33(2):232–4.

Application of Minimally Invasive Surgery in Paediatric Oncology

77

Thomas Blanc, Luca Pio, and Sabine Sarnacki

77.1 Introduction

Childhood cancers represent 1% of all cancers. This equates to a paediatric cancer incidence of 122 cases per million children in the United States or 1800 new patients each year (700 between the ages of 15 and 19 years) in France. As a result of advances in treatment, almost 80% of children and adolescent who receive a diagnosis of cancer become long-term survivors [1]. Efforts are therefore directed towards decreasing sequels and improving quality of life. In the surgical field, this includes less mutilating procedure such as nephron- or ovarian-sparing surgery, fertility preservation procedures and minimally invasive surgery (MIS). The well-recognized advantage of MIS that reduces parietal injury and risk of wound infections and favours fast-track rehabilitation is an important factor to consider for cancer patients requiring a long-lasting multimodal treatment strategy.

Indications could be divided in four main areas: staging, biopsy, supportive care and resection. Since the first report of Holcomb et al. in 1995 of a series of children with thoracic and abdominal cancer undergoing biopsy thanks to MIS [2], many authors confirmed then the feasibility and accuracy of MIS not only for diagnosis purposes but also for resection of children solid cancers. This approach developed however more slowly for essentially three reasons:

1. Indications are few as most of children cancers are embryonic tumours with a huge size at diagnosis and even after size reduction by neoadjuvant chemotherapy.
2. Paediatric oncologists feared incomplete resection and most of all peritoneal dissemination with higher rate recurrence as it was described in adults.
3. Paediatric surgeons involved historically in children cancer were not those that were the pioneers of MIS, and it took some time to merge both expertises.

The use of MIS in paediatric oncology is now a part of the tools offered to cure children from cancer and should be discussed when appropriate, provided the surgery follows the same basic oncologic than those applied to open surgery. Although the literature is profuse and generally underlines the feasibility, advantages and limits of this approach [3–5], randomized prospective clinical trials are lacking to elaborate worldwide-accepted guidelines [6]. Reports of tumour graft on site ports are currently very few [7] but should be considered as a potential risk when performing MIS in paediatric oncology.

T. Blanc · L. Pio · S. Sarnacki (✉)
Pediatric Surgery and Urology Department, AP-HP, Hopital Necker Enfants Malades, Université Paris Descartes, Sorbonne Paris Cité, Paris, France
e-mail: sabine.sarnacki@aphp.fr

C. Esposito et al. (eds.), *ESPES Manual of Pediatric Minimally Invasive Surgery*,
https://doi.org/10.1007/978-3-030-00964-9_77

77.2 Case Selection and Indications

In the absence of official guidelines, the indication for minimally invasive diagnostic biopsy or ablative surgery is generally considered and approved by an interdisciplinary panel, including paediatric oncologists, surgeons, radiologists, radiotherapists and pathologists. The expertise of the surgical team should gather knowledge of children cancer treatment strategies and surgical skills not only with MIS but also with open procedures. The main obvious contraindications for MIS in paediatric oncology are huge and fragile tumour carrying a high risk of tumour spillage, extensive previous surgery resulting in dense intra-abdominal or thoracic adhesions and severe respiratory impairment. Tumour spillage results indeed in intensified chemotherapy regimens and radiotherapy in these children with a high risk of recurrence impairing their prognosis. It is thus mandatory not to hesitate to convert to an open procedure if there is any doubt in the quality of resection or any risk of spillage or complication that may delay the post-operative recovery and thus the pursue of treatment.

The main tumours for which minimally invasive resection are not debated are those that can be fragmented during open procedure: neuroectodermal tumours (neuroblastoma, ganglioneuroblastoma and ganglioneuroma), pheochromocytoma, paraganglioma and benign tumours. In contrast, MIS for tumours that cannot be fragmented such as Wilms tumours, adrenocortical tumours, malignant ovarian tumours and solid pseudopapillary tumour or Frantz tumour remain a matter of debate.

77.3 Abdominal Tumours

77.3.1 Technical Notes

From the technical point of view, different approaches may be considered: transperitoneal approach (laparoscopy) or retroperitoneal approach (lateral and prone), mostly depending on the localization and the size of the tumour and the experience of the surgeon [5]. Laparoscopic approach is generally preferred because of a larger working space and more familiar anatomic landmarks, which are crucial to the surgeon. Limits of the retroperitoneal approach lie in the absence of the ability to explore the abdominal cavity. In the context of malignancy, the first step of any procedure is to make a proper staging which comprises the exploration of the parietal peritoneum and Douglas cul-de-sac, a step greatly facilitated by the MIS approach. Whenever recommended, lymph node sampling should precede tumour excision, as tissues may retract following tumour ablation and limit lymph node exposure.

Once completely dissected, tumours are most commonly removed from the abdomen in an endoscopic bag by enlarging the umbilical port site or through a suprapubic incision. This step of the procedure should be considered as important as the dissection steps in order to avoid bag rupture and tumour spillage, whatever the nature of the tumour. The specific technical issues for adrenal, renal and pancreatic surgery are described in the respective chapters of this book.

77.3.2 Neuroblastoma and Adrenal Tumours

Neuroblastomas (NBs) are the most common extracranial solid tumours in children. They mostly arise from the abdomen (adrenal gland 48%, extra-adrenal retroperitoneum 25%), less frequently from the chest (16%) and rarely from the pelvis (3%) or the neck (3%). These tumours are associated with remarkable biological heterogeneity and outcome. Some NBs may undergo spontaneous regression; some are cured by surgery alone or after chemo-reduction, while others have an extremely aggressive behaviour with metastases and recurrences despite intensive treatments. The main indications of MIS in NBs treatment are currently:

77.3.2.1 Tumour Biopsy

Procurement of tumour tissue is mandatory to confirm the diagnosis, define the histological type (favourable or not) and the genetic alterations (MYCN status and other anomalies) and assign the patient in the appropriate treatment group. Although percutaneous biopsy is the less invasive approach to obtain tumour tissue, a minimally invasive approach is of great help when the tumour location is not favourable for a percutaneous approach or when a huge amount of tissue is required.

77.3.2.2 Tumour Resection

The introduction of image-defined risk factors (IDRFs) in the clinical practice has brought more objective criteria to define the surgical risk of tumour removal. In the absence of IDRF, regardless the size of the tumour, MIS has been established as safe alternative to open ablative surgery essentially in adrenal tumours and thoracic neuroblastoma arising from the paravertebral parasympathetic chain [8] (Fig. 77.1).

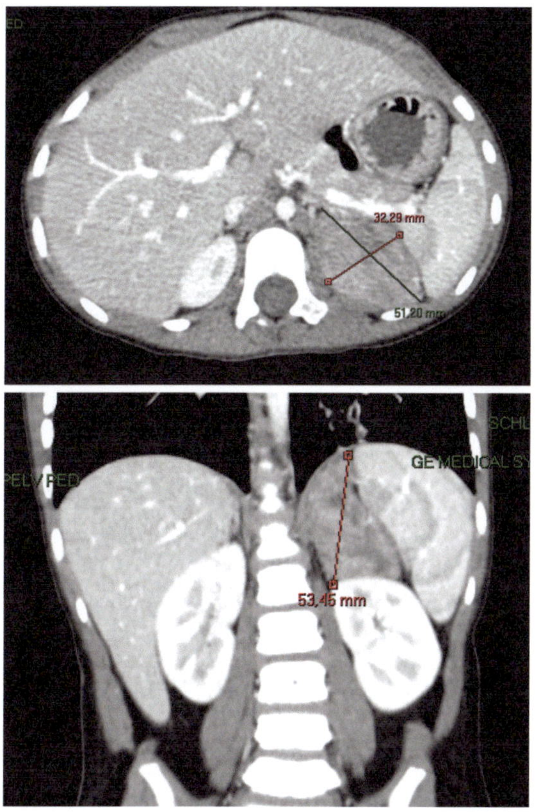

Fig. 77.1 Adrenal neuroblastoma without image-defined risk factors (no contact with renal vessels): a good indication for MIS

The first reports on MIS included a high percentage of infants diagnosed perinatally with an adrenal tumour. Regarding the high rate of tumour spontaneous regression and/or maturation in this population, an expectant observation is currently recommended, provided that the patient has no life-threatening symptoms and that the tumour is of favourable biology and not increasing in size. When persisting after 12 months with no IDRFs, these adrenal tumours are good candidates for surgical resection with MIS. In contrast, when IDRFs are persisting after this wait-and-see strategy, the question of surgery in tumour with good biology is still debated whatever the surgical approach, open or MIS. The presence of IDRFs in most of the other abdominal extra-adrenal locations of NBs explained that MIS has been poorly reported for these locations. In the thorax, NBs arising from the paravertebral parasympathetic chain appeared as the best indication for MIS. MIS is particularly interesting in mature neurogenic tumours such as ganglioneuroblastoma and ganglioneuroma in the thorax but also in the abdomen or the pelvis as the benefit of surgery for those tumours is still debated [4, 5].

Adrenocortical tumours are rare tumours, representing 0.2% of all paediatric malignancies, i.e. 0.1–0.4 out of one million. Complete excision is the treatment of choice, as they usually do not respond to chemo- or radiotherapy. The risk of spillage is considerably high due to the friability of the tumour's capsule and impairs notably the prognosis of these very aggressive tumours. Biopsy is thus formally contraindicated, and although surgery may appear not difficult when the tumour is small and localized to the adrenal gland, laparoscopic resection should be discouraged when clinical presentation and imaging favour this diagnosis.

Pheochromocytoma and paraganglioma are rare catecholamine-secreting tumours in children, benign in approximately 90% of cases. Regarding the possible cardiac impact of the associated hypertension, a preoperative preparation of the patient is usually mandatory. Surgical resection is the main treatment. The advantage of MIS on open procedure is well recognized, as it allows less manipulation of the lesion, less

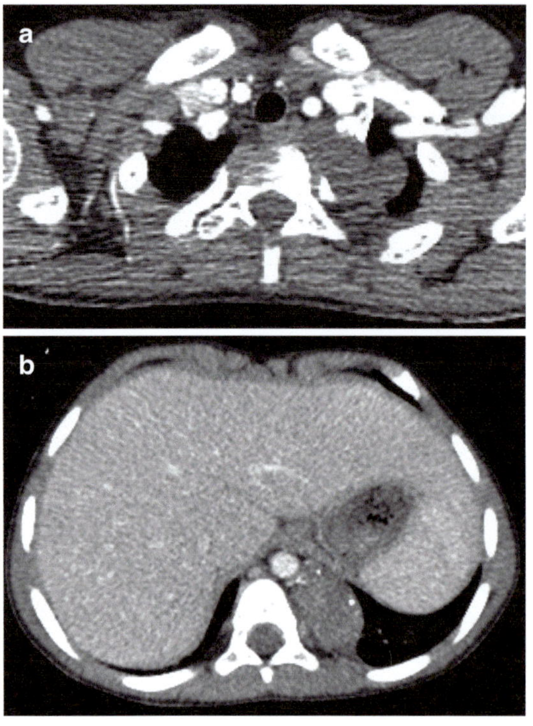

Fig. 77.2 MIS delivers easy access to upper (**a**) and lower (**b**) paravertebral neuroblastoma

delivery of catecholamines during the procedure and thus less tensional instability (Fig. 77.2). Although only case reports are documented, MIS is an accepted procedure for pheochromocytoma, especially when bilateral.

77.3.3 Renal Tumours

Wilms tumour or nephroblastoma is the most common malignant renal tumour of childhood, representing 90% of all malignant renal tumours. Complete surgical resection, without spillage, associated with a sufficient lymph node sampling (at least six) is the main goal of surgical treatment and strongly predicts final outcome. Intraoperative tumour spillage influences the multimodality treatment intensity as it upgrades the local staging to stage III and requires thus post-operative irradiation of the whole abdominal cavity, worsening the overall prognosis. Insufficient lymph node sampling may also lead to under staging and risk of recurrence and/or metastasis. Limited working space, risk of tumour rupture and difficulties in correct lymph node sampling are factors that explain that MIS may greatly affect the safety of the procedure especially in large tumours. Based on a multicentric study of 24 patients, Varlet et al. concluded that only lesion that is not extending beyond the midline may be potential candidate for MIS, whereas the presence of inferior vena cava or renal thrombosis, adhesions to other organs and initial tumour rupture would strongly contraindicate such an approach [9]. A recent series combined with a complete review of the literature identified 104 cases of laparoscopic transperitoneal radical nephrectomy (LTRN) with an incidence of local recurrence of 3.8%, a number lower than the one observed in European series (e.g. with neoadjuvant chemotherapy) with open surgery. The authors also underlined that tumours amenable to minimally invasive surgery are smaller, with higher numbers of low stage and standard histology [10]. Finally nephron-sparing surgery (NSS) should be preferentially considered when the tumour is small, as it preserves renal function.

Other malignant non-Wilms renal tumours: They consist of rare subgroups including clear cell sarcoma of the kidney (CCSK), renal cell carcinoma (RCC), malignant rhabdoid tumours of the kidney (MRTK), congenital mesoblastic nephroma (CMN) and few others, even rarer tumours. Complete radical resection together with extended lymph nodes dissection is the cornerstone of treatment for most of them. They are currently a contraindication of MIS.

77.3.4 Ovarian Tumours

Ovarian tumours in children and adolescents consist mainly in germ cell tumours (GCT), including a benign condition, the mature teratoma, which is the most commonly encountered and malignant tumours (yolk sac tumour, choriocarcinoma, teratoma, gonadoblastoma, dysgerminoma). The other ovarian tumour types are benign epithelial tumours (serous and mucinous cystadenoma) and sex cord-stromal tumours, mainly represented by juvenile granulosa cell tumour (JGCT) and Sertoli-Leydig cell tumours, both highly malignant. In most of the cases, surgery will be the only treatment, and the prognosis will be good, provided the surgery is done adequately. If a malignant tumour is ruptured during surgery, adjuvant chemotherapy will be required with its own morbidity (especially hearing loss with the cisplatin-derived drugs included in most of the protocols). Thus the main challenge is to recognize a benign condition that requires an ovarian-sparing procedure to minimize the risk of long-term ovarian failure and infertility from a malignant tumour where a complete ovariectomy/adnexectomy and a proper inspection of the peritoneal cavity are mandatory. In this context, laparoscopy is of great help for an appropriate staging by allowing a complete inspection of the peritoneum and omentum but should be used very carefully for ovarian tumour surgical treatment as the malignant or benign nature of these lesions is not always easy to determine (malignant non-secreting tumours) [11]. Some teams preferred to approach any ovarian lesion by a suspubic approach, especially for ovarian-sparing surgery, as it is safe and ensures an optimal sparing of the remaining ovarian parenchyma in benign teratoma or cystadenoma. Finally laparoscopy is recognized as the best approach for fertility preservation procedures such as ovarian transposition for patients requiring pelvic radiation or ovarian harvesting for cryopreservation in patients receiving sterilizing treatments.

77.3.5 Pancreatic Tumours

Tumours of the pancreas are rare in children and cover different pathologies of benign (serous or mucinous cystadenoma), malignant (pancreatoblastoma, carcinoma) and borderline type (solid pseudopapillary tumour or Frantz tumour, endocrine tumours). Pancreatoblastoma is mainly seen in young children less than 10 years of age and Frantz tumour in older ones. Complete tumour excision in the absence of rupture is of utmost importance in the treatment of those malignancies and decisive for the outcome. While the impact of tumour rupture is still debated in Frantz tumours, incomplete resection clearly increases the risk of recurrence [12]. Concerns with MIS for pancreatic tumours in children are mainly directed towards the requested experience in all advanced surgical techniques of pancreatic surgery including the Whipple procedure. However, spleen-preserving distal pancreatectomy and central pancreatectomy with pancreaticogastrostomy for pseudopapillary tumours have been described.

77.3.6 Liver Tumours

Liver tumours in childhood (hepatoblastoma and hepatocellular carcinoma) are rare tumours. Complete tumour resection is the key factor for survival. Most of the studies dealing with the role of MIS in liver tumours report on resection of benign lesions such as focal nodular hyperplasia, hamartoma, haemangioma or dysontogenetic cysts. Minimally invasive resection for malignant tumours is more rarely reported [13] and should certainly be developed with highly trained surgeons, like adult liver surgeons.

77.3.7 Lymph Node Sampling

Paratesticular rhabdomyosarcomas or GCT of the testis may metastasize to the retroperitoneal lymph nodes. MIS staging sampling performed by retroperitoneoscopy or laparoscopy has been described.

77.4 Mediastinal Tumours and Lung Metastasis

Thoracic MIS procedures should follow the same oncologic rules described for abdominal tumours.

The main indications are biopsy or resection of ***mediastinal tumours*** and particularly neurogenic tumours arising from the paravertebral sympathetic chain [8]. Airway and/or lung compression, increased intrathoracic pressure and intraoperative carbon dioxide uptake may however prevent the use of MIS, especially in small children and infants. Germ cell tumours, located in the anterior or medium mediastinum, are usually infiltrating lesions with close relationship with vascular structures not easy to manage with a MIS approach. Complete surgical resection is mandatory and MIS is not a good option to achieve this goal. Hodgkin and non-Hodgkin lymphoma, representing 6–7% of all paediatric malignancies, generally originate from the anterior mediastinal thymic compartment, causing relevant tracheal compression with a high risk of intraoperative anaesthesiological complications. Percutaneous or anterior thoracotomy is considered as best options for a representative tumour biopsy for diagnostic workup and risk stratification if no peripheral accessible lymph nodes are accessible.

Regarding *lung lesions*, a thoracoscopic approach could be proposed when the aim of the procedure is to resect superficial tumours which are easy to identify. Preoperative tattooing or harpooning of lung lesions to overcome the lack of tactile abilities and the inability to visualize intraparenchymal lesions (the most common being coils, coil wires, colour dye or radionuclide as well as minimally invasive thoracoscopic ultrasound) has been proposed [14] to help identification for MIS resection, but these technics are currently not completely reliable. Finally, lung lesions are mainly metastasis of osteosarcoma, Ewing sarcoma or Wilms tumours, which usually required the whole palpation of the inspected lung to retrieve and resect them all.

The technical points of thoracoscopy for mediastinal or lung lesions are developed in the respective chapters of this book.

77.5 Supportive Care

Supportive care procedures include gastrostomy for enteral feeding, fertility preservation procedures [15] and techniques of bowel protection for irradiation treatment using sigmoid as a hammock [16].

77.6 Outcome and Discussion

The fear of tumour spillage, previously reported in adult cancers, was a brake for the development of MIS in paediatric oncology. The advantages of MIS in providing sufficient tumour tissue for pathological and molecular biology analysis are now well recognized as well as many aspects of the supportive care requested by cancer patients such as preservation fertility methods. Neuroblastoma was critical for the development of MIS in surgical resection as fragmentation is unavoidable in many cases in open surgery and does not seem to impair prognosis. The recent introduction of nephroblastoma as a potential indication, with strict criteria of inclusion, of MIS is certainly reflecting the favourable experience generally acquired with minimally invasive approaches in paediatric oncology [17]. There is however not a single randomized and controlled clinical trials to ascertain the differences in outcome between MIS and open approach with respect to the overall and event-free survival.

Appropriate patient selection, detailed evaluation of surgical risk factors and conformity to oncological principles with a good experience not only in MIS but also in paediatric oncology surgery are thus mandatory to run a MIS program in paediatric oncology. Conversion should be performed more easily than with non-malignant conditions in order to prevent unexpected spillage or complication that will upgrade tumour staging and thus treatment burden, delay postoperative adjuvant chemotherapy or radiotherapy and potentially compromise survival.

Future directions already explored in the paediatric field including enhanced pre- or perioperative 3D visualization, perioperative fluorescent imaging for the identification of tumour location and margins and robotic surgery will certainly secure and improve the development of MIS in paediatric oncology (Fig. 77.3). Robot-assisted solid tumour resection procedures are now regularly reported demonstrating the feasibility and reliability of this approach [18]. European and international collaborations are specifically needed to develop safe and efficient strategies

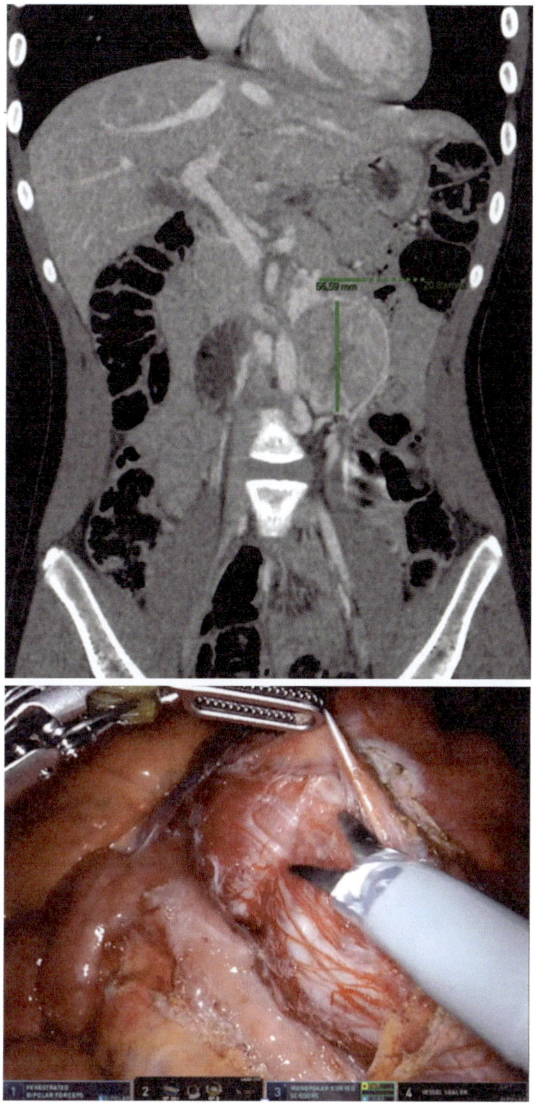

Fig. 77.3 Robot-assisted surgery offers 3D vision and enhanced dexterity that allow resection of an abdominal paraganglioma

and to define indication and limits of robot-assisted surgery for paediatric cancers.

77.7 Conclusions

MIS, regardless of the different techniques—thoracoscopy, laparoscopy, retroperitoneoscopy and robot-assisted—is increasingly being used as surgical approach in children with cancer and will certainly have a definitive place in the future in this field. Unfortunately, although case control studies have shown its non-inferiority to open approach, neither randomized clinical trials nor worldwide-accepted guidelines to date have clearly demonstrated its routine applicability. The decision whether to use MIS or not is therefore generally demanded to an interdisciplinary panel and a meticulous patient selection. An expertise in MIS and surgical oncology is essential for operating surgeons and treating centres to guarantee acceptable treatment outcomes. Efforts from European and international paediatric oncology surgery panels should be addressed to edit guidelines for MIS for each tumour group. Collaboration between centres specializing in MIS and paediatric oncology should be set up to produce high-quality randomized controlled trials comparing MIS to open surgery.

References

1. Grabow D, Kaiser M, Hjorth L, et al. The PanCareSurFup cohort of 83,333 five-year survivors of childhood cancer: a cohort from 12 European countries. Eur J Epidemiol. 2018;33:335–49.
2. Holcomb GW 3rd, Tomita SS, Haase GM, et al. Minimally invasive surgery in children with cancer. Cancer. 1995;76:121–8.
3. Spurbeck WW, Davidoff AM, Lobe TE, et al. Minimally invasive surgery in pediatric cancer patients. Ann Surg Oncol. 2004;11:340–3.
4. Cecchetto G, Riccipetitoni G, Inserra A, et al. Minimally invasive surgery in paediatric oncology: proposal of recommendations. Pediatr Med Chir. 2010;32:197–201.
5. Fuchs J. The role of minimally invasive surgery in pediatric solid tumors. Pediatr Surg Int. 2015;31:213–28.
6. van Dalen EC, de Lijster MS, Leijssen LGJ, et al. Minimally invasive surgery versus open surgery for the treatment of solid abdominal and thoracic neoplasms in children (review). Cochrane Database Syst Rev. 2015;(1):CD008403.
7. Pentek F, Schulte JH, Schweiger B, et al. Development of port-site metastases following thoracoscopic resection of a neuroblastoma. Pediatr Blood Cancer. 2016;63:149–51.
8. Irtan S, Brisse HJ, Minard-Colin V, et al. Minimally invasive surgery of neuroblastic tumors in children: indications depend on anatomical location and image-defined risk factors. Pediatr Blood Cancer. 2015;62:257–61.

9. Varlet F, Stephan JL, Guye E, et al. Laparoscopic radical nephrectomy for unilateral renal cancer in children. Surg Laparosc Endosc Percutan Tech. 2009;19:148–52.
10. Bouty A, Burnand K, Nightingale M, et al. What is the risk of local recurrence after laparoscopic transperitoneal radical nephrectomy in children with Wilms tumours? Analysis of a local series and review of the literature. J Pediatr Urol. 2018;14(4):327.e1–7.
11. Sarnacki S, Brisse H. Surgery of ovarian tumors in children. Horm Res Paediatr. 2011;75(3):220–4.
12. Irtan S, Galmiche-Rolland L, Elie C, et al. Recurrence of solid pseudopapillary neoplasms of the pancreas: results of a nationwide study of risk factors and treatment modalities. Pediatr Blood Cancer. 2016;63:1515–21.
13. Veenstra MA, Koffron AJ. Minimally-invasive liver resection in pediatric patients: initial experience and outcomes. HPB. 2016;18(6):518–22.
14. Parida L, Fernandez-Pineda I, Uffman J, et al. Thoracoscopic resection of computed tomography-localized lung nodules in children. J Pediatr Surg. 2013;48:750–6.
15. Sarnacki S. Ovarian tissue cryopreservation in children with cancer. Lancet Oncol. 2014;15(10):1049–50.
16. Irtan S, Mascard E, Bolle S, Brugières L, Sarnacki S. The small bowel in its hammock: how to avoid irradiation thanks to the sigmoid. J Laparoendosc Adv Surg Tech A. 2015;25(1):77–80.
17. Ezekian B, Englum BR, Gulack BC, et al. Comparing oncologic outcomes after minimally invasive and open surgery for pediatric neuroblastoma and Wilms tumor. Pediatr Blood Cancer. 2018;65(1).
18. Meignan P, Ballouhey Q, Lejeune J, et al. Robotic-assisted laparoscopic surgery for pediatric tumors: a bicenter experience. J Robot Surg. 2018;12(3):501–8.

FSC
www.fsc.org
MIX
Papier aus verantwortungsvollen Quellen
Paper from responsible sources
FSC® C105338

If you have any concerns about our products,
you can contact us on
ProductSafety@springernature.com

In case Publisher is established outside the EU,
the EU authorized representative is:
Springer Nature Customer Service Center GmbH
Europaplatz 3, 69115 Heidelberg, Germany

Printed by Libri Plureos GmbH
in Hamburg, Germany